D1251797

THE COGNITIVE
ELECTROPHYSIOLOGY
OF MIND AND BRAIN

THE COGNITIVE ELECTROPHYSIOLOGY OF MIND AND BRAIN

Edited by

ALBERTO ZANI
Institute of Neuroscience and Bioimaging
CNR
Milan, Italy

ALICE MADO PROVERBIO
Department of Psychology
University of Milano-Bicocca
Milan, Italy

With a Foreword by
MICHAEL I. POSNER
Director, Sackler Institute for Developmental Psychobiology
Weill Medical College of Cornell University, New York

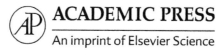

ACADEMIC PRESS
An imprint of Elsevier Science

Amsterdam   Boston   London   New York   Oxford   Paris   San Diego   San Francisco   Singapore   Sydney   Tokyo

Academic Press
An imprint of Elsevier Science.
525 B Street, Suite 1900, San Diego, California 92101-4495, USA
http://www.academicpress.com

Academic Press
84 Theobald's Road, London WC1X 8RR, UK
http://www.academicpress.com

Library of Congress Catalog Card Number: 200210853

International Standard Book Number: 0-12-775421-0

PRINTED IN THE UNITED STATES OF AMERICA
02 03 04 05 06 07 MM 9 8 7 6 5 4 3 2 1

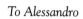

To Alessandro

Contents

B. AFFECTIVE AND DEVELOPMENTAL PERSPECTIVES OF NEURAL COGNITION

SECTION III

NEURAL MECHANISMS OF SELECTIVE ATTENTION

11. Steady-State VEP and Attentional Visual Processing

Francesco Di Russo, Wolfgang A. Teder-Sälejärvi, and Steven A. Hillyard

12. Visual Selective Attention to Object Features

Alice Mado Proverbio and Alberto Zani

SECTION IV

CLINICAL AND APPLIED PERSPECTIVES

13. Event-Related EEG Potential Research in Neurological Patients

Rolf Verleger

14. Mismatch Negativity: A Probe to Auditory Perception and Cognition in Basic and Clinical Research

Risto Näätänen, Elvira Brattico, and Mari Tervaniemi

APPENDIXES

A PRIMER OF BRAIN RESEARCH TECHNIQUES AND CLINICAL SYNDROMES

Appendix A
Recording and Neurochemical Methods: From Molecules to Systems

Gabriele Biella, Alice Mado Proverbio, and Alberto Zani

Appendix B
A Synopsis of Neurological Diseases
Rolf Verleger

Appendix C
State-of-the-Art Equipment for Electroencephalographic and Magnetoencephalographic Investigation of the Brain and Cognition
Alberto Zani and Alice Mado Proverbio

Appendix D
Recording and Analysis of High-Density Electromagnetic Signals of the Brain
Alberto Zani and Alice Mado Proverbio

Contributors

C. J. Aine New Mexico VA Health Care System and Departments of Radiology, Neurology, and Neuroscience, University of New Mexico School of Medicine, Albuquerque, New Mexico 87018

Gabriele Biella Institute of Neuroscience and Bioimaging, Consiglio Nazionale delle Ricerche, 20090 Segrate (Milan), Italy

Elvira Brattico Cognitive Brain Research Unit, Department of Psychology, FIN-00014 University of Helsinki, Finland

Roberto Cabeza Center for Cognitive Neuroscience, Duke University, Durham, North Carolina 27708

Francesco Di Russo Department of Neurosciences, University of California, San Diego, La Jolla, California 92093; and IRCCS Fondazione Santa Lucia, 306 00174 Rome, Italy

Kara D. Federmeier Department of Cognitive Science, University of California, San Diego, La Jolla, California 92093

Steven A. Hillyard Department of Neurosciences, University of California, San Diego, La Jolla, California 92093

Robert Kluender Department of Cognitive Science, University of California, San Diego, La Jolla, California 92093

Marta Kutas Departments of Cognitive Science and Neurosciences, University of California, San Diego, La Jolla, California 92093

Phan Luu Electrical Geodesics, Inc., University of Oregon, Eugene, Oregon 97403

George R. Mangun Center for Cognitive Neuroscience, Duke University, Durham, North Carolina 27708

Teresa V. Mitchell Brain Imaging and Analysis Center, Duke University Medical Center, Durham, North Carolina 27710

Risto Näätänen Cognitive Brain Research Unit, Department of Psychology, FIN-00014 University of Helsinki, Finland

Helen J. Neville Department of Psychology, University of Oregon, Eugene, Oregon 97403

Lars Nyberg Department of Psychology, Umeå University

Alice Mado Proverbio Department of Psychology, University of Milano-Bicocca, 20126 Milan, Italy; and Institute of Neuroscience and Bioimaging, Consiglio Nazionale delle Ricerche, 20090 Segrate (Milan), Italy

Helen Sharpe School of Psychology, Cardiff University, Cardiff CF10 3YG, Wales, United Kingdom

Wolfgang Skrandies Institute of Physiology, Justus-Liebig University, 35392 Giessen, Germany

J. M. Stephen New Mexico VA Health Care System and Department of Radiology, University of New Mexico School of Medicine, Albuquerque, New Mexico 87018

Wolfgang A. Teder-Sälejärvi Department of Neurosciences, University of California, San Diego, La Jolla, California 92093

Mari Tervaniemi Cognitive Brain Research Unit, Department of Psychology, FIN-00014 University of Helsinki, Finland

Don M. Tucker Electrical Geodesics, Inc., University of Oregon, Eugene, Oregon 97403

Rolf Verleger Department of Neurology, University Clinic, D23538 Lübeck, Germany

Edward L. Wilding School of Psychology, Cardiff University, Cardiff CF10 3YG, Wales, United Kingdom

Alberto Zani Institute of Neuroscience and Bioimaging, Consiglio Nazionale delle Ricerche, 20090 Segrate (Milan), Italy

Acknowledgments

We express our heartfelt gratitude to Johannes Menzel, Senior Publishing Editor, Neuroscience, of Elsevier Science/Academic Press, who from the very beginning believed in the project and encouraged us strongly. His unflagging good spirits made him a joy to work with, and his concern for quality kept us on our toes.

Also many thanks are due to Cindy Minor for supervising the gathering of chapter manuscripts and for paying careful attention to detail. Without her assistance, this complex project would never have gotten off the ground. Both Johannes Menzel and Cindy Minor were staunch supporters for the realization of the book.

To Mike Posner, a peerless, unflagging pioneer in indicating new tracks for the uncovering of how mind and brain are strictly intermingled, and who willingly wrote the foreword to the book, we offer our great respect and admiration. We also thank the three anonymous reviewers, who gave such a positive appraisal of our book proposal and its table of contents, and the distinguished panel of international contributors. We are deeply indebted to all the contributors who, we feel, played a most relevant role in making this book a reality. We thank them for contributing the outstanding chapters gathered in the book.

We are also indebted for the generous financial support given by the Institute of Neuroscience and Bioimaging (INB) of the National Research Council (CNR), Milan (Italy), and the Department of Psychology of the University of Milano-Bicocca. We thank Minna Huotilainen and Fred Previc, who willingly gave their permission for the reproduction of their illustrations. In addition, we thank Kathy Nida, Production Editor for Academic Press, and Shirley Tan, of Best-Set Typesetters, as well as all those of the staff of Academic Press who helped us, in any way at all, during the development of the project itself.

For the photos of the ERP Lab we thank Luciano Chiumento for the shooting and Luisa Aquino, who kindly volunteered to pose during the shooting itself. Thanks are also due to Ian McGilvray for his help in re-editing some chapters of the book.

Special thanks to Dr. Rachel C. Stenner who, through her creative rewriting, contributed greatly to the clarity and fluency of a significant part of our writings. Furthermore, the constant support of our collaborators and the kindness they showed at all times, despite their being somewhat neglected, has been much appreciated.

Finally, we acknowledge, with our most heartfelt and affectionate thanks, our families, who gave of themselves unstintingly when we needed them and who showed great patience, especially little Alessandro for his understandable lack of it given his tender years and for the quality time that was inevitably lost to him now and then.

Foreword

ELECTRICAL PROBES OF MIND AND BRAIN

The Cognitive Electrophysiology of Mine and Brain makes explicit that scalp electrical recordings have joined other methods as a means of understanding the connections between brain and mind. Only seven years ago, I wrote a foreword to a new volume, *Electrophysiology of Mind* (Rugg and Coles, 1995). That book summarized the use of electrical recording as a chronometric tool to describe the time course of mental operations, but no explicit effort was made to relate these findings to other approaches to neuroimaging. In that foreword, I suggested that the future of scalp electrical recording lay in firm connections to hemodynamic imaging methods such as PET and fMRI. Acceptance of the full import of these connections is still inhibited. However, in my view and those of most of the authors of this volume, it is time to face the consequences of localization of generators in neural tissue, by making efforts to use electrical recording methods to probe the time course of anatomical areas recruited in performing cognitive functions.

The effort to understand the origins and significance of the brain's electrical and magnetic signals is detailed in Chapter 2.

The methods for linking them to underlying generators in the brain are described in several of the chapters; these efforts are active areas of research (e.g., Dale et al., 2000). A number of algorithms are already available as commercial packages, and new ideas, like those described in Chapters 5 and 11, are being developed. Within the visual system, there has been very detailed validation linking these generators to retinotopic maps found in several visual areas. For complex skills, the evidence is less complete, but because tasks like visual imagery, reading, and number processing have yielded widely separated generators, it has proven possible to provide detailed analysis of their time course from scalp electrical recordings (Abdullaev and Posner, 2000; Dehaene, 1996; Posner and McCandliss, 1999; Raij, 1999).

Even if researchers reading this book are convinced that electrical recordings can play a role in probing the organization of neural networks involved in cognition, it does not mean that all controversies are settled. In fact, the controversy may be more severe, because if scalp electrodes are to be integrated with lesion studies, cellular recording, and hemodynamic imaging as a means of probing both mind and brain, we will have to be serious about reasoning from the combination of these methods.

Chapter 3 provides a very useful summary of many findings that indicate different cognitive function (e.g., working memory and attention) often recruit the same brain area. The authors are surely correct that cognitive psychology textbook chapter titles are not an appropriate guide to brain localization. However, before we conclude that different operations activate the same brain area, we need to be more clear about what makes a difference in mental operations. For example, theories of working memory assume the involvement of attentional networks, so it would be surprising not to find attention areas active in working memory tasks, but it is rather easy to design an attention task that does not involve working memory. We also need to be more explicit about what the same brain area means (i.e., the extent of overlap needed to assume identity). Finally we need to know when in the task a particular area is active. Both perception and imagery tasks may activate prestriate visual areas, but the latter may do so only after activation of higher association areas.

The use of electrical recordings is important for tracing the time course of brain activity and for indexing communication between neural areas. This book shows how such recordings can be useful in analyzing generators of the electrical signals in real time as is done in chapters on language (Chapter 6), memory (Chapter 7), executive function (Chapter 8), and attention (Chapters 10, 11, and 12). These chapters also discuss event related potentials, while steady state electrical potentials are discussed in Chapters 4 and 11, and some concerns with the use of oscillations and correlations within particular frequency bands as a means of probing communication between neural areas are discussed in Chapters 5 and 8.

The editors have also made a significant attempt to give new readers the background necessary to understand the material contained in the volume. Chapter 1 deals with general theoretical issues and

Chapter 2 reviews how electrical and magnetic signals arise from neural tissue and get conducted to the sensors from which they are recorded. Appendixes A—F provide a primer of brain recording techniques as applied to normal persons and those suffering from neurological disorders.

The visual system, including visual attention (Chapters 4, 5, 8, 10, 11, and 12), has been the best area for the close integration of hemodynamic, lesion, and EEG work. In my view, the results have been very impressive. A few years ago, it was puzzling that different areas of the parietal and occipital lobes were active during attention tasks. However, by use of event related fMRI methods it now seems clear that the superior parietal lobe is most related to orienting (e.g., voluntary shifts of attention), while the temporal parietal junction is most important for processing novel or unexpected events. Lesions of the TOJ and surrounding areas are also closely related to the neurological phenomena of extinction and neglect. The occipital sites, which are related to the processing of target identity, while not a part of the attention systems per se, can, like most brain areas, be amplified during an attentive act. Detailed analysis of the orienting network tends to bring into harmony the study of lesions, hemodynamic imaging, and electrical recording.

Cognitive neuroscience involves functional anatomy, circuitry, plasticity, and pathology. All these topics are well represented within the volume. Although most chapters deal with circuitry (i.e., time course of processing), chapters on memory, vision, development, and self-regulation provide substantial backgrounds in how the brain changes with experience and maturation. Human brain development is becoming an increasingly important field of research (see Chapter 9 and Posner, Rothbart, Farah and Bruer, 2001). For example, new methods are now available for examining the development of white matter pathways in the human brain by use of diffusion tensor MRI. This could open up the prospect of using measures of the development of coherence between distant electrode sites as a means of probing the earliest functional use of particular white matter pathways. In addition to Chapter 9, which deals with some forms of atypical development, a whole section of the volume is devoted to applications to neurological patients (Chapter 13) and clinical application of mismatch negativity.

This volume sets research with the brain's electrical and magnetic signals squarely within the large and growing tool kit of methods that have opened up the black box and made the human brain accessible to detailed investigation. What is the next step? A goal must be to move beyond the box score data summaries found in Chapter 3, to reveal the principles through which brain areas are assigned to functions and get assembled into circuits. We are starting to have the requisite clues to do this for visual attention and some high level skills like reading and numeracy. It will be a great challenge, but reading this book and absorbing its many lessons should give the researchers of the next generation a good start.

References

Abdullaev, Y. G., and Posner, M. I. (1998). Event-related brain potential imaging of semantic encoding during processing single words. *Neuroimage* **7**, 1–13.

Dale, A. M., Liu, A. K., Fischi, B. R., Ruckner, R., Beliveau, J. W., Lewine, J. D., and Halgren, E. (2000). Dynamic statistical parameter mapping: Combining fMRI and MEG for high resolution cortical activity. *Neuron* **26**, 55–67.

Dehaene, S. (1996). The organization of brain activation in number comparison: Event related potentials and the additive factors method. *J. Cog. Neurosci.* **8**, 47–68.

Posner, M. I., and McCandliss, B. D. (1999). Brain circuitry during reading. *In* "Converging Methods for Understanding Reading and Dyslexia" R. Klein and P. McMullen, eds.), pp. 305–337. MIT Press, Cambridge, MA.

Posner, M. I., Rothbart, M. K., Farah, M., and Bruer, J. (eds) (2001). Human brain development. *Dev. Sci.* **4/3**, 253–384.

Raij, T. (1999). Patterns of brain activity during visual imagery of letters. *J. Cog. Neurosci.* **11**(3), 282–299.

Rugg, M. D., and Coles, M. G. H. (eds.) (1995). "Electrophysiology of Mind." Oxford Univ. Press.

Michael Posner
Sackler Institute
University of Oregon

A COGNITIVE FRAMEWORK FOR AN INTEGRATIVE PSYCHOPHYSIOLOGICAL APPROACH TO THE STUDY OF MIND AND BRAIN

1

Cognitive Electrophysiology of Mind and Brain

Alberto Zani and Alice Mado Proverbio

INTRODUCTION

The event-related potentials (ERPs) of the brain are wave forms reflecting brain voltage fluctuations in time. These wave forms consist of a series of positive and negative voltage deflections relative to some base line activity prior to the onset of the event. Under different conditions, changes may be observed in the morphology of the wave forms (e.g., the presence or absence of certain peaks), the latency, duration, or amplitude (size) of one or more of the peaks, or their distribution over the scalp. ERPs are useful measures for studying mind and brain functions because they are continuous, multidimensional signals. Specifically, ERPs give a direct estimate of what a significant part of the brain is doing just before, during, and after an event of interest, even if this is prolonged. ERPs can indicate not only that two conditions are different, but also whether, for example, there is a quantitative change in the timing and/or intensity of a process or a qualitative change as reflected by a different morphology or scalp distribution of the wave forms. For all these reasons, ERPs are well established as powerful tools for studying physiological and cognitive functions of the brain.

ERPs AND COGNITIVE THEORY

The so-called cognitive revolution (Baars, 1986) that has permeated research on the mind in psychology and the neurosciences has led to widespread recognition that cognition and the knowledge that derives from it, rather than being an accumulation of sensory experiences, is a constructive process that requires the verification of hypotheses influenced by previous knowledge, past experience, and current aims, as well as emotional and motivational states. Cognitive theory led not only to the rejection of the mind–brain dualism (Mecacci and Zani, 1982; Finger, 1994), but also to firm establishment of the notion that the nature of the mind is determined to a large extent by the neurofunctional architecture of the brain. An important corollary of this concept is the idea that in order to understand the mind it is essential to study and understand the brain (Gazzaniga, 1984, 1995; Posner and DiGirolamo, 2000).

Understanding the mind and brain does not in any way mean understanding conscious processes—quite the contrary, because to a large extent it means investigating nonconscious neural processes. This fact suggested to researchers of the stature

3

of Le Doux (1996) that the unconscious is real, and the renown Gazzaniga (1998) stated that "many experiments highlight how the brain acts earlier than we realize." This occurs at different hierarchical levels within the complex entity of the mind–brain, ranging from intra- and inter-cellular ion exchanges at the microcellular level to the flow of information, at the macrosystem level, along the different functional circuits underlying the very function of the brain and the mind. On the other hand, at a macrosystem level, uncon-scious function is manifested throughout almost all spheres of the mind, starting from the basic operations of analyzing physical characteristics of stimuli by our sensory system, to recording past events or making decisions.

We do not believe that this is surprising if we consider results of modern research on the brain; contemporary studies demon-strate the existence of processes of uncon-scious or subliminal knowledge and perception that influence a manifested behavior, or the capacity of the brain to "filter" or suppress the processing of stimuli (this argument is dealt with more fully in Section III of this volume, on processes of attention). This capacity to filter, studied by Freud, who used the term "repression" to describe it, allows us to be concious of specific thoughts and percep-tions, but not others, apparently under free will and by choice.

In consideration of the relevance of this substantial unconscious component of the mind and, indeed above all, the emotions, it can only be concluded that a heuristi-cally valid cognitive theory of the mind is one that considers the mind's rational and cognitive aspects, which are maintained by the activity of the neocortex, inseparable from the emotive and irrational aspects, expressed by the amygdala and the limbic anterior cingulate cortex (Bush et al., 2000; see also Chapter 8, this volume). This conclusion is also supported by the close relationship existing between thought pro-cesses and emotional processes, suggested by authoritative researchers of the brain such as Le Doux (1996) and Damasio (1994). According to this logic, the brain is seen as a so-called living system. A system, despite being the sum of various parts, each with its specific function, acts as a whole in which each function inevitably influences the other.

Furthermore, it must be remembered that whatever conception of the mind is adopted, it is not heuristically correct to consider this latter as an immutable entity. In fact, the mind must be considered in dynamic terms, that is, as undergoing con-tinuous variations on the basis of evolutive processes and experience (Berlucchi and Aglioti, 1997). It is essential to remember that the functional processes that distin-guish the mind vary as a function of the ontogenetic development of the individual —depending, as a consequence, on the diversified maturation of cerebral structure —and as a function of the individual's learning processes and specific experience gained for the stage of development reached (Nelson and Luciana, 2001; see also Chapter 9, this volume).

Cognitive electrophysiology is a very well-established field of science (Heinze et al., 1994; Kutas and Dale, 1997). The new technologies used to pursue the investiga-tion of mind and brain, with the theoretical backing of the cognitive sciences, have developed at a dizzying speed over the recent "decade of the brain." As a research tool, cognitive electrophysiology may provide relevant contributions to both cog-nitive and brain sciences, putting together new knowledge about humans as inte-grated sociobiological individuals. This ambitious task implies an integration of neurofunctional concepts and basic or more complex cognitive concepts, such as those proposed in cognitive sciences (Wilson and Keil, 1999). Unlike most elec-trophysiological research, mired down by data collection and "correlation state-ments," to the detriment of theorization, the main assumption of cognitively oriented electrophysiological research is that cognition is implemented in the brain through physiological changes. An implicit corollary of this assumption is that electrophysiological measures, i.e., ERP components, may be taken as manifestations, and not simply as correlates, of these intervening processes of the flow of information processing (McCarthy and Donchin, 1979).

Indeed, arguments may be, and indeed often are, raised against this theoretical view in the name of "physiological objectivity." However, we are aware that these statements arise from questionable adherence, in many cases without any awareness, to operational meaning theory. The procedure of giving meaning to concepts inductively on the basis of measures provides an outmoded brand of operationism that may have functioned well for theoretically developed sciences, such as physics, proceeding in the framework of the Popperian view of scientific progress, but which has been only detrimental to atheoretical electrophysiological research. Indeed, the difficulties often met in defining any intrinsic and immutable property of a physiological response, changing as a function of the conditions of its occurrence, make the latter loosely defined in conceptual terms. This failure to find a specific response definition is a problematic criterion for delineating a psychological process for the correlational approach.

To cope with the spatiotemporal overlap in scalp-recorded manifestations of underlying cerebral processes, and with the problems in determining their physiological generators, cognitive electrophysiologists identify ERP components, i.e., the cerebral responses, as the portions of a recorded wave form that can be independently changed by experimental variables—task condition, state, subject strategy, etc. ERP components are not viewed as "structural markers" per se, but as "psychological tools," as is any other psychological measure, e.g., reaction times.

The relationships between these "tools" and cognitive processing are deduced by means of an "assumed" criterion that locates these physiological responses in accordance with hypothesized constraints about their position and function within ongoing activity. These constraints are mediated by well-defined theories of human cognition and information processing (Donchin, 1982, 1984a).

In seeking to clarify these procedural steps, let us take a concept such as learning, viewed from the psychological or behavioral level, and let us try to show how this concept may fruitfully drive electrophysiological experiments. Both at the levels of cognition and brain neurofunction three different, major principles of learning have been coherently identified: (1) knowing what is out in the world, to be used in later recognition and recall (2) knowing what goes with, or follows, what, and (3) knowing how to respond or what to do, given the drive and the situation. The interweaving of these three kinds of knowledge is manifested as complex voluntary action and skilled performance. In many respects these principles underlie the acquisition and deployment of procedures that manipulate the knowledge structures (Bransford et al., 1999). A very relevant topic relative to these procedures is the distinction between so-called controlled and automatic procedures. Skill learning is thought to be characterized by a slow transition from dominance by controlled processes to dominance by automatic processes. However, this transition has been shown to take place only for tasks for which consistent—i.e., repetitive and predictable—information is available. Taking this theoretical framework as a starting point for psychophysiological research on learning, it may be predicted that any spatiotemporal changes in ERP components (amplitude and latency) that may occur with learning should only be observed in tasks providing such consistent information (Kramer and Strayer,

1988; Sirevaag *et al.*, 1989). In the past decades, evidence strongly supporting this prediction has been accumulated in ERP literature relative to all the best known components, especially the contigent negative variation (CNV) and the so-called late positive complex (LPC), i.e., N2, P300, and slow wave (see, Proulx and Picton, 1980; Kramer *et al.*, 1986). Thanks to its inconsistent features, the "oddball" task is a simple but flexible experimental task that has helped to provide evidence, either as such or in the context of a probe-based dual-task paradigm, for the limited capacity of controlled processes and the spatiotemporal stability of ERP components.

ERPs AND THE BRAIN

Traditionally, for more than 100 years cognitive and neurophysiological processes in humans have been studied by psychophysical and behavioral methods. Modern neurosciences offer several hemodynamic, anatomofunctional, and electrophysiological methods to further investigations of the mind and brain. Nevertheless, only noninvasive whole-system procedures can be used to examine humans (see Appendix A, this volume, for a synopsis of molecular and systemic research methods). Because neurophysiological processing takes place in fractions of a second, one of the most feasible tools is to record brain electrofunctional activity (see, e.g., Heinze *et al.*, 1994; Rugg and Coles, 1995). The advantages of electrophysiological signals, or ERPs, lie in their very high time resolution—in the order of milliseconds—and their reliable sensitivity in detecting functional changes of brain activity. The high temporal resolution and noninvasiveness of this method privilege its use over brain imaging techniques such as computed tomography (CT), positron emission tomography (PET), or functional magnetic resonance imaging (fMRI), as well as over the behavioral measures most used in traditional neuropsychological studies. Thanks to these advantages, event-related brain potentials may reveal steps in sensory–cognitive information processing occurring very rapidly within the brain. Furthermore, unlike behavioral and neuroimaging techniques, ERPs may reveal details of functional organization, and timing of the activation, of regional areas of anatomically distributed functional systems of the brain involved in cognitive skills as well as in executive capacities.

Volume conduction and lack of three-dimensional reality do, however, mean that these brain signals are of more limited use than neuroimaging techniques for examining where in the brain processes take place. Nevertheless, localization processes carried out using these signals may be made more sound through source-modeling algorithms.

There is no doubt that modern neuroimaging techniques have dramatically increased our knowledge of the brain and the mind (Posner and Raichle, 1994; Rugg, 1998; Cabeza and Kingstone, 2001). As with ERPs, studies carried out with these techniques focus on an individual's brain when it is involved in carrying out a particular mental task: memorizing a list of words, distinguishing some objects from others that are similar but not the same, directing attention toward objects presented in a particular part of the visual field, etc. The theory underlying all these studies is that the areas of the brain that are found to be most active during the tasks are those that are crucial for the various types of mental activity.

However, simple mapping of the sites of mental processes can indicate only where in the brain a given functional activation takes place but, at present, can in no way explain the mechanisms of the mind. How do we recognize objects and faces, how do we recall the memory of experiences and things, how do we direct our attention to objects and the surrounding space, etc.? These complex and extraordinary mental mechanisms still remain uncharted territory.

No spatial or temporal resolution, however good, can localize something of which we have only superficial knowledge. In fact, in order to be able to "localize" a given cognitive state or mental process (for example, "remembering something") in the brain we must know clearly what the state or process is and what the functional subprocesses are that invariably lead to one cognitive state and not another. If we do not know what these subprocesses are, or whether they vary in different conditions, we cannot reliably localize them in the brain.

It is not at all difficult to find examples in the literature to illustrate what we mean. The reader is referred to Chapter 7 in this volume for an impressive review showing how different the cerebral localizations of activity can be during episodic mnemonic analysis of figurative and linguistic information, according to the different type/state of analysis carried out by subjects (e.g., familiarity, encoding effort, recognition). Furthermore, there is no lack of examples of different localizations in different studies by different scientists for a similar form of mental activity, such as spatial attention. For example, Mangun and colleagues repeatedly reported activation of the fusiform gyrus with PET imaging, and of this same gyrus together with the medial occipital gyrus, when imaged with fMRI, during attention to a relevant space location (see the exhaustive review by Mangun in Chapter 10), whereas Corbetta and colleagues (see Corbetta, 1998) reported a localized activity in the parietal lobe, a region of the cortex classically associated with the control of spatial attention, in addition to the more dorsolateral occipital regions. It is not inconceivable that to cope with differences in the spatial tasks across these studies, different cognitive processes, and thus, different regions of the volunteers' brains, must have been activated during what was

reported by the authors as apparently the same mental activity.

The difficulty in differentiating cognition from brain localization is not, however, unique to neuroimaging and electrophysiological studies. Unfortunately, it is also difficult in most traditional clinical neuropsychological research. Consider, for instance, research on hemineglect or cortical blindness, or any other clinical syndrome. Although robust, direct postmortem and neuroimaging evidence is available for the anatomical localization of brain lesions from which these syndromes derive, only controversial theories can be advanced to explain which processes are lacking, compared to normal cognition, in these patients' cognitive processing and thus to explain their symptomatology. Examples of opposing theories can be found in Köhler and Moscovitch's (1997) outstanding review on unconscious visual processing.

To complicate the picture further, localization research is often pushed to an extreme, frequently without being soundly based on the theory of the mind or the functional architecture of the brain. There are now many authoritative investigators speaking out against this approach to research, and it will probably emerge as more of a hindrance than a help for understanding the mind and brain. For example, according to Frith and Friston (1997), most neuroimaging studies concentrate exclusively on subtraction techniques and on functional segregation to associate a given area with a given function. However, according to Frith and Friston, in order to build an accurate map of the mind, it is crucial to understand the functional interconnectivity of the centers and pathways of the brain by investigating the correlations between these different anatomofunctional entities.

This problem is felt, shared, and creatively developed in the excellent review by Cabeza and Nyberg in Chapter 3. Not by chance did they give their chapter the title "Seeing the Forest through the Trees: The Cross-Function Approach to Imaging Cognition"; they identify "the trees" as the single cognitive functions on which many imaging studies focus their concern, with loss of sight the whole—"the forest"—represented by the fact that, on the one hand, many brain areas are involved in many cognitive functions, and, on the other, that cognition is not actually subdivided into distinct modular cognitive processes, as artificially proposed in cognitive science textbooks for explanatory purposes.

Fuster (2000) is of the same opinion, and authoritatively reports that "common sense, psychophysics, and experimental psychology provide ample evidence that all cognitive functions are interdependent. ...Also interdependent must be, of course, their neural foundations." And, cautioning the reader about some of the problems with the neuromodular principle of cognition, Fuster advances the concept of a "distributed cortical network" according to which performance in cognitive tasks, or, more specifically, tasks of executive control functions, is not solely mediated via localized areas of the brain, but by many regional brain areas that are dispersed throughout the brain, although being strictly linked to each other, and activated in a divergent and convergent way at different times. Again in Fuster's (2000) words, "practically any cortical neuron or neuronal assembly, or module, can be part of many networks. A network can serve several cognitive functions, which consists of neuronal interactions within and between cortical networks." The close resemblance between this carefully worded and articulate definition and the nowadays forgotten "functional system" theory of brain neurofunctional architecture, first advanced by the great Russian neuropsychologist Alexander Lurija (Lurija, 1962, 1976), will, we believe, have hardly escaped anyone.

In the light of these considerations, we believe that it is correct to think that the moment has returned for researchers to dedicate more of their forces to studying the mechanisms inherent to human cognition in order to reach a fuller understanding not merely of the brain, of which in a broad sense we know quite a lot, but rather the mind, that is, its higher and more arcane product, of which we are still profoundly ignorant.

For decades, aware of the limited capacity of ERPs to localize intracerebral processes of cognition, cognitive electrophysiologists have continued their research in the firm belief that the brain's electromagnetic signals spread over the scalp during electrofunctional activation are precious for understanding the ways with which the brain changes with experience and knowledge. Furthermore, they have shared the belief that the nature and mechanisms of the neural processes of cognitive and emotional reorganization are objectively and reliably codified by the different components of the ERPs and event-related fields (ERFs) (Donchin, 1979, 1984b; Hillyard and Picton, 1979; Zani, 1988; Hillyard, 1993; Näätänen and Ilmoniemi, 1994; Rugg and Coles, 1995; Kutas and Dale, 1997).

It was in this conceptual "framework" that the idea was advanced that ERPs could make an important contribution to our understanding of the cerebral mechanisms of knowledge (Kutas and Hillyard, 1984; Heinze et al., 1994). And it is following this idea that the ERPs, rather than being considered a now obsolete method in comparison with the currently available techniques, are still used as a direct, quantifiable measure of processes of knowledge, both conscious and unconscious, and as such are still used to produce and validate models of the mind rather than to provide generic "correlates" of poorly defined psychological constructs. This will become extremely clear in the prestigious articles written by renowned researchers collected together in this book.

In conclusion, it seems that using ERPs, in combination with other available techniques, as quantifiable measures of cognitive and affective processes of the brain, the cognitive electrophysiologist can help test existing theories on the human mind and also can propose newer and more heuristic ones. In order to be efficient in this task of identifying mental processes arising from the brain, it is essential to work in the context of well-founded theories and with sophisticated methodology capable of distinguishing between these theories.

THIS BOOK—OVERVIEW

The chapters of this book—prepared by a panel of international neuroscientists and electrophysiologists—provide state-of-the-art reviews of the latest developments in the study of the relationships between mind and brain as investigated by event-related potentials and event-related fields. Some indications are explored of how these signals may be combined with the high spatial resolution of the hemodynamic signals of the brain, such as those acquired through positron emission tomography and functional magnetic resonance imaging, in order to come closer to the goal of localizing cognition within the brain.

The book is systematically organized into thematic sections. The three chapters in the first section cover the theoretical and methodological framework of investigating the human mind through the recording of electrical, magnetic, and hemodynamic signals of the brain. In Chapter 1 we have raised the point that the study of cognition can benefit enormously from the use of brain electrical and magnetic activity. Efforts are being made to demonstrate that these benefits will derive mostly from theoretically oriented electrophysiological research in the framework of cognitive sciences and neurosciences. Chapter 2 focuses on the morphology of visual, audi-

tory, and somatosensory wave forms of electric potentials and magnetic fields of the brain, and also on the functional significance of these electrophysiological indices in relation to the basic and higher domains of cognition. Furthermore, the intracranial electro ionic origins of these scalp-recorded physiological measures are described, with indications for solving the "direct" and "inverse" problems of localizing their electromagnetic dipoles within the brain.

Chapter 3 (Cabeza and Nyberg) offers an original theoretical cross-function framework for guiding hemodynamic functional imaging of brain and cognition. This framework provides the foremost constraints to functional interpretations, particularly when assuming the so-called sharing view, that is, the view that the same brain region is recruited by different cognitive functions. In the authors' words, these constraints "help us overcome function-chauvinism and see the 'big picture.' In other words, cross-function comparisons allow us to see the forest [what many functional studies have in common] through the trees [the single cognitive domains investigated by single studies]."

The second section (Chapters 4–9) systematically covers electromagnetic research on a representative sample of the neural domains of human cognition. Chapter 4 (Skrandies) illustrates how the recording of brain electrical activity in combination with knowledge on the human visual system may be employed to study visual information processing in healthy volunteers as well as in patients with selective visual deficiencies. Data are presented on different experimental questions related to human visual perception, including contrast and stereoscopic vision as well as perceptual learning.

Chapter 5 (Aine and Stephen) deals with magnetoencephalography (MEG) mapping of the ventral and dorsal streams in human visual cortex. MEG cues, proving that isoluminant, central field stimuli preferentially excite the ventral stream structures and, alternatively, that peripheral stimuli alternating at high rates preferentially activate the dorsal stream, are systematically addressed. Furthermore, the focus is on present progress in our understanding of brain cortical areas involved in higher visual processing, such as recognition memory, as investigated by means of MEG, and the future direction of MEG research in this field is discussed.

Chapter 6 (Federmeier, Kluender, and Kutas) reviews ERP studies on language. Rather than simply presenting a collection of various processes, throughout the chapter the authors illustrate the viewpoint that the goals of electrophysiological investigations of language, as well as the goals of research exploring language processing with other tools, are to fashion an understanding of how the various processes involved in language comprehension and production are coordinated to yield the message-level apprehension we attain from reading or listening to speech. As stated in Chapter 6, "linguists, psycholinguists, and neurolinguists alike strive to understand how the brain 'sees' language—because, in turn, language is such an important facet of how humans 'see' their world."

Chapter 7 (Wilding and Sharpe) is devoted to memory processes that constitute another very important domain of human cognition. Indeed, memory has been a subject of fascination to psychologists and other brain scientists for over a century. Recently, the study of the role of different brain areas in memory has received a boost from new techniques and changing pretheoretical orientations. The authors offer an original review of the bulk of electrophysiological studies on retrieval and encoding processes underlying episodic memory. Commendably, they do not simply share knowledge from ongoing research, but identify some acute outstanding problems in this field of investigation, indicating its likely future developments.

Chapter 8 (Luu and Tucker) is intended to close the misleading gap that exists in the "cognitive" approach to brain function and architecture between a pure cognitive functional processing of the brain and its emotional counterpart, which is of such importance in producing thinking and behavior, both in normal and emotionally disordered people. With such a goal, the authors deal specifically with mental processes involved in emotion, motivation, and reward, reviewing studies in this field from a modern neuroscience-based viewpoint.

Chapter 9 (Mitchell and Neville) addresses "neuroplasticity," a dominant research theme in neuroscience at present. Neuroplasticity usually refers to some change in the nervous system as a function of age and/or experience. This contribution reviews studies on the effects of age and experience on the development of neurocognitive systems. A broad survey and synthesis are provided of essential data on normal brain and cognitive development, as well as on development after early deafness, blindness, or following delays in language acquisition. The authors provide insights into and ideas on the complexity and diversity of contemporary brain neuroplasticity research in humans.

The three chapters gathered in the third section are concerned with visual attention. Chapter 10 (Mangun) and Chapter 11 (Di Russo, Teder-Sälejärvi, and Hillyard) mostly address neural mechanisms of spatial attention. Chapter 10 reviews findings indicating how human spatial attention involves top-down processes that influence the gain of sensory transmission early in the visual cortex. Chapter 11 deals with steady-state cortical processing of the brain that reveals slow-rising changes in cortical reactivity to the outer world. First, the authors provide an overview of this processing mode in the visual modality. Then they present a review of experimental findings of modulations of this processing mode with selective attending of spatial and, to a lesser extent, nonspatial features (color, shape, etc.) of visual information, in line with the previous chapter. Unlike Chapters 10 and 11, Chapter 12 (Proverbio and Zani) concentrates on feature-based and object-based selection mechanisms of the brain as investigated with ERPs. An overview is provided of studies showing the close interconnections across the anterior and posterior attention systems. In addition, a review is made of studies reporting the differential activation of the "Where" and "What" systems of the visual brain in conditions in which stimulus attributes have to be separately and/or conjointly attended. Efforts are made to demonstrate the task-related relative segregation and complex interactions of the aforementioned systems during the separate or conjoint processing of stimulus attributes.

The final two chapters comprising the fourth section are concerned with clinical and applied perspectives of ERP research. Chapter 13 (Verleger) provides an exhaustive overview of ERP studies on neuropsychological syndromes. The detailed description given of these syndromes is subdivided into three main categories. The result is a unique, up-to-date, and wide-ranging discussion of these disorders that draws on biology, genetics, neuropsychology, clinical presentation, and treatment. Chapter 14 (Näätänen, Brattico, and Tervaniemi) introduces the mismatch negativity (MMN), a component of auditory ERPs reflecting the brain's automatic response to any discriminable change in auditory stimulation. Because the MMN can be measured even in the absence of attention and without any task requirements, it is particularly suitable for investigating several clinical populations as well as infants. Moreover, the MMN provides a unique index of the subject's accuracy in the processing of speech and musical sounds. It can be used, for example, to unravel the neural determinants of language skills and musical expertise.

In addition to the specialist review chapters, a fifth section of this book collects together a number of appendixes containing the primers of the theoretical and methodological matters—including some simple-level mathematical material—treated in the specialist chapters. These appendixes are intended for the benefit of nonexperts (such as psychology and medical students), as well as experts in other neighboring fields. These appendixes have been included in order to clarify, in simple but detailed terms, the basics of molecular and systemic methods of investigating the nervous system (Appendix A), as well as neuropsychological clinical practice (Appendix B). They also provide the fundamentals of electromagnetic recording and data analysis and laboratory setup (Appendixes C and D), and topographic and dipole mapping methods (Appendix E). Last but not least, the invasiveness and the spatial and temporal resolution of electromagnetic techniques, as compared to other techniques, are given (Appendix F).

References

Baars, B. J. (1986). "The Cognitive Revolution in Psychology." Guilford, New York.

Berlucchi, G., and Aglioti, S. (1997. The body in the brain: Neural bases of corporeal awareness. *Trends Neurosci.* **20**, 560–564.

Bransford, J. D., Brown, A. L., and Cocking, R. R. (1999). "How People Learn. Brain, Mind, Experience, and School." National Academy of Sciences, New York.

Bush, G., Luu, P., and Posner, M. I. (2000). Cognitive and emotional influences in anterior cingulate cortex. *Trends Cogn. Sci.* **4**, 215–222.

Cabeza, R., and Kingstone, A. (2001). "Handbook of Functional Neuroimaging of Cognition." MIT Press, Cambridge, Massachusetts.

Corbetta, M. (1998). Functional anatomy of visual attention in the human brain: Studies with positron emission tomography. *In* "The Attentive Brain" (R. Parasuraman, ed.), pp. 95–122. MIT Press, Cambridge, Massachusetts.

Damasio, A. R. (1994). "Descartes' Error: Emotion, Reason, and the Human Brain." Avon Books, New York.

Donchin, E. (1979). Event-related brain potentials: A tool in the study of human information processing. *In* "Evoked Brain Potentials and Behavior" (H. Begleiter, ed.), pp. 13–88. Plenum Press, New York and London.

Donchin, E. (1982). The relevance of dissociations and the irrelevance of dissociationism: A reply to Scwartz and Pritchard. *Psychophysiology* **19**, 457–463.

Donchin, E. (1984a). Dissociation between electrophysiology and behavior—A disaster or a challenge? *In* "Cognitive Psychophysiology. Event-related Potentials and the Study of Cognition" (E. Donchin, ed.), pp. 107–118. Lawrence Erlbaum Assoc., Hillsdale, New Jersey.

Donchin, E. (1984b). Cognitive psychophysiology. *In* "Event-related Potentials and the Study of Cognition" (E. Donchin, ed.), pp. 107–118. Lawrence Erlbaum Assoc. Hillsdale, New Jersey.

Finger, S. (1994). "Origins of Neuroscience." Oxford University Press, New York.

Frith, C. D., and Friston, K. J. (1997). Studying brain function with neuroimaging. *In* "Cognitive Neuroscience" (M. Rugg, ed.), pp. 169–195. Psychology Press, London.

Fuster, J. M. (2000). The module: Crisis of a paradigm. *Neuron* **26**, 51–53.

Gazzaniga, M. S. (ed.) (1984). "Handbook of Cognitive Neuroscience." Plenum Press, Cambridge.

Gazzaniga, M. S. (ed.) (1995). "The Cognitive Neurosciences." MIT Press, Cambridge, Massachusetts.

Gazzaniga, M. S. (1998). "The Mind's Past." University of California Press, Berkeley and Los Angeles.

Heinze, H.-J., Münte, T. F., and Mangun, G. R. (1994). "Cognitive Electrophysiology." Birkhäuser, Boston, Basel, and Berlin.

Hillyard, S. A. (1993). Electrical and magnetic brain recordings: Contributions to cognitive neuroscience. *Curr. Opin. Neurobiol.* **3**, 217–224.

Hillyard, S. A., and Picton, T. W. (1987). Electrophysiology of cognition. *In* "Handbook of Physiology: Section 1, The Nervous System: Higher Brain Functions" (V. B. Mountcastle, ed.), Vol. 5, Part 2, pp. 519–584. American Physiological Society, Baltimore.

Köhler, S., and Moscovitch, M. (1997). Unconscious visual processing in neuropsychological syndromes: A survey of the literature and evaluation of models of consciousness. *In* "Cognitive Neuroscience" (M. Rugg, ed.), pp. 305–373. Psychology Press, London.

Kramer, A. F., and Strayer, D. L. (1988). Assessing the development of automatic processing: An application of dual-task and event-related brain potential methodologies. *Biol. Psychol.* **26**, 231–267.

Kramer, A. F., Schneider, W., Fisk, A., and Donchin, E. (1986). The effects of practice and task structure on components of event-related brain potentials. *Psychophysiology* **23**, 33–47.

Kutas, M., and Dale, A. (1997). Electrical and magnetic reading of mental functions. *In* "Cognitive Neuroscience" (M. D. Rugg, ed.), pp. 197–242. Psychology Press, Taylor & Francis Group, Hove, East Sussex, UK.

Kutas, M., and Hillyard, S. A. (1984). Event-related potentials in cognitive science. *In* "Handbook of Cognitive Neuroscience" (M. S. Gazzaniga, ed.), pp. 387–409. Plenum Press, New York.

Le Doux, J. E. (1996). "The Emotional Brain." Simon and Schuster, New York.

Lurija, A. R. (1962). Vysšie korkovye funkcii čeloveka [The Superior Cortical Functions in Man]. Moscow University (MGU), Moscow.

Lurija, A. R. (1976). "The Working Brain. An Introduction to Neuropsychology." Penguin Books, Harmondworth.

McCarthy, G., and Donchin, E. (1979). Event-related potentials—manifestations of cognitive activity. *In* "Bayer Symposium VII, Brain Function in Old Age" (F. Hoffmeister and C. Muller, eds.), pp. 318–335. Springer-Verlag, New York.

Mecacci, L., and Zani, A. (1982)."Theories of the Brain. Since the Ninth Century Up to Today" [in Italian]. Loescher, Torino.

Näätänen, R., and Ilmoniemi, R. J. (1994). Magnetoencephalography in studies of human cognitive brain function. *Trends Neurosci.* **17**, 389–395.

Nelson, C. A., and Luciana, M. (eds.) (2001). "Handbook of Developmental Cognitive Neuroscience." MIT Press, Cambridge, Massachusetts.

Posner, M. I., and DiGirolamo, G. J. (2000). Cognitive neuroscience: Origins and promise. *Psychol. Bull.* **126**, 873–889.

Posner, M. I., and Raichle, M. E. (1994). "Images of Mind." W. H. Freeman, New York.

Proulx, G. B., and Picton, T. W. (1980). The CNV during cognitive learning and extinction. *In* "Motivation, Motor and Sensory Processes of the Brain: Electrical Potentials, Behaviour and Clinical Use" (H. H. Kornhuber, and L. Deecke, eds), pp. 309–313. Elsevier, Amsterdam.

Rugg, M. D. (1998). Functional neuroimaging in cognitive neuroscience. *In* "The Neurocognition of Language" (C. M. Brown and P. Hagoort, eds.), pp. 15–36. Oxford University Press, Oxford.

Rugg, M. D., and Coles, M. G. H. (1995). The ERP and cognitive psychology: Conceptual issues. *In* "Electrophysiology of Mind: Event-related Brain Potentials and Cognition" (M. D. Rugg and M. G. H. Coles, eds.), pp.27–39. Oxford University Press, Oxford.

Sirevaag, E. J., Kramer, A. F., Coles, M. G. H., and Donchin, E. (1989). Resource reciprocity: An event-related brain potential analysis. *Acta Psychol.* **70**, 77–97.

Wilson, R. A., and Keil, F. C. (1999). "The MIT Encyclopaedia of the Cognitive Sciences." MIT Press, Cambridge, Massachusetts.

Zani, A. (1988). Event-related brain potentials as a point of entry into the integrated analysis of the cognitive and affective bases of perceptual and aesthetic experiences. *In* "X International Colloquium on Empirical Aesthetics," pp. 90–100. Corda Fratres, Barcelona (ME).

2

Electromagnetic Manifestations of Mind and Brain

Alice Mado Proverbio and Alberto Zani

ELECTROENCEPHALOGRAM AND MAGNETOENCEPHALOGRAM

The cognitive activity that accompanies functional activation of the brain is reflected in a series of physiological transformations; these can be recorded by a variety of techniques of varying invasiveness, ranging from single-unit recordings to hemodynamic and electromagnetic techniques (Hugdhal, 1993).

From an electrofunctional point of view, the activity of the brain essentially translates into (1) wave-formed electromagnetic fields or potentials, which constitute the electroencephalogram and the magnetoencephalogram and (2) transient changes in the electromagnetic fields caused by nerve impulses induced by external stimuli or independent mental events, which constitute the *event-related potentials* (ERPs) and *event-related fields* (ERFs), respectively. It is not the aim of this review to discuss the electroencephalogram (EEG). The reader interested in the EEG and the rhythmical waves that distinguish it, as well as its origins in the cerebral cortex or in processes regulating these waves (*pacemaker*) in the thalamic nuclei, is referred to the excellent works by Buzsaki (1991) and Silberstein (1995a,b), as well as the impressive review by Nunez *et al.* (2001).

In this chapter we discuss the principles underlying the nature of the electromagnetic signal, including a description of the intracortical sources of the potentials recorded from scalp surface, as well as the methods of analyzing and identifying the best known components of these signals based on their functional properties. For further information on neurofunctional changes other than the strictly electrophysiological ones (namely, ERPs), and on the techniques by which these can be recorded, the reader is referred to Chapters 5 and 14, for a description of magnetoencephalographic studies on the mechanisms of analyzing visual and auditory information, respectively. Chapter 3, on the other hand, carefully examines the cross-functional approach to hemodynamic neuroimaging of cognition.

Electroionic Origins of Electromagnetic Signals

The changes in electrical potential recorded on the scalp are generated by the sum of the excitatory and inhibitory postsynaptic potentials (EPSPs and IPSPs) of the nerve cells, which must be oriented in a certain way. The EEG technique can measure only the potentials of cells arranged in organized layers and whose

13

apical dendrites are oriented perpendicularly to the surface of the cortex (as are, for example, pyramidal cells or the hypercolumns of the visual cortex). The bioelectric potential that can be recorded at the surface is nothing other than the difference in potential between the basal part and the apical part of the active neurons that are oriented in that direction, producing an infinitely low-intensity flow of current. In the example shown in Fig. 1a, the EPSPs that converge on the pyramidal neurons through the direct afferent fibers that end in the upper part of the apical dendrites cause a flow of charged ions between points at different potentials within and outside the neurons. In other words, positive ions entering the cell produce a transmembrane electrical current (as shown in Fig. 1b). Once the positive ions have entered the cell, following the concentration and electrical charge gradient, they propagate from the subsynaptic area to the rest of the neuron (Fig. 1c). When the EPSP has involved the distal part of the apical dendrite, as shown in Fig. 1, the flow of current is greater starting from the apical part nearest to the synapse toward the cell body, rather than in the opposite direction, because the resistance to this flow is less. The flow of positive ions entering the cell progressively neutralizes the negative ions inside the extracellular somatodendritic membrane (Fig. 1d). Outside, on the other hand, the positive ions that have entered the cell are substituted by ion flow directed toward the synaptic region along the extracellular space (cases c and d in Fig. 1).

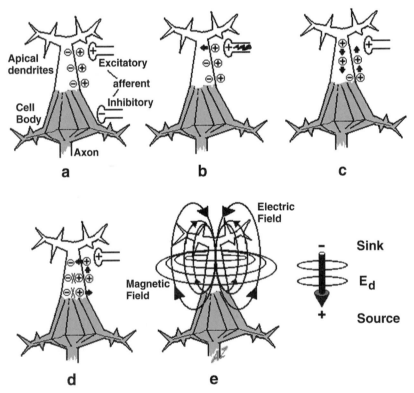

FIGURE 1 Electrofunctional activity of a pyramidal neuron: the relative transmembrane ion flows and electromagnetic induction phenomena. (a–e) Subsequent stages of electroionic alterations between the cell body and the apical dendrites of the neuron induced by postsynaptic excitatory potentials and the generation of reverberating flows of current, which generate the fields of potential or equivalent electromagnetic dipoles. The large vertical, cylindrical arrow pointing downward indicates the electromagnetic dipole (E_d) with its relative sink and source.

These flows particularly involve the ions released by the neutralization of the charge of negative ions arranged along the internal surface of cell membrane. The flow of the current perpendicular (or radial) to the apical dendrite is accompanied by a magnetic field that propagates orthogonally (or tangentially) to the flow of current along the extracellular somatodendritic membrane (Fig. 1e). This set of electroionic functional alterations thus generates the so-called *fields of electromagnetic potentials* or *electromagnetic dipoles*. Alternatively, they are defined as *single equivalent dipoles*. In correspondence with the intracortical area where the excitatory (or generator) post-synaptic potential is generated, a negative potential (the so-called *sink*, or minimum) is recorded, whereas in correspondence with the "outflow" of the current on the scalp a positive potential (the so-called *source*, or maximum) is recorded (Fig. 1). The outflow indicates the dispersion of the flow of intracerebral current on the surface of the scalp after it has crossed the cerebrospinal fluid, the meninges, and the bony structures of the skull (Fig. 2). In the case of inhibitory postsynaptic potential, the relationship between the site of the synapses and the polarity of the recording is inverted.

As can be seen in Fig. 2, electrofunctional activation of the pyramidal cells oriented perpendicularly to the surface of the skull—that is, those located in the dorsal gyri of the encephalus—can be recorded on the scalp in the form of an EEG or ERPs, because it generates so-called *open fields*. In contrast, because of the morphology and the directional arrangement of the dendrites of the cell assembly units (some neuronal assembly units in the brain stem and telencephalon, e.g., the hippocampus, are organized concentrically), some intracerebral potentials finish by canceling each other or by being too weak to be recorded by electrodes far away from them. This is the reason that they are called *closed fields* (Fig. 2).

For further details on the neuronal electroionic bases of cerebral electromagnetic fields the reader is referred to the influential articles by Katznelson (1981) and Pilgreen (1995), and the outstanding and more recent surveys by Kutas and Dale (1997) and Kutas *et al.* (1999).

The Electromagnetic Dipoles

Given that the electroencephalogram (EEG) is generated by electrical activity that derives from neuronal interactions, the distribution of the EEG signals on the scalp contains information on the localization of the underlying electrical sources. It must not, however, be thought that the electrical source is more or less exactly underneath the electrode that records the strongest intensity signal. Even in the cases in which this is in fact the situation, no information is given on the depth of the source within the skull. In many cases, however, the electrode is not recording electrical sources from directly below its location, because the electrical sources of the brain generate a dipolar distribution of potentials, thus the minimum (sink) and the maximum (source) of the distribution of the potential do not necessarily coincide with the localization of the source. As a further complication, in the cases in which more than one source is activated (multiple equivalent dipoles), the maximum of one source can be cancelled by the minimum of another. A similar logic also applies in the case of magnetoencephalography (MEG), which measures the very weak magnetic fields produced by neuronal electrical activity of the brain. These signals are in the order of femtoteslas (10^{-15} T) (Peters and De Munck, 1990; Scherg, 1992). In order to be able to appreciate just how weak these signals are, consider that 1 T, which measures the strength of magnetic induction, is equivalent (in gauss) to about 0.6 G, and that the Earth's magnetic field is in the order of 0.3–0.6 G (depending on the latitude). On the basis

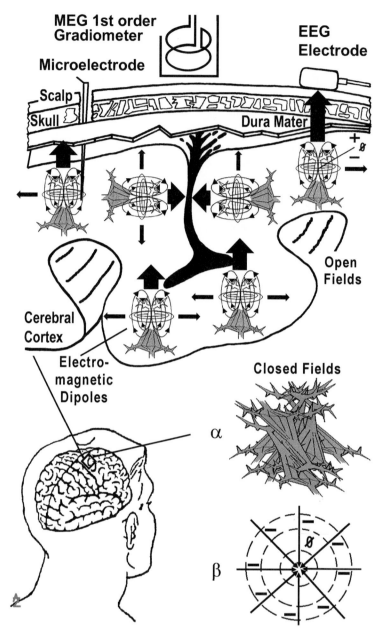

FIGURE 2 Simplified diagram of the cortical generators of electromagnetic fields and both intracerebral and surface recordings of the signals derived from them. **Top:** Enlarged detail of a section below the scalp, skull, and meninges, depicting a cerebral cortical convolution with one of its characteristic sulci formed by the folding of the cortical mantle. The section also shows some pyramidal neurons with their apical dendritic prolongations, oriented perpendicularly or horizontally, depending on their position in the folds of the cortex. These neurons produce open fields. The thick, dark arrows represent the direction of propagation of the electrical counterpart of the dipole; the smaller arrows indicate the direction of propagation of its magnetic counterpart. In the superficial areas of the cortex, the propagation of the electrical dipoles of the pyramidal neurons is radial to the brain and head. An electroencephalogram (EEG) electrode (shown on the right of the scalp) is therefore able to pick up this propagated current and reflect it in the form of an electroencephalogram. Only part of the electrical activity of the neurons arranged perpendicularly deep in the bottom of the sulci is picked up by the electrode. Thus, this part of the cerebral electrofunctional activation is not appropriately represented in the EEG. The same electrode

of this rough equation, the magnetic fields of the brain are about one billionth less strong than the Earth's magnetic field.

The Direct and Inverse Problem

We have so far seen that the neurons that transmit signals to the synapses act as electromagnetic dipoles that constitute intracortical generators of the EEG and the MEG. The reason why these sources are represented by dipoles is that, in an activated synapse, electrical current flows from a localized source to a nearby minimum. In mathematical terms, a dipole is the simplest description of this geometric flow. It can be described by a *vector*, indicated by an arrow that points from maximum to minimum. The length of the arrow indicates the intensity (or strength) of the source.

Overall, the dipole is characterized by six parameters: three of position (x, y, and z) on a three-dimensional plane, two that fix the orientation, and one that represents its intensity (De Munck *et al.*, 1988). These dipoles are situated in a conductor (brain tissue) and set into movement the free charges (electrons and ions) present in the conductor. The amount of movement of the charges (that is, the electrical current) depends on the conductivity of the medium. When many neurons are simultaneously activated with a unidirectional orientation, these produce measurable signals in the form of EEG and MEG activity.

It is important to note that even if the electrical activity of the brain starts at one point, the resulting EEG can be measured all over the scalp. In other words, the conductive medium (generally defined, the *volume conductor*) diffuses the localized electrical activity throughout its volume (DeMunck *et al.*, 1988). To a certain extent, this can be likened to seismic activity in that an earthquake occurring at its epicenter can be recorded on the Earth's surface a considerable distance away from the epicenter, with ever decreasing intensity (Allison, 1984); this same analogy links the activity of electrophysiologists and seismologists. If there is more than one source activated simultaneously in the brain, each electrode measures a contribution from all the sources. In order to separate these sources it is fundamentally important to study the spread of the conductance on the basis of the volume— or in other words, to resolve the so-called *direct problem.*

This problem consists in providing the distribution of the potential (or of the magnetic field outside the head) on the scalp for a given electrical source located within the head. The reason why this problem cannot be ignored is that the head consists of different compartments, each with different conductance and geometry. Each compartment affects the electrical and magnetic fields generated by the source. The most important compartments are the white matter (nerve fibers), the gray

---

FIGURE 2 (*continued*) is, however, insensitive (i.e., "blind") to the dipole flows occurring in the neurons in the vertical parts of the walls of the cortical sulci. This is because, as indicated by the thick, horizontal arrows, these flows move in parallel or tangentially to the surface of the cortex. The situation for the magnetic component of the dipoles is, normally, the reverse. The magnetic dipoles of the neurons of the superficial areas of the cortical convolutions are not, in fact, picked up by the sensor of magnetic activity (indicated in the figure as "MEG 1st order gradiometer") because, as can be seen, the dipole and the magnetic flow are tangential to the skull. The gradiometer does, however, efficiently pick up magnetic fields, even of infinitesimally small strength, coming from neurons arranged horizontally on the vertical area of the opposing walls of the cortical sulci. It is not, however, able to pick up the magnetic fields generated by neurons arranged perpendicularly to the base of the sulci. This set of signals can be efficiently recorded by an intracortical microelectrode placed near the neuronal membrane. **Bottom:** An example of neuronal units arranged concentrically (α) and a closed field (β) thus derived because of the convergent dipolar flows.

matter (neuronal bodies), the cerebrospinal fluid, the skull, and the skin. Most of these tissues are anisotropic conductors. This means that the electrical current depends not only on the conductivity and the amplitude of the applied potential, but also on the direction of the gradient of the potential. This type of current conduction, which has been demonstrated to occur in the skull, cortex, and white matter, further complicates calculations of electrical potentials and magnetic fields (Peters and De Munck, 1990).

In any case, it is important that the head is roughly spherical and that the compartments form a series of concentric spherical layers. With the geometry it is possible to calculate the distribution of potentials using a fast mathematical algorithm, even if some of the conduction is anisotropic. This model is normally called the *multisphere model*. It is completely characterized by the external radius, the radial conductivity, and the tangential conductivity of each layer.

The *three-spheres model*, often used and reported in literature, is a special case of the multisphere model. In this model the head is taken to be a homogeneous sphere. It is considered to have an external spherical layer of poor conductive capacity (in practice, being isotropic), and an interior, which is the brain. The model is characterized by three parameters: the internal and external radii of the cranium, and its conductivity (relative to the homogeneous sphere). This is, therefore, a much simpler model than the general spherical model. However, disregarding the anisotropy of the skull and the conductivity distorted by other parameters could lead to large errors in estimating the parameters of a source. Furthermore, the simplification does not provide a faster algorithm for calculating the potential. It is, therefore, better to use the multisphere model.

It is important to remember that there is a marked difference between MEG and EEG as far as concerns the effect of conduc-

tivity changes of the signal measured. If the head were a perfect sphere, made up of perfect concentric spheres, the magnetic field generated by the electrical sources of the conductor would be independent of the rays that intersect the various layers of the sphere and of the conductivity of these layers. Thus MEG has the advantage over EEG of eliminating possible systematic errors in source localizing caused by the use of inaccurate parameters of conductivity. Another advantage is the amount of diffusion produced by the conductor, which is much less with MEG than with EEG, thus resulting in a better spatial resolution. The problem, however, is that the MEG is insensitive to radial dipoles. In other words, a dipole directed along a line that crosses the center of the sphere (that is, the radius) does not spread a magnetic field outside the sphere (see Fig. 2), and thus this type of source can never be recorded using MEG equipment (Peters and De Munck, 1990; Del Gratta and Romani, 1999). Strictly speaking, however, these characteristics of the MEG are valid within the class of models based on exact spheres.

In practice, it can be emphasized that the MEG predominantly provides a representation of dipoles of neural activation arranged perpendicularly in the cortical sulci, whereas EEG provides a profile of cortical activation above all by measuring the dipoles radial to the cortical gyri. It will, therefore, be clear that only combined recordings of electrical and magnetic flows will be able to provide an exhaustive and accurate localization of functional activity of the cortex of the brain.

Independently of this, as has been seen, the source of a dipole can be considered to be described by six parameters, of which three denote position and three denote orientation. There are various coordinate systems to translate the series of values of these parameters into a three-dimensional vector in space. All the coordinate systems are derived from Cartesian coordinates,

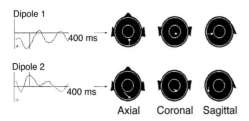

Axial　Coronal　Sagittal

FIGURE 3 Equivalent dipoles. Diagram of the hypothesized localization of the electrical dipoles of visual ERPs in three planes. The temporal functions of the sources, calculated by principal component analysis, are shown on the left. The vertical lines overlying the wave forms indicate the latency (~110 msec) with which the two different dipoles are calculated. On the right, the localization of the two dipoles within the three-sphere model of the head can be observed in the different axial, coronal, and sagittal planes. The white circles in these sections indicate the site of the dipole. The lines extending from them indicate the direction of the flow of the dipole.

consisting of three perpendicular axes: x, y, and z. In all these systems the angles are measured in degrees and the distances are measured in fractions of the radius of the head, or in centimeters. A diagram of the dipole, with its identifying characteristics, is shown in Fig. 3.

From a practical point of view, electrophysiologists and magnetophysiologists trying to localize neural processes find themselves working in the difficult situation in which the cerebral potentials and magnetic fields are known, because they have been recorded, but their intracerebral origins are still to be determined. In order to gain this information, they must resolve the so-called *inverse problem*. It is clear that this is easier to say than to do because in order to find these sources, exactly what is being searched for must be described as precisely as possible. Fortunately, given that, as seen above, there are good reasons to assume that the brain's electrical sources can be described efficiently by mathematical dipoles (De Munck *et al.*, 1988), the series of possible responses is considerably reduced. This is because each dipole has only six unknown parameters.

If it is assumed that a specific peak of the potential that occurs in all recordings

can be attributed to a dominant source, only six parameters need to be estimated in order to resolve the spatiotemporal modeling of this source. Normally, the estimate is based on the mathematical criterion of *least squares*. This requires collecting the group of parameters of the dipole that best explain the measurements obtained—that is, the group of parameters that minimize the sum of the squared deviations between the real measurements and those of the model.

In practice, with this procedure, resolving the inverse problem corresponds, more or less, to nothing other than resolving the direct problem by applying a mathematical equation that allows a satisfactory minimum to be found starting from the many different groups of parameters. The group of parameters yielding the minimum value is the solution to the inverse problem and constitutes the source of the investigated dipole (Peters and De Munck, 1990).

Principal Component Analysis

In the context of spatiotemporal modeling, in order to estimate the minimum number of sources and speed up the computations, a mathematical technique known as *principal component analysis* (PCA) is applied. The minimum number of sources depends largely on the estimate of the relationship between signal and noise, which can be inaccurate (for more details on the advantages and limitations of this mathematical technique, see Appendix E, this volume).

Localization of the Dipole and the Reference Electrode

In order to localize the sources, it is not necessary to have a site hypothetically "silent" from an electrical point of view to act as a reference electrode. Given that the head can be considered as an isolated conductor with finite dimensions and a group of sources that produce potentials on the surface of the conductor, the potentials recorded consist of the differences in potentials between active electrodes and the reference electrode and not absolute values. This has an effect on the morphology of the signals (for more information on this subject see Appendixes D and E).

Indeed, the reference electrode could be among the grid of electrodes used, as long as its position is known with the same precision with which the positions of the other electrodes are known. In the inverse model this condition is taken into consideration by treating the measurements not as absolute potentials but rather as differences in potentials between active electrodes, and the reference electrode prior to the computation of the sum of the squared errors. This does not mean that the choice of reference does not affect the results. In fact, for each possible reference, a different sum of the squares is obtained, which, in principle, could lead to a different minimum of the dipole. Great care is, therefore, required on this point (Peters and De Munck, 1990).

EVENT-RELATED POTENTIALS

ERPs are based on the electrophysiological recording of brain potentials synchronized with the presentation of external sensory stimuli such as light flashes, words, faces, etc., as well as the occurrence of internal cognitive events such as decision making or selective attention processes (Hillyard *et al.*, 1978; Hillyard and Kutas, 1983; Picton and Hillyard, 1988). In the first theoretical treatise the former potentials were called *exogenous* because they were produced or evoked by external stimuli, whereas the latter were defined *endogenous* because they were "emitted" even in the absence of any physical stimulus, and were linked to cognitive processing of information in which the individual was occupied. The potentials

intermediate between these two types, more of a perceptive type than a sensory type (such as visual N1), were called *mesogenous* (Hillyard and Kutas, 1983). In reality this distinction between exogenous and endogenous potentials is no longer considered to be valid because it has been discovered that sensory potentials are also strongly modified by higher cognitive processes such as attention (for further details on this topic refer to Chapters 10–12, this volume). Naturally, the first sensory components of the ERPs (exogenous) are much more strongly influenced by sensory-physical factors (such as stimulus luminance, spatial frequency, eccentricity) than are the later components, which reflect higher order mental processes linked to thought and emotions.

Unlike the electroencephalogram, made up of "spontaneous" fluctuations of electrical activity in the brain—linked, in a broad sense, to variations in the state of general activation (e.g., sleep–wake, different arousal states)—ERPs represent transient changes of potentials in the form of a series of negative and positive deflections measurable only with the technique of synchronization between the event and the potential that it produces. Besides the potentials synchronized with a stimulus administered or omitted, it is also possible to record potentials synchronized with the individual's motor response, using this latter as the synchronization event and averaging the EEG traces relative to a certain number of trials with a backward trend for a certain period of time with respect to it. In this way brain activity occurring during decisional processes and motor programming preceding the response can be studied.

In general, evoked potentials, whether these are visual, auditory, or somatosensory, are wave forms characterized by a series of positive or negative deflections whose polarity is often indicated by the letters P and N, respectively, followed by increasing numbers denoting the temporal progression of their appearance. Although to some extent incorrect, these deflections are sometimes called "components." In reality, it is correct to speak of components only when the functional properties of a certain response are known together with the other characteristics, such as the topographic distribution. For example, according to Donchin (1979) it is appropriate to speak of the ("endogenous") ERP component when this varies systematically as a function of the cognitive context. Each bioelectrical potential recorded on the surface can be considered the manifestation of nervous activity associated with specific stages of transmission and processing of information within the nervous system. Measuring the various parameters of the ERP components, numerous indications can be obtained on the velocity and efficiency with which the processing of information occurs, on the processing resources required by each of the stages of the processing, and on the levels of mental load and attention invested in each of these. But, above all, compared with the other neuroimaging techniques, the ERPs are able to provide very precise information, with a resolution of milliseconds, on the time course of the various processing stages. In order to measure the amplitude of the evoked potentials in microvolts (μV), the so-called *base line*, or isoelectric line, must be calculated by measuring the mean value of the EEG in a given time window (normally 100 msec), which precedes the onset of the stimulus and which represents the absolute amplitude of the nervous system response in neutral conditions or during rest. This value is hypothetically considered as a zero amplitude response and every variation in positive or negative potential is measured with respect to this zero amplitude.

Alternatively the peak-to-peak amplitude can be obtained by calculating the distance between one positive peak and the subsequent negative one. In both cases, the amplitude is considered, in a broad sense,

to be the expression of the entity of the activation of the cell assembly units and the processing carried out on the stimulus. In other words, the greater the amplitude, the greater the number of activated neuronal units, the more elaborate the processing carried out on the stimulus at that particular stage. The exception to this rule is the so-called *probe* technique used by some investigators in research paradigms based on recordings of the ERPs in response to irrelevant stimuli administered to volunteers while they perform primary tasks. While the volunteer is occupied in tasks that are increasingly difficult to perform, the stimuli presented have the function of "probing" the level of mental work required by that task. It is probably obvious that in this case the implicit assumption is the opposite of the preceding: the greater the amplitude of the components recorded in response to the irrelevant stimuli, the greater the state of processing being used on these latter, the less the "cost" of the mental work required to carry out the "primary" task. It is reasonable to think that this method can be used to obtain information on processing resources, be they controlled or automated, "saved" by the individual during the experimental protocol to tackle concomitant tasks that might be administered to the individual (Isreal *et al.*, 1980; Papanicolau and Johnston, 1984).

In linear terms, on the other hand, the time interval between the stimulus (or the moment in which this should have been presented, because in reality it has been "omitted") and the appearance of each of the different components indicates the latency of these latter, normally expressed in milliseconds. The longer this interval, the later the activation of a particular stage of reflex information processing of the measured component is considered to be. For example, a component with a positive polarity appearing about 300 msec after the delivery or omission of a stimulus is defined P300.

The functional properties of the major ERP components so far known are described in the following discussions. This description is divided according to the different sensory modalities. As will be seen, there are considerable differences between the modalities in the components that reflect early sensory processing.

Auditory Evoked Potentials

Different wave forms generated by auditory stimuli can be distinguished on the basis of the latency of their appearance. Each potential reflects the response of different districts of the auditory pathways, has a different latency of appearance, and offers different possibilities for the study of information processing (Picton and Hillyard, 1988; Kutas and Dale, 1997) and for clinical and diagnostic aims (Gibson, 1980; McCandles, 1987).

Brain Stem and Middle Latency Potentials

Brain stem potentials, a group of components with a short latency, appear between 1 and 10 msec after administration of an auditory stimulus. These components are exclusive to acoustic stimuli and consist of six positive waves recorded at the central region of the head or the vertex (Cz); they are identified by Roman numerals of increasing size (I–VI), as can be seen in Fig. 4. They are surface reflections of sequential activation evoked by the acoustic stimuli in different centers and auditory pathways of the brain stem, that part of the central nervous system between the spinal cord and the encephalon, and are thus defined *brain stem potentials* (*BSPs*). In detail, these "exogenous" potentials are an expression of the sequential activity of the auditory nerve, the cochlear nuclei, the superior olives, the lateral lemniscus, the inferior colliculus, and the medial geniculate nucleus. The first, the third, and the fifth of these wave responses can be measured without problems or ambiguity in the majority of subjects examined and the reproducibility of the wave forms is constant. Because of this relationship between the wave form and the underlying nerve structures, the brain stem evoked potentials are without doubt the method of choice for (1) studying the mechanisms of processing auditory information at a very early level (e.g., Zani, 1989; Giraud *et al.*, 2000; Galbraith *et al.*, 2000) and (2) establishing

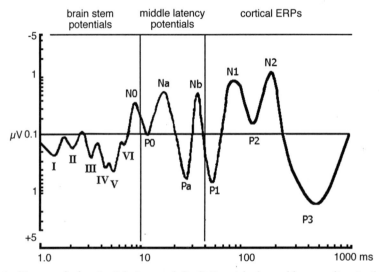

FIGURE 4 Auditory evoked potentials in an adult, distinguished roughly according to the poststimulus latency and the neural source of the different components.

Wave V peak latency   **Age**

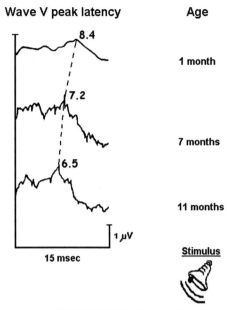

8.4

1 month

7.2

7 months

6.5

11 months

1 µV

15 msec

Stimulus

60 dB, 2000 Hz, 2 msec duration

FIGURE 5 Brain stem evoked potentials in response to tones of 60 dB intensity, recorded from neonates of various ages. The latency of the V component (expressed in milliseconds) changes with age, reflecting the degree of biological maturation.

the functional integrity of the auditory apparatus or the level of functional disorder in uncollaborative subjects (such as young children). Given the noninvasive nature of the technique of evoked potentials, the BSPs are very useful in ascertaining the degree of maturation of nerve pathways at various ages and, above all, in neonates, as can be seen in Fig. 5. The latencies of these components, and in particular that of the V wave, do in fact change with age and consequently with the degree of biological maturation. Starting from 1 to $1\frac{1}{2}$ months of age, the relationship between the intensity of the stimulus and the latency of the peak is similar to that found in adults. It is, therefore, understandable how these BSPs constitute a valuable method for early diagnosis of auditory defects and congenital deafness, thus allowing correspondingly early intensive rehabilitation interventions.

The so-called *middle latency potentials* appear between about 10 and 50 msec after

the stimulus onset (as shown in the second box in Fig. 4) (Picton *et al.*, 1974) and probably reflect neural activity of the thalamic nuclei, as well as the initial stages of arrival in the temporal region of the auditory cortex. These potentials, too, are useful for audiological analyses, but knowledge on their specific functions is scarce. It seems that they are an expression of the response of the auditory system to specific frequencies of presentation of the stimulus (that is, the number of repetitions of the stimulus in a given unit of time). They can be correctly identified in the wave forms recorded from children, but even if they can be used efficiently to analyze the auditory capacity of children, the reliability of the results obtained is less than that afforded by the brain stem potentials (McCandles, 1987; Gibson, 1980).

Cortical Auditory Potentials

The cortical components of auditory potentials form part of the class of ERP components, and apart from the first responses of sensory/perceptive type among which the N1 and the P2 are prominent (Picton and Hillyard, 1988), they are very similar to those elicited in the visual modality, and are schematically presented in the third box in Fig. 4. The first two components appear between 60 and 250 msec after the stimulus has been administered and reflect the activity generated in the cortex by the primary and associative areas of the temporal and parietal lobes of the cerebral hemispheres. These potentials seem to reflect analysis of the physical characteristics of a stimulus—for example, its intensity, frequency, pitch, timbre. In situations in which the individual is involved in cognitive tasks that, for example, require processes of allocation of attention or discrimination of stimulus material, these components become superimposed by negative potentials that modulate their amplitude. These oscillations are called attention-related negativity or *processing negativity* (Hansen and Hillyard,

1980; Näätätnen, 1982; Näätätnen *et al.*, 1985). The so-called negative difference (Nd) is the negative difference wave obtained by subtracting ERPs to irrelevant stimuli from those to task-relevant stimuli. There is evidence that Nd contains an early phase (Nde) with a central maximum (sensory specific), and a later phase (Ndl) with a more anterior distribution.

One very characteristic component of the auditory ERP, because it is not present in the other sensory modalities, is the so-called mismatch negativity (MMN), identified by Risto Näätänen (Näätänen *et al.*, 1978), to which a whole chapter of this book is dedicated. The MMN generally represents the response of the brain to any detectable difference in a repetitive acoustic stimulus and has a very wide range of uses in both clinical and experimental settings (see Ch. 14).

Late Components and the P300

The so-called late or cognitive components of the ERPs appear between 250 msec and 1 sec after the stimulus (Picton and Hillyard, 1988). Although they have a fairly supramodal character, they are not completely nonspecific. There is, in fact, experimental evidence of topographical differences according to the sensory modality considered. These components include the so-called P300, a family of components with positive polarity that appear from about 250 msec onward after the stimulus. They include a P3a, prominent on the frontal area of the brain in response to an unexpected novelty, which suggests an orientation reflex by the individual, and also a P3b, prominent on the parietal areas of the brain in response to stimuli that, even if known, are of unlikely probability of being presented, requiring reiteration of the process of categorization (Ruchkin *et al.*, 1987). Furthermore, they include a slow positive component, the *slow wave*, appearing at about 600–700 msec and continuing sometimes even beyond 1 sec.

These components reflect processes of cognitive updating, of activation of working memory, and of comparison with models stored in the memory. They are, therefore, strongly dependent on past experience, the individual's expectations, and semantic evaluation of the stimulus. It is precisely for this reason that they also appear in the case of a lack of presentation (omission) of an expected stimulus, thus justifying their designation as "endogenous" components (Ruchkin *et al.*, 1988). In more detail, if, as the result of the process of categorizing a stimulus, a discordance with the individual's own interior "model" is perceived, a process of "contextual cognitive updating" takes place, reflected by the P300. The hypothesized "subroutine" (Donchin, 1981) or the so-called dedicated processor (Donchin *et al.*, 1973), of which these components are thought to be the surface expression, would therefore be invoked by the system any time that it obtains information that requires a revision of hypotheses or models of the surrounding environment. These are, therefore, formed only after the individual clearly recognizes to which category to attribute the stimulus. An obvious extension of this is that these components are also expressions of the ability to discriminate the stimulus. In practice they are a function of the *a posteriori* certainty of having correctly received and interpreted the stimulus.

Speaking of processes of contextual updating or memory recovery is not antithetical to the distinctions proposed between *automated and controlled processes* in information processing (Hoffman, 1990; Rösler and Manzey, 1986). This conceptualization is based on the assumption that there are two qualitatively different modalities of processing that characterize our nervous system. *Automated processes* are carried out without the individual's attention and indeed the individual is not conscious of performing them. Furthermore, they do not interfere with other automated activities carried out at the same time by the nervous system. For example, all those processes that synthesize a percept starting from the sensory input or that transform a plan of action into a real movement can be automated. Examples of automated processes in daily life are all those complex motor actions that we carry out without any apparent effort in adult life (such as eating spaghetti, unbuttoning a shirt, brushing our teeth, driving a car) and that allow us to speak or carry out other activities at the same time without any difficulty. Nevertheless, these are very difficult and complex to reproduce for a small child or anyone who has not had adequate training. Another characteristic of the *automated processes* is that they are carried out without a control that we could define as conscious or voluntary, to the point that they can be unintentional—for example, when we dial one telephone number instead of another when our mind is occupied with other things. In contrast, *controlled processes* are voluntary and indeed cannot take place without direct control of the conscience. These interfere with other controlled cognitive activities because they are dependent on a central system (presumably frontal) with a limited capacity. The controlled processes take longer to carry out compared to the automated processes. On the other hand, controlled processes can be changed and altered and applied in new and different situations that could not be efficiently managed by the automated processes. Examples of controlled processes are learning new material or difficult motor sequences. For example, dialing a telephone number never previously used requires attention to the task and does not allow other tasks requiring attention to be carried out simultaneously.

Analyzing the properties of the P300 in the framework of this theory, it can be shown that the P300 is always evoked with a notable amplitude when the situation requires controlled processing, whereas it has a minimal amplitude or is absent when the situation can be managed automati-

cally. Contextual updating, therefore, is an example of a situation that requires adoption of a controlled strategy in a situation in which the processing of information, which proceeded up to that point in an automated way, no longer permits automation because the resulting stimuli are different from the model stored in the memory.

This explains some contradictory results in the scientific literature. Some studies found a correlation between P300 and reaction times (Roth *et al.*, 1978), whereas others, with rigorously controlled studies, found no association between the two (e.g., Karlin *et al.*, 1971). This contradiction was resolved by the repeated demonstration that the latency of the P300 depends only on the processes of classifying the stimulus and is, to a large extent, independent of the selection of the motor response and the time to carry it out. For example, it was shown (Kutas *et al.*, 1977) that in a situation requiring precision and accuracy in evaluating a stimulus, the selection of the response depends on the process of categorizing the stimulus, and, thus, the reaction times (RTs) and the latency of the P300 appear to be strongly correlated. In contrast, if the speed of response is privileged, the response can be made before the stimulus has been completely evaluated and thus the two measures result as only being weakly correlated or indeed not correlated at all. Thus, generally speaking, although the RTs depend on many processes between the stimulus and the response, including selection of a plan of action and processes of performing the response, the latency of the P300 depends largely on the processes of evaluating the stimulus. Valuable data supporting this theoretical model were provided by studies based on Sternberg's paradigm of additive factors. In some of these (McCarthy and Donchin, 1981; Magliero *et al.*, 1984), both the discriminability of the stimulus (easy or difficult) and the response processes (compatible or incompatible with the stimulus) were made to vary. The result was that although the latency of the P300 depended only on the discriminability of the stimulus, the RTs depended in an additive manner on both the discriminability of the stimulus and the compatibility between the stimulus and response.

Besides categorization processes, the P300 has been strongly associated with working and short-term memory processes. For example, in an electrophysiological study by Kleins et al. (1984) it emerged that this component represented processes of access to the representation of sounds in the auditory working memory. This study compared the ERPs recorded in two groups of musicians, one with absolute pitch, the other without this ability. The ear with absolute pitch allows its owner to identify the absolute pitch of pure tones in the absence of reference stimuli. The results showed that both groups had a positive component (between 300 and 600 msec poststimulus) over the parietal area during a visual "oddball" task. During an auditory oddball task, however, this component was present only in the control group and its amplitude was greatly reduced or indeed not present in the group of musicians with absolute pitch. The authors' hypothesis was that these latter have a permanent reference of all tones and do not need to make continual comparisons of information and thus activation of short-term memory mechanisms expressed by the P300 component.

In another electrophysiological study by Nielsen-Bohlman and Knight (1994), the P300 was associated with processes of short-term maintenance of mental representation. This study consisted of a task of recognizing pictorial images of familiar objects that could have been presented in the previous 1.2 sec (immediate interval), in the previous 1.2 to 4 sec (short interval), or more than 5 sec earlier (5–158 seconds, long interval). The ERP results showed a frontal P3a and a parietal P3b in concomi-

tance with the recognition of stimuli presented after a short interval, and a mesial temporal N400 for stimuli presented immediately or after a long interval. According to the authors, the P300 could indicate activation of mechanisms of access to the working memory guided by the frontal area, whereas the N400 could reflect activation of the mesial temporal cortex involved in long-term memory.

Alternatively, and also on the basis of ERP and RT data that demonstrate the decreasing P300 and the prolongation of the RT with the increasingly long interval, it could be hypothesized that the P300 observed in this study reflects in any case the certainty of the recognition and thus processes of categorization rather than of memory.

Motor Potentials

Stimulus-locked motor potentials are formed from variations of brain electrical potentials that occur when an individual's attention is directed to planning an action in relation to a sequence of stimuli. This action can be a decision process, a motor action, or inhibition of a possible motor action. In these situations a large expectation negativity develops, which is called *contingent negative variation* (CNV) [see also Fabiani et al. (2000) and Brunia and Van Boxtel (2000) for a description of motor potentials]. This deflection is considered to be the expression of processes of preparation and orientation in view of performing a required response to the task (see an example in Fig. 6).

A series of two negative and two positive components, defined as a whole as "motor and premotor potentials" distinguished by CNV and direct expression of the performance of motor actions, belong to the same family. In fact, the motor and premotor potentials are obtained by synchronizing the EEG with the onset of the electromyographic activity. By recording the EEG and EMG simultaneously and without interruptions, the start of the first

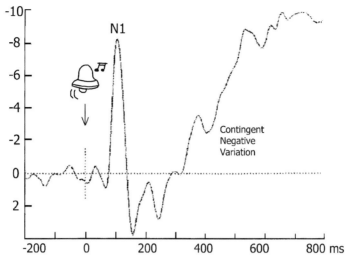

FIGURE 6 Grand-average auditory potential evoked by a 1000-Hz pure tone of 100-msec duration, and recorded from the midline central site Cz. In this experiment (Proverbio, 1993), the auditory stimulus acted as a warning tone, alerting the subject to the appearance of a visual target stimulus to which the subjects had to respond. Note the prominent cortical N1 and P2 followed by an increasing negativity lasting for the more than 600 msec; this is the contingent negative variation.

muscle *spike* is used as the synchronization event to average the EEG trace, both in the time preceding and subsequent to it for a given interval. It is, therefore, understandable that these can be recorded only for an intentional act carried out by the individual, completely independently of any stimulus. The first negative component that precedes the start of muscle activity is known as *readiness potential* (*Bereitschaftpotentiale*, in German). This deflection, which evolves symmetrically over both cerebral hemispheres for up to 500 msec before the start of the motor activity, becomes asymmetrically greater over the motor areas of the hemisphere contralateral to the limb to be moved from 500 msec onward. It appears to reflect the general preparation, or motivation, of a voluntary motor action. It is followed by a small positive deflection, called P1 and defined as "premotor positivity," which develops starting from 150 msec before the start of the movement (or rather the onset of EMG, because between this and the motor action there is a delay of 250 msec, on average). It has been suggested that this expresses the sending of the order of the

motor program. The wave form then continues with a negative deflection, called N2, defined as the "motor potential," and is particularly pronounced over the motor areas. Finally, this is followed by the so-called reafference potential, or P2 (Deecke *et al.*, 1984; Kristeva *et al.*, 1990). This description should, however, be considered a simplification because there is a much richer and complex division of the potentials [see Brunia and Van Boxtel (2000) for an exhaustive review].

Visual Evoked Potentials

The visual evoked potentials (VEPs) are distinguished from the auditory evoked potentials predominantly by their morphology and by the fact that it is not possible, or only to a very limited extent, to observe the evoked responses derived from subcortical structures such as the superior colliculus or lateral geniculate nucleus of thalamus. Therefore, they consist of fewer waves, namely, those deriving from the activity of the cerebral cortex.

The study of VEPs has elicited great interest since the very earliest electrophysiological techniques were realized to be instruments to identify anomalies or pathologies of the visual system (e.g., Celesia and Daly, 1977). These techniques remain an irreplaceable tool for studying alterations in the mechanisms of visual processing. For the past 25 years, thanks to the development of cognitive electrophysiology and cognitive neuroscience, researchers have not merely concentrated on the first stages of sensory analysis, traditionally studied by VEPs (Jeffreys, 1970), but also on the subsequent stages of information processing and on the way in which higher cognitive processes (such as attention, emotions, motivation, memory, and cognition) can affect visual processing (e.g., Neville *et al.*, 1982; Duncan-Johnson

and Donchin, 1982). Therefore, in modern studies the term "VEPs" has been replaced by or combined with the concept of visual ERPs (e.g., Friedman *et al.*, 1978; Shulman-Galambos and Galambos, 1978).

Here we briefly describe the main sensory components of visual ERPs, which modern literature has shown to be affected by higher cognitive processes. This topic is dealt with specifically in Chapters 10 and 12, which are devoted to visual selective attention mechanisms. Therefore, the old distinction between exogenous and endogenous components (e.g., Picton and Hillyard, 1988) will not be referred to in this discussion.

Figure 7 shows human VEPs elicited by a black and white luminance-modulated grating with a spatial frequency of 6 cycles per degree. The grating was presented to

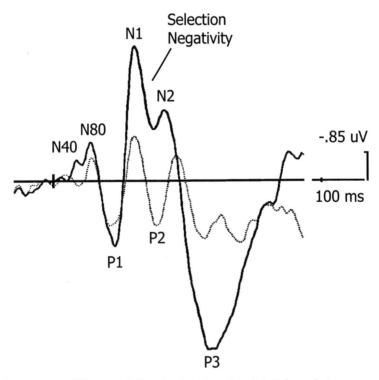

FIGURE 7 Grand-average ERPs recorded at the right lateral occipital electrode in response to gratings of 6 cycles/degree presented to the fovea during a task of selective attention for spatial frequency. The two superimposed lines indicate different conditions of attention of the observer, depending on the type of stimulus seen: the solid line represents cerebral activity evoked by gratings of the relevant spatial frequency, whereas the dotted line represents the cerebral response to the same stimuli when irrelevant.

the central visual field with a *pattern onset*[1] modality, randomly intermixed with gratings of different spatial frequencies. The solid line represents the cerebral activity evoked by the same grating when its spatial frequency was relevant, whereas the dotted line represents the evoked response to the same grating when irrelevant. The potentials are grand averages and were recorded at the right lateral occipital site. At this location a characteristic series of negative and positive deflections can be seen, reflecting the different stages of analysis of the visual information. The first peak around 40 msec is not always seen because its amplitude is modest and it emerges only when the signal-to-noise ratio is optimal. In this case it has a negative polarity and reflects a stage of subcortical analysis (probably thalamic). The second peak is called N80, or P80 when it presents with the opposite polarity, and reflects the earliest stages of processing of visual inputs in the primary visual area (striate cortex or area 17). It is also known as C1, which stands for the first component of VEPs (Jeffreys, 1971, 1977; Drasdo, 1980). This early component, together with the subsequent P1, has a variable amplitude and latency according to the spatial frequency of the stimulus. In

particular, low spatial frequencies (e.g., 1.5 cycles/degree) elicit a bigger and faster P1, whereas higher spatial frequencies (e.g., 12 cycles/degree) elicit a more modest and later P1 and large early negativities (Bodis-Wollner *et al.*, 1992; Hudnell *et al.*, 1990; Previc, 1988; Proverbio *et al.*, 1996; Skrandies, 1984; Zani and Proverbio, 1995, 1997). These two components are very sensitive to physical parameters of the stimulus (Lesevre, 1982) and vary greatly in function of the quadrant of stimulation, its luminance, contrast, retinal location (Clark and Hillyard, 1995), width of the visual field, orientation (Proverbio *et al.*, 2002b), and color, as well as spatial frequency (Aine *et al.*, 1990). It has been hypothesized that the C1 (or PN/80), which is topographically and functionally separable from the P1, represents activity of the *parvocellular visual system*,[2] devoted to analysis of color and high-frequency pattern (Livingstone and Hubel, 1988), whereas P1 represents the activity of the *magnocellular system*, devoted to analysis of achromatic, low-frequency patterns (Kulikowski *et al.*, 1989; Paulus and Plendl, 1988; Zani and Proverbio, 1995). One is overrepresented in the fovea, thus conferring the visual acuity necessary for *photopic vision*; the other constitutes the majority of peripheral ganglia cells and allows, for example, immediate appreciation of a shadow moving at the observer's shoulder (*scotopic vision*). In an ERP study showing hemispheric asymmetries in evoked activity during passive viewing of sinusoidal spatial frequency gratings (Proverbio *et al.*, 1996), *scalp current density* mapping (see Appendix D for details on this procedure) provided evidence of a progressive shift of focus of the maximum amplitude of the N80 from the right hemisphere to the left

---

[1] The recording of an evoked potential using the *pattern onset* modality occurs in synchrony with the *onset* (or start) of the stimulus, generally followed by its disappearance (or pattern offset). This gives rise to a transient cerebral response, which is a contingent response from the brain followed by a return to prestimulus base line "activity." When the stimuli are presented very closely together in time, thus not allowing a return to base line, a so-called stable (or steady-state) evoked response is produced. The same type of response occurs when the configuration of stimuli remaining fixed on the screen alter over time [for example, a checkerboard with black and white squares or differently colored squares, whose constituent elements rhythmically, at a preestablished velocity (e.g., 3 Hz) take on the opposite color: white–black, black–white, etc.], a technique defined as pattern inversion (or pattern reversal). For a fuller treatment of evoked potentials in response to *pattern reversal* the reader is referred to Silberstein (1995b) and to Chapter 11, this volume.

---

[2] In particular, reflecting activity of the ganglia cells from the lateral geniculate body of the thalamus and afferents to the striate visual cortex (area 17).

one as the spatial frequency increased. These data support the hypothesis of a hemispherical asymmetry in spatial frequency processing independent of higher order cognitive factors (Hellige, 1993; Hughes *et al.*, 1996; Proverbio *et al.*, 1997a, 1998). Other properties of this component, with particular reference to the neural generators and modulation by superior cognitive factors such as attention, are described in Chapter 12 (this volume).

The third positive peak is the P1 component of VEPs, which has a latency of about 100 to 140 msec. This is supposed to derive from the evoked activity of the extrastriate visual cortex (Lesevre and Joseph, 1979; Heinze *et al.*, 1994; Mangun *et al.*, 2001; Ossenblock and Spekreijse, 1991; Proverbio *et al.*, 1996; Zani and Proverbio, 1995, 1997) and often shows a right hemispheric asymmetry. P1 component analysis is crucial for studies on space-based selective attention mechanisms. Its amplitude is strongly affected by attention and expectancy factors. For example, if an observer expects that a certain stimulus will appear at a given space location (for example, that a mouse will come out of a mousehole) the visual system processes all the stimuli relative to that retinal location with more emphasis and accuracy. This activates a larger number of neurons that fire with greater strength as soon as they receive the subcortical inputs, producing larger bioelectrical potentials with a shorter latency. The greater efficiency of the sensory analysis, as well as of the classification processes and motor programming, mean that the reaction times to the stimulus are faster (the mouse will be caught). Observing the amplitude of the visual P1, it is possible to establish a gradient of activation in function of the different levels of attention and expectation of the observer.

Returning to the ERP in Fig. 7, the P1 sensory component is followed by a series of negative deflections, N1 and N2, both strongly affected by attention. As can be seen in the figure (see also Chapters 10–12, on attention), selective attention toward a given category of visual stimuli is manifested by an increase in the negativity recorded over the posterior region of the scalp between 150 and 300 msec after the stimulus; this is called *selection negativity* (Harter and Aine, 1984) or *processing negativity* (Näätänen, 1982). This large negativity is followed by the P300 positive component, which we have already discussed thoroughly—this, too, strongly influenced by attention, cognitive, and motivational factors of various types.

Linguistic Potentials

On the basis of the rich literature on this subject (e.g., Kutas and Van Petten, 1994; Kutas *et al.*, 1999; Osterhout, 1994; Osterhout and Holcomb, 1995; Van Petten, 1995), various different ERP components have been identified, each with their own topography and functional characteristics. The observation and analysis of these in certain experimental paradigms allow us to investigate the different processing stages of mechanisms of understanding language in humans. Given the obvious production of muscle artifacts during speech, oral production of language is not generally used in studies with this method. Analysis of the different components of the ERPs, described extremely well in Chapter 6, has allowed identification (roughly speaking) of a stage of grapheme/orthographic (in reading) or phonological (in speech processing) analysis, a stage of semantic/lexical analysis, a stage of analysis of the structure of the phrase, and a more sophisticated stage of syntactic analysis. The technique of ERPs enables a certain temporal course to be established for the various processes, but naturally many of these occur in parallel and are accompanied by numerous integration processes that put together the information in a compatible way, piece by piece, as it becomes available on the basis of context and previous knowledge.

On the basis of event-related brain potential studies we are able, for example, to establish that semantic analysis and integration processes take place about 400 msec poststimulus, as reflected by the N400 component, a centroparietal negativity whose properties have been widely characterized (Kutas and Hillyard, 1980; Kutas and Van Petten, 1994). On the other hand, phrase structure assignment and syntactic integration are assumed to be reflected by an early left anterior negativity (ELAN) with a latency of about 100–300 msec, a left anterior negativity (LAN) with a latency of about 300–500 msec, and a late centroparietal positivity (P600), also called *syntactic positive shift* (Osterhout and Holcomb, 1992, 1993; Hahne and Friederici, 1999; Friederici *et al.*, 1999; Münte *et al.*, 1998). The ELAN is thought to reflect a first-pass parsing process and to be very sensitive to word category, being guided by phrase structure rules. The later negativity (LAN), overlapping in time with semantic N400, is thought to reflect morphosyntactic analysis. This late positivity might reflect relatively controlled language-related processes (Hahne and Friederici, 1999) sensitive to inflectional information (Gunter and Friederici, 1999) and associated with secondary syntactic processes such as sentence reanalysis and repair (Friederici, 1997), or processes to inhibit incorrect representation due to difficulty with syntactic integration (Kaan *et al.*, 2000).

Figure 8 shows an example of these linguistic components derived from data obtained in our laboratory in an experiment in which volunteers were required to evaluate the correctness of visually presented phrases (Proverbio *et al.*, 2002a). In the example shown below, the ERPs were recorded at the onset of the last word, which could be correct or incorrect and/or incongruous with respect to the previous context:

Correct sentence: *She was frightened by his NASTINESS*

Semantically incongruent: *The structure of the city was too ENVIOUS*

Syntactically incongruent: *All the windows were CONVICTION*

In the upper part of Fig. 8, grand-average ERPs recorded from the frontal sites are displayed as a function of correctness of the terminal word. We can see that semantically + syntactically incongruent words elicit a large negativity around 400 msec poststimulus, which is the N400 component originally identified by Marta Kutas (Kutas and Hillyard, 1980; Kutas and Van Petten, 1988). This negative response generally indicates word recognition and semantic processing, as well as the brain response to contextually unexpected items (Kutas and Kluender, 1994). It is generated by semantically anomalous words, or at any rate words not expected by the subject—that is, at low *cloze probability* (probability that a given word will be used to finish the sentence); for a more in-depth discussion of the functional

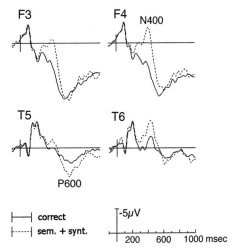

FIGURE 8 Examples of grand-average ($N = 9$) ERPs recorded at left and right frontal and posterior temporal sites in response to correct (solid line) or semantically + syntactically incongruent terminal words (dashed line). Note the large anterior negativity (N400) in response to semantic incongruence, and the delayed left temporal positivity (P615) in response to syntactic incongruence (adapted and modified from Proverbio *et al.*, 2002a).

significance of this see Chapter 6 (this volume).

The lower part of Fig. 8 shows grand-average ERPs recorded from the posterior temporal sites, where it is possible to see the onset of a late positive component (P600) for the phrases that are also syntactically incorrect. A late centroparietal positivity with a latency varying between 600 and 900 msec has been described in the literature as the response to syntactic incongruence, *syntactic positive shift* (SPS) (Hagoort *et al.*, 1993), and/or processes of reviewing the interpretation of a phrase (Mecklinger *et al.*, 1995). The two components N400 and P600 indicate, also in terms of temporal latency, that the linguistic processing is occurring at two levels: a *semantic* level with analysis of significance on the basis of context and a *syntactic* level with analysis of the relationships between the parts of the phrase on the basis of the grammatical rules of the language. Semantic analysis thus seems to take place about 400 msec after auditory or visual presentation of a word, but it can be seen how the N400 peak in reality represents the culmination of a process (access to the lexicon) that has begun gradually several tens of milliseconds earlier.

The first stage of processing visually presented words consists of a sensory analysis of their physical features, such as luminance, orientation, size, color, contrast, and spatial frequency. Identification of the characters as having linguistic significance (orthographic analysis) takes place about 150 msec after the onset of the stimulus in the occipitotemporal area (lingual gyrus and left and right fusiform gyri), as shown in a magnetoencephalographic study by Kuriki *et al.* (1988). On the other hand, with a PET study, Petersen and colleagues (1988) identified a visual area specialized in recognizing the graphic form of words (*visual word form system*) in the left medial extrastriate cortex of the occipital lobe. In their study, strong activation of this region was seen during the reading of words or pseudowords (nonexistent words, but ones that obeyed the orthographic rules of the given language), but this activation was absent for nonwords (ill-formed letter strings) or false font strings. These first findings were confirmed by subsequent studies that identified the area devoted to recognition of real letters in the posterior fusiform gyrus (Allison *et al.*, 1994) and in the occipitotemporal and inferior occipital sulci (Puce *et al.*, 1996). The left hemisphere's specialization of the region devoted to letter analysis was very recently demonstrated by neuroimaging studies (Polk *et al.*, 2002).

The first stages of graphemic analysis and recognition of the above-described words correspond to the appearance of the N1 evoked component with a latency between 150 and 200 msec (Bentin *et al.*, 1999). Subsequently, the N2 indicates a stage of phonological type analysis of the information—that is, analysis related to the sounds of the language, both with the auditory and visual modalities of presentation. For example, in the ERP study by Connolly and Phillips (1994), auditory–phonemic type linguistic violations produced a negative response called phonological *mismatch negativity* (MMN) around 270–300 msec after the onset of the word. This component in reality responds automatically to any discriminable difference between two auditory stimuli (e.g., pure sounds, chords, linguistic stimuli) even in the absence of attention (Näätänen, 1992, 1995) and is described in depth in Chapter 14.

In a study in our laboratory (Proverbio *et al.*, 1997b, 1999), subjects performed a phonological decision task on parts of words or syllables without sense (trigrams) briefly presented to the central visual field. The ERPs showed a large negative response to phonological incongruence (nontargetness) starting from about 250 msec poststimulus. Figure 9 shows grand-average ERPs to targets (syllables whose grapheme/phoneme conversion produced

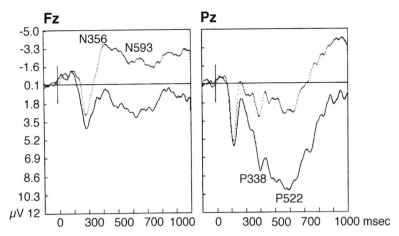

FIGURE 9 Examples of grand-average ERPs elicited by visually presented syllables during a phonologic decision task, and recorded at frontal (Fz) and parietal (Pz) midline sites. The solid and dashed lines represent the potentials elicited, respectively, by the syllables that included or did not include the target sounds (adapted from Proverbio *et al.*, 1999).

the phonological form expected by subjects) and nontargets (syllables incompatible with the expected phonological form) recorded at frontal (FZ) and parietal (PZ) sites. It is interesting to note that over the anterior area there was a negative deflection in response to phonologically incorrect syllables, with two peaks around 350 and 600 msec, whereas over the posterior area correct syllables produced a huge positivity, with two peaks around 340 (P300) and 520 msec (late positivity). Given that the participants had to respond to both targets and nontargets by pressing one of two response keys with either the index or middle finger, any difference between the two wave forms can be attributed to recognition of a phonological incongruence that generates a phonological *mismatch negativity* similar to that found in the auditory–phonetic modality.

SOMATOSENSORY EVOKED POTENTIALS

The *somatosensory evoked potentials* (SEPs), reflect the activity of cortical regions of somatosensory projections, and thus, in the initial stages, of the functional-

ity of the somatesthetic systems. Most of the components that indicate the different stages of both sensory and cognitive processing of the somatesthetic inputs are shown in Fig. 10a. The positive components P10, P12, P13, and P14, not represented in the figure and indicating the very early latency of the first phases of the processing, are thought to reflect, respectively, discharge of the peripheral nerve, arrival in the dorsal root of the spinal cord, and then arrival in the mesencephalon (13–14 msec). On the other hand there are indications that the P15 (see Fig. 10b) could be generated in the medial lemniscus, or in the thalamus (Allison, 1984). The N20, the P20, and the P25 are thought to reflect activity of the primary somatosensory cortex. All of the other components up to P100 reflect potentials generated in the primary somatosensory cortex or surrounding areas. Desmedt and Robertson (1977) demonstrated that the N140 and the P190, also called *vertex potentials*, are strongly influenced by attention. Indeed, during tasks of selective attention, a large somatosensory *processing negativity* (Näätänen and Michie, 1979) develops, which is very similar to that described for the auditory modality. More recent electro-

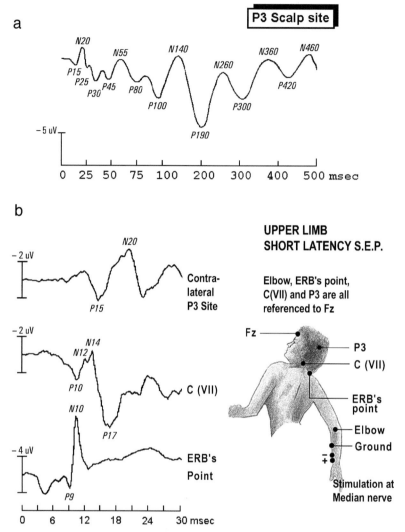

FIGURE 10 Diagram of somatosensory evoked potentials. (a) Theoretical example of a wave form recorded over the left parietal area (P3) in response to electric shocks to the right median nerve in a young adult; (b) prominent early components of the wave form of the somatosensory evoked potential (SEP) obtained recording at Erb's point, or the midclavicular point, from the cervical vertebrae, and from the contralateral cortex, respectively.

physiologic studies have provided evidence of attention-related modulation of somatosensory potentials already at the level of the early cortical P40 component. This component is, in fact, more positive for relevant stimuli than for irrelevant stimuli over the areas of the scalp contralateral to the stimulated limb (Desmedt and Tomberg, 1989; Garcia-Larrea *et al.*, 1991; see also Näätänen, 1992).

EVENT-RELATED FIELDS

The notable development of neuromagnetometry, which is the recording of brain magnetic fields, has led to the identification of a set of components of different prominence and polarity in wave forms, which distinguish the magnetic responses, or event-related fields, elicited by stimuli in the various sensory modalities. In the following discussion we provide some brief descriptions of the nature and functional characteristics of these components. We are, of course, completely aware that these descriptions are far from being exhaustive.

Auditory Event-Related Fields

Similar to the findings of the auditory ERP, the first deflection shown by an auditory ERF wave form is an early positive component defined as P50m (see Fig. 11). This component appears in particular when a click is used instead of tones. It is followed by a prominent N100m, whose generator seems to lie in the supratemporal auditory cortex. The amplitudes of both are greater over the auditory cortex of the hemisphere contralateral to the stimulated ear (Hari *et al.*, 1987). It was found that the source of the N100m has different locations within the auditory cortex; the locations are a function of the frequency of the transient tones administered. These results indicate that the auditory cortex has a tonotopic organization (Romani *et al.*, 1982). This type of functional organization was also suggested by sustained (*steady-state*) auditory stimuli (Elberling *et al.*, 1982).

The N100m component is followed by a P200m. Rif *et al.* (1991) reported that paying attention to tones administered at a constant interval of 405 msec modifies the wave forms starting precisely from the P200m. Indeed, the authors found a notable reduction in the amplitude of the P200m caused by the superimposition of the magnetic analog (i.e., SNm) of selection negativity (Näätänen, 1982). However, in a more recent study, Woldorff *et al.* (1993) demonstrated that attention modulates the brain auditory magnetic responses much earlier than indicated by the results cited above. Using an attention-requiring task in which the participants had to concentrate on tones presented rapidly to one ear while ignoring those presented to the other ear,

they found that when the tones were relevant, they elicited fields of a greater amplitude than when they were irrelevant, as early as 20 msec after the stimulus. On the basis of the measurement of fMRI-recorded brain activity in this same study, the authors were also able to indicate that the generators of these very early auditory attention effects were localized in the supratemporal plane of the temporal lobe.

Visual Event-Related Fields

As can be seen in Fig. 11, the wave form of the visual magnetic fields (*visual evoked fields*, VEFs) is characterized by a prominent P1m component, the peak of which appears after a latency between 100 and 150 msec. This is followed by an N1m and a P2m. A full treatment of the functional properties of these components is beyond the scope of this chapter. For this the reader is referred to the impressive review

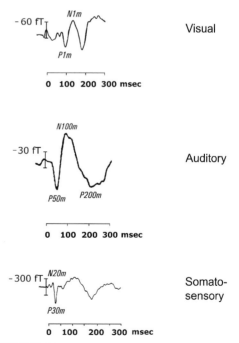

FIGURE 11 Diagram of the magnetic wave forms illustrating the components most discussed in the literature as a function of sensory modality. Note the different scales [in femtoteslas (fT)] of the wave forms.

in Chapter 5, on MEG studies of visual cognition.

We restrict discussion here to a couple of short and very sketchy notes on the P1m component. There are experimental results in the literature demonstrating that this component varies as a function of the threshold of contrast, and of the temporal and spatial frequencies of the visual stimulus. For example, there is evidence that with increased temporal frequency, low spatial frequency gratings elicit magnetic P1m of greater amplitude than do high spatial frequency gratings (e.g., Okada *et al.*, 1982). Furthermore, and most importantly, there are indications that paying selective attention to a point in space or to the physical characteristics of the stimulus (e.g., spatial frequency) increases the amplitude of this early magnetic response (Aine *et al.*, 1995), analogous to the findings of Zani and Proverbio (1995, 1997) for its electrical counterpart, the P1, of the ERPs.

Somatosensory Event-Related Fields

In neurologically healthy individuals, electrical stimulation of the median nerve in the wrist induces an early magnetic response in the contralateral primary somatosensory cortex, SI, detectable by 20 msec after the stimulation. This response has a negative polarity and is therefore indicated as N20m (Fig. 11). It should be emphasized, however, that the polarity of this response changes as the recording electrode is moved from the perisylvian area up to the vertex of the parietal postcentral gyrus. This early component is followed by the P30m.

The latency of appearance of both these components is much delayed in patients with multiple sclerosis. Furthermore, in such patients the responses recorded with a latency of about 50–80 msec for the area representing the hand, within the SI, are abnormally large (Karhu *et al.*, 1982).

The responses on the ipsilateral somatosensory cortex are very different and vary according to whether an electric shock is used to stimulate the median nerve (upper limb) or the peroneal nerve (lower limb). In the former case, the first magnetic response observable in the SEF wave forms has a poststimulus latency of about 90–95 msec. In the latter case, the peak latency of the first response is later at about 110–125 msec (Hari *et al.*, 1984; Hari, 1994). It has been suggested (Hari *et al.*, 1984) that the magnetic flow of these components reflects the functional modifications in the secondary somatosensory cortex, SII.

References

Aine, C. J., Bodis-Wollner, I., and George, J. S. (1990). Spatial frequency segregation and evidence for multiple sources. *In* "Advances in Neurology. Magnetoencephalography" (S. Sato, ed.), pp. 141–155. Raven Press, New York.

Aine, C. J., Supek, S., and George, J. S. (1995). Temporal dynamics of visual evoked neuromagnetic sources: Effects of stimulus parameters and selective attention. *Int. J. Neurosci.* **80**, 79–104.

Allison, T. (1984). Recording and interpreting event-related potentials. *In* "Cognitive Psychophysiology. Event-related Potentials and the Study of Cognition" (E. Donchin, ed.), pp. 1–36. Lawrence Erlbaum Assoc., Hillsdale, New Jersey.

Allison, T., McCarthy, G., Nobre, A., Puce, A., and Belger, A. (1994). Human extrastriate visual cortex and the perception of faces, words, numbers, and colors. *Cerebral Cortex* **4**, 544–554.

Bentin, S., Mouchetant-Rostaing, Y., Giard, M. H., *et al.* (1999). ERP manifestations of processing printed words at different psycholinguistic levels: Time course and scalp distribution. *J. Cogn. Neurosci.* **11**, 235–260.

Bodis-Wollner, I., Brinnan, J. R., Nicoll, J., Frkovic, S., and Mylin, L. (1992). A short latency cortical component of the foveal VEP is revealed by hemifield stimulation. *Electroencephalogr. Clin. Neurophysiol.* **84**, 201–205.

Brunia, C. H. M., and Van Boxtel, G. J. M. (2000). Motor preparation. *In* "Handbook of Psychophysiology" (J. T. Cacioppo, L. G. Tassinary, and G. G. Berntson, eds.), 2nd Ed., pp. 507–532. Cambridge University Press, Cambridge.

Buzsaki, G. (1991). The thalamic clock: Emergent network properties. *Neuroscience* **41**, 351–364.

Celesia, G. G., and Daly, R. F. (1977). Visual electroencephalographic computer analysis (VECA). A new electrophysiologic test for the diagnosis of optic nerve lesions. *Neurology* **27**(7), 637–641

Clark, V. P., and Hillyard S. A. (1995). Identification of early visual evoked potential generators by retinotopic and topographic analyses. *Human Brain Mapping* **2**, 170–187.

Connolly, J. F., and Phillips, N. A. (1994). Event-related potential components reflect phonological and semantic processing of the terminal word of spoken sentences. J. Cogn. Neurosci. 3, pp. 256–266.

Deecke, L., Bashore, T., Brunia, C. H., Grunewald-Zuberbier, E., and Grunewald, G. (1984). Movement-associated potentials and motor control. *Ann. N.Y. Acad. Sci.* **425**, 398–428.

Del Gratta, C., and Romani, G. L. (1999). MEG: Principles, methods, and applications, *Biomed. Technik* **44**, Suppl. 2, pp. 11–23.

De Munck, J. C. (1990). The estimation of time varying dipoles on the basis of VEP. *Electroencephalogr. Clin. Neurophysiol.* **77**, 156–160.

De Munck, J. C., Van Dijk, B. W., and Spekreijse, H. (1988). Mathematical dipoles are adequate to describe realistic generators of human brain activity. *IEEE Trans. Biomed. Eng.* **11**, 960–966.

Desmedt, J. E., and Robertson, D. (1977). Differential enhancement of early and late components of the cerebral somatosensory evoked potentials during forced-paced cognitive tasks in man. *J. Physiol.* **271**, 761–782.

Desmedt, T. J., and Tomberg, C. (1989). Mapping early somatosensory evoked potentials in selective attention: Critical evaluations of control conditions used for titrating by difference the cognitive P30, P40, P100 and N140. *Electroencephalogr. Clin. Neurophysiol.* **74**, 321–346.

Donchin, E. (1979). Event-related brain potentials in the study of human information processing. *In* "Evoked Brain Potentials and Behaviour" (H. Begleiter, ed.), pp. 13–88, Plenum Press, New York.

Donchin, E. (1981). Surprise!...Surprise! *Psychophysiology* **9**, 493–513.

Donchin, E., Kubovy, M., Kutas, M., Johnson, R., Jr., and Hernin, G. F. (1973). Graded changes in evoked response (P300) amplitude as a function of cognitive activity. *Perception Psychophys.* **14**, 319–324.

Drasdo, N. (1980). Cortical potentials evoked by pattern presentation in the foveal region. *In* "Evoked Potentials" (C. Barber, ed.), pp. 167–174. MTP Press, Falcon House, Lancaster, England.

Duncan-Johnson, C. C., and Donchin, E. (1982). The P300 component of the event-related brain potential as an index of information processing. *Biol. Psychol.* **14**, 1–52.

Elberling, C., Bak, C., Kofoed, B., Lebech, J., and Saermark, K. (1982). Auditory magnetic fields. *Scand. Audiol.* **11**, 61–65.

Fabiani, M., Gratton, G., and Coles, M.G. H. (2000). Event-related brain potentials. Methods, theory and applications. *In* "Handbook of Psychophysiology" (J. T. Cacioppo, L. G. Tassinary, and G. G. Berntson, eds.), 2nd Ed., pp. 27–52. Cambridge University Press, Cambridge.

Friederici, A.D. (1997). Neurophysiological aspects of language processing. *Clin. Neurosci.* **4**, 64–72.

Friederici, A.D., Steinhauer, K., and Frisch. S. (1999). Lexical integration: Sequential effects of syntactic and semantic information. *Memory Cogn.* **27**, 438–453.

Friedman, D., Vaughan, H. G., Erlen-Meyer-Kimling, L. (1978). Stimulus and response related components of the late positive complex in visual discrimination tasks. *Elecroencephalogr. Clin. Neurophysiol.* **45**, 319–330.

Galbraith, G. C., Threadgill, M. R., Hemsley, J., Salour, K., Songdej, N., Ton, J., and Cheung, L. (2000). Putative measure of peripheral and brainstem frequency-following in humans. *Neurosci. Lett.* **6**, 123–127.

Garcia-Larrea, L., Bastuji, H., and Mauguier, E. F. (1991). Mapping study of somatosensory evoked potentials during selective spatial attention. *Electroencephalogr. Clin. Neurophysiol.* **80**, 201–214.

Gibson, W. P. R. (1980). The auditory evoked potential (AEP). *In* "Evoked Potentials" (C. Barber, ed.), pp. 43–54. MIP Press, Falcon House, Lancaster, England.

Giraud, A. L., Lorenzi, C, Ashburner, J., Wable, J., Johnsrude, I., Frackowiak, R., and Kleinschmidt, A. (2000). Representation of the temporal envelope of sounds in the human brain. *J. Neurophysiol.* **84**, 588–598.

Gunter, T.C., and Friederici, A.D. (1999). Concerning the automaticity of syntactic processing. *Psychophysiology* **36**, 126–137.

Hagoort, P., Brown, C., and Groothusen, J. (1993). The syntactic positive shift (SPS) as an ERP measure of syntactic processing. *Lang. Cogn. Processes* **8**, 439–483.

Hahne, A., and Friederici, A. D. (1999). Electrophysiological evidence for two steps in syntactic analysis. Early automatic and late controlled processes. *J. Cogn. Neurosci.* **11**, 194–205.

Hansen, J. C., and Hillyard, S. A. (1980). Endogenous brain potentials associated with selective auditory attention. *Elecroencephalogr. Clin. Neurophysiol.* **49**, 277–290.

Hari, R. (1994). Magnetoencephalography in the study of human brain functions. *In* "Cognitive Electrophysiology" (H. J. Heinze, T. F. Münte, and G. R. Mangun, eds.), pp. 368–378. Birkhäuser, Boston.

Hari, R., Reinikainen, K., Kaukoranta, E., Hamalainen, M., Ilmoniemi, R., Penttinen, A., Salminen, J., and Teszner, D. (1984). Somatosensory evoked cerebral magnetic fields from SI and SII in man. *Elecroencephalogr. Clin. Neurophysiol.* **57**, 254–263.

Hari, R., Pelizzone, M., Mäkelä, J. P., Hällström, J., Leinonen, L., and Lounasamaa, O. V. (1987). Neuromagnetic responses of the human auditory cortex to on- and off-sets of noise burst. *Audiology* **25**, 31–43.

Harter, M. R., and Aine, C. J. (1984), Brain mechanisms of visual selective attention. *In* "Varieties of Attention" (R. Parasuraman, and R. Davies, eds.), pp. 293–321. Academic Press, New York.

Heinze, H. J., Mangun, G. R., Burchert, W., Hinrichs, H., Scholze, M., Münte, T. F., Gös, A., Johannes, S., Scherg, M., Hundeshagen, H., Gazzaniga, M. S., and Hillyard, S. A. (1994). Combined spatial and temporal imaging of spatial selective attention in humans. *Nature* **372**, 543–546 .

Hellige, J. B. (1993). "Hemispheric Asymmetries. What's Right and What's Left." Harvard University Press, Cambridge.

Hillyard, S. A., and Kutas, M. (1983). Electrophysiology of cognitive processing. *Annu. Rev. Psychol.* **34**, 33–61.

Hillyard, S. A., Picton, T. W., and Regan, D. M. (1978). Sensation, perception, and attention: Analysis using ERPs. *In* "Event-related Brain Potentials in Man" (E. Callaway, P. Tueting, and S. Koslow, eds.), pp. 223–322. Academic Press, New York.

Hoffman, J. E. (1990). ERP and automatic and controlled processing. *In* "Event-related Brain Potentials. Basic Issues and Applications" (J. W. Rohrbaugh, R. Parasuraman, and R. Johnson, Jr., eds), pp. 145–156. Oxford University Press, Oxford.

Hudnell, H. K., Boyes, W. K., and Otto D. A. (1990). Stationary pattern adaptation and the early components in human visual evoked potentials. *Electroencephalogr. Clin. Neurophysiol.* **77**, 190–193.

Hugdhal, K. (1993). Psychophysiology. "The Mind–Body Perspective". Harvard University Press, Cambridge, Massachusetts.

Hughes, H. C., Nozawa, G., and Kitterle, F. (1996). Global precedence, spatial frequency channels and the statistics of natural images. *J. Cogn. Neurosci.* **8**, 197–230.

Isreal, J. B, Chesney, G. L., Wickens, C. D., and Donchin, E. (1980). P300 and tracking difficulty: Evidence for multiple resources in dual-task performance. *Psychophysiology* **17**, 259–273.

Jeffreys, D. A. (1970). Striate and extra-striate origins of pattern-related visual evoked potential (VEP) components. *J. Physiol.* **211** (Suppl.), 29.

Jeffreys, D. A. (1971). Cortical source localizations of pattern related visual evoked potentials recorded from the human scalp. *Nature* **229**, 502–504.

Jeffreys, D. A. (1977). The physiological significance of pattern visual evoked potentials. *In* "Visual Evoked Potentials in Man" (J. E. Demedt, ed.), pp. 134–167. Clarendon, Oxford.

Kaan, E., Harris, A., Gibson, E., and Holcomb, P. (2000). The P600 as an index of syntactic integration difficulty. *Lang. Cogn. Processes* **15**, 159–201.

Karhu, J., Hari, R., Mäkelä, J. P., Hottunen, J., and Knuutila J. (1982). Somatosensory evoked magnetic fields in multiple sclerosis. *Electroencephalogr. Clin. Neurophysiol.* **83**, 192–200.

Karlin, L., Mariz, M. J., Brauth, S. E, and Mardkoff, A. M. (1971). Auditory evoked potentials, motor potentials and reaction times. *Electroencephalogr. Clin. Neurophysiol.* **31**, 129–136.

Katznelson, R. D. (1981). EEG recording, electrode placement, and aspects of generator localization. *In* "Electric Fields of the Brain. The Neurophysics of EEG" (P. L. Nunez, ed.), pp. 176–213. Oxford University Press, New York and Oxford.

Kleins, M., Coles, M. G. H., and Donchin, E. (1984). People with absolute pitch process tones without producing a P300. *Science* **224**, 1306–1309.

Kristeva, R., Cheyne, D., Lang, W., Lindinger, G., and Deecke L. (1990). Movement-related potentials accompanying unilateral and bilateral finger movements with different inertial loads. *EEG Clin. Neurophysiol.* **75**, 410–418.

Kulikowski, J. J., Murray, I. J., and Perry, N. R. A. (1989). Electrophysiological correlates of chromatic-opponent and achromatic stimulation in man. *Color Vision Defici.* **9**, 145–153.

Kuriki, S., Takeuchi, F., and Hirata, Y. (1988). Neural processing of words in the human extrastriate visual cortex. *Cogn. Brain Res.* **6**, 193–203.

Kutas, M., and Dale, A. (1997). Electrical and magnetic reading of mental functions. *In* "Cognitive Neuroscience" (M. D. Rugg, ed.), pp. 197–242. Psychology Press, Taylor & Francis Group, Hove, East Sussex, UK.

Kutas, M., and Hillyard, S. A. (1980). Reading senseless sentences: Brain potentials reflect semantic incongruity. *Science* **207**, 203–205.

Kutas, M., and Kluender, R. (1994). What is who violating? A reconsideration of linguistic violations in light of event-related brain potentials. *In* "Cognitive Electrophysiology" (H. J. Heinze, T. F. Münte, and G. R. Mangun, eds.), pp. 183–210. Birkhäuser, Boston.

Kutas, M., and Van Petten, C. (1988). Event–related brain potentials studies of language. *In* "Advances in Psychophysiology" (P. K. Ackles, J. R. Jennings, and M. G. H. Coles, Eds.), Vol. 3, pp. 139–188. JAI Press Inc., Greenwich, Connecticut.

Kutas, M., and Van Petten, C. K. (1994). Psycholinguistics electrified: Event–related brain potential investigations. *In* "Handbook of Psycholinguistics" (M. A. Gernsbacher, ed.), pp. 83–143. Academic Press, San Diego.

Kutas, M., McCarthy, G., and Donchin, E. (1977). Augmenting mental chronometry: The P300 as a measure for stimulus evaluation time. *Science* **197**, 792–795.

Kutas, M., Federmeier, K. D., and Sereno, M. I. (1999). Current approaches to mapping language in electromagnetic space. *In* "The Neurocognition of

Language" (C. M. Brown and P. Hagoort, eds.), pp. 359–392. Oxford University Press, Oxford.

Lesèvre, N. (1982). Chronotopographical analysis of the human evoked potential in relation to visual field data from normal individuals and hemianoptic patients. *Ann. N.Y. Acad. Sci."*, **388**, 635–641.

Lesevre, N., and Joseph, J. P. (1979). Modifications of the pattern-evoked potential (PEP) in relation to the stimulated part of the visual field (clues for the most probable origin of each component*).* *Electroencephalogr. Clin. Neurophysiol.* **47**, 183–203.

Livingstone, M. S., and Hubel D. H. (1988). Segregation of color, form, movement and depth: Anatomy, physiology and perception. *Science* **240**, 740–749.

Magliero, A., Bashore, T. R., Coles, M. G. H., and Donchin, E. (1984). On the dependence of P300 latency on stimulus evaluation processes. *Psychophysiology* **21**, 171–186.

Mangun, G.R., Hinrichs, H., Scholz, M., Mueller-Gaertner, H.W., Herzog, H., Krause, B.J., Tellman, L., Kemna, L., and Heinze H. J. (2001). Integrating electrophysiology and neuroimaging of spatial selective attention to simple isolated visual stimuli. *Vision Res.* **41**, 1423–1435.

McCandles, G. A. (1987). Electrophysiological measurements in the assessment of the young child. *In* "Childhood Deafness: Causation, Assessment and Management" (F. H. Bess, ed.), pp. 161–169. Grune & Stratton, New York, San Francisco, London.

McCarthy, G., and Donchin. F. (1981). A metric for thought. A comparison of P300 latency and reaction time. *Science* **211**, 77–80.

Mecklinger, A., Schriefers, H., Steinhauer, K., and Friederici A. D. (1995). Processing relative clauses varying on synctactic and semantic dimensions: An analysis with event-related potentials. *Memory and Cogn.* **23**, 477–494.

Münte, T. F., Heinze, H. J., Matzke, M., Wieringa, B. M., and Johannes, S. (1998). Brain potentials and syntactic violations revisited: No evidence for specificity of the syntactic positive shift. *Neuropsychologia* **36**, 217–226.

Näätänen, R. (1982). Processing negativity: An evoked-potential reflection of selective attention. *Psychol. Bull.* **92**, 605–640.

Näätänen, R. (1992). *"Attention and Brain Function."* Erlbaum, London.

Näätänen, R. (1995*).* The mismatch negativity—A powerful tool for cognitive neuroscience. *Ear Hearing* **16**, 6–18.

Näätänen, R., and Michie, P. T. (1979). Early selective attention effects on the evoked potentials. A critical review and reinterpretation. *Biol. Psychol.* **8**, 81–136.

Näätänen, R., Gaillard, A. W. K., and Mantisalo, S. (1978). Early selective-attention effect reinterpreted. *Acta Psychol.* **42**, 313–329.

Näätänen, R., Alho, K., and Sams, M. (1985). Selective information processing and event-related brain potentials. *In* "Psychophysiological Approaches to Human Information Processing" (F. Klix, R. Näätänen, and R. Zimmer, eds.), pp. 49–83. Elsevier, Amsterdam.

Neville, H., Snyder, E., Woods, D., and Galambos, R. (1982). Recognition and surprise alter the human visual evoked response. *Proc. Natl. Acad. Sci. U.S.A.* **79**, 2121–2123.

Nielsen-Bohlman, L., and Knight, R. (1994). Electrophysiological dissociation of rapid memory mechanisms in humans. *Neuroreport* **1221**, 1517–1521.

Nunez, P. L., Brett, M. W., and Silberstein, R. B. (2001). Spatial-temporal structures of human alpha rhythms: Theory, microcurrent sources, multiscale measurements, and global binding of local networks. *Human Brain Mapping* **13**, 125–164.

Okada, Y. C., Kaufman, C., Brenner, D., and Williamson, S. S. (1982). Modulation transfer functions of the human visual system revealed by magnetic field measurements, *Vision Res.* **22**, 319–333.

Ossenblock, P., and Spekreijse, H. (1991). The extrastriate generators of the EP to checkerboard onset. A source localization approach. *Electroencephalogr. Clin. Neurophysiol.* **80**, 181– 193.

Osterhout, L. (1994). Event-related brain potentials as tools for comprehending language comprehension. *In* "Perspectives on Sentence Processing" (J. Charles Clifton, L. Frazier, and K. Rayner, eds.), pp. 15–44. Lawrence Erlbaum Assoc., Hillsdale, New Jersey.

Osterhout, L., and Holcomb, P. J. (1992). Event-related brain potentials elicited by syntactic anomaly. *J. Memory Lang.* **31**(6), 785–806.

Osterhout, L., and Holcomb, P. J. (1993). Event-related potentials and syntactic anomaly: Evidence of anomaly detection during the perception of continuous speech. *Lang. Cogn. Processes* **8**, 413–437.

Osterhout, L., and Holcomb, P. J. (1995). Event related potentials and language comprehension. *In* "Electrophysiology of Mind: Event-Related Brain Potentials and Cognition" (M. D. Rugg, and M. G. H. Coles, eds.), Vol. 25, pp. 171–215. Oxford University Press, Oxford.

Papanicolau, A. C., and Johnston, J. (1984). Probe evoked potentials: Theory, method and applications. *Int. J. Neurosci.* **24**, 107–131.

Paulus, W. M., and Plendl, H. (1988). Spatial dissociation of early and late colour evoked components. *Electroencephalogr. Clin. Neurophysiol.* **71**, 81–88.

Peters, M. J., and De Munck, J. C. (1990). On the forward and the inverse problem for EEG and MEG. *In* "Auditory Evoked Magnetic Fields and Electric Potentials, Advances in Audiology" (F. Grandori, M. Hoke, and G. L. Romani, eds.), Vol. 6, pp. 70–102. Karger, Basel.

Petersen, S. E., Fox, P. T., Posner, M. I., Mintun, M., and Raichle M. E. (1988). Positron emission tomography studies of the processing of single words. *J. Cogn. Neurosci.* **1**, 153–170.

Picton, T. W., and Hillyard, S. A. (1988). Endogenous event-related potentials. *In* "Handbook of Electroencephalography and Clinical Neurophysiology" (T. W. Picton, ed.), Vol. 3, pp. 361–426. Elsevier, Amsterdam.

Picton, T. W., Hillyard, S. A., Krautsz, H. I., and Galambos, R. (1974). Human auditory evoked potentials. I. Evaluation of components. *Electroencephalogr. Clin. Neurophysiol.* **36**, 179–190.

Pilgreen, K. L. (1995). Physiological, medical, and cognitive correlates of electroencephalography. *In* "Neocortical Dynamics and Human EEG Rhythms" (P. L. Nunez, ed.), pp. 195–248. Oxford University Press, New York and Oxford.

Polk, T. A., Stallcup, M., Aguirre, G. K., Alsop, D. C., D'Esposito, M., Detre, A. J., and Farah M. J. (2002). Neural specialization for letter recognition. *J. Cogn. Neurosci.* **14**,145–159.

Previc, F. H. (1988). The neurophysiological significance of the N1 and P1 components of the visual evoked potential. *Clin. Visual Sci.* **3**, 195–202.

Proverbio, A. M. (1993). The role of left and right hemisphere in sustained and selective attention. Ph.D. Doctoral Thesis. University of Padua.

Proverbio, A. M., Zani, A., and Avella, C. (1996). Differential activation of multiple current sources of foveal VEPs as a function of spatial frequency. *BrainTopogr.* **9**, 59–69.

Proverbio, A. M., Zani, A., and Avella, C. (1997a). Hemispheric asymmetries for spatial frequency discrimination in a selective attention task. *Brain Cogn.* **34**, 311–320.

Proverbio, A. M., Lilli, S., Zani, A., and Semenza, C. (1997b). Neural basis of common vs. proper name retrieval: An electrophysiological investigation, *Brain Lang.* **60**, 31–33.

Proverbio, A. M., Minniti, A., and Zani, A. (1998). Electrophysiological evidence of a perceptual precedence of global vs. local visual information. *Cogn. Brain Res.* **6**, 321–334.

Proverbio, A. M., Lilli, S., and Zani, A. (1999). ERP mapping of brain activation during phonological processing. *Biomed. Technik* **44**, Suppl. 2, 178–180.

Proverbio, A. M., Cok B., and Zani A. (2002a). Electrophysiological measures of language processing in bilinguals. *J. Cogn. Neurosci.* (in press).

Proverbio, A. M., Esposito, P., and Zani, A. (2002b). Early involvement of temporal area in attentional selection of grating orientation: An ERP study. *Cogn. Brain Res.* **13**, 139–151.

Puce, A., Allison, T., Asgari, M., Gore, J. C., and McCarthy, G. (1996). Differential sensitivity of human visual cortex to faces, letter strings, and textures: A functional magnetic resonance imaging study. *J. Neurosci.* **16**, 5205–5215.

Rif, J., Hari, R., Hämäläinen, M., and Sams, S. A. (1991). Auditory attention affects two diffrent areas in the human auditory cortex. *Electroencephalogr. Clin. Neurophysiol.* **79**, 464–472.

Romani, G. L., Williamson, S. S., and Kaufman, L. (1982). Tonotopic organization of the human auditory cortex. *Science* **216**, 1339–1340.

Rösler, F., and Manzey, D. (1986). Automatization of cognitive operations as reflected in event-related brain potentials: Methodological considerations and data. *In* "Human Memory and Cognitive Capabilities. Mechanisms and Performances" (F. Klix, and H. Hagendorf , eds.), pp. 659–673. Elseviers, Amsterdam.

Roth, W., Ford, J. M., and Kopell, B. S. (1978). Long-latency evoked potentials and reaction times. *Psychophysiology* **15**, 17–23.

Ruchkin, D. S., Sutton, S., and Mahaffey, D. (1987). Functional differences between members of the P300 complex: P3a and P3b. *Psychophysiology* **24**, 87–103.

Ruchkin, D. S., Johnson, R., Jr., Mahaffey, D., and Sutton, S. (1988). Toward a functional categorization of slow waves. *Psychophysiology* **25**, 339–353.

Scherg, M. (1992). Functional imaging and localization of electromagnetic brain activity, *Brain Topogr.* **5**, 103–111.

Shulman-Galambos, C., and Galambos, R. (1978). Cortical responses from adults and infants in complex visual stimuli. *Electroencephalogr. Clin. Neurophysiol.* **45**, 425–35.

Silberstein, R. B. (1995a). Neuromodulation of neocortical dynamics. *In* "Neocortical Dynamics and Human EEG rhythms" (P. Nunez, ed.), pp. 591–627. Oxford University Press, New York.

Silberstein, R. B. (1995b). Steady-state visually evoked potentials, brain resonances, and cognitive processes. *In* "Neocortical Dynamics and Human EEG Rhythms" (P. Nunez, ed.), pp. 272–303. Oxford University Press, New York.

Skrandies, W. (1984). Scalp potential fields evoked by grating stimuli: Effects of spatial frequency and orientation. *Electroencephalogr. Clin. Neurophysiol.* **58**, 325–332.

Van Petten, C. (1995). Words and sentences: Event-related brain potential measures. *Psychophysiology* **32**, 511–525.

Woldorff, M. G., Gallen, C. C., Hampson, S. A., Hillyard, S. A., Pantev, C., Sobel, D., and Bloom, C. G. (1993). Modulation of early processing in human auditory cortex during auditory selective attention. *Proc. Natl. Acad. Sci.* **90**, 8722–8726.

Zani, A. (1989). Brain evoked responses reflect information processing changes with the menstrual cycle in young female athletes. *J. Sport Med. Physical Fitne*ss **29**,113–121.

Zani, A., and Proverbio, A. M. (1995). ERP signs of early selective attention effects to check size. *Electroencephalogr. Clin. Neurophysiol.* **95**, 277–292.

Zani, A., and Proverbio, A. M. (1997). Attention modulation of short latency ERPs by selective attention to conjunction of spatial frequency and location. *J. Psychophysiol.* **11**, 21–32.

3

Seeing the Forest through the Trees: The Cross-Function Approach to Imaging Cognition

Roberto Cabeza and Lars Nyberg

INTRODUCTION

During the past decade, the field of functional neuroimaging of cognition has grown exponentially. From a handful of studies in the early 1990s, this research domain expanded to more than 800 studies by the early 2000s. Today, positron emission tomography (PET) and functional MRI (fMRI) studies cover almost every aspect of human cognition, from motion perception to moral reasoning. If each study is seen as a tree, the field has grown from minimal vegetation to a luxuriant tropical forest in less than 10 years. Yet, functional neuroimaging researchers sometimes focus exclusively on their own cognitive domain and do not see the forest through the trees. The goal of the present chapter is to call attention to the forest—that is, to what many functional neuroimaging studies of cognition have in common.

When we say that most researchers are focused on the trees, we refer to the fact that the vast majority of functional neuroimaging studies investigate a single cognitive function, such as attention, working memory, or episodic memory. Yet, with the accumulation of functional neuroimaging data, it has become obvious that the brain is not organized like a cognitive psychology textbook, with dedicated systems for perception, attention, working memory, episodic memory, and so forth. Instead, the neural correlates of cognitive functions overlap considerably, with each brain region being involved in a variety of cognitive functions. What cognitive processes do these common regions mediate? By comparing patterns of brain activity across different cognitive functions, answers to this question can be generated.

The matrix in Fig. 1 illustrates the difference between the traditional within-function approach and the cross-function approach we are advocating in this chapter. Let us assume that in functional neuroimaging studies Cognitive Function A typically is associated with activations in Brain Regions 1 and 3, Cognitive Function B with activations in Brain Regions 2 and 3, and Cognitive Function C with activations in Brain Regions 1 and 2. In the standard within-function approach, functional neuroimaging researchers are primarily concerned with one cognitive function and interpret activations in relation to this par-

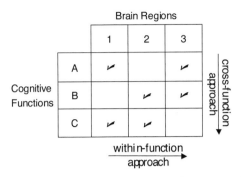

FIGURE 1 Illustration of within-function and cross-function approaches to functional neuroimaging.

ticular function. Thus, in a situation such as the one depicted in Fig. 1, researchers of Function A would attribute the activation of Region 1 to a certain aspect of Function A, whereas researchers of Function C would attribute the activation of the same region to a certain aspect of Function C. For instance, left ventrolateral prefrontal cortex activations have been attributed to language processes by language researchers, to working memory processes by working memory researchers, to semantic memory processes by semantic memory researchers, and so forth (Cabeza and Nyberg, 2000). In contrast with the within-function approach, the cross-function approach focuses on the columns of the matrix rather than on the rows, and asks questions about the functional role of a brain region (e.g., Region 1) that is recruited by different cognitive functions (e.g., Functions A and C).

Thus, the basic question the cross-function approach asks concerns why the same brain region is recruited by different cognitive functions. There are at least three possible answers to this question. First, according to a *sharing view*, the common region is involved in cognitive operations that are recruited by different cognitive functions. In the case of Fig. 1, the sharing view would argue that Region 1 mediates processes that are engaged both by Function A and by Function C. A *reduction-*

istic interpretation of the sharing view would say that shared operations "belong" to one of the two functions, and are "borrowed" by the other function. For example, prefrontal cortex (PFC) regions activated both by episodic memory and by working memory could mediate working memory processes that are also tapped by episodic memory (e.g., Wagner, *et al.*, 1998a). In contrast, an *abstractive interpretation* of the sharing view would argue that the shared processes should be described in more abstract terms than either of the two functions. For instance, dorsolateral PFC regions common to episodic and working memory could reflect general monitoring operations that were tapped by both functions (e.g., Cabeza *et al.*, 2002a).

Second, according to a *subdivision view*, when different functions activate the same region, the region actually consists of several subregions that are differentially involved in each of the functions. In the case of Fig. 1, the subdivision view would argue that Function A and Function C activate different subregions of Region 1 (e.g., Subregion 1a and Subregion 1c). From this point of view, the goal of the cross-function approach would not be to identify a common process shared by different functions, but to dissociate the functions of each subregion by increasing the spatial resolution of functional neuroimaging techniques and/or the specificity of experimental manipulations. Much of the functional neuroimaging work on visual recognition favors the subdivision view, and researchers in this area have identified subregions on the ventral surface of the temporal lobes that are specialized in recognizing faces, places, animals, and tools (for reviews, see Kanwisher *et al.*, 2001; Martin, 2001). It should be noted, however, that the subdivision view does not necessarily imply modularity, because one may argue that a region can be divided into subregions without assuming that these subregions have the properties typically attributed to neurocognitive modules, such as domain specificity, cognitive impenetrability, shallow output, etc. (Fodor, 1983).

Third, according to a network view, the finding that the same region is activated by several functions does not imply that the common region performs the same cognitive operations in all the functions. On the contrary, this view assumes that the cognitive operations performed by a brain region depend on the interactions between the region and the rest of the brain, and because these interactions change across functions, so do the operations performed by the region (McIntosh, 1999; Nyberg and McIntosh, 2000). In the case of Fig. 1, the network view would argue that Region 1 performs different operations in Functions A and C, because during Function A it interacts with Region 3, whereas during Function C it interacts with Region 2. An extreme version of the network view would say that—with the exception of primary sensory and motor cortices—brain regions are not specialized in particular cognitive process, and their operations are completely determined by network interactions. A moderate version of the network view would state that there is a broad specialization, but the specific operations performed by a region are determined by network interactions. For example, Region 1 may have a broad specialization in fast online computations, but these computations may be applied to speech processing during a language task or to rotating an object during an imagery task. It should be noted that the idea that brain regions have broad specializations is close to the abstractive interpretation of the sharing view.

Regardless of what view one endorses—the three views are not incompatible and may be combined in different ways—it seems clear that in order to understand why the same brain regions are activated by a variety of cognitive functions one must go beyond the standard within-function approach and adopt a cross-function approach. The cross-function approach has two basic methods, and both are described in the present chapter. One method is to conduct a metaanalysis combining the results of studies that originally investigated a single cognitive function (Cabeza and Nyberg, 2000; Christoff and Gabrieli, 2000; Duncan and Owen, 2000; Fletcher and Henson, 2001). Another method is to conduct functional neuroimaging studies that compare different cognitive functions directly within-subjects (Braver et al., 2001; Cabeza et al., 2002a,b; LaBar et al., 1999; Nyberg et al., 2002a,b; Ranganath and D'Esposito, 2001). The present chapter describes both methods: first, we report a cross-study metaanalysis, and then we review the results of the first crop of studies that compare different functions within-subject.

COMPARING DIFFERENT COGNITIVE FUNCTIONS ACROSS STUDIES

This section reports a metaanalysis of functional neuroimaging data. First, we describe the methods of the metaanalysis, including the characteristics of the data set, the rationale for the classification employed, and the calculation of activation frequency. Then, we describe and discuss the results of the metaanalysis for prefrontal, midline, parietal, temporal, and medial temporal regions.

Methods

From the data set of a previous large-scale metaanalysis (Cabeza and Nyberg, 2000), we selected 136 studies in five cognitive domains: (1) attention, (2) perception, (3) working memory, (4) semantic memory retrieval and episodic memory encoding, and (5) episodic memory retrieval. The rationale for considering semantic memory retrieval and episodic memory encoding within the same category is that these two processes tend to

TABLE 1 Number of Activations (Reported Peaks) in 136 PET/fMRI Studies According to Cognitive Function and Stimulus Involved

Function	Stimulus			
	Verbal	Object	Spatial	Total
Attention	37	60	83	180
Perception	106	109	27	242
Working memory	238	85	177	500
Semantic retrieval/episodic encoding	171	124	60	355
Episodic retrieval	216	49	45	310
Total	768	427	392	1587

co-occur and are very difficult to differentiate: semantic retrieval involves incidental episodic encoding, and intentional episodic encoding involves incidental semantic retrieval (for a discussion, see Nyberg *et al.*, 1996a; Tulving *et al.*, 1994). Consistent with this idea, semantic retrieval and episodic encoding tend to show very similar activation patterns, except in medial temporal lobe (MTL) regions (see below).

As Table 1 shows, for each cognitive domain, we classified activations according to whether the study involved verbal, object, or spatial stimuli. There were slight differences in the types of stimuli used in each domain, however. For verbal stimuli, the Working Memory domain included both words and numerical stimuli. In the Attention domain, studies in the verbal category used the Stroop task, and hence are characterized not only by their verbal nature but by the conflict-monitoring operations tapped by this task as well. In the Perception domain, the verbal category corresponded to word-reading studies in which overt verbal responses were absent or subtracted out by the control task. Differences in the spatial category existed as well. The memory conditions also included imagery operations and the semantic retrieval category included letter rotation studies.

As in our previous metaanalysis (Cabeza and Nyberg, 2000), we used

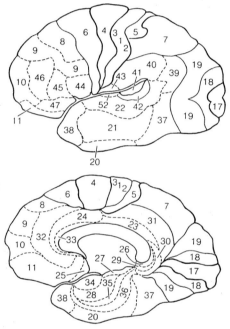

FIGURE 2 Brodmann areas. From Elliott (1964). "Textbook of Neuroanatomy," with permission of Lippincott Williams & Wilkins.

Brodmann areas (BAs) as the unit of analysis (see Fig. 2). Some BAs (e.g., 3/1/2, 4, 5, 33, 43, 38) were excluded because they showed very few activations, and some areas were collapsed together (BAs 41 and 42; BAs 30 and 31) to simplify analyses. Medial temporal lobe regions were treated as a unit because the overall area is small and the localization of activations in different regions is not always clear. Due to space limitations, we do not report or discuss the results for occipital regions, basal ganglia, thalamic, and cerebellar regions.

In our previous metaanalysis (Cabeza and Nyberg, 2000), we identified typical activation patterns for each cognitive function using a qualitative evaluation of the frequency of activations across studies. Although we emphasized representative activations, we also noted exceptions to the general pattern and discussed specific findings and studies. By contrast, in the present metaanalysis, we used a quantitative measure of activation frequency and focused on aggregate results without discussion of individual studies. The quantitative measure employed is the number of activations reported in each BA or brain

region in the studies reviewed. The number of activations is defined by the number of different coordinates reported, with some studies reporting more than one coordinate in each BA. The rationale for using this measure is that the numbers of coordinates reported tended to be positively correlated with the size of the activations, and hence, this measure provides an indirect index of both frequency and relative size of the activations. The numbers of activations in each brain region were separately analyzed for each cognitive function and stimulus type (see Figs. 2–7). Because the total number of activations varied across cognitive domains and stimulus type, we express the number of activations as a percentage of the number of activations in each cell in

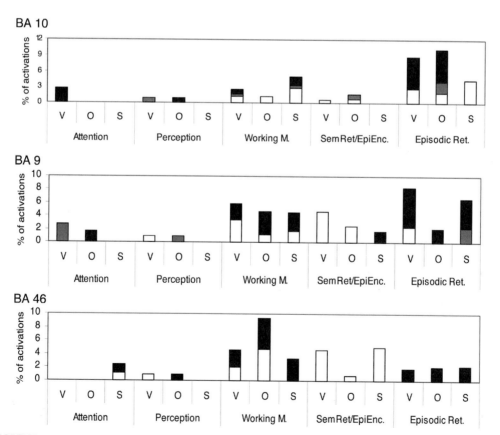

FIGURE 3   Percentage of activations in anterior and dorsolateral prefrontal regions in five cognitive domains. BA, Brodmann area; V, verbal; O, object; S, spatial.

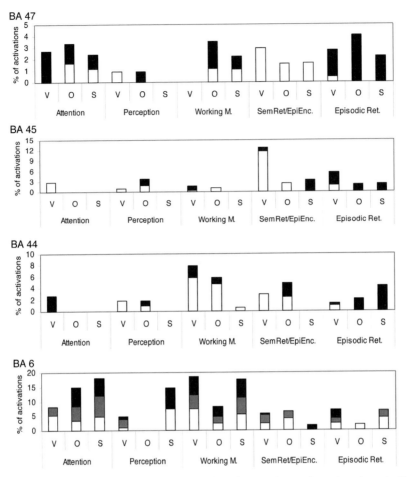

FIGURE 4 Percentage of activations in ventrolateral and posterior prefrontal regions in five cognitive domains. BA, Brodmann area; V, verbal; O, object; S, spatial.

Table 1. Although using percentages provides a straightforward method to compare across category/stimuli cells, these percentages should be considered with caution in the case of cells with few activations (e.g., spatial perception), because they may reflect the peculiarities of the few studies in the cell rather than a general pattern.

Results

Prefrontal Regions

The distribution of activations in the prefrontal cortex for the five cognitive functions is shown in Figs. 3 and 4. The lat-eralization of activation for semantic retrieval/episodic encoding and for episodic retrieval was consistent with the hemispheric encoding/retrieval asymmetry (HERA) model (Nyberg *et al.*, 1996a, 1998; Tulving *et al.*, 1994), which postulated that the left PFC is differentially more involved in retrieving information from semantic memory and in simultaneously encoding novel aspects of this information into episodic memory, whereas the right PFC is differentially more involved in retrieving information from episodic memory. At the same time, the lateralization of PFC activity was also affected by stimulus type: right-lateralized activations during semantic retrieval/episodic encoding usually occurred for nonverbal materials and left-lateralized activations during episodic retrieval usually occurred for verbal materials. Thus, the lateralization of PFC activity depends both on processes (Nyberg *et al.*, 1996a, 1998) and stimuli (e.g., Kelley *et al.*, 1998; McDermot *et al.*, 1999; Wagner *et al.*, 1998b).

Turning to the activation pattern for different PFC subregions, Fig. 3 shows the frequency of activation for anterior (BA 10) and dorsolateral (BAs 9 and 46) PFC regions. Anterior PFC (BA 10) activations were frequent for episodic memory retrieval, particularly in the right hemisphere. Frontopolar activity during episodic retrieval has been attributed to the generation and maintenance of the mental set of episodic retrieval, or *episodic retrieval mode* (Cabeza *et al.*, 1997; Düzel *et al.*, 1999; Lepage *et al.*, 2000; Nyberg *et al.*, 1995). This idea is supported by evidence that activity in BA 10 remains constant across different levels of episodic retrieval performance (Nyberg *et al.*, 1995) and different types of episodic retrieval tasks (Cabeza *et al.*, 1997) and is sustained throughout the retrieval task (Düzel *et al.*, 1999). Although not shown in Fig. 3, activations in BA 10 are also frequent during problem solving (Cabeza and Nyberg, 2000), suggesting that this region has a more general role of monitoring internally generated information (Christoff and Gabrieli, 2000). Dorsolateral PFC (BAs 9 and 46) activations were frequent for working memory, semantic retrieval/ episodic encoding, and episodic retrieval (see Fig. 3). A sharing account of this overlap would be that semantic retrieval/episodic encoding and episodic retrieval depend on working memory (reductionistic interpretation) or that the three functions depend on monitoring operations (abstractive interpretation). However, sharing accounts cannot easily explain why the lateralization of dorsolateral PFC changes across functions, tending to be bilateral for working memory, left lateralized for semantic retrieval/episodic encoding, and right lateralized for episodic retrieval (see Fig. 3). The subdivision view could argue that this different lateralization pattern reflects the existence of different subregions within dorsolateral PFC, whereas the network view could argue that the function of dorsolateral PFC, as well as its lateralization, is determined by its interactions with other brain regions (e.g., parietal cortex in for working memory, left temporal cortex for semantic retrieval/episodic encoding).

Figure 4 shows the frequency of activations in ventrolateral (BAs 47 and 45), ventral/posterior (BA 44), and posterior (BA 6) PFC regions. BA 47 activations were lateralized similarly to dorsolateral PFC, but unlike dorsolateral PFC activations, they were also frequent not only for memory domains but also for the attention domain. This pattern suggests that BA 47 is involved in processes that are shared by working, semantic, and episodic memory as well as by attention tasks. In contrast, BA 45 seems to be more specific to semantic retrieval/episodic encoding, particularly in the left hemisphere and for verbal stimuli, consistent with the idea that this region is involved in semantic processing (Gabrieli *et al.*, 1998; Poldrack *et al.*, 1999). Like BAs 47 and 45, BA 44 also shows left-lateralized activation during semantic retrieval/episodic encoding, but unlike BAs 47 and 45, left BA 44 is often activated during verbal working memory tasks. This pattern is in keeping with the notion that left BA 44, which overlaps with Broca's area, is involved in phonological maintenance and rehearsal (for a review, see Smith and Jonides, 1999). Thus, the present results are consistent with the notion that the anterior part of the left inferior frontal gyrus (BAs 47 and 45) is involved in semantic processing, whereas the posterior part (BA 44) is involved in phonological working memory (Kapur *et al.*, 1996; Poldrack *et al.*, 1999). Yet, left BA 44 activations have also been found in working memory studies that employed faces and meaningless shapes (Cabeza and Nyberg, 2000), suggesting that the function of this region is not strictly verbal. The role of right BA 44—the homolog of Broca's area in the right hemisphere—is also unclear. Finally, the distribution of activations in posterior PFC (BA 6) looks quite different than the ones previously described. Activation overlaps in BA 6 are difficult to interpret because this is a very large Brodmann area that probably comprises two or more different functional subregions. The inferior part of BA 6 is close to Broca's area, and some of the left BA 6 activations during verbal working memory and semantic retrieval may reflect phonological rehearsal. In contrast, more dorsal parts of BA 6 may be more related to attentional and working memory processes.

Midline Regions

Figure 5 shows the frequency of activations in midline regions, including the anterior cingulate cortex (BAs 32 and 24) and the precuneus (BA 31). Central cingulate activations are not depicted because they were scarce, but they show a pattern similar to those in the anterior cingulate. Anterior cingulate activations were frequent during attention (e.g., Stroop tasks), working memory, and episodic retrieval. The role of the anterior cingulate in cognition has been attributed to initiation of action (Posner and Petersen, 1990) and to conflict monitoring (for a review, see Botvinick et al., 2001), among other processes (for a review, see Devinsky et al., 1995). The initiation-of-action hypothesis accounts well for activations during demanding cognitive tasks, such as working memory and episodic retrieval, whereas the conflict-monitoring

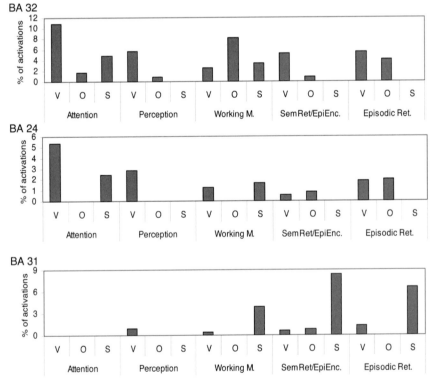

FIGURE 5 Percentage of activations in midline regions in five cognitive domains. BA, Brodmann area; V, verbal; O, object; S, spatial.

hypothesis provides a better account for anterior cingulate activations during Stroop tasks (see verbal attention in Fig. 5). Obviously, these two views are not incompatible: the anterior cingulate cortex could both initiate appropriate responses and suppress inappropriate ones (Paus *et al.*, 1993). Given the heterogeneous structure and complex connectivity of the anterior cingulate (Devinsky *et al.*, 1995), it is quite possible that different processes are tapped depending on the particular subregion engaged [subdivision view, e.g., Bush *et al.*, (2002)] and its interactions with the rest of the brain (network view).

Precuneus activations in BA 31 showed a very different functional pattern compared to those in the anterior cingulate cortex. They were not frequent during Stroop or object working memory tasks,

and were more specifically associated with the processing of spatial information in working memory, semantic retrieval/episodic encoding, and episodic retrieval tasks. The association between the precuneus region and memory for spatial stimuli fits well with the idea that this region is involved in imagery (Fletcher *et al.*, 1995; Shallice *et al.*, 1994), although evidence against this hypothesis has been reported (Buckner *et al.*, 1996; Krause *et al.*, 1999). The present results also link the precuneus to the processing of spatial information, which is a link that has been discussed relatively little in the functional neuroimaging literature.

Parietal Regions

Figure 6 shows the frequency of activations in parietal regions (BAs 7, 40, and 39).

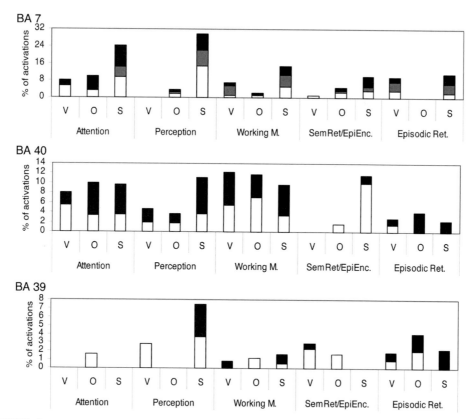

FIGURE 6 Percentage of activations in parietal regions in five cognitive domains. BA, Brodmann area; V, verbal; O, object; S, spatial.

BA 7 activations were frequent during attention, perception, and working memory, and also common during semantic retrieval/episodic encoding tasks involving spatial stimuli. This pattern fits well with the idea that this region is part of a dorsal pathway involved in spatial perception (Ungerleider and Mishkin, 1982). However, BA 7 is also activated by verbal attention, working memory, and episodic retrieval studies, and it is unclear how the spatial-processing hypothesis can account for these activations. Also, the spatial-processing hypothesis cannot easily account for activations in BA 40, which are frequent for attention, perception, and working memory, regardless of stimuli. Working memory activations in left BA 40 have been attributed to the storage of verbal information in working memory (Awh *et al.*, 1996; for a review, see D'Esposito, 2001; Jonides *et al.*, 1998; Paulesu *et al.*, 1993). The involvement of this region in spatial semantic retrieval could be related to a verbal component in some of these studies [e.g., letter rotation (Alivisatos, 1997); encoding the location of nameable objects (Owen, 1996)]. Finally, BA 39 activations seem to reflect both a spatial and verbal processing component. Left BA 39 activations in verbal perception studies may reflect the link between the left angular gyrus and graphemic/phonological processing (for a review, see Binder and Price, 2001).

Temporal Regions

Figure 7 shows the frequency of activations in lateral temporal regions: BAs 22, 21, 20, and 37. Activations in left BA 22 were much more frequent for verbal than for object and spatial stimuli, suggesting they are primarily associated with language processing. Left BA 22 overlaps with Wernicke's area, which has been strongly linked to language comprehension in research with aphasic patients (Benson, 1988). In contrast, left BA 21 activations were frequent not only for verbal but also for object stimuli. From a sharing--abstractive point of view, this pattern suggests that BA 21 is involved in a process common to processing verbal and object stimuli, such as meaning-based analyses. Finally, consistent with its location along the ventral pathway for object processing (Ungerleider and Mishkin, 1982), activations in BAs 20 and 37 were more frequent when objects were used as stimuli. Thus, the distribution of activations over the lateral surface of the left temporal lobes, from the superior to the inferior temporal gyri, can be described as a gradient from verbal to object processing, with more abstract (stimulus-independent) semantic processing in the middle.

Medial Temporal Lobes

Finally, Fig. 8 shows the frequency of activations in the medial temporal lobes. These activations were frequent during episodic memory encoding and retrieval, consistent with the evidence that lesions in this area impair episodic memory functions (for a review, see Squire, 1992). The role of the MTL in episodic memory has been attributed to binding (Henke *et al.*, 1997; Lepage *et al.*, 2000) and novelty detection (Tulving *et al.*, 1996) during encoding, and to trace recovery (Cabeza *et al.*, 2001; Nyberg, *et al.*, 1996b) and recollection (Eldridge *et al.*, 2000; Schacter *et al.*, 1996a) during retrieval (for a review, see Cohen *et al.*, 1999). The MTL has been also linked to spatial processing (Maguire *et al.*, 1998; O'Keefe and Nadel, 1978), but this idea cannot be easily explain the relative lack of MTL activations during spatial attention, spatial perception, and spatial working memory. In contrast, MTL activations during attention and perception tasks were frequent when object stimuli were employed (see Fig. 8). This pattern fits well with the notion that the MTL is an anterior part of the ventral pathway for object processing. It is unclear if the episodic memory and object-processing roles of MTL can be subsumed under a more

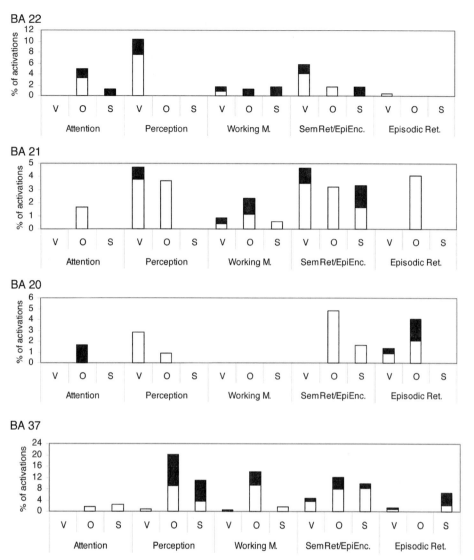

FIGURE 7   Percentage of activations in temporal regions in five cognitive domains. BA, Brodmann area; V, verbal; O, object; S, spatial.

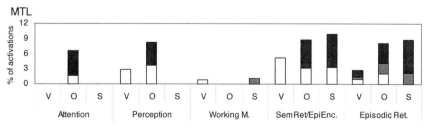

FIGURE 8   Percentage of activations in medial temporal lobe regions in five cognitive domains. BA, Brodmann area; V, verbal; O, object; S, spatial.

general function (sharing view), whether they involve different subregions of MTL (subdivision view), or whether they reflect different interactions between MTL and the rest of the brain (network view).

Summary

Table 2 summarizes the results previously displayed in Figs. 3–8. For each brain region (e.g., BA 10), the presence of a symbol indicates that the frequency of activations for a stimuli/function combination (e.g., verbal episodic retrieval) was above the average for the region, and the size of the symbol indicates whether the frequency was slightly above average, high, or very high. The symbols indicate how activations are lateralized (black symbol, right lateralized; white symbol, left lateralized; rosette, bilateral; diamonds, midline) when the frequency in one hemisphere was at least twice the frequency in the other hemisphere.

As illustrated by Table 2, anterior PFC activations in BA 10 were particularly frequent during episodic memory retrieval tasks. These activations have been attributed to episodic retrieval mode (Cabeza et al., 1997; Düzel et al., 1999; Lepage et al., 2000; Nyberg et al., 1995), but the involvement of anterior PFC in problem solving (Cabeza and Nyberg, 2000) suggests this region has a general role in monitoring internally generated information (Christoff and Gabrieli, 2000). Dorsolateral PFC activations in BAs 9 and 46 were very frequent during working memory, semantic retrieval/episodic encoding, and episodic retrieval tasks, possibly reflecting working memory (Wagner, 1999) or monitoring (Cabeza et al., 2002a) operations. Ventrolateral PFC activations in BA 47 were also common during attention tasks. In the left hemisphere, BA 45 activations were particularly frequent during verbal semantic retrieval/episodic encoding tasks, and BA 44 activations were frequent during verbal working memory tasks. This pattern is consistent with the idea that the anterior part of the left inferior

frontal gyrus is involved in semantic processing and the posterior part (i.e., Broca's area) is involved in phonological rehearsal (Kapur et al., 1996; Poldrack et al., 1999). Finally, posterior PFC activations in BA 6 were most frequent during attention and working memory tasks.

Midline activations include those in anterior cingulate (BAs 32 and 24) and precuneus (BA 31) regions. Anterior cingulate activations were common for all functions, but—consistent with the conflict-monitoring hypothesis (for a review, see Botvinick et al., 2001)—they were particularly frequent for Stroop tasks (verbal attention category). In contrast, precuneus activations were especially frequent for spatial memory tasks. Although the precuneus has been associated with imagery (Fletcher et al., 1995; Shallice et al., 1994), a specific link with spatial processing has been discussed very little in the literature.

Table 2 also shows the frequency of activation in parietal, temporal, and MTL regions. Parietal activations in BA 7 were common for all functions, and—consistent with the ventral/dorsal pathway distinction (Ungerleider and Mishkin, 1982)—they were often found during spatial tasks. In contrast, parietal activations in BA 40 were particularly frequent during attention and working memory tasks regardless of the stimuli. BA 39 activations were often found in the left hemisphere during verbal perception (reading) and verbal semantic retrieval/episodic encoding tasks, possibly reflecting the role of the left angular gyrus in language processing (for a review, see Binder and Price, 2001). Temporal activations in the left hemisphere can be described as a gradient from verbal processing in the superior temporal gyrus (BA 21) to object processing in the inferior temporal gyrus (BAs 20 and 37), with more abstract semantic processing in the middle (BA 22). Finally, MTL activations were common during long-term memory and episodic and semantic tasks, consistent with the involvement of the MTL in declarative memory (Squire, 1992). They were also

Table 2   Typical Activation Patterns in PET and fMRI Studies of Five Cognitive Functions[a]

Function	Prefrontal							Midline			Parietal			Temporal				
	10	9	46	47	45	44	6	32	24	31	7	40	39	22	21	20	37	MTL
Attention																		
Verbal	●				●	○	●	❖	❖			✿						
Object				✿			✿				✿	✿		✿		●		●
Spatial				✿			✿	❖	❖		✿	✿						
Perception																		
Verbal								❖	❖					○	○	○	○	
Object					✿										○		✿	✿
Spatial							✿				✿	✿	✿				✿	
Working memory																		
Verbal		✿	✿		○	✿			❖			✿						
Object		●	✿	✿	○			❖				✿		✿			✿	
Spatial	✿	✿	●				✿		❖	❖	✿	✿						
Semant retriev/episod encod																		
Verbal	○	○	○	○	○			❖				○	○	○				○
Object				✿									○	○	○	✿		✿
Spatial		○	●						❖		✿	○		✿	○	○		✿
Episodic retrieval																		
Verbal	●	●		●	✿			❖	❖		✿				✿			
Object	●	●		●	●			❖	❖				✿		○	✿		✿
Spatial	○	●		●		●				❖	✿		●				✿	●

[a] *Notes*: ○, Left lateral; ●, right lateral; ✿, bilateral lateral; ❖, midline. For each brain region (e.g., BA 10), a symbol is shown if the frequency of activations for a particular stimulus cognitive function cell (e.g., verbal episodic retrieval) was higher than the average frequency for the region. The size of the symbol approximately corresponds to the relative proportion of activations for each function compared to the rest of the functions. Activations are shown as lateralized when the frequency for one hemisphere was at least double that in the other hemisphere. MTL, Medial temporal lobes.

associated with object perception and attention, suggesting that the MTL is the anterior part of the ventral pathway for object processing (Ungerleider and Mishkin, 1982)

COMPARING DIFFERENT COGNITIVE FUNCTIONS WITHIN SUBJECTS

Although cross-function comparisons in large-scale metaanalyses of imaging data like the one previously described (see also, Cabeza and Nyberg, 2000; Christoff and Gabrieli, 2000; Duncan and Owen, 2000) can help identify regions that show activation overlap across functions, their results are usually confounded with differences in stimuli, tasks, and imaging methods. Although these differences could be considered an advantage from a sharing point of view (because activation overlaps reflect similarities in processes rather than similarities in methods), they are a disadvantage from a subdivision point of view (location differences may reflect methodological differences rather than functional differences). More generally, the problem of cross-study comparisons is that they only allow qualitative statements about the involvement of a certain region in various functions but not quantitative statistical measures of the strength of these activations across functions. Thus, activations that appear to differ across functions may actually be similar (e.g., a threshold effect), and activations that appear similar across functions may actually be different (e.g., activation intensity). Thus, in order to determine accurately similarities and differences in activation across different functions it is critical to compare these functions directly, within-subjects, and under similar experimental conditions.

Only a few functional neuroimaging studies have tried such direct within-subject comparisons. One reason for this scarcity is historical: because most cognitive researchers specialize in a single cognitive function, it is only natural that they maintained this specialization when they started conducting functional neuroimaging studies. In addition, functional neuroimaging researchers inherited a long list of research questions about each particular function from cognitive psychology, and this list of questions kept them focused for many years on their favorite function. Another reason for the dearth of cross-function studies is that these studies are particularly difficult to design. First, the paradigms used to investigate different cognitive functions tend to be dissimilar (e.g., the cuing paradigm used to study attention vs. the old/new recognition paradigm used to study episodic retrieval), and it is challenging to design tasks for two different functions that have a similar structure in terms of stimuli, responses, and timing. Thus, trying to compare different functions may appear sometimes as trying to "compare apples and oranges." It should be noted, however, that if one does

not compare apples and oranges, one may miss the fact that they are both round and sweet fruits. Second, some functions are inherently more difficult than others. For example, in the case of working memory and episodic memory, if the memory load is kept constant (e.g., one word), then retrieval from working memory is always easier than retrieval from long-term memory. In these situations, one is faced with the dilemma of matching experimental conditions at the expense of having differences in task difficulty or matching task difficulty at the expense of introducing differences in experimental conditions. Despite all these problems, successful direct cross-function studies can be designed, and they offer unique insights into the role of different brain regions across various functions.

The next two sections review comparisons of different functions within-subjects (see Table 3). The first section reviews studies that used blocked fMRI and PET designs, and the second section reviews studies that employed event-related fMRI designs. An advantage of blocked designs for cross-function comparisons is that they measure both item- and state-related activity. Item-related activity refers to transient changes associated with cognitive operations specific to particular items within the task (e.g., old vs. new stimuli in a memory test), whereas state-related activity refers to sustained changes associated with mental states that are characteristic of the task (Donaldson *et al.*, 2001; Düzel *et al.*, 1999). Because different functions can resemble each other or differ both in terms of item-related or state-related activity, it is convenient that blocked designs measure both of them at the same time. Event-related fMRI designs have several advantages for cross-function research. Importantly, these designs provide separate measures of different task components, such as the encoding, maintenance, and retrieval components of working memory tasks. Also, they allow separate analyses of trials associated with successful vs. unsuccessful behavioral responses, thereby providing a better control for differences in task difficulty across functions.

Blocked Studies

LaBar et al. (1999)

One of the first functional neuroimaging studies that directly compared different cognitive functions within-subjects is probably the study by LaBar *et al.* (1999), which contrasted verbal working memory and visuospatial attention using fMRI. This study compared a working memory task without a spatial attention component (a letter two-back task) to a spatial attention task without a working memory component (a Posner cuing paradigm in which the cue remained on until the target was presented). Each task was compared to its own control task, and common regions were identified with a conjunction analysis.

As shown in Table 3, the conjunction analysis identified a common network of brain regions for verbal working memory and spatial attention, including posterior/dorsomedial PFC (BA 6), parietal (BAs 7/40), and left temporal regions. This overlap in posterior PFC and parietal regions is consistent with the results of the foregoing metaanalysis (see spatial attention and verbal working memory in Table 2). In the LaBar *et al.* study, the verbal working memory tasks involved shifts between external (letters on display) and internal (letters in working memory) frames of reference, whereas the spatial attention task involved shifts to different locations in space. Thus, the authors proposed that the common network reflects shifts in attentional focus, irrespective of whether the shifts occur over space, time, or other cognitive domains.

In addition to conjunction analyses, LaBar *et al.* compared verbal working memory and spatial attention directly—after subtracting out their respective control conditions (see Table 3). Working memory was associated with activations in supplementary motor area (SMA), left opercular PFC (BA 44), precuneus, and inferior parietal regions (right BA 40), whereas spatial attention was associated with occipitotemporal and extrastriate cortex. The finding that SMA was more activated for verbal than for spatial stimuli is intriguing because this region was previously associated with spatial processing (e.g., Courtney *et al.*, 1998). The finding that Broca's area (left BA 44) was more activated for working memory than for spatial attention is consistent with the metaanalysis reported in this chapter (see Table 2)

Braver et al. (2001)

The blocked fMRI study by Braver *et al.* (2001) compared PFC activations during working memory (two-back task), episodic encoding (intentional learning), and episodic retrieval (old/new recognition). Each task was investigated using words and unfamiliar faces. The authors made three predictions. (1) Dorsolateral PFC should be selectively activated by the working memory task. According to Braver *et al.*, dorsolateral PFC "is critically important for tasks requiring active maintenance over intervening items and/or the monitoring and manipulation of maintained information," and these processes are not engaged during episodic memory encoding or retrieval. (2) Regardless of the task, ventrolateral PFC activity should be left lateralized for verbal materials and right lateralized for spatial materials (e.g., Kelley *et al.*, 1998; McDermott *et al.*, 1999). (3) Frontopolar PFC should be selectively activated by episodic memory retrieval. The authors based this prediction on the aforementioned idea that anterior PFC regions are involved in episodic retrieval mode (e.g., Lepage *et al.*, 2000; Nyberg *et al.*, 1995).

The results confirmed the first two predictions but not the third. Dorsolateral

TABLE 3   Results of PET/fMRI Studies That Compared Different Cognitive Functions Within-Subjects[a]

Study/comparison	Prefrontal							Midline			Parietal			Temporal				MTL
	10	9	46	47	45	44	6	32	24	31	7	40	39	22	21	20	37	
Blocked paradigms																		
LaBar et al. (1999)																		
Both WM and spatial attention							✻				✻	✻			○		○	
WM > spatial attention						○	✻				✻	●					✻	
Spatial attention > WM																		
Braver et al. (2001): PFC																		
WM > other tasks	○		✻	●			●											
Episodic enc. > other tasks[b]					○													
Episodic ret. > other tasks[b]	◆			●														
Nyberg et al. (2002): task PLS																		
Exp. 1																		
Both WM and episodic ret.				●		○				◆	✻	✻			○			
Episodic ret. > other tasks		○			○		●			◆	○	✻			○			
Semantic ret. > other tasks		✻				○					◆	○						
WM > other tasks	○		✻		○		✻					✻			○		●	
Exp. 2																		
Both autobio. memory and sem. ret.					○													
Nyberg et al. (2002): seed PLS																		
WM, episod. ret., and sem. ret.								◆										

Activation pattern

Event-related paradigms

Ranganath *et al.* (2002): PFC; Ranganath and D'Esposito (2001): MTL

   Both WM enc. and episodic enc.

   Both WM ret. and episodic ret.

   WM > episodic m.

   Episodic m. > WM

Cabeza *et al.* (2002)

   Both WM and episodic ret.

   Episodic ret. > WM

   WM > episodic ret.

Cabeza *et al.* (2002)

   Both episodic ret. and visual attention

   Episodic ret. > visual attention

   Visual attention > episodic ret.

[a] Notes: ○, Left lateral; ●, right lateral; l, bilateral lateral;l, midline; Exp, experiment; enc., encoding; ret., retrieval; sem., semantic; WM, working memory; MTL, medial temporal lobes.

[b] The activation did not meet the significance criteria used for other contrasts.

PFC regions were activated during working memory but not during episodic encoding or retrieval. Although this finding confirms the first prediction of Braver *et al.*, it is surprising because dozens of PET and fMRI studies of episodic memory encoding and retrieval have reported significant activations in dorsolateral PFC regions (Cabeza and Nyberg, 2000). The second prediction that ventrolateral PFC regions should be lateralized according to materials (left for words, right for faces) for both working and episodic memory was confirmed, suggesting that this lateralization pattern is a function-independent phenomenon. Finally, because anterior PFC was not differentially activated by episodic memory retrieval, the third prediction was not confirmed. On the contrary, a left anterior PFC (BA 10) was more activated for working memory than for episodic encoding and retrieval. This may have happened because the episodic retrieval task involved only retrieval processes whereas the working memory task (two-back) involved encoding, maintenance processes, and retrieval processes. Thus, it is possible that the working memory task was more complex and involved greater time-on-task activity than did the episodic encoding and retrieval tasks. Because blocked designs cannot distinguish encoding, maintenance, and retrieval phases of working memory, they do not allow an appropriate comparison between episodic retrieval and the retrieval phase of working memory.

Nyberg et al. (2002a,b)

In two PET experiments, the neural correlates of working memory, semantic memory, and episodic memory were compared (Nyberg *et al.*, 2002a). Across the two experiments, three measures were used for each of the examined memory systems. Results were analyzed using multivariate statistical technique (partial least squares; PLS) (McIntosh *et al.*, 1996) that can identify the combinations of experimental conditions that account for most variance in the brain images. In Experiment 1, both working memory and episodic retrieval were associated with activations in right anterior PFC, precuneus/cuneus, and bilateral parietal regions (see Table 3). In keeping with the results of Braver *et al.* (2001), right BA 47 was more activated for episodic retrieval than for working memory. Consistent with the metaanalysis previously reported, left PFC (BAs 9, 45, and 44) was differentially activated by semantic retrieval tasks, and posterior PFC (BA 6), by working memory tasks (see Table 3). Experiment 2 yielded an unexpected finding: an autobiographical memory task, which can be classified as episodic, activated a set of regions similar to that activated by semantic retrieval tasks, including left ventrolateral PFC. We suggested that the cued word retrieval used in the task elicited general semantic retrieval, and therefore had a shared pattern of brain activity with tests of semantic retrieval.

In a follow-up study (Nyberg *et al.*, 2002b), the frontal regions common to working memory, episodic retrieval, and semantic retrieval were identified and the functional connectivity of these regions and the rest of the brain was investigated across tasks (e.g., McIntosh *et al.*, 1997). This undertaking is closely related to the network view discussed in the Introduction, and to our knowledge this is the first study to consider connectivity analyses in cross-function comparisons. Three frontal regions were identified: left anterior PFC (BA 10), left ventrolateral PFC (BA 45), and dorsal anterior cingulate cortex (BA 32) (see Table 3). Of the three common regions, only the ventrolateral PFC region showed a shared pattern of functional connectivity. Thus, despite the fact that the anterior cingulate and anterior PFC regions were consistently activated across working memory, episodic retrieval, and semantic retrieval, they apparently played different roles in each of these functions. In contrast, the left ventrolateral region appeared to play the same role across the three memory functions, consistent with the idea that this region is involved in semantic generation (Fletcher and Henson, 2001) and active retrieval (Owen *et al.*, 2000) processes.

Event-Related fMRI Studies

Ranganath and D'Esposito (2001) and Ranganath et al. (2002)

Ranganath and collaborators (Ranganath and D'Esposito, 2001; Ranganath *et al.*, 2002), compared brain activity during the encoding and retrieval phases of working memory and episodic memory. In PFC (Ranganath *et al.*, 2002), bilateral posterior (BA 6) and ventrolateral (BAs 44, 45, and 47) regions were activated during both encoding and retrieval phases of both working memory and episodic memory. Additionally, bilateral dorsolateral PFC regions (BAs 9, and 46) and left anterior PFC region (BA 10/46) were activated during the retrieval phase but not during the encoding phase of both functions (see Table 3). A left ventrolateral PFC region (BA 47) was more activated during episodic retrieval than during working memory retrieval, but this region did not show a significant difference with respect to base line in either condition. Thus, working memory and episodic memory recruited similar PFC regions, including a left anterior PFC region that was associated with the retrieval phase of both functions. According to the authors, the left anterior PFC activation reflected the "online" monitoring and evaluation of specific memory characteristics during retrieval.

In MTL regions, the study yielded a very interesting finding: whereas the hippocampus was activated during the maintenance phase of the working memory task, the parahippocampal gyrus was activated during the encoding and retrieval phases of both working memory and episodic memory (Ranganath and D'Esposito, 2001). A second experiment

replicated these results, and additionally showed that both hippocampal and parahippocampal activations were greater for novel than for familiar faces (Ranganath and D'Esposito, 2001). The authors argued that both regions play a role in episodic memory (e.g., Aggleton and Brown, 1999). To explain why the hippocampus was not significantly activated during episodic encoding and retrieval tasks, the authors suggested that the hippocampus may use sparse representations (e.g., Fried *et al.*, 1997), and as a result, its transient activity during episodic encoding and retrieval may be difficult to detect. In contrast, prolonged hippocampal activity may be easier to detect during working memory tasks, or during episodic tasks involving sustained recollective processing (e.g., Eldridge *et al.*, 2000). More generally, the authors argued that their results cast doubts on the idea that working memory and episodic memory depend on distinct neural correlates, and endorsed the notion that working memory maintenance is the outcome of controlled activation of episodic memory networks (e.g., Fuster, 1995).

Cabeza et al. (2002a)

In this study by Cabeza *et al.*, (2002a), the neural correlates of episodic retrieval and working memory for verbal materials were compared. The trials of both tasks consisted of two phases (Phase 1 and Phase 2). In the episodic retrieval trials, Phase 1 consisted of an instruction to think back to a previous study episode, and Phase 2 consisted of a retrieval cue, to which subjects made a Remember–Know–New recognition response. Phase 1 was expected to elicit retrieval mode activity, and Phase 2 was expected to elicit cue-specific retrieval activity. In working memory trials, Phase 1 consisted of a memory set of four words in two columns, and Phase 2 consisted of a word probe, to which subjects made a Left–Right–New response. Thus, Phase 1 measured working memory encoding and maintenance activity, and Phase 2 measured working memory retrieval activity.

The fMRI data yielded two main findings (see Table 3). First, there were similarities and differences in PFC activity across tasks: (1) a left dorsolateral region (BA 9) was similarly activated for working memory and episodic retrieval tasks, (2) anterior (BA 10) and ventrolateral (BAs 47 and 45) regions were more activated for episodic retrieval, and (3) Broca's (left BA 44) and posterior/dorsal (BAs 44 and 6) regions were more activated for working memory (see Table 3). The first finding of overlapping dorsolateral PFC activity for episodic retrieval and working memory is consistent with the aforementioned results by Ranganath et al. (2002). Dorsolateral prefrontal activations have been attributed to monitoring in both episodic retrieval and working memory studies, and the results were consistent with this idea. The second finding of anterior PFC activation during episodic retrieval was consistent with the hypothesis that this region is involved in retrieval mode (Cabeza and Nyberg, 2000; Düzel et al., 1999; Lepage et al., 2000; Nyberg et al., 1995). In keeping with this idea, the anterior PFC activation started during Phase 1, before the presentation of the retrieval cue, and was sustained throughout the trial (see Fig. 9). This timecourse could explain why Braver et al. (2001) and Ranganath et al. (2002) failed to detect differential anterior PFC activity

during episodic retrieval because those studies did not differentiate between retrieval mode and cue-specific aspects of episodic retrieval. Greater ventrolateral PFC activity for episodic retrieval than for working memory is consistent with the results of Braver et al. (2001) and Nyberg et al. (2002a). The fact that this activation occurred during Phase 2 following the recognition cue (see Fig. 9) fits well with the notion that this region is involved in the specification of episodic retrieval cues (Henson et al., 1999). Finally, the third finding, that Broca's area was differentially engaged during working memory, is consistent with the results of LaBar et al. (1999), and the fact that this activation was maximal during the maintenance phase of working memory harmonizes with the idea that this region mediates phonological rehearsal (for a review, see Smith and Jonides, 1999).

The second main result of the study was the unexpected finding that anterior MTL was activated during both episodic retrieval and working memory. Although consistent with the aforementioned study by Ranganath and D'Esposito (2001), this finding is surprising because MTL has been strongly associated with episodic retrieval but not with working memory. We speculated that the MTL overlap might reflect the indexing functions of this region, which could play a role not only during the access of stored long-term memory traces but also during the mainte-

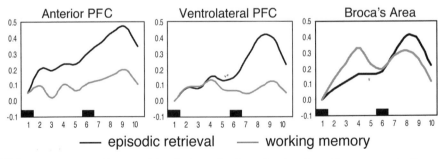

FIGURE 9 Time courses of brain activity during episodic retrieval and working memory in three prefrontal regions (after Cabeza et al., 2002a).

nance of short-term memory representations. As discussed below, however, more recent findings show that anterior MTL is also activated during an attention task without a mnemonic component, suggesting that the representations indexed by MTL are not necessarily mnemonic.

Cabeza et al. (2002b)

In an event-related fMRI study, the neural correlates of episodic memory retrieval and visual attention were compared. The motivation for comparing these two functions was that many of the brain regions typically activated during episodic retrieval tasks (for reviews, see Cabeza, 1999; Rugg and Henson, 2002), such as prefrontal, parietal, anterior cingulate, and thalamic areas, are also frequently activated during visual attention tasks (for reviews, see Handy et al., 2001; Kanwisher and Wojciulik, 2000). Thus, although the involvement of these regions during episodic retrieval has been attributed to episodic retrieval processes (e.g., postretrieval monitoring), it may actually reflect attentional operations. To investigate this idea, the previously described episodic retrieval task with retrieval mode and cue-specific retrieval phases (Cabeza et al., 2002a) was compared to a visual attention task with an important sustained attention component. In the visual attention task, participants stared at a letter in the center of the screen to determine whether it blipped once, twice, or never during a 12-sec interval.

The study yielded three main findings. First, consistent with previous functional neuroimaging evidence, the study identified a common frontoparietal–cingulate–thalamic network for episodic retrieval and visual attention. This finding suggests that many of the PFC and parietal activations frequently found during episodic retrieval reflect basic attentional processes rather than complex mnemonic operations. Actually, some of the memory-related interpretations proposed in episodic retrieval

studies can be easily rephrased in terms of simpler attentional processes. For example, right dorsolateral PFC activations during episodic retrieval have been attributed to postretrieval monitoring (Henson et al., 1999), but because monitoring involves sustained attention and sustained attention is associated with right PFC activations (for reviews, see Coull, 1998; Sarter et al., 2001), then right PFC activations during episodic retrieval may be described as sustained attention to the retrieval output.

Second, several subregions were differentially involved in episodic retrieval vs. visual attention. For example, left PFC was more activated for episodic retrieval than for visual attention, possibly reflecting semantically guided information production, whereas right PFC was more activated for visual attention than for episodic retrieval, possibly reflecting monitoring processes (Cabeza et al., 2002c). Consistent with Cabeza et al. (2002a), anterior PFC (BA 10) was differentially involved in episodic retrieval, possibly reflecting retrieval mode. The precuneus and neighboring regions were more activated for episodic retrieval than for visual attention, suggesting that these areas are involved in processing internally generated information.

Finally, the study yielded an unexpected finding: anterior MTL regions were similarly activated during episodic retrieval and during visual attention (see Fig. 10). If one assumes that MTL has an indexing function (e.g., MClelland et al., 1995), then this finding suggests that MTL indexes not only episodic memory and working memory representations (Cabeza et al., 2002a), but also perceptual representations. In other words, anterior MTL may index representations in the focus of consciousness, regardless of whether the representations originate in episodic memory, working memory, or the senses. This idea is consistent with Moscovitch's proposal that MTL is a module specialized in automatically registering the conscious experience

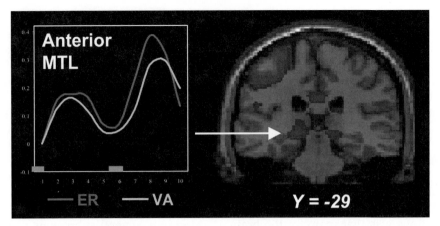

FIGURE 10 Time courses of brain activity during episodic retrieval (ER) and visual attention (VA) in a left anterior medial temporal lobe region. Reprinted from *Neuropsychologia*; R. Cabeza, F. Dolcos, S. Prince, H. Rice, D. Weissman, and L. Nyberg; Attention-related activity during episodic memory retrieval: A cross-function fMRI study. Copyright 2002, with permission from Elsevier Science.

(Moscovitch, 1992). Also, the idea is coherent with evidence that MTL activity during episodic retrieval differs for old items associated with different forms of consciousness (remembering vs. knowing) (Eldridge *et al.*, 2000) but is similar for old and new items associated with similar forms of consciousness (veridical vs. illusory recognition) (Cabeza, *et al.*, 2001; Schacter *et al.*, 1996b). Because MTL lesions do not usually impair working memory and attention tasks, but sometimes disrupt implicit tasks (e.g., Chun and Phelps, 1999), one has to conclude that MTL activity may reflect processing the contents of consciousness but is neither necessary nor sufficient for this processing.

CONCLUSIONS

To summarize the main findings of comparing different cognitive functions across studies (Figs. 3–8, Table 2) and within-subjects (Table 3), we performed the drastic simplification shown in Table 4. First, we collapsed over verbal, object, and spatial stimuli because the modulatory effects of stimulus type can be summarized in two simple statements: differences between object and spatial stimuli generally follow

the ventral/dorsal pathway distinction (Ungerleider and Mishkin, 1982), and differences between verbal and nonverbal stimuli follow hypothetical hemisphere specializations (e.g., Milner, 1971). Second, we considered only activation overlaps supported by both cross-study (Table 2) and within-subjects (Table 3) analyses. Thus, Table 4 does not include the perception domain, which has not been investigated by direct cross-function studies. Finally, we focused on the most consistent activation patterns and did not emphasize exceptions to these patterns or theoretical controversies.

As illustrated by Table 4, anterior PFC (BA 10) plays a prominent role in episodic retrieval and, to a lesser degree, in working memory. The involvement of this region in episodic retrieval is consistent with the retrieval mode hypothesis (Cabeza *et al.*, 2002a) and the overlap between episodic retrieval and working memory (Nyberg *et al.*, 2002a; Ranganath *et al.*, 2002) is consistent with a more general role in monitoring internally generated information (Christoff and Gabrieli, 2000). Dorsolateral PFC (BA 9/46) is most strongly associated with working memory and episodic retrieval, possibly reflecting a role in monitoring (Cabeza *et al.*, 2002a). Anterior ventrolateral PFC (BA 47/45) is also involved in

Region/Brodmann area

TABLE 4 Common Regions for Four Cognitive Functions and Their Hypothetical Roles in Cognition[a]

Function	PFC					ACC: 32, 24	Precun.: 31	Pariet: 40, 7	Temp.: 21	MTL
	Ant.: 10	DL: 9, 46	aVL: 47, 45	pVLp: 44	postDors: 6					
Attention	1, 3, 4, 5		1, 7		1,2,7	1,7		1,2,7		1,7
Working memory	1, 4, 5	1, 3, 4, 5, 6	1, 4, 5, 6	1, 2, 5, 6	1, 3, 4, 5, 6	1, 4, 5, 6	1, 4	1, 4, 5, 6	1, 4	5, 6
Epi. enc./sem. ret.		1, 4	1, 4, 5	1, 4, 5		1, 4				1
Episodic retrieval	1, 4, 5, 6, 7	1, 4, 5, 6, 7	1, 4, 5, 6, 7			1, 4, 5, 6, 7	1, 4, 6, 7	1, 4, 5, 7	1, 4, 7	1, 5, 6
Hypothetical processes	Retrieval mode and /or monitoring of internally generated information	Monitoring	Semantic processing and inhibitory control	In left hemisphere: phonological rehearsal	Top-down selection	Initiation of action and/ or conflict monitoring	Orienting attention to internally generated information	Shifts of attention among external or internal events	Semantic processing	Indexing of representations within the focus of consciousness

[a] *Abbreviations*: epi., episodic; enc., encoding; ret., retrieval; sem., semantic; PFC, prefrontal cortex; ACC, anterior cingulate; precun., precuneus; pariet., parietal cortex; temp., temporal cortex; MTL, medial temporal lobes; ant., anterior; DL, dorsolateral; aVL, anterior ventrolateral; pVLp, posterior ventrolateral-posterior; postDors, posterior dorsal. Symbols have the same meaning as in Tables 2 and 3; the symbol size approximately corresponds to the relative proportion of activations for each function compared to the rest of the functions. The numbers adjacent to the symbols refer to the following studies: 1, present metanalysis (see Table 2); 2, LaBar *et al.* (1999); 3, Braver *et al.* (2001); 4, Nyberg *et al.* (2002a, b); 5, Ranganath and D'Esposito (2001) and Ranganath *et al.* (2002); 6, Cabeza *et al.* (2002a); 7, Cabeza *et al.* (2002b).

working memory and episodic retrieval, but in the left hemisphere it plays a major role in episodic encoding/semantic retrieval, possibly reflecting semantic processing (e.g., Gabrieli et al., 1998). Ventrolateral PFC is also known to play an important role in inhibitory control (D'Esposito et al., 1999; Jonides et al., 1998), and this function could account for its involvement in Stroop tasks. In the left hemisphere, posterior ventrolateral PFC (BA 44) is strongly associated with verbal working memory, consistent with a hypothetical role in phonological rehearsal (Cabeza et al., 2002a; Kapur et al., 1996; Poldrack et al., 1999). Finally, posterior–dorsal PFC (dorsal BA 6) seem primarily associated with attention and working memory, consistent with a hypothetical role in top-down selection (Corbetta and Shulman, 2002)

Table 4 shows that whereas parietal regions (BAs 40 and 7) were primarily associated with attention and working memory, left temporal regions (particularly BA 21) were primarily associated with semantic and episodic memory. The involvement of parietal regions in attention and working memory, as well as in episodic retrieval, can be explained if one assumes that these regions are involved in shifting attention not only among external events (spatial and nonspatial attention), but also among internal events (working memory and episodic retrieval). The involvement of left temporal regions in both semantic and episodic memory tasks (Nyberg et al., 2002a) can be explained by a general role in semantic processing.

Finally, the MTL seems to be involved in all four cognitive functions. Although the cross-study metaanalysis did not link MTL to working memory, two cross-function fMRI studies found the MTL to be activated for both episodic retrieval and working memory (Cabeza et al., 2002a; Ranganath and D'Esposito, 2001). Overlapping MTL activations for episodic retrieval and visual attention have been found and suggest that this region indexes

representation within the focus of consciousness (Cabeza et al., 2002b). This hypothesis fits well a popular cognitive neuroscience model (Moscovitch, 1992) and can account for the involvement of these regions in several different cognitive functions.

As noted above, Table 4 shows an extremely simplified (almost simplistic) description of typical activation patterns, which does not acknowledge exceptions to the patterns or theoretical controversies about the functions of different brain regions. For example, although anterior PFC tends to play a more important role in episodic retrieval than in working memory, Ranganath et al. (2002) found similar anterior PFC activity across these functions and Braver et al. (2001) found greater activity for working memory. Even if the findings of Ranganath et al. reflect a lack of power and the results of Braver et al. reflect the lack of differentiation between working memory encoding and retrieval, further research is clearly warranted. Also, there are inconsistencies about the lateralization of overlapping PFC activations. For instance, overlapping anterior PFC activations for episodic retrieval and working memory have been found in the right hemisphere (Nyberg et al., 2002a), in the left hemisphere (Ranganath et al., 2002), and bilaterally (Cabeza et al., 2002a). Moreover, Table 4 collapsed over regions is likely to have different roles in cognition, such as inferior (BA 40) and posterior (BA 7) parietal regions. For example, we have found that the posterior parietal cortex was similarly involved in working memory and episodic retrieval, whereas the anterior parietal cortex in the left hemisphere was differentially involved in working memory (Cabeza et al., 2002a; see also Ranganath et al., 2002). If there is disagreement about the activation patterns in Table 4, there is of course much more disagreement about the theoretical interpretations of these activations. For instance, a fMRI study (Bush et al., 2002) pointed out that if one considers only research with human subjects, the list of cognitive processes attributed to the anterior cingulate cortex include the following: attention-for-action/target selection, motivational valence assignment, motor response selection, error detection/performance monitoring, competition monitoring, anticipation, working memory, novelty detection, and reward assessment. Cross-function comparisons could help decide among these different functional interpretations

Cross-function comparisons provide important constraints to functional interpretations, particularly if one assumes the sharing view. For example, although we have attributed MTL activity to the recovery of episodic memory traces (e.g., Cabeza et al., 2001; Nyberg et al., 1996b), the involvement of these regions in attention, working memory, and semantic memory suggests a much more general function in cognition. Cross-function comparisons work against the natural tendency to interpret activations in terms of our favorite cognitive function (episodic memory in our case). They help us to overcome function chauvinism and to see the "big picture." In other words, cross-function comparisons allow us to see the forest through the trees.

References

Aggleton, J. P., and Brown, M. W. (1999). Episodic memory, amnesia, and the hippocampal-anterior thalamic axis. *Behav. Brain Sci.* **22**(425–289).

Awh, E., Jonides, J., Smith, E. E., Schumacher, E. H., et al. (1996). Dissociation of storage and rehearsal in verbal working memory: Evidence from positron emission tomography. *Psychol. Sci.* **7**(1), 25–31.

Benson, D. F. (1988). Classical syndromes of aphasia. *In* "Handbook of Neuropsychology" (F. Foller and J. Grafman, eds.), Vol. 1, pp. 267–280. Elsevier, Amsterdam.

Binder, J. R., and Price, C. J. (2001). Functional neuroimaging of language. *In* "Handbook of Functional Neuroimaging of Cognition" (R. Cabeza and A. Kingstone, eds.), pp. 187–251. MIT Press, Cambridge, Massachussetts.

Botvinick, M. M., Braver, T. S., Barch, D. M., Carter, C. S., and Cohen, J. D. (2001). Conflict monitoring and cognitive control. *Psychol. Rev.* **108**(3), 624–652.

Braver, T. S., Barch, D. M., Kelley, W. M., Buckner, R. L., Cohen, N. J., Miezin, F. M., Snyder, A. Z., Ollinger, J. M., Akbudak, E., Conturo, T. E., and Petersen, S. E. (2001). Direct comparison of prefrontal cortex regions engaged by working and long-term memory tasks. *Neuroimage* **14**, 48–59.

Buckner, R. L., Raichle, M. E., Miezin, F. M., and Petersen, S. E. (1996). Functional anatomic studies of memory retrieval for auditory words and visual pictures. *J. Neurosci.* **16**(19), 6219–6235.

Bush, G., Vogt, B. A., Holmes, J., Dale, A. M., Grave, D., Jenike, M. A., and Rosen, B. R. (2002). Dorsal anterior cingulate cortex: A role in reward-based decision making. *Proc. Natl. Acad. Sci. U.SA.* **99**, 523–528.

Cabeza, R. (1999). Functional neuroimaging of episodic memory retrieval. In "Memory, Consciousness, and the Brain: The Tallinn Conference" (E. Tulving, ed.), pp. 76–90. The Psychology Press, Philadelphia.

Cabeza, R., and Nyberg, L. (2000). Imaging Cognition II: An empirical review of 275 PET and fMRI studies. *J. Cogn. Neurosci.* **12**, 1–47.

Cabeza, R., Kapur, S., Craik, F. I. M., McIntosh, A. R., Houle, S., and Tulving, E. (1997). Functional neuroanatomy of recall and recognition: A PET study of episodic memory. *J. Cogn. Neurosci.* **9**(2), 254–265.

Cabeza, R., Rao, S. M., Wagner, A. D., Mayer, A. R., and Schacter, D. L. (2001). Can medial temporal lobe regions distinguish true from false? An event-related fMRI study of veridical and illusory recognition memory. *Proc. Natl. Acad. Sci. U.S.A.* **98**, 4805–4810.

Cabeza, R., Dolcos, F., Graham, R., and Nyberg, L. (2002a). Similarities and differences in the neural correlates of episodic memory retrieval and working memory. *Neuroimage* **16**, 317–330.

Cabeza, R., Dolcos, F., Prince, S., Rice, H., Weissman, D., and Nyberg, L. (2002b). Attention-related activity during episodic memory retrieval: A cross-function fMRI study. *Neuropsychologia.* In press.

Cabeza, R., Kester, J., and Anderson, N. D. (2002c). Lateralization of prefrontal cortex activity during episodic memory retrieval: Evidence for the generate-recognize hypothesis. Submitted.

Christoff, K., and Gabrieli, J. D. E. (2000). The frontopolar cortex and human cognition: Evidence for a rostrocaudal hierarchical organization within the human prefrontal cortex. *Psychobiology* **28**, 168–186.

Chun, M. M., and Phelps, E. A. (1999). Memory deficits for implicit contextual information in amnesic subjects with hippocampal damage. *Nat. Neurosci.* **2**, 844–847.

Cohen, N. J., Ryan, J., Hunt, C., Romine, L., Wszalek, T., and Nash, C. (1999). Hippocampal system and declarative (relational) memory: Summarizing the data from functional neuroimaging studies. *Hippocampus* **9**, 83–98.

Corbetta, M., and Shulman, G. L. (2002). Control of goal-directed and stimulus-driven attention in the brain. *Nat. Rev.* **3**, 201–215.

Coull, J. T. (1998). Neural correlates of attention and arousal: Insights from electrophysiology, functional neuroimaging and psychopharmacology. *Prog. Neurobiol.* **55**, 343–361.

Courtney, S. M., Petit, L., Maisog, J. M., Ungerleider, L. G., and Haxby, J. V. (1998). An area specialized for spatial working memory in human frontal cortex. *Science* **279**, 1347–1351.

D'Esposito, M. (2001). Functional neuroimaging of working memory. *In* "Handbook of functional neuroimaging of cognition" (R. Cabeza and A. Kingstone, eds.), pp. 293–327. MIT Press, Cambridge, Massachusetts.

D'Esposito, M., Postle, B. R., Jonides, J., and Smith, E. E. (1999). The neural substrate and temporal dynamics of interference effects in working memory as revealed by event-related functional MRI. *Proc. Natl. Acad. Sci. U.S.A.* **96**, 7541–7519.

Devinsky, O., Morrell, M. J., and Vogt, B. A. (1995). Contributions of anterior cingulate cortex to behaviour. *Brain* **118**, 279–306.

Donaldson, D. I., Petersen, S. E., Ollinger, J. M., and Buckner, R. L. (2001). Dissociating state and item components of recognition memory using fMRI. *Neuroimage* **13**, 129–142.

Duncan, J., and Owen, A. M. (2000). Common regions of the human frontal lobe recruited by diverse cognitive demands. *Trends Cogn. Sci.* **23**, 473–483.

Düzel, E., Cabeza, R., Picton, T. W., Yonelinas, A. P., Scheich, H., Heinze, H.-J., and Tulving, E. (1999). Task- and item-related processes in memory retrieval: A combined PET and ERP study. *Proc. Natl. Acad. Sci. U.S.A.* **96**, 1794–1799.

Eldridge, L. L., Knowlton, B. J., Furmanski, C. S., Bookheimer, S. Y., and Engle, S. A. (2000). Remembering episodes: A selective role for the hippocampus during retrieval. *Nat. Neurosci.* **3**(11), 1149–1152.

Elliott, H. (1964). "Textbook of Neuroanatomy." Lippincott, Philadelphia.

Fletcher, P. C., and Henson, R. N. A. (2001). Frontal lobes and human memory: Insights from functional neuroimaging. *Brain* **124**, 849–881.

Fletcher, P. C., Frith, C. D., Grasby, P. M., Shallice, T., Frackowiak, R. S. J., and Dolan, R. J. (1995). Brain systems for encoding and retrieval of auditory–verbal memory: An *in vivo* study in humans. *Brain* **118**, 401–416.

Fodor, J. (1983). "The Modularity of Mind" MIT/Bradford Press, Cambridge, Massachusetts.

Fried, I., MacDonald, K. A., and Wilson, C. L. (1997). Single neuron activity in human hippocampus and amygdala during recognition of faces and objects. *Neuron* **18**, 753–765.

Fuster, J. M. (1995). "Memory in the Cerebral Cortex." MIT Press, Cambridge, Massachusetts.

Gabrieli, J. D., Poldrack, R. A., and Desmond, J. E. (1998). The role of left prefrontal cortex in language and memory. *Proc. Natl. Acad. Sci. U.S.A.* **95**(3), 906–913.

Handy, T. C., Hopfinger, J. B., and Mangun, G. R. (2001). Functional neuroimaging of attention. *In* "Handbook of Functional Neuroimaging of Cognition" (R. Cabeza and A. Kingstone, eds.), pp. 75–108. MIT Press, Cambridge, Massachusetts.

Henke, K., Buck, A., Weber, B., and Wieser, H. G. (1997). Human hippocampus establishes associations in memory. *Hippocampus* **7**(3), 249–256.

Henson, R. N. A., Shallice, T., and Dolan, R. J. (1999). Right prefrontal cortex and episodic memory retrieval: A functional MRI test of the monitoring hypothesis. *Brain* **122**, 1367–1381.

Jonides, J., Smith, E. E., Marshuetz, C., Koeppe, R. A., and Reuter-Lorenz, P. A. (1998). Inhibition in verbal working memory revealed by brain activation. *Proc. Natl. Acad. Sci. U.S.A.* **95**(14), 8410–8413.

Kanwisher, N., and Wojciulik, E. (2000). Visual attention: Insights from brain imaging. *Nat. Rev.* **1**, 91–100.

Kanwisher, N., Downing, P., Epstein, R., and Kourtzi, Z. (2001). Functional neuroimaging of visual recognition. *In* "Handbook of Functional Neuroimaging of Cognition." (R. Cabeza and A. Kingstone, eds.), pp. 109–151. MIT Press, Cambridge, Massachusetts.

Kapur, S., Tulving, E., Cabeza, R., McIntosh, A. R., Houle, S., and Craik, F. I. (1996). The neural correlates of intentional learning of verbal materials: A PET study in humans. *Cogn. Brain Res.* **4**(4), 243–249.

Kelley, W. M., Miezin, F. M., McDermott, K. B., Buckner, R. L., Raichle, M. E., Cohen, N. J., Ollinger, J. M., Akbudak, E., Conturo, T. E., Snyder, A. Z., and Petersen, S. E. (1998). Hemispheric specialization in human dorsal frontal cortex and medial temporal lobe for verbal and nonverbal memory encoding. *Neuron* **20**(5), 927–936.

Krause, B. J., Schmidt, D., Mottaghy, F. M., Taylor, J., Halsband, U., Herzog, H., Tellmann, L., and Müller-Gärtner, H.-W. (1999). Episodic retrieval activates the precuneus irrespective of the imagery content of word pair associates: A PET study. *Brain* **122**, 225–263.

LaBar, K. S., Gitelman, D. R., Parrish, T. B., and Mesulam, M. (1999). Neuroanatomic overlap of working memory and spatial attention networks: A functional MRI comparison within subjects. *Neuroimage* **10**(6), 695–704.

Lepage, M., Ghaffar, O., Nyberg, L., and Tulving, E. (2000). Prefrontal cortex and episodic memory retrieval mode. *Proc. Natl. Acad. Sci. U.S.A.* **97**(1), 506–511.

Maguire, E. A., Frith, C. D., Burgess, N., Donnett, J. G., and O'Keefe, J. A. (1998). Knowing where things are: Parahippocampal involvement in encoding object locations in virtual large-scale space. *J. Cogn. Neurosci.* **10**(1), 61–76.

Martin, A. (2001). Functional neuroimaging of semantic memory. *In* "Handbook of Functional Neuroimaging of Cognition." (R. Cabeza and A. Kingstone, eds.), pp. 153–186. MIT Press, Cambridge, Massachusetts.

McDermot, K. B., Buckner, R. L., Petersen, S. E., Kelley, W. M., and Sanders, A. L. (1999). Set and code-specific activation in the frontal cortex: An fMRI study of encoding and retrieval of faces and words. *J. Cogn. Neurosci.* **11**, 631–640.

McDermott, K. B., Buckner, R. L., Petersen, S. E., Kelley, W. M., and Sanders, A. L. (1999). Set- and code-specific activation in frontal cortex: an fMRI study of encoding and retrieval of faces and words. *J. Cogn. Neurosci.* **11**(6), 631–640.

McClelland, J. L., McNaughton, B. L., and O'Reilly, R. C. (1995). Why there are complementary learning systems in the hippocampus and neocortex: Insights from the successes and failures of connectionist models of learning and memory. *Psychol. Rev.* **102**, 419–457.

McIntosh, A. R. (1999). Mapping cognition to the brain through neural interactions. *Memory* **7**, 523–548.

McIntosh, A. R., Nyberg, L., Bookstein, F. L., and Tulving, E. (1997). Differential functional connectivity of prefrontal and medial temporal cortices during episodic memory retrieval. *Hum. Brain Mapping* **5**, 323–327.

Milner, B. (1971). Interhemispheric differences in the localization of psychological processes in man. *Br. Med. Bull.* **27**, 272–277.

Moscovitch, M. (1992). Memory and working-with-memory: A component process model based on modules and central systems. *J. Cogn. Neurosci.* **4**(3), 257–267.

Nyberg, L., and McIntosh, A. R. (2000). Functional neuroimaging: Network analyses. *In* "Handbook of Functional Neuroimaging of Cognition" R. Cabeza and A. Kingstone, eds.), pp. 49–72. MIT Press, Cambridge, Massachusetts.

Nyberg, L., Tulving, E., Habib, R., Nilsson, L.-G., Kapur, S., Houle, S., Cabeza, R., and McIntosh, A. R. (1995). Functional brain maps of retrieval mode and recovery of episodic information. *NeuroReport* **7**, 249–252.

Nyberg, L., Cabeza, R., and Tulving, E. (1996a). PET studies of encoding and retrieval: The HERA model. *Psychonom. Bull. Rev.* **3**(2), 135–148.

Nyberg, L., McIntosh, A. R., Houle, S., Nilson, L.-G., and Tulving, E. (1996b). Activation of medial temporal structures during episodic memory retrieval. *Nature* **380**(6576), 715–717.

Nyberg, L., Cabeza, R., and Tulving, E. (1998). Asymmetric frontal activation during episodic memory: What kind of specificity? *Trends Cogn. Sci.* **2**, 419–420.

Nyberg, L., Forkstam, C., Petersson, K. M., Cabeza, R., and Ingvar, M. (2002a). Brain imaging of human memory systems: Between-systems similarities and within-system differences. *Cogn. Brain Res.* **13**, 281–292.

Nyberg, L., Marklund, P., Persson, J., Cabeza, R., Forkstam, C., Petersson, K. M., and Ingvar, M. (2002b). Common prefrontal activations during working memory, episodic memory, and semantic memory. Submitted.

O'Keefe, J. A., and Nadel, L. (1978). "The Hippocampus as a Cognitive Map." Oxford, London.

Owen, A. M., Lee, A. C. H., and Williams, E. J. (2000). Dissociating aspects of verbal working emmory within the human frontal lobe: Further evidence for a "process-specific" model of lateral frontal organization. *Psychobiology* **28**, 146–155.

Paulesu, E., Frith, C. D., and Frackowiak, R. S. J. (1993). The neural correlates of the verbal component of working memory. *Nature* **362**, 342–345.

Paus, T., Petrides, M., Evans, A. C., and Meyer, E. (1993). Role of the human anterior cingulate cortex in control of oculomotor, manual, and speech responses: A positron emission tomography study. *J. Neurophysiol.* **70**, 453–469.

Poldrack, R. A., Wagner, A. D., Prull, M. W., Desmond, J. E., Glover, G. H., and Gabrieli, J. D. E. (1999). Functional specialization for semantic and phonological processing in the left inferior prefrontal cortex. *Neuroimage* **10**(1), 15–35.

Posner, M. I., and Petersen, S. E. (1990). The attention system of the human brain. *Annu. Rev. Neurosci.* **13**, 25–42.

Ranganath, C., and D'Esposito, M. (2001). Medial temporal lobe activity associated with active maintenance of novel information. *Neuron* **31**, 865–873.

Ranganath, C., Johnson, M. K., and D'Esposito, M. (2002). Temporal dynamics of prefrontal activity during working and long-term memory. Submitted.

Rugg, M. D., and Henson, R. N. A. (2002). Episodic memory retrieval: An (event-related) functional neuroimaging perspective. *In* "The Cognitive Neuroscience of Memory Encoding and Retrieval" (A. E. Parker, E. L. Wilding, and T. Bussey, eds.), Psychology Press, Hove, UK. In press.

Sarter, M., Givens, B., and Bruno, J. P. (2001). The cognitive neuroscience of sustained attention: Where top-down meets bottom-up. *Brain Res. Rev.* **35**, 146–160.

Schacter, D. L., Alpert, N. M., Savage, C. R., Rauch, S. L., and Albert, M. S. (1996a). Conscious recollection and the human hippocampal formation: Evidence from positron emission tomography. *Proc. Natl. Acad. Sci. U.S.A.* **93**, 321–325.

Schacter, D. L., Reiman, E., Curran, T., Yun, L. S., Bandy, D., McDermott, K. B., and Roediger, H. L., 3rd. (1996b). Neuroanatomical correlates of veridical and illusory recognition memory: Evidence from positron emission tomography. *Neuron* **17**(2), 267–274.

Shallice, T., Fletcher, P., Frith, C. D., Grasby, P., Frackowiak, R. S. J., and Dolan, R. J. (1994). Brain regions associated with acquisition and retrieval of verbal episodic memory. *Nature* **368**(6472),633–635.

Smith, E. E., and Jonides, J. (1999). Storage and executive processes in the frontal lobes. *Science* **283**(1657–1661).

Squire, L. R. (1992). Memory and the hippocampus: A synthesis from findings with rats, monkeys, and humans. *Psychol. Rev.* **99**, 195–231.

Tulving, E. (1983). "Elements of Episodic Memory." Oxford University Press, Oxford.

Tulving, E., Kapur, S., Craik, F. I. M., Moscovitch, M., and Houle, S. (1994). Hemispheric encoding/retrieval asymmetry in episodic memory: Positron emission tomography findings. *Proc. Natl. Acad. Sci. U.S.A.* **91**, 2016–2020.

Tulving, E., Markowitsch, H. J., Craik, F. I. M., Habib, R., and Houle, S. (1996). Novelty and familiarity activations in PET studies of memory encoding and retrieval. *Cereb. Cortex* **6**(1), 71–79.

Ungerleider, L. G., and Mishkin, M. (1982). Two cortical visual systems. *In* "Analysis of Visual Behavior" (D. J. Ingle, M. A. Goodale, and R. J. W. Mansfield, eds.), pp. 549–589. MIT Press, Cambridge, Massachusetts.

Wagner, A. D. (1999). Working memory contributions to human learning and remembering. *Neuron* **22**, 19–22.

Wagner, A. D., Desmond, J. E., Glover, G., and Gabrieli, J. D. E. (1998a). Prefrontal cortex and recognition memory: Functional-MRI evidence for context-dependent retrieval processes. *Brain* **121**, 1985–2002.

Wagner, A. D., Poldrack, R. A., Eldridge, L. L., Desmond, J. E., Glover, G. H., and Gabrieli, J. D. E. (1998b). Material-specific lateralization of prefrontal activation during episodic encoding and retrieval. *NeuroReport* **9**, 3711–3717.

COGNITIVE AND AFFECTIVE PROCESSING OF THE BRAIN

A. VISION, PERCEPTION, LANGUAGE, AND MEMORY

4

Evoked Potentials Studies of Visual Information Processing

Wolfgang Skrandies

INTRODUCTION

Sensory and perceptual processes of the human mind have been extensively studied in the past by psychophysical methods. Modern neurosciences offer several anatomical and physiological methods to complement such studies by analyzing the neurophysiological correlates of sensory information processing (Kandel *et al.*, 2000). In animal experiments, neuronal mechanisms are investigated using invasive biochemical, anatomical, and neurophysiological methods that tag activity and processes within various structures of the nervous system. For the examination of human subjects, in general only noninvasive procedures can be used. Because human information processing takes place in fractions of a second, one of the most feasible methods constitutes the recording of brain electrical activity. The strengths of electrophysiological methods lie in their very high time resolution (in the order of milliseconds) and their sensitivity to detect functional changes of global brain states and of nervous activity. The high temporal resolution as well as their noninvasive nature constitute a significant advantage of these methods over brain imaging techniques [computer topography (CT), positron emission tomography (PET), or functional magnetic resonance imaging (fMRI)], and evoked brain activity data reveal steps in sensory information processing that occur very rapidly. Comparison of imaging and neurophysiological methods shows that there is a reasonable but imperfect correlation between electrophysiological data and hemodynamic responses measured by fMRI (George *et al.*, 1995).

For the study of perception and cognition, measures with very high temporal resolution are needed. This is reflected by the fact that brain mechanisms related to perception are fast (note that motor reaction to visual stimuli occurs in a fraction of a second), and that individual steps in information processing are associated with rapid changes of the spatiotemporal characteristics of spontaneous and evoked electrical brain activity. In addition, the binding of stimulus features by the cooperation of distinct neural assemblies has been proposed to be mediated through high-frequency oscillation and its coherence of neuronal activation in different parts of the brain (Singer, 1999).

The present chapter illustrates how the recording of brain electrical activity in combination with knowledge of the human visual system may be employed to study information processing in healthy volunteers as well as in patients with selective visual deficiency. Data are presented on different experimental questions related to human visual perception, including contrast and stereoscopic vision as well as perceptual learning.

Psychophysical procedures are inherently subjective because the dependent variable consists of the verbal response or motor reaction to a physical stimulus of the subject under study. Thus, the subject's willingness and ability to cooperate in the examination determines the result of the experiment. We also draw attention to the fact that psychophysical results always reflect the final outcome of the complete chain of information processing involving sensory transduction in specialized receptor organs (Corey and Roper, 1992), subcortical and cortical processes, as well as higher, cognitive strategies. This mostly prevents the identification and direct interpretation of behavioral data in terms of isolated steps of sensory processing.

Electrophysiological recordings constitute a supplement to such psychophysical methods, whereby the electrical activity of large neuronal populations is obtained noninvasively via electroencephalograms (EEGs) or evoked and event-related potentials; these may be used to quantify neuronal correlates of perceptual and cognitive processes and relate them to anatomical structures and functional systems of the human central nervous system.

NEUROPHYSIOLOGICAL BASES OF EVOKED ELECTRICAL BRAIN ACTIVITY

Neurons communicate by transmitting to their neighbors membrane potential changes in their synaptic endings, and they are able to connect different structures by sending over long distance in the brain information in the form of frequency-modulated action potentials of constant amplitude. In animal experiments, it is possible to record such activity directly inside of neurons or in their vicinity, whereas human studies have to rely on recordings from the intact skull. Due to the fact that scalp-recorded activity has amplitudes in the order of only microvolts (μV), for technical reasons it was not until about 70 years ago that EEG recordings became possible (Berger, 1929). For the interpretation of such data it is important to keep in mind that we are dealing with mass activity originating from large neuronal populations, spreading by volume conduction to the scalp. The electrodes commonly used are very large (about 10 mm in diameter) as compared to the dimension of individual neurons (about 20 μm in diameter), which implies that the area of a single electrode corresponds to that of about 250,000 neurons. The spatial integration of electrical nervous activity is even larger considering the fact that activity simultaneously originating in distant neuronal structures is always picked up by the recording electrodes (Skrandies et al., 1978).

In contrast to the spontaneous EEG of relatively large amplitude, stimulus-related brain activity is much weaker, and may be revealed only by some processing of the data. More than 100 years ago sensory evoked potentials had been recorded by the English physiologist Caton, (1875) directly from the cortical surface of rabbit and monkey brains, whereas the recording of human evoked potentials became feasible only after the advent of electronic and computerized signal-processing capabilities in the 1950s and 1960s.

Evoked potentials are systematic changes of the EEG induced by incoming information to the brain. Every sensory stimulus elicits electrical activity that is projected by selective and specialized afferent fiber systems to the corresponding cortical sensory areas, where it induces changes of the ongoing electrical activity. These changes depend on (1) the function state of the brain (information processing is different during various sleep stages and in different states of wakefulness), (2) the specific meaning and importance of a given stimulus (attention and cognitive set of the subject determine the way stimuli are processed), and (3) the physical stimulus parameters and sensory thresholds of the organism (which also influence the subject's sensory capability to perceive stimuli).

A single sensory stimulus evokes brain activity of only very small amplitude; although the ongoing EEG has amplitudes in the order of up to 150 μV, evoked brain activity reaches amplitudes between only 0.1 and 20 μV, and such small changes cannot be detected in the spontaneous EEG. Signal averaging enables identification of evoked activity: the same stimulus is presented repeatedly, and typically EEG segments of 10–1000 msec in length, following each stimulus presentation, are averaged. Stimulus-related brain activity looks similar in repeated trials, whereas the spontaneous EEG shows a randomized amplitude distribution over time.

Figure 1 illustrates how visual evoked potentials (VEPs) are obtained by averaging. From animal experiments it is known that neurons in the mammalian visual cortex can be activated optimally by contrast changes. In order to obtain the data illustrated in Fig. 1, at time 0 msec the contrast of a checkerboard pattern is reversed, and the EEG segment following stimulation is recorded for an epoch of 1000 msec. This procedure is repeated at a rate of 2 Hz, thus two stimuli occur during the recording epoch. The contrast reversal elicits an occipitally positive component with a latency of about 100 msec that, however, cannot be seen in the raw EEG. With the averaging of only a few trials it is obvious that large, independent potential fluctuations occur with positive and negative polarity at random (see upper two curves in Fig. 1); with further averaging their mean value tends toward 0 μV. On the other hand, all stimulus-related, time-locked VEP activity shows consistent

polarities over the recording epoch, and a stable potential configuration emerges after summation of several single potentials. This can be seen for both contrast reversals that occur every 500 msec (stimulus onset is indicated in Fig. 1 by the solid vertical lines at 0 and 500 msec). The averaging of 32 single potentials yields a VEP wave form with a consistent positive component with a latency of about 100 msec (indicated by dashed lines in Fig. 1), and additional stimulus presentations result in

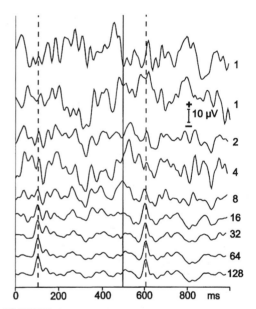

FIGURE 1   Averaging of evoked EEG potentials: every 500 msec the contrast of a checkerboard pattern presented electronically on a monitor is reversed (denoted by vertical lines), and the EEG is recorded over the occipital brain areas for an epoch of 1000 msec. The numbers on the right indicate the number of trials averaged, and it is obvious that in the spontaneous EEG (upper two curves) no consistent pattern of electrical brain activity can be detected. The averaging of the EEG following a different number of stimulus presentations (n = 2, 4, 8, 16, 32, 64, 128) shows how stimulus-dependent activity emerges, whereas independent potential fluctuations with positive and negative polarity occurring at random cancel each other. A positive component with a latency of about 110 msec marked by the dashed vertical line, can be seen after 32 individual sweeps. Note that the VEP amplitude reaches about 15 μV, whereas the stimulus-independent EEG is in the order of 20 to 30 μV.

a further decrease in variability of the recorded signal. Evoked components are commonly denoted by their relative polarity (positive, P; negative, N) followed by the number of milliseconds of their approximate latency. Thus, Fig. 1 displays the so-called P100 component of the VEP.

The latencies and amplitudes of evoked potential components as well as the number of stimulus presentations needed to obtain a stable evoked brain response are dependent on the physical stimulus parameters as well as on the sensory modality: the amplitudes of the so-called brain stem auditory evoked potentials are in the order of 0.2–1.0 μV, thus 1500–2000 single evoked responses have to be used (Jewett *et al.*, 1970). The small amplitudes are due to the fact that the neuronal elements activated are located in the brain stem structures of the auditory pathway, and thus are far away from the recording electrodes on the scalp. Along a similar line, fewer cortical neurons are selectively sensitive to visual horizontally disparate stimuli than they are to contrast changes, and 300–600 trials are needed to obtain a VEP elicited by stereoscopic stimuli (see later discussion on stereoscopic perception).

Evoked brain activity consists of a sequence of components that are interpreted to reflect steps in information processing; these must be determined by quantitative methods (Lehmann and Skrandies, 1980; Skrandies, 1987). Such components occur at times of high neural activity accompanied by strong electrical fields, and large potential differences are seen in the recorded wave forms. The main parameters extracted from evoked brain activity are component latencies (time between stimulus presentation and the occurrence of a given component indicating neural processing times), amplitude (strength of the evoked electrical field, indicating the degree of synchronous neuronal activation), and amplitude topogra-

phy, which may give some indication of the neuronal populations involved in the processing of a given stimulus.

It is important to note that mapping of electrical activity does not make it possible directly to draw conclusions on the exact neuroanatomical locations of the intracranial sources. Neuronal mass activity produces electrical fields that spread via volume conduction throughout the brain, and these can be recorded at locations distant from the generating source. This has been shown in a study on various stages of the cat visual system, whereby single unit activity and field potentials were compared and the spread of electrical activity was evident throughout the brain (Skrandies *et al.*, 1978). Thus, model source computations on scalp-recorded data always have to rest on certain explicit (and sometimes implicit) assumptions concerning the number, location, and spatial extent of dipoles as well as the homogeneity and geometry of the intracranial media in order to arrive at physiologically meaningful solutions (Koles, 1998). It is also obvious that the "inverse problem" of how to determine the sources of potentials in a conductive medium, when the scalp potential field is given, has no unique solution (Von Helmholtz, 1853). The computation of equivalent dipoles thus must be regarded as a further step of data reduction. The multidimensional scalp data space consisting of potential measurements from many electrode locations may be explained or modeled by an equivalent dipole data space with typically fewer dimensions. It is evident that such a data reduction has to be performed for each poststimulus time point separately, whereby the solution reflects the instantaneous source configuration.

As will be shown in the next section, direct interpretations of scalp potential fields in terms of intracranial neuronal generator locations may be misleading. This is due to the fact that the inverse problem, and source localizations, should mainly be viewed as models that explain the scalp-recorded activity.

Visually elicited activity may be recorded noninvasively, both at the level of the retina as electroretinogram (ERG) and from the visual cortex as visual evoked potential. Here the focus is concentrated on VEP activity, and the reader is referred elsewhere for a more detailed description of electroretinographical methods in basic research and in clinical settings (Armington, 1974; Heckenlively and Arden, 1991). Skrandies and Leipert (1988) give some instructive examples on how the combination of cortical and retinal electrophysiological recordings allows the topological identification and diagnosis of the causes of visual field defects in neuroophthalmologic patients.

MULTICHANNEL RECORDING AND TOPOGRAPHIC MAPPING

EEG activity derives from an electrical field, the characteristics of which vary with time and space. Thus, the position of recording electrodes on the scalp determines the pattern of the recorded activity; multichannel recordings of EEGs and evoked potentials enable topographical analysis of the electrical fields of the brain as they are reconstructed from many spatial sampling points. [For details of topographical analysis of EEG data, see also Skrandies (2002) and Appendix E, this volume.]

Figure 2 illustrates the scalp distribution of evoked potential fields between 60 and 190 msec obtained from 30 electrodes, with contrast reversing stimuli presented to different retinal areas. The upper row in Fig. 2 shows maps of activity evoked by stimuli presented to the left hemiretina; the bottom map series shows activity elicited by visual stimuli presented to the right retinal half. The maps in the middle row illustrate the activity evoked when the same stimulus was foveated by the subject, and one can see that the major positive component that occurs at a latency of 110 msec shows a symmetrical distribution over the occipital areas. When lateralized stimuli are presented to the subject, it is obvious that the evoked potential fields show a strong lateralization of activity depending on retinal stimulus location. In humans, the retinal projections to the visual cortex are very orderly, resulting in a retinotopic cortical representation of the visual field. Due to the decussation of the ganglion cell fibers originating from the nasal retina in the optic chiasm, each visual half-field projects to the contralateral visual cortex. Thus, with lateralized

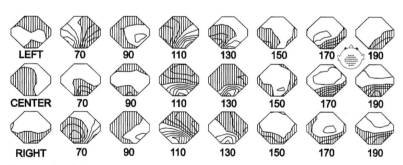

FIGURE 2 Topographical distribution of potential fields between 60 and 190 msec at 10-msec intervals evoked by contrast reversal stimuli presented to different retinal areas. Recordings were obtained simultaneously from 30 electrodes distributed over the head (note head scheme in inset). Checkerboard reversal stimuli were presented to the left or right hemiretina or with central fixation of the subject. In all map series a major positive component occurs with a latency of 110 msec with a symmetrical occipital distribution for central stimuli, and with a lateralized distribution for lateral stimuli. Equipotential lines in steps of 2 μV; hatched areas are negative with respect to the average reference.

stimulation, neurons are activated in the visual cortex ipsilateral to the retinal half that receives the stimulus. Inspection of the potential distributions in Fig. 2 reveals, however, that the evoked potential data appear to show a different picture: with lateral half-field stimulation we see an occipital positive component occurring between 100 and 120 msec after stimulation that is largest over the contralateral hemisphere (maps series in Fig. 2, top and bottom). This effect is called "paradoxical lateralization" of the VEP. From earlier work it is known that visual stimuli presented in the lateral half-fields yield a complex pattern of asymmetric distributions of evoked potential components on the scalp: ipsilateral and contralateral component locations have been described, and the direction and amount of scalp potential lateralization appears to depend critically on the physical stimulus parameters (Skrandies and Lehman, 1982). Of course, the lateralization of evoked potential components is different from hemispheric specialization effects.

One aim of electrophysiological recordings of human brain activity is the identification of the underlying sources in the brain. Information is processed in circumscribed areas of the central nervous system, and spontaneous activity also originates from specific brain structures. Thus, it appears of consequence to try to explain the topography of scalp distribution patterns in terms of anatomical localization of neuronal generators. To arrive at valid interpretations of scalp-recorded data is no trivial task: a fundamental and severe complication constitutes the so-called "inverse" problem that cannot be uniquely solved. Any given surface distribution of electrical activity can be explained by an endless variety of intracranial neural source distributions that produce an identical surface map. Thus, there is no unique numerical solution when model sources are determined, but knowledge of the anatomy and

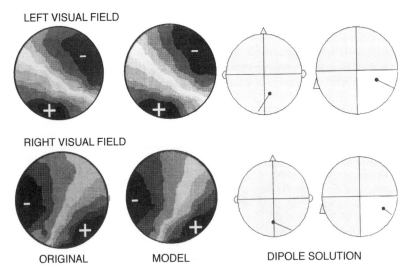

LEFT VISUAL FIELD

RIGHT VISUAL FIELD

ORIGINAL   MODEL   DIPOLE SOLUTION

FIGURE 3   Original and reconstructed potential fields evoked by stimuli in the left or right visual field at component latency (110 msec for left, 105 msec for right visual field stimuli). Original maps represent the original potential distribution; the model maps are the surface distribution computed from the model dipoles. The great similarity between the recomputed and original potential fields indicates that the model dipoles are able to explain most of the variance in the data (more than 95% for each data set). The head schemes with the results of model dipole computations are shown from above or from the left side. Dots mark the locations of the dipole, the lines indicate dipole orientation and strength. Recordings are in 30 channels, with electrodes evenly distributed between the inion and 25% of the nasion–inion distance (see scheme in Fig. 2).

physiology of brain systems allows deduction of a meaningful source localization (see below and Fig. 3). We note that this still implies that *model* sources are determined and this aspect needs to be considered when interpreting evoked potential or EEG data (Skrandies, 2002).

Data such as those illustrated in Fig. 2 indicate that the scalp locations of strongest electrical activity do not necessarily coincide with the intracranial localization of the neuronal generators, and most attention should be drawn to the areas where steep potential gradients occur. This will now be illustrated with results from dipole location computations. With mathematical approaches it is possible to compute the electric potential distribution on the surface of a homogeneous conducting sphere surrounded by air, which is due to a point current dipole inside the sphere (cf. Pascual *et al.*, 1990). In addition, it appears reasonable to assume the head to be represented best by a concentric three-shell model (Ary *et al.*, 1981). Other methods for localization of sources of electrical brain activity consider more complex anatomical (realistic head model) and physiological (distributed sources) information, as is illustrated by the merging of data from imaging methods and electrophysiological data (Fuchs *et al.*, 1998; George *et al.*, 1995; Koles, 1998; Pascual-Marqui *et al.*, 1994; Skrandies, 2002).

The results of such a source localization computation for lateralized visual evoked potential fields are given in Fig. 3. In order to control for positional errors, prior to computation all electrode locations have been quantified by digitizing their positions in three dimensions on the subject's head. This information, along with the positional information on the major anatomical landmarks of the head, was used for computation of best-fit dipole localizations. Figure 3 illustrates the dipole source location of a component occurring between 105 and 110 msec latency after the presentation of a visual stimulus in the left

or right visual half-field. Component latency was determined by the computation of maximal field strength as the mean standard deviation within the field at each time point [i.e., global field power (GFP)] (Lehmann and Skrandies, 1980; Skrandies, 1987) (see also Appendix E, this volume).

The evoked potential fields at component latency [110 msec for stimuli presented in the left visual field (i.e., on the right hemiretina; upper part of Fig. 3), 105 msec for stimulation of the right visual field (i.e., on the left hemiretina; lower part of Fig. 3)] are illustrated in the maps on the left side of Fig. 3. As seen before, lateral visual stimuli result in a "paradoxical" lateralization, with potential maxima occurring contralateral to the retinal half stimulated. The results of the dipole computation are given as source localizations in the schematic head as seen from above or from the left side. Despite the lateralization of high peaks of activity over the contralateral hemisphere, the model sources are located in the hemisphere ipsilateral to the hemiretina stimulated. This is in line with the anatomy of the visual cortex whereby the retinal projections arrive in the calcarine fissure in the medial part of the ipsilateral occipital cortex. Electrodes over the contralateral hemisphere, however, appear to be located optimally to record most of the activity originating from the calcarine cortex. This observation has been confirmed by intracranial recordings in human patients (Lehmann *et al.*, 1982), and it also explains why the retinal extension of the stimulus determines the amount of lateralization of the evoked brain activity (Skrandies and Lehmann, 1982).

We must stress the point that such dipole computations result in a *model* that best explains the electrical field recorded on the scalp, but due to the inverse problem discussed above, there is no unique solution for such computations. Anatomical locations of the neuronal sources determined may be quite different if the same data have to be fit by more than one dipole or if different assumptions about conductivity and head geometry are made. On the other hand, the "model" maps computed from the dipole source solution (the so-called forward solution) are very similar to the measured data of our example: for both data sets illustrated in Fig. 3, more than 95% of the variance is explained. This indicates that the data reduction achieved by the model dipole computation yields reasonable results. It is important to keep in mind that the absolute locations of the potential maxima or minima in the field do not necessarily reflect the location of the underlying generators (this fact has led to confusion in the EEG literature, and for visual evoked activity this phenomenon became known as "paradoxical lateralization"). Rather, the location of steepest potential gradients in the scalp fields is a more adequate parameter, indicating the intracranial source locations. This is evident when the potential distribution maps and the location of the model dipoles are inspected in Fig. 3.

STEADY-STATE VEPs: INFLUENCE OF STIMULATION FREQUENCY

The data illustrated in Fig. 1 and 2 were elicited by a checkerboard pattern reversing in contrast at a rate of 2 reversals/sec,

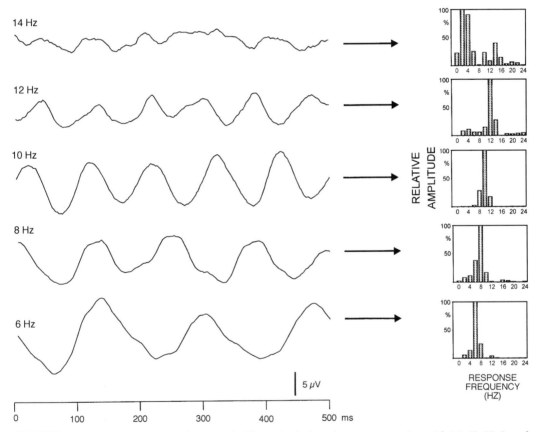

FIGURE 4 Visual potential wave forms evoked by a checkerboard pattern reversing with 14, 12, 10, 8, and 6 reversals/sec. Note how response frequencies follow stimulation frequency. On the right the normalized amplitude spectra are shown stemming from a fast Fourier transform computation. For each condition the amplitude corresponding to the stimulation frequency is plotted. Data recorded from O_z versus a reference at F_z.

and two responses occur in 1 sec. With increasing stimulation frequency the brain responses follow the reversal rates because each single stimulus elicits time-locked brain activity, and subsequent components overlap. This is shown in Fig. 4, where VEP activity was recorded while a checkerboard stimulus was reversed in contrast at 6, 8, 10, 12, or 14 reversals/sec.

All VEP wave forms are highly correlated with the stimulation frequency: e.g., for 6 reversals/sec three components occur within 500 msec, and 8 reversals/sec elicit four components, etc. This means that every contrast reversal is followed by evoked activity in the visual cortex. Such potentials are also called "steady-state" VEPs because it is assumed that repetitive stimulation results in a continuous stream of steady responses. It is also obvious that different frequencies yield brain responses of different strengths. Note that amplitudes are largest with the stimulus changing at 6 reversals/sec, and there is some amplitude tuning for the higher frequencies, with a relative maximum occurring for a stimulation frequency of 10 reversals/sec. Frequency analysis may be used to quantify amplitudes in given frequency bands and also to detect brain responses in noisy signals. Conventionally, this is done by computing a fast Fourier transform (FFT) on the VEP amplitudes, resulting in a description of the data in the frequency domain. As is evident from the wave forms in Fig. 4, low stimulation rates evoke time-locked activity as can be determined by visual inspection of the VEPs for frequencies up to a rate of 12 reversals/sec. On the other hand, it looks like there is no stimulus-related activity when the subject observes a checkerboard pattern changing at 14 reversals/sec.

The results of a frequency analysis, however, reveal that also with 14 reversals/sec significant stimulus-related VEP activity may be detected (see spectra in Fig. 4). Although its amplitude is rather small and the VEP wave form is largely dominated by lower frequencies, there occurs a clear peak at 14 Hz when the power spectra resulting in a frequency analysis are consulted (see Fig. 4, right side). Thus, prior knowledge of the temporal course of stimulation allows one to detect brain activity related to the processing of visual input.

Stimulation with high temporal frequencies may also be employed in order to study the time resolution and refractory periods of the human visual system. With double-flash stimulation (two flashes occurring at intervals in the order of milliseconds) Skrandies and Raile (1989) demonstrated that both retinal and cortical activity may be recorded with such stimuli. Most interestingly, even when the subject was not able to perceive two flashes, the evoked neuronal activity showed two responses. In addition, there were significant differences of retinal and cortical structures in temporal resolution capabilities: with intervals below 40 msec only very few subjects displayed a VEP response to the second flash, whereas the electroretinogram yielded two separate responses to a double flash even with an interval of only 10 msec. Differences between retinal and cortical processing are further supported by the fact that there appears to exist no direct relationship between the amplitudes and latencies of retinal and cortical potentials (Skrandies and Raile, 1989) indicating that knowledge of electrophysiological parameters in the retina does not allow prediction of how cortical potentials will be influenced by the variation of stimulus parameters.

PERCEPTUAL LEARNING, NEURAL PLASTICITY, AND HIGHER COGNITIVE PROCESSES

Cognitive effects also affect evoked brain activity, which depends on the information processing during a task. Factors such as attention, motivation, or expectancy as well as the occurrence probability of stimuli determine the pattern of electrical brain activity. The presentation of task-relevant information yields so-called endogenous components, commonly occurring with large latencies of more than 300 msec. In general, such components are elicited only when the stimulus is relevant for a task and the subject attends to the stimuli. An identical stimulus presented without task relevancy is not followed by this kind of activity. These endogenous components are interpreted to reflect higher, cognitive information-processing steps (see also Gazzianiga *et al.*, 1998; Picton, 1988; Skrandies, 1995).

One may find that attentional processes also influence earlier components. In a study on visual information processing the randomized presentation of relevant and irrelevant alphanumeric and geometric stimuli yielded significant differences in evoked components at a latency of only about 100 msec, in addition to the expected effects occurring at much longer latencies (Skrandies *et al.*, 1984). This indicates that rather early information-processing steps, probably in primary visual cortical areas, are influenced when the subject is involved in a pattern discrimination task [see Skrandies (1983) for a more detailed description]. Such data are in line with the report by Zani and Proverbio (1995), who illustrated the effect of selective attention to the size of checks (squares) on early VEP components.

In addition, there are systematic changes in the scalp topography of event-related brain activity during processing of language stimuli (Skrandies, 1998). According to the "semantic differential technique" the affective meaning of words can be quantified in statistically defined, independent dimensions, in which every word is uniquely located in three dimensions—evaluation (good/bad), potency (strong/weak), and activity (active–passive). These dimensions are very stable and culture independent (Osgood *et al.*, 1975). It is important to note that visual processing of words yields a scalp topography of the P100 component which is *globally* similar to checkerboard evoked brain activity. With more detailed topographical analysis, however, small but significant differences appeared when the locations of the positive and negative centers of gravity (so-called centroids; for details see Appendix E) were compared (Skrandies, 1998).

When brain activity evoked by different semantic word classes was analyzed, significant effects were not restricted to late "cognitive" components, but brain activity at early latencies (corresponding to the P100 component) was affected by semantic meaning of the stimuli. These data show how visually evoked brain activity is modulated by the meaning of the stimuli at early processing stages (see Skrandies, 1998). In a similar way, it has been illustrated that attention affects early steps of visual processing (Skrandies *et al.*, 1984). Thus, the influence of attention and cognitive parameters on activation of the visual cortex can be studied electrophysiologically by recordings of VEP activity.

Similarly, there are effects on brain electrical activity that accompany learning processes. From psychophysical experiments it is known that performance of a number of perceptual tasks improves as a result of training, not only during the ontogenetic development in early childhood but also in adults, reflected by perceptual improvements in sensory discrimination ability (Fiorentini and Berardi, 1981; Gibson, 1953). Similarly, neurophysiological studies on the cortical plasticity in adult animals have established that the representation of sensory functions in cortical areas is not hard wired, and it can change as a function of repeated stimulus processing. Selective deafferentiation is the most drastic alteration of adequate sensory input: the interruption of peripheral somatosensory afferences is followed by an extensive rewiring of cortical projections in the somatosensory cerebral cortex

(Merzenich *et al.*, 1984). Such modifications were also found in animals trained for perceptual discrimination, whereby functional changes of cortical mechanisms have been documented with invasive neurophysiological methods; there is a correlation between functional changes observed in single-unit responses and sensory discrimination performance in adult monkeys observed with somatosensory stimuli (Recanzone *et al.*, 1992) as well as in auditory frequency-discrimination tasks (Recanzone *et al.*, 1993). For the mammalian visual system, functional changes in receptive field organization of cortical neuronal assemblies were demonstrated (Gilbert and Wiesel, 1992).

Electrophysiological correlates of improved discrimination performance of special visual stimuli have been reported by Skrandies and Fahle (1994) and by Skrandies *et al.* (2001). The human visual system is able to resolve stimuli with an accuracy that is much better than the spacing of individual photoreceptors in the retina: the small offset of line stimuli (so-called vernier targets) in the order of only a few seconds of arc may be detected by normal human subjects, yielding much higher than usual visual acuity coined ("hyperacuity") (see overview in Westheimer, 1982). The repeated presentation of such visual vernier targets during an experimental session is accompanied by a significant improvement in sensory thresholds within less than half an hour of training. This learning is stimulus specific, based on the demonstration that there is no transfer of improved performance when the orientation of the stimuli is changed by 90° (Poggio *et al.*, 1992). Thus, there are no attention effects, and the subject does not learn simply to adjust to the experimental procedure, but rather very specific information-processing strategies improve by training. In different populations of healthy adults, Skrandies and Fahle (1994) and Skrandies *et al.* (1996) consistently found that the mean performance

improved significantly within about half an hour of passive training. Such improvements in performance derived from psychophysical testing are paralleled by significant alterations of electrical brain activity. Analysis of potential distributions recorded over the occipital areas of the subjects during the learning phase revealed highly significant changes. These effects were reflected by differences in the topography of the scalp potential distributions, with short latencies below 100 msec as well as at latencies extending to over 500 msec.

Figure 5 illustrates the mean potential fields of 10 subjects at 250 msec latency evoked by the first or second block of 600 presentations of vertical or horizontal vernier targets. Note the very small amplitude of the brain electrical response to such weak stimuli. This is commonly observed also with three-dimensional visual stimuli that selectively activate only a small population of neurons in the human visual cortex (see below). From Fig. 5 it is obvious that for both stimulus orientations the scalp potential fields that are elicited after learning are very different from those evoked by the same stimulus before learning. Before the training the potential fields are shallow, and display only little activity. After training a strong negative component over the occipital areas can be seen. The direct statistical comparisons computed as paired *t*-tests between maps turn out to be highly significant, indicating the occurrence of different electrical brain activity after learning (see significance probability maps illustrated in Fig. 5). These differences cannot be explained by a different time course of evoked activity in the two conditions, as has been shown in a number of different studies (Skrandies and Fahle, 1994; Skrandies *et al.*, 1996, 2001). Learning of a vertical vernier target and learning of a horizontal target are both followed by similar electrophysiological changes, although differences in electrical activity,

HORIZONTAL   VERTICAL

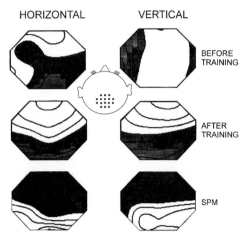

BEFORE TRAINING

AFTER TRAINING

SPM

FIGURE 5 Mean evoked potential fields of 10 subjects at 250 msec latency evoked by the first (before training) or second block of 600 presentations (after training) of visual hyperacuity targets. The results of corresponding *t*-tests are illustrated on the bottom as significance probability maps (SPM). The left-hand maps show the data obtained with horizontal stimuli; the right-hand maps display the fields evoked by vertical stimuli. Note pronounced and highly significant changes in topography after learning, which correlates with significant improvements of sensory thresholds. Recordings are from 16 electrodes over the occipital areas (note head scheme in inset); shaded areas are negative with respect to the average reference; steps are in 0.1 μV for the potential fields; steps are in 1.0 *t*-values units for the *t*-maps. Data from Skrandies and Fahle (1994).

depending on the orientation of grating stimuli, have been reported (Skrandies, 1984). Similarly, in our psychophysical experiments we could verify that improvements in performance over time are independent of the orientation of the stimulus (Skrandies and Fahle, 1994; Skrandies *et al.*, 1996), although with vertical vernier stimuli, in general, sensory thresholds are smaller than with horizontal stimuli (Skrandies *et al.*, 2001).

We note that at certain latencies similar field configurations occurred, and mainly field strength increased after training (e.g., at 50, 350, or 550 msec), whereas at other times the evoked potential fields were completely and significantly different, as illustrated in Fig. 5. This suggests that the activation of new neuronal populations by an identical

stimulus is induced after perceptual learning. In Fig. 5, the data from a component elicited by vernier stimuli at 250 msec latency are illustrated, showing large differences in the pattern of electrical brain activity. We note that such significant differences in electrical brain activity occurred not only at this time point but also over extended periods of the recording epoch (Skrandies and Fahle, 1994; Skrandies *et al.*, 1996, 2001). These results suggest that after training intracranial neuronal generator populations were activated in a different way by an identical visual stimulus. It is important that in both psychophysical and electrophysiological experiments significant effects of perceptual learning were obtained with a similar time course. The high correlation between the change in perceptual performance and the change of stimulus-related brain potential topography as a function of practice, as well as the spatiotemporal pattern of neuronal activation with steep gradients over the primary visual cortex, corroborates the notion that perceptual learning occurs at an "early" level of visual processing. This interpretation is in line with the fact that neurons in the striate cortex respond to the presentation of vernier offset stimuli (Swindale and Cynader, 1986).

In summary, significant effects of perceptual learning can be obtained in both psychophysical and electrophysiological experiments with a similar time course—within about half an hour. The covariation of the subjective sensory and neurophysiological results illustrates that more efficient perceptual processing is paralleled by activation changes, mainly over the primary visual cortex, suggesting that implicit learning may occur at a relatively early level of perceptual processing. The neurophysiological data recorded noninvasively from large neuronal assemblies of human subjects simultaneously during perceptual processing reflect the dynamic changes going on at the cortical level (Darian-Smith and Gilbert, 1995).

Similar learning takes place with three-dimensional perception. Random-dot stereograms (RDSs) have been used in studies for many years (Julesz, 1971; Bergua and Skrandies, 2000), and these stimuli contain only binocular horizontal disparity as depth cue to be extracted by the visual system. Three-dimensional information contained and hidden in RDSs is not easy to see. Similar stimuli are the so-called autostereograms, printed in the well-known "Magic-Eye" books; in these it is obvious that naive observers must learn to perceive a three-dimensional structure. With RDS stimuli most normal subjects also need several seconds or even longer to identify stereoscopic targets, and this response time drops significantly with practice (O'Toole and Kersten, 1992). Skrandies and Jedynak (1999) have shown in a combined psychophysical and electrophysiological study that more than half of the 16 subjects tested learned to see stereoscopic targets after 8 min of training. It is important to note that significant improvements in sensory discrimination occur even after viewing only stimuli below perceptual threshold. These observations are in line with previous studies on subliminal perception and implicit learning in normal subjects (Berry and Dienes, 1993) and "blind sight" in brain-damaged patients (Weiskrantz *et al.*, 1974; Zihl, 1980), which also suggests that perceptual processing and learning are possible without conscious awareness. On a cortical level, this learning was accompanied by topographic changes in the electrophysiological pattern of activation of neural assemblies in the visual cortex, where the center of activity shifted toward the right hemisphere. Subjects who did not improve in perception displayed no such effects (Skrandies and Jedynak, 1999).

STEREOSCOPIC PERCEPTION AND EVOKED POTENTIALS: PHYSIOLOGICAL BASIS AND CLINICAL APPLICATION

Binocular and depth perception have been examined for many years and are being studied today by employing computer-generated random-dot stereograms. A historical account of the invention and development of random-dot stimuli has been given by Bergua and Skrandies (2000).

Three-dimensional depth perception is based in part on the fact that our two eyes see the environment from slightly different viewpoints, and depth information is extracted from the horizontal disparity of visual stimuli on the two retinas. Slight differences in the image viewpoints—horizontal disparity—are the crucial cue for depth perception. Because the input into the two eyes remains separated up to the level of the visual cortex (Bishop, 1973; Gonzalez and Peres, 1998), evoked brain activity generated exclusively by cortical structures may be investigated when random-dot stereograms (Julesz, 1971) are presented binocularly. Such RDS stimuli do not contain any contrast information, and can be used to investigate three-dimensional vision in isolation. Commonly, such stimuli are presented dynamically at high frequency by modern computer graphics (Skrandies, 2001). The perception of these stereograms depends on the fusion of two nonidentical, horizontally disparate inputs in the visual cortex, and under monocular viewing conditions a dynamic RDS (dRDS) stimulus cannot be perceived stereoscopically. The neuronal correlates of these processes are cortical neurons selectively responsive to disparate binocular stimuli; these as have been found in the monkey visual cortex (Hubel and Wiesel, 1970; Von der Heydt *et al.*, 1981).

For experimental studies of human vision, the use of dRDSs offers the possibility to investigate selectively cortical processing of visual information. With random-dot displays any desired three-dimensional form can be created: e.g., a three-dimensional checkerboard pattern is produced when each eye sees a different array of randomly arranged dots, and one of the patterns is horizontally displaced in such a way that the area of each individual check square contains crossed binocular disparity. After binocular fusion, these areas will stand out in front of the plane of fixation, and a study participant will perceive a checkerboard pattern hovering in front of the monitor. The time-locked averaging of electrical brain activity is triggered by the sudden change in horizontal disparity, but independent stimulation of the two eyes may be achieved by employing polarizing foils or anaglyphs (red and green dots in combination with red/green goggles), or by liquid crystal diode shutter glasses. With such glasses, dRDSs are presented as monocular half-images alternating at the refresh rate of the monitor, and the glasses are electronically synchronized with the monitor frequency so that every second image is seen by one eye only. For practical application, the different methods yield very similar perceptual effects, they are employed only in order to route independent information to the left and the right eye.

Figure 6 illustrates evoked potentials recorded from a healthy young adult. Checkerboard reversal stimuli with contrast borders were presented either monocularly to the left and right eyes (lowest two curves) or binocularly (second curve). It is obvious that differences in component latencies can be seen when VEPs evoked by monocular and binocular stimulation are compared: stimulation of both the left and right eyes yields latencies of 113 msec, whereas binocularly evoked brain activity displays a component latency of only 103 msec. Such binocular summation effects have been described before, illustrating that latencies or amplitudes of the evoked potential are significantly different when binocular and monocular conditions are compared (e.g., Nakayama *et al.*, 1982; Skrandies, 1993). The physiological correlate for such findings is the fact that many neurons of the mammalian visual cortex are influenced by input from both

eyes (Gonzalea and Perez, 1998), and vision with two eyes and monocular vision result in different perceptions. Binocular fusion of disparate retinal images yields stereopsis (see below), and vision with two eyes enlarges the visual field. In psychophysical experiments it was shown that with binocular stimuli higher contrast sensitivity is obtained, as compared with monocular targets (Campbell and Green, 1965).

Figure 6 also shows stereoscopic VEPs that were elicited by the presentation of a three-dimensional checkerboard pattern: red/green anaglyph dynamic RDS patterns that were generated every 20 msec by special hardware were presented on a color monitor. By using red/green spectacles, each eye saw only a portion of the dots displayed, and the green pattern was horizontally displaced in such a way that the subject could perceive a checkerboard

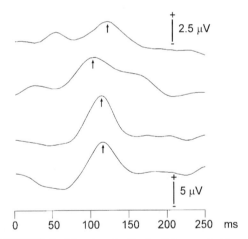

FIGURE 6 Visual evoked potentials recorded from the occipital areas of a healthy subject; obtained with the reversal in depth of a stereoscopic checkerboard pattern with horizontal disparities changing by 13.8 min of visual angle (top), or with binocular (second curve) or monocular contrast reversal stimuli (lower two curves). Major components are marked by arrows. Note shorter latencies for binocular (103 msec) as compared to monocular stimulation (113 msec). With three-dimensional stimuli, amplitudes are small, thus the stereo VEP is scaled differently (see vertical calibration bar). Reference electrode at F_z; occipital positive is up.

pattern standing in front of the plane of the monitor. Disparities were changed locally every 256 msec by 13.8 min of visual angle, resulting in the percept of a three-dimensional checkerboard pattern that stood in front of the monitor and reversed in depth. Stereoscopic evoked activity yields evoked components with latencies very similar to those due to contrast evoked brain activity, whereas stereoscopically elicited amplitudes were significantly smaller. This is evident in Fig. 6, and has been described repeatedly (Skrandies, 1986, 1991, 2001; Skrandies and Vomberg, 1985), suggesting that the afferent binocular information flow to the human visual cortex is of similar velocity for processing of both dynamic RDS patterns and contrast borders. On the other hand, three-dimensional stimuli are significantly less effective in exciting many visual neurons synchronously, which is in line with the assumption that there are many more neurons sensitive to contrast changes than there are neurons selectively sensitive to binocular disparate stimuli. In addition, topographic comparisons of stereoscopic and contrast evoked potential fields suggest that disparate retinal stimuli are processed preferentially by neuronal populations outside area 17 (Skrandies, 1986, 1991, 1997; Skrandies and Vomberg, 1985), which is consistent with results obtained with single-unit recordings in cats and monkeys (Hubel and Wiesel, 1970; Von der Heydt, 1981).

Within certain physiological limits, increasing disparities lead to the perception of increasing depth, and one would expect some optimal disparity range when depth perception is strongest. Thus, stereoscopic evoked brain activity also depends on the horizontal disparity of the RDS stimulus, and significant effects of horizontal disparities on brain electrical activity are observed (Skrandies, 1997).

Figure 7A illustrates the topographical data recorded in 30 channels over the occipital areas with dynamic RDS stimuli of different disparities, ranging from 7 to 24.5 min of arc. Stimulation frequency was 6 Hz, and stimulus-locked brain activity was obtained with all disparity values. The maps in Fig. 7A are the responses occurring at stimulation frequency. With large or small disparities, potential field strength was rather small, whereas the largest responses were obtained with intermediate disparities, as is evident from the fewer field lines in Fig. 7A. This observation illustrates that there is a functional disparity tuning of cortical activation: low and high disparities yield less synchronized neural activity as compared to intermediate disparities. This tuning of response strength is in line with studies on single neurons in the monkey visual cortex (Gonzalez and Perez, 1998; Hubel and Wiesel, 1970). In addition, significant differences were observed in dRDS evoked brain activity when central and lateral stimulus locations were compared. With lateral stimuli (extending from the fovea to 17.1° eccentricity), maximal amplitudes were obtained at larger disparities than with central stimuli (Fig. 7B): with RDS stimuli presented to foveal areas, the largest amplitudes occurred with mean disparities of 10.5 min of arc, whereas with lateral stimuli, sensitivity was largest with stimuli of 14 min of arc (Skrandies, 1997). These observations indicate that more peripheral and lateral areas are less sensitive to disparity information, supporting data on disparity thresholds for fusion where for patent and qualitative stereopsis as well as stereo, thresholds increase with retinal eccentricity (Ogle, 1962).

Further analysis of the data also reveals that there are not only differences between central and eccentric stimulation, but that there are also pronounced differences between brain activity evoked with stereo stimuli presented in the left or right visual field (Fig. 7B). Stimuli located in the right visual field show a tuning function with a clear response peak at 14 min of arc disparity. Neuronal response strength is

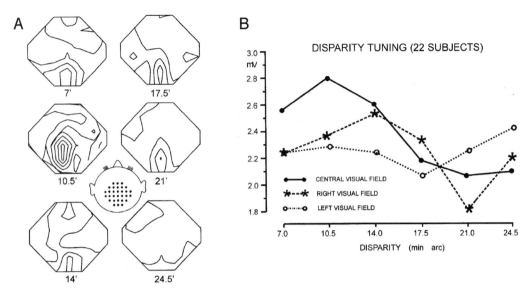

FIGURE 7 (A) Scalp distributions of power of the 6-Hz band recorded in 30 channels (electrode locations as indicated by head scheme). Disparity varied between 7 and 24.5 min of arc, stimulation frequency was 6 depth reversals/sec. Individual maps are shown for stimuli of different disparity; numbers in the figure refer to disparity values, lines are in steps of 0.5 μV. Note different response strength with different disparities. (B) Mean field strength computed on 30 channels of the responses in the 6-Hz band as a function of horizontal disparity of the stimulus between 7 and 24.5 min of arc. Note differences in absolute strength between central (solid line) and lateralized stimuli. As ANOVA revealed, disparity tuning is significantly different for dynamic RDS stimuli occurring in the right (dashed line) or left visual field (dotted line). Mean values computed from data on 22 subjects. Data from Skrandies (1997).

significantly reduced for higher and lower disparities, as is reflected by smaller amplitudes of brain electrical activity. Surprisingly, with stimuli presented in the left visual field the brain responses lack this tuning function: here all horizontal disparities appear to be processed in a similar way, and there is no peak in the tuning curve. In a population of 22 test subjects there was no preference for a certain disparity of the RDS stimuli, and an analysis of variance confirmed a significant interaction between visual field location and disparity. These results are independent of the location of the recording site, because recording electrodes over the left and right hemispheres yield very similar results (Skrandies, 1997). The lack of disparity tuning of VEP responses with stimuli in the left visual field is explained by high intersubject variability of amplitudes in this stimulus condition. In the case of large-amplitude variation between subjects, the tuning effect is expected to disappear. Thus, the basic difference between the processing of disparity information in the left and right visual fields may be explained by the smaller variation and higher consistency of brain activity elicited by three-dimensional stimuli presented to foveal areas or parafoveal areas extending toward the right visual field, indicating differences in global processing of three-dimensional information.

Knowledge of the influence of the horizontal disparity of VEP activity may be useful for the clinical application of recordings of stereoscopically evoked brain activity. In psychophysical and electrophysiological experiments, we compared patients with selective disturbance of stereoscopic vision and healthy young adults (Vomberg and Skrandies, 1985; Skrandies, 1995, 2001). It is important to note that meaningful comparisons are possible only with patients who have normal visual acuity in both eyes and who possess other normal visual functions (color vision, visual fields, contrast sensitivity). It is comprehensible that these are rare cases because the patients have no subjective symptoms and experience only very little disturbance.

The data displayed in Fig. 8 illustrate evoked potentials recorded from a subject with microstrabism. The conventional VEPs elicited by contrast reversal stimulation of the left and right eyes or binocularly, show amplitudes and latencies in the normal range. As in the healthy subject, with binocular stimuli, significantly shorter component latencies (108 msec) are observed as compared with monocular stimulation (115 msec). However, with dRDS stimuli, quite a different picture emerges: when a stereogram with a hori-

zontal disparity of 13.8 min of visual angle is presented, the major VEP component displays a reduced amplitude as well as a latency prolongation by more than 20 msec, resulting in a component latency of about 140 msec. These data suggest that there is some deficiency that affects only stereovision in this patient, leaving the processing of contrast information intact. This is in agreement with the fact that this patient had increased psychophysical thresholds for three-dimensional stimuli. With an increase of horizontal disparity ("more depth"), the pathological VEP activity may become normal: a dRDS pattern with a horizontal disparity of 27.6 min of visual angle elicits brain activity with normal component latencies (113 msec) and amplitudes that are similar to those of the healthy subject (compare the upper curves of Figs. 6 and 8).

Related electrophysiological results have been described by Vomberg and Skrandies (1985) and Skrandies (1995, 2001) in groups of patients with various degrees of stereovision deficiency but normal binocular visual acuity: there is a high correlation between disparity thresholds that were determined psychophysically and electrophysiologically in a group of patients with various degrees of stereovision deficiency but normal binocular visual acuity.

Such results indicate that the recording of brain activity evoked by three-dimensional stimuli may be employed to objectively determine stereovision capability. Another application is the monitoring of visual development in infants: similar to many other sensory functions, depth perception is no innate capacity but has to be learned in the first months of life. This has also been demonstrated in evoked potential studies in which, with contrast stimuli, evoked brain activity is recordable in neonates; using RDS stimuli, stimulus-related brain activity is elicited only after about 4 months of age. The critical period of stereovision development as determined electrophysiologically is in the

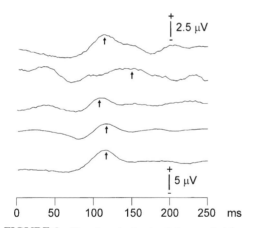

FIGURE 8 Visual evoked potentials recorded from the occipital areas of a patient with microstrabism. The upper two curves illustrate stereoscopic VEPs elicited by the reversal in depth of a stereoscopic checkerboard pattern with horizontal disparities of 27.6 or 13.8 min of visual angle. The third curve was obtained with binocular, and the lowest two curves with monocular, contrast reversal stimuli. Major components are marked by an arrow. Note latency prolongation with small disparities, and normal latencies with large horizontal disparities. With three-dimensional stimuli, amplitudes are small, thus the stereo VEP is scaled differently (see calibration bar). Reference electrode at F_z; occipital positive is up.

order of 10 and 19 weeks of age, which is somewhat earlier than when it is determined by behavioral methods (Petrig *et al.*, 1981).

CLINICAL APPLICATIONS IN NEUROLOGY AND OPHTHALMOLOGY

The classical application of VEP measurements for clinical purposes is its contribution to the diagnosis of multiple sclerosis (MS). The main characteristic of this disease is the patchy demyelination of afferent and efferent nerve fibers distributed all over the nervous system, and the patients have neurological symptoms that cannot be explained by a single lesion. Myelin is an insulating sheath, found on most axons, that increases conduction velocity (cf. Kandel *et al.*, 2000), thus, electrophysiologically, latency prolongations are expected when demyelination occurs. In many patients the visual system is affected at an early state of the disease, and one finds patients with pathological VEP results who, however, do not display any subjective visual symptoms (i.e., they have normal visual acuity and visual fields). An optic neuritis occurs frequently at a very early stage of the disease, which in general is followed by a recovery after several weeks, whereas other symptoms—hemiparesis, ataxia, and sensory disturbances—may be seen only after some years. The diagnosis of MS is warranted only if several independent lesions can be quantified, or if several repeated attacks of similar neurological symptoms occur over time. Thus, with pathological VEP measurements clinically silent lesions can be detected in patients with no visual symptoms, and this may contribute to a final diagnosis of MS. For more information on pathophysiological and clinical details of MS the reader is referred to Bauer *et al.*, (1980) and McKhann (1982).

Other applications of VEP measurements in ophthalmology and neurology comprise the documentation of visual development in infants (as discussed in the section on stereoscopic vision) as well as the topologic localization of disturbances in the visual system (Heckenlively and Arden, 1991). The combined recordings of VEP and ERG activity allow localization of lesions in the afferent visual pathway in patients with visual field defects. Skrandies and Leipert (1988) could demonstrate a significant relationship between pathological electrical acivity and the site of the lesion in a group of neuro-ophthalmological patients. After lesions of the optic nerve or optic tract, ERG changes appear in parallel to a retrograde degeneration of the axons of the retinal ganglion cells. On the other hand, in adult patients with cortical lesions, no electrophysiological sign of subsequent retinal alterations can be found. This has also been demonstrated in controlled lesion experiments performed on adult cats (see Skrandies and Leipert, 1988). In summary, such data illustrate the topodiagnostic possibilities of the combination of various electrophysiological recordings in patients with defective vision. Due to their noninvasive nature and their sensitivity to functional (and not only structural and anatomical) changes, these methods are commonly applied for a wide variety of diagnostic questions.

CONCLUSION

Classical psychophysics allows study of integrative, subjective aspects of sensory information processing, but electrophysiological experiments give us tools for the assessment of neuronal mechanisms at various levels of the central nervous system. In addition to the visual processes described in this chapter, various sensory modalities may be investigated with only minimal active cooperation of the subject, and primary sensory evoked brain activity is largely independent of cognitive processing strategies.

High temporal resolution inherent in electrophysiological recordings helps to reveal steps in information processing occurring in fractions of a second. For functional analyses of sensory processes this is a significant advantage over brain imaging techniques such as computer topography, positron emission tomography, or magnetic resonance imaging, the strengths of which are the exact anatomical three-dimensional identification of structures of the central nervous system. For MRI, substantial improvements in time resolution are in reach, as reports on "functional MRI" suggest (cf., Belliveau *et al.*, 1991; Frackowiak *et al.*, 1997). However, the direct relationship between neuronal activation and local hemodynamic changes that occur on a much cruder time scale still remains unclear (George *et al.*, 1995). Although it has been demonstrated that functions of the human visual cortex may be successfully studied by fMRI (Wandell, 1999), due to the huge cost of the equipment and the technical operating expense, however, one may predict that in most cases the access to such techniques will be restricted to medical centers specialized for clinical diagnosis, and in general it will not be available on a routine basis for workers in the fields of sensory physiology or experimental psychology. On the other hand, electrophysiological recording of brain electrical activity is relatively easy to perform, and it has widespread applications in the fields of human basic and clinical neurophysiology as well as in cognitive neuroscience (Gazzanigga *et al.*, 1998).

The noninvasive recording of evoked potentials constitutes a powerful supplement to psychophysical testing, and it may reveal steps of information processing with a high resolution in the time domain. As has been illustrated in this chapter, electrophysiological measures may also be employed for functionally localizing certain effects in the central nervous system, as is also evident from the clinical applications of auditory brain stem potentials, electroretinography, and visual evoked brain activity. On the other hand, it is important to keep in mind that direct interpretations of electrical brain activity in terms of absolute anatomical localization of neuronal generator populations are not warranted. Careful experimental planning as well as profound knowledge on the anatomical and neurophysiological bases of perceptual processes are mandatory in order to arrive at a meaningful interpretation of the recorded data. Thus, a combination of psychophysical and electrophysiological methods in controlled experiments holds the promise for further insight into the mechanisms of sensory information processing in the human brain in the future.

Acknowledgment

Supported in part by Deutsche Forschungsgemeinschaft, DFG SK 26/8-3.

References

Armington, J. C. (1974). "The Electroretinogram." Academic Press, New York.

Ary, J. P., Klein, S. A. and Fender, D. H. (1981), Location of sources of evoked scalp potentials: Corrections for skull and scalp thickness. *IEEE Trans. Biomed. Eng.* **BME-28**, 447–452.

Bauer, H. J. , Poser, S., and Ritter, G. (eds.) (1980). "Progress in Multiple Sclerosis Research." Springer, Berlin.

Belliveau, J. W., Kennedy, D. D., Kinstry, R. C., Buchbinder, B. R., Weisskoff, R. M., Cohen, M. S., Venea, J. M., Brady, T. J., and Rosen, B. R. (1991). Functional mapping of the human visual cortex by magnetic resonance imaging. *Science* **245**, 716–719.

Berger, H. (1929). Über das Elektrenkephalogramm des Menschen. I. Mitteilung. *Arch. Psychiat. Nervenkr.* **87**, 527–570.

Bergua, A., and Skrandies, W. (2000). An early antecedent to modern random dot stereograms— "The Secret Stereoscopic Writing" of Ramón y Cajal. *Int. J. Psychophysiol.* **36**, 69–72.

Berry, D., and Dienes, Z. (1993). "Implicit Learning. Theoretical and Empirical Issues." Lawrence Erlbaum Assoc., Hillsdale, New Jersey.

Bishop, P. O. (1973). Neurophysiology of binocular single vision and stereopsis. *In* "Handbook of Sensory Physiology" (R. Jung, ed.), *(VII/3A)*, pp. 255–305. Springer, Berlin.

Campbell, F. W., and Green, D. G. (1965). Monocular versus binocular visual acuity. *Nature* **208**, 191–192.

Caton, R. (1875). The electric currents of the brain. *Br. Med. J.* **2**, 278.

Corey, D. P., and Roper, S. D. (eds.) (1992). "Sensory Transduction." The Rockefeller University Press, New York.

Cormack, L. K., Stevenson, S. B., and Schor, C. M. (1993). Disparity-tuned channels of the human visual system. *Vis. Neurosci.* **10**, 585–596.

Darian-Smith, C., and Gilbert, C. D. (1995). Topographic reorganization in the striate cortex of the adult cat and monkey is cortically mediated. *J. Neurosci.* **15**, 1631–1647

Fiorentini, A., and Berardi, N. (1981). Perceptual learning specific for orientation and spatial frequency. *Nature* **287**, 43–44.

Frackowiak, R. S. J., Friston, K. J., Frith, C. D., Dolan, R. J., and Mazziotta, J. C. (1997). "Human Brain Function." Academic Press, San Diego.

Fuchs, M., Drenckhahn, R., Wischmann, H. A., and Wagner, M. (1998). An improved boundary element method for realistic volume-conductor modeling. *IEEE Trans. Biomed. Eng.* **45**, 980–997.

Gazzaniga, M., Ivry, R., and Mangun, G. R. (1998). "Cognitive Neuroscience: The Biology of the Mind." Norton, New York.

George, J. S., Aine, C. J., Mosher, J. C., Schmidt, D. M., Ranken, D. M., Schlitt, H. A., Wood, C. C., Lewine, J. D., Sanders, J. A., and Belliveau, J. W. (1995). Mapping function in the human brain with magnetoencephalography, anatomical magnetic resonance imaging, and functional magnetic resonance imaging. *J. Clin. Neurophysiol.* **12**, 406–431.

Gibson, E. J. (1953). Improvement in perceptual judgements as a function of controlled practice or training. *Psychol. Bull.* **50**, 401–430.

GIlbert, C. D., and Wiesel, T. N. (1992). Receptive field dynamics in adult primary visual cortex. *Nature* **356**, 150–152.

Gonzalez, F., and Perez, R. (1998). Neural mechanisms underlying stereoscopic vision. *Prog. Neurobiol.* **55**, 191–224.

Heckenlively, J. R., and Arden, G. B. (eds.) (1991). "Principles and Practice of Clinical Electrophysiology of Vision." Mosby, Year Book Inc., St. Louis.

Hubel, D. H., and Wiesel, T. N. (1970). Cells sensitive to binocular depth in area 18 of the macaque monkey cortex. *Nature* **225**, 41–42.

Jewett, D. L., Romano, M. N., and Williston, J. S. (1970). Human auditory evoked potentials: Possible brainstem components detected on the scalp. *Science* **167**, 1517–1518.

Julesz, B. (1971). "Foundations of Cyclopean Perception." The University of Chicago Press, Chicago.

Kandel, E. R., Schwartz, J. H., and Jessel, T. M. (2000). "Principles of Neural Science," 4th Ed. McGraw-Hill, New York.

Koles, Z. J. (1998). Trends in EEG source localization. *Electroencephalogr. Clin. Neurophysiol.* **106**, 127–137.

Lehmann, D., and Skrandies, W. (1980). Reference-free identification of components of checkerboard-evoked multichannel potential fields. *Electroencephalogr. Clin. Neurophysiol.* **48**, 609–621.

Lehmann, D., Darcey, T. M., and Skrandies, W. (1982). Intracerebral and scalp fields evoked by hemiretinal checkerboard reversal, and modelling of their dipole generators. *In* "Clinical Applications of Evoked Potentials in Neurology." (J. Courjon, F. Mauguière, and M. Révol, eds.), pp. 41–48. Raven Press, New York.

McKhann, G. M. (1982). Multiple sclerosis. *Annu. Rev. Neurosci.* **5**, 219–239.

Merzenich, M. M., Nelson, R. J., Stryker, M. P., Cynader, M. S., Schoppmann, A., and Zook, J. M. (1984). Somatosensory cortical map changes following digit amputation in adult monkeys. *J. Comp. Neurol.* **224**, 591–605.

Nakayama, K., Apkarian, P., and Tyler, C. W. (1982). Spatial frequency limitations in binocular neurons: Visual evoked potential evidence. *Ann. N.Y. Acad. Sci.* **388**, 610–614.

Ogle, N. K. (1962). The optical space sense. *In* "The Eye" (H. Davson, ed.), Vol.4, pp. 211–432. Academic Press, New York.

Osgood, C. E., May, W. H., and Miron, M. S. (1975). "Cross-cultural Universals of Affective Meaning." University of Illinois Press, Urbana, Illinois.

O'Toole, A. J., and Kersten, D. J. (1992). Learning to see random-dot stereograms. *Perception* **21**, 227–243.

Pascual, R., Biscay, R., and Valdes, P. (1990). The physical basis of electrophysiological brain imaging: Exploratory techniques for source localization and waveshape analysis of functional components of electrical brain activity. *In* "Machinery of the Mind—Data, Theory, and Speculations about Higher Brain Function," (E. R. John, ed.), pp. 435–459. Birkhäuser, Boston.

Pascual-Marqui, R. D., Michel, C. M., and Lehmann, D. (1994). Low resolution electromagnetic tomography: A new method for localizing electrical activity in the brain. *Int. J. Psychophysiol.* **18**, 49–65.

Petrig, B., Julesz, B., Kropfl, W., Baumgartner, G., and Anliker, M. (1981). Development of stereopsis and cortical binocularity in human infants. *Science* **213**, 1402–1405.

Picton, T. W. (ed.) (1988). "Handbook of Electroencephalography and Clinical Neurophysiology, Revised Series, Vol. 3, Human Related Potentials." Elsevier, Amsterdam.

Poggio, T., Fahle, M., and Edelman, S. (1992). Fast perceptual learning in visual hyperacuity. *Science* **256**, 1018–1021.

Recanzone, G. H., Merzenich, M. M., and Schreiner, C. E. (1992). Changes in the distributed temporal response properties of SI cortical neurons reflect improvements in performance on a temporally based tactile discrimination task. *J. Neurophysiol.* **67**, 1071–1091.

Recanzone, G. H., Schreiner, C. E., and Merzenich, M. M. (1993). Plasticity in the frequency representation of primary auditory cortex following discrimination training in adult owl monkeys. *J. Neurosci.* **13**, 87–103.

Singer, W. (1999). Neuronal synchrony: A versatile code for the definition of relations? *Neuron* **24**, 49–65.

Skrandies, W. (1983). Information processing and evoked potentials: Topography of early and late components. *Adv. Biol. Psychiatr,* **13**, 1–12.

Skrandies, W. (1984). Scalp potential fields evoked by grating stimuli: Effects of spatial frequency and orientation. *Electroencephalogr. Clin. Neurophysiol.* **58**, 325–332.

Skrandies, W. (1986). Visual evoked potential topography: Methods and results. *In* "Topographic Mapping of Brain Electrical Activity," (F. H. Duffy, ed.), pp. 7–28 Butterworths, Boston.

Skrandies, W. (1987). The upper and lower visual field of man: Electrophysiological and functional differences. *Prog. Sens. Physiol.* **8**, 1–93.

Skrandies, W. (1991). Contrast and stereoscopic visual stimuli yield lateralized scalp potential fields associated with different neural generators. *Electroencephalogr. Clin. Neurophysiol.* **78**, 274–283.

Skrandies, W. (1993). Monocular and binocular neuronal activity in human visual cortex revealed by electrical brain activity mapping. *Exp. Brain Res.* **93**, 516–520.

Skrandies, W. (1995). Visual information processing: Topography of brain electrical activity. *Biol. Psychol.* **40**, 1–15.

Skrandies, W. (1997). Depth perception and evoked brain activity: The influence of horizontal disparity. *Vis. Neurosci.* **14**, 527–532.

Skrandies, W. (1998). Evoked potential correlates of semantic meaning: A brain mapping study. Cogn. Brain Res. **6**, 173–183.

Skrandies, W. (2001). The processing of stereoscopic information in human visual cortex: Psychophysical and electrophysiological evidence. *Clin. Electroencephalogr.* **32**, 152–159.

Skrandies, W. (2002) EEG topography. *In* "The Encyclopedia of Imaging Science and Technology," (J. P. Hornak, ed.). John Wiley & Sons, New York (in press).

Skrandies, W., and Fahle, M. (1994). Neurophysiological correlates of perceptual learning in the human brain. *Brain Topogr.* **7**, 163–168.

Skrandies, W., and Jedynak, A. (1999). Learning to see 3-D: Psychophysical thresholds and electrical brain topography. *NeuroReport* **10**, 249–253.

Skrandies, W., and Lehmann, D. (1982). Spatial principal components of multichannel maps evoked by lateral visual half-field stimuli. *Electroencephalogr. Clin. Neurophysiol.* **54**, 662–667.

Skrandies, W., and Leipert, K. P. (1988). Visual field defects are not accompanied by electrophysiological evidence of transsynaptic retrograde degeneration. *Clin. Vis. Sci.* **3**, 45–57.

Skrandies, W., and Raile, A. (1989). Cortical and retinal refractory periods in human visual system. *Int. J. Neurosci.* **44**, 185–195.

Skrandies, W., and Vomberg, H. E. (1985). Stereoscopic stimuli activate different cortical neurons in man: Electrophysiological evidence. *Int. J. Psychophysiol.* **2**, 293–296.

Skrandies, W., Wässle, H., and Peichl, L. (1978). Are field potentials an appropriate method for demonstrating connections in the brain? *Exp. Neurol.* **60**, 509–521.

Skrandies, W., Chapman, R. M., McCrary, J. W., and Chapman J. A. (1984). Distribution of latent components related to information processing. *Ann. N.Y. Acad. Sci.* **425**, 271–277.

Skrandies, W., Lang, G., and Jedynak, A. (1996). Sensory thresholds and neurophysiological correlates of human perceptual learning. *Spatial Vis.* **9**, 475–489.

Skrandies, W., Jedynak, A., and Fahle, M. (2001) Perceptual learning: Psychophysical thresholds and electrical brain topography. *Int. J. Psychophysiol.* **41**, 119–129

Swindale, N. V., and Cynader, M. S. (1986). Vernier acuity of neurons in cat visual cortex. *Nature* **319**, 591–593.

Vomberg, H. E., and Skrandies, W. (1985). Untersuchung des Stereosehens im Zufallspunkt-muster-VECP: Normbefunde und klinische Anwendung. *Klin. Monatsbl. Augenheilkd.* **187**, 205–208.

Von der Heydt, R., Hänni, P., Dürsteler, M., and Peterhans, E. (1981). Neuronal responses to stereoscopic stimuli in the alert monkey—A comparison between striate and prestriate cortex. *Pflügers Arch.* **391**, R34.

Von Helmholtz, H. (1853). Über einige Gesetze der Vertheilung elektrischer Ströme in körperlichen Leitern, mit Anwendung auf die thierelektrischen Versuche. *Ann. Phys. Chem.* **29**, 211–233, 353–377.

Wandell, B. (1999). Computational neuroimaging of human visual cortex. *Annu. Rev. Neurosci.* **22**, 145–173

Weiskrantz, L., Warrington, E. K., Sanders, M. D., and Marshall, J. (1974). Visual capacity in the hemianopic field following a restricted occipital ablation. *Brain* **97**, 709–728.

Westheimer, G. (1982). Visual hyperacuity. *Prog. Sens. Physiol.* **1**, 1–30.

Zani, A., and Proverbio, A. M. (1995). ERP signs of early selective attention effects to check size. *Electroencephalogr. Clin. Neurophysiol.* **95**, 277–292.

Zihl, J. (1980)."Blindsight": Improvement of visually guided eye movements by systematic practice in patients with cerebral blindness. *Neuropsychologia* **18**, 71–77.

5

MEG Studies of Visual Processing

C. J. Aine and J. M. Stephen

INTRODUCTION

Numerous magnetoencephalographic (MEG) investigations of the functional organization of the human visual system have been conducted since 1968, when Cohen from MIT made the first recordings of neuromagnetic fields associated with alpha rhythms (Cohen, 1968). In 1972, Cohen recorded spontaneous brain activity using a single-channel superconducting quantum interference device (SQUID) in a shielded room (Cohen, 1972), and by 1975, visual evoked responses to a strobe flash were acquired (Teyler *et al.*, 1975). Williamson and Kaufman at NYU began conducting a number of visual and auditory evoked response studies using a seven-channel system (two channels were used for noise rejection) in the following years (e.g., Brenner *et al.*, 1975; Williamson *et al.*, 1978; Kaufman and Williamson, 1980). Currently, MEG systems contain 64–306 sensors, providing whole-head coverage.

MEG can provide sensitive temporal information about sensory and cognitive functions (on the order of milliseconds) and can provide good spatial resolution as well. Hemodynamic measures (e.g., functional magnetic resonance imaging and positron emission tomography), although

providing good spatial resolution, have a lower temporal resolution (seconds and tens of seconds, respectively) that is inadequate for documenting changes in conduction velocities or neural processing times. MEG methods provide some benefits for data analysis compared to event-related potential (ERP) methods in terms of visualizing the data and ease in localizing the sources. In the first case, because MEG signals are generated from intracellular currents (Okada *et al.*, 1997; Tesche *et al.*, 1988; Wu and Okada, 1998), the skull is virtually transparent to magnetic fields (Barth *et al.*, 1986; Okada *et al.*, 1999a,b), and because MEG measurements are reference free, the field distributions at the surface of the head are more focal, making it easier to visualize general source locations from the surface patterns. In the second case, because the skull is virtually transparent to magnetic fields, simple head models (e.g., homogeneous spherical conductive medium) may be used for source localization of MEG data (Hämäläinen and Sarvas, 1987, 1989; Cuffin, 1990). Therefore, the field of MEG is in a unique position to draw from both the single- and multiunit studies in monkeys and the hemodynamic studies of functional neuroimaging. The most serious limitation of MEG and electroencephalographic (EEG) methods is the

93

nonuniqueness of the solutions (i.e., a number of different spatial configurations of sources within the brain can create the same field pattern at the surface of the head).

Early MEG investigations of the visual system attempted to corroborate findings between noninvasive MEG measures and invasive studies in monkeys, because much of the knowledge of the visual system had been gained from these anatomical, lesional, and electrophysiological studies. Invasive studies reveal a number of different areas in monkey brain that contain different representations of the visual field, which process information in slightly different ways (Zeki, 1978). For example, visual area 4 (V4) in monkeys contains a heavy representation of the central visual field and a large proportion of color selective cells, whereas the medial temporal area (MT) emphasizes peripheral vision and is quite sensitive to motion (Zeki, 1973, 1978, 1980; Maunsell and Van Essen, 1983; Albright, 1984). Felleman and Van Essen (1991) have identified 32 different visual areas in monkey brains, although some of these areas are still under debate. Most early MEG studies of basic vision focused on examining properties (e.g., spatial frequency/temporal frequency tuning functions and retinotopic organization) of single visual areas (e.g., V1, V4, or MT). A review of these studies indicates that by carefully selecting stimulus parameters (e.g., field position, color, size, and motion) it is possible to identify and characterize several different visual areas in the human brain.

More recently, MEG studies have examined cognitive issues such as the representation of language processes in the brain, as well as memory and imagery (e.g., Salmelin et al., 1994; Michel et al., 1994; Kuriki et al., 1996; Eulitz et al., 1996; Koyama et al., 1998; Zouridakis et al., 1998; Walla et al., 2001; Iwaki et al., 1999). Studies of language and imagery rely less on invasive results in monkeys for indirect valida-tion but depend more on results from other functional neuroimaging methods, such as positron emission tomography (PET) and functional magnetic resonance imaging (fMRI) for corroboration. But even contemporary views of higher cognitive functions (i.e., memory) draw on knowledge gleaned from invasive studies of primate sensory/perceptual systems to some extent, which emphasize that a number of different neural systems participate in the representation of an object or event (Squire, 1986; Kosslyn, 1988). Although there is overwhelming evidence that feature integration relies on convergent hierarchical processing, i.e., the visual system can be viewed as a series of processing stages that represent a progressive increase in complexity of neu-ronal representations (e.g., Zeki, 1978; Van Essen, 1985; Van Essen and Maunsell, 1983; De Yoe et al., 1994), there is also overwhelming evidence for the existence of at least two functionally specialized processing streams in the visual system ("dorsal" and "ventral") operating in parallel (e.g., Ungerleider and Mishkin, 1982; Ungerleider, 1995; Van Essen and Maunsell, 1983; Merigan and Maunsell, 1993; De Yoe and Van Essen, 1988). Many investigators currently believe that information concerning the attributes of stimuli is not stored as a unified percept in a single cortical location, but rather, appears to be stored in a distributed cortical system in which information about specific features is stored close to the regions of cortex that mediate the perception of those features (e.g., Ungerleider, 1995; Mesulam, 1998; Goldman-Rakic, 1988). The issue of how features and attributes of stimuli become integrated across widespread cortical regions has been of intense interest and debate. By capitalizing on the temporal resolution of neuromagnetic measures in conjunction with anatomical MRI, insights into the connectivity patterns of the different cortical regions (i.e., functional systems or networks) can be obtained.

The MEG studies reviewed in this chapter represent steps toward the general goal of a noninvasive delineation of visual information-processing pathways in the human brain. The following general topics are examined: (1) retinotopic organization, (2) basic visual functions within or across visual areas, (3) synchronization or oscillatory behavior, (4) higher order processes that may alter the flow of information through the visual system (e.g., selective attention), and (5) general issues. This review is not intended to be comprehensive in the sense of referencing all visual MEG studies conducted during the past 30 years. Instead, we provide a conceptual physiological/anatomical framework for each of the subject headings provided above and discuss representative MEG studies published in journals, relative to each of these subject headings.

IDENTIFICATION OF VISUAL AREAS AND RETINOTOPY

Visual information flows from retina to cortex through two primary pathways. The tectopulvinar system in monkeys projects from the retina to the superior colliculus, pulvinar, or lateral posterior nucleus of the thalamus, to predominantly extrastriate areas such as parietal cortex (Schneider, 1969; Rodieck, 1979; Van Essen, 1979; Wilson, 1978). In contrast, the phylogenetically newer geniculostriate system, the focus of this review, is the one most frequently studied using neuroimaging methods. In monkeys, the geniculostriate system projects from the retina to the lateral geniculate nucleus (LGN) of the thalamus, and from the LGN to layer IV of visual cortical area 1 (V1), the primary visual cortex. V1 contains a point-to-point representation of the entire contralateral visual hemifield (Rodieck, 1979; Van Essen, 1979; Felleman and Van Essen, 1991). Visually responsive cortex projects from V1 to additional areas within the occipital lobe

(e.g., V2, V3, V3A, VP) and to large portions of the temporal (e.g., V4, TEO, TE) and parietal lobes (MT, MST, STP, PO, VIP, LIP). Many of the visual areas contained within these regions have a topographic mapping of the contralateral visual hemifield; however, some areas have either a very crude retinotopic representation (i.e., point-to-point projection of the visual field onto striate and extrastriate cortex) or none at all. Visual areas in monkeys have been identified using any of the following criteria: (1) retinotopic organization, (2) anatomical connections, (3) neuronal response properties, (4) architectonics, and (5) behavioral deficits resulting from ablation (Maunsell and Newsome, 1987; Zeki, 1978). The general strategy employed for noninvasive studies attempting to identify visual areas in humans has relied heavily on two of the criteria mentioned above: (1) evidence of distinct retinotopic organization and (2) functional specialization (e.g., motion selective, color selective).

Several event-related potential studies attempted to examine the field representation of V1 in humans. Jeffreys and Axford (1972a,b), for example, have suggested that the field representation of V1 is organized into four basic quadrants (cruciform model); this division results from the intersection of the longitudinal and calcarine fissures (i.e., they form the vertical and horizontal axes of the cruciform). The right field projects to the left hemisphere and the left field projects to the right hemisphere. Similarly, the lower visual field projects to the upper bank of the calcarine fissure and the upper field projects to the lower bank of the calcarine fissure. Unfortunately, although many ERP studies in humans have routinely noted robust effects of retinal location on amplitude, wave shape, and polarity on the 100-msec response to stimuli, there has been considerable disagreement concerning the neural generators of the evoked responses (Michael and Halliday, 1971; Drasdo, 1980; Lesevre and Joseph, 1979; Butler et al.,

1987; Maier *et al.*, 1987; Darcey *et al.*, 1980). The temporal overlap of activities from multiple cortical areas presents a clear challenge for ERP methods. Activity from more than one visual area can summate and contribute to a single peak in the wave form, making it difficult to infer discrete cortical generators from the scalp distributions alone (Jeffreys and Axford, 1972a,b). Although mathematical models for source localization have been available for ERP measures, only limited attempts have been made to localize sources using ERPs. Inconsistencies between ERP studies also arose from differences in (1) stimulus parameters, (2) reference electrode locations, and (3) the number of electrode locations utilized in the study (Regan, 1989).

Early MEG studies examining retinotopy used only a few sensors for recording the magnetic fields and did not identify the structures generating the fields measured at the surface of the head (i.e., they did not superimpose the calculated source locations onto MRIs). Maclin *et al.*, (1983) presented a contrast reversed (13-Hz) sinusoidal grating in the right visual field and masked off portions of this stimulus to create the appearance of either a semicircular area of adjustable outer radius, or a semiannular area of adjustable inner and outer radii. They found that the depth of the source (inferred to be primary visual cortex) increased with greater eccentricity of the stimulus, consistent with the cruciform model.

Ahlfors and colleagues (1992) used checkerboard octants placed in eight central locations (octant sectors within a 1.8° radius circle) or eight parafoveal locations in octant sectors of an annulus with an inner radius of 1.8° and an outer radius of 3.8°. Larger stimuli were presented to the parafoveal locations due to the cortical magnification factor, i.e., larger stimuli are needed in the periphery to activate the same amount of tissue in primary visual cortex that is activated by smaller stimuli in the central field (e.g., Rovamo and Virsu,

1979; Perry and Cowey, 1985). These investigators also used smaller stimuli (<2°) than were used in previous visual studies because of the assumption of point current dipoles used in dipole modeling; the use of large stimuli would violate the basic assumption that the modeled source is a point source, because large stimuli activate extended regions of tissue in cortex. A single-dipole model and a minimum norm method were applied to the 80-msec deflection, which revealed activity contralateral to the field of stimulation. However, the results did not reveal clear order for upper versus lower field stimulation (i.e., activity evoked by the upper field stimuli were not located below active regions associated with lower field stimuli, respectively). In addition, they reported that most responses to parafoveal stimuli were superior to the corresponding foveal stimuli, and the depths of the sources were approximately equal. In general, these results did not correspond well with the classical cruciform model, except for the contralateral projections. These investigators also noted considerable differences in the pattern of the minimum norm results (i.e., orientation of net current flow) across subjects and studies. Again, source locations were not superimposed on MRIs to visualize the generators of these signals, and due to the infancy of multidipole models at that time, they used a single-dipole model to account for activity at 80 msec even though they acknowledged that there was evidence suggesting that at least two sources must have been active at that time.

Aine and colleagues (1996) attempted to map the borders of different human visual areas using methods similar to those applied in monkey studies. The boundaries of different visual areas within a single hemisphere may be outlined by focusing on the representations of the vertical and horizontal meridia in the visual field, because these locations typically project to the edges of cortical areas (Cragg, 1969;

Zeki, 1969, 1978; Van Essen *et al.*, 1982; Van Essen, 1985). Callosal fibers terminate preferentially in regions representing the vertical midline of the visual field, and an examination of their distribution has led to the identification of different visual areas in nonhuman primates (Cragg, 1969; Zeki, 1969, 1978; Van Essen *et al.*, 1982) and in human autopsy specimens (Clarke and Miklossy, 1990). Aine *et al.* (1996) placed small circular sinusoids (ranging in size from 0.4 to 1° for central versus more eccentric field placements) in seven different positions along the lower vertical meridian and right horizontal meridian. Stimuli were located off the meridia by 0.5° and were scaled according to the cortical magnification factor. A seven-channel system was positioned over 10–15 different head surface locations covering occipital, occipitoparietal, and occipito-temporal regions. Multidipole spatiotemporal models were applied to various time intervals ranging from 80 to 165 msec post-stimulus.

The results of Aine and colleagues confirm the general features of the classical retinotopic model for V1: (1) lower field stimuli generally activated regions in the upper bank of the calcarine fissure and (2) V1 sources were more anterior for eccentric placements along the vertical meridian. However, there was a discrepancy between their results and the classical model for that portion of the V1 retinotopic map corresponding to eccentric placements below the horizontal meridian, following its extent. With the use of small stimuli, it was clear that the most eccentric placements of the stimuli along the horizontal meridian did not project onto the upper bank, as predicted by the classical model. It is generally assumed that the representation of the horizontal meridian lies precisely at the base (i.e., lateral extent) of the calcarine fissure, but the data of Aine *et al.* showed that the representation of the horizontal meridian in some cases deviates downward from a posterior to anterior

direction or lies primarily in the lower bank for some individuals. It turns out that extensive anatomical studies of human V1 show that the anterior boundary of V1 is ordinarily found in the lower lip of the fissure (Polyak, 1957), unlike the cruciform model. These results are a reminder that the classical model represents an ideal case and that most human anatomical data indicate extreme variability across subjects and that the calcarine fissure per se is not synonymous with V1 (Polyak, 1957; Stensaas *et al.*, 1974).

Although Aine and colleagues (1996) identified multiple visual areas, including occipitoparietal, occipitotemporal, and ipsilateral occipital activity, the retinotopic organization of these areas was not determined. Supek and colleagues (1999), however, did examine retinotopic organization of the occipitoparietal and occipitotemporal regions, as one of their goals, by placing small difference of gaussians stimuli (DOGs) in the lower right visual field, just to the right of the vertical meridian. Again, a seven-channel system was moved over several locations of the head surface and multidipole spatiotemporal models were applied to the data spanning an 80- to 170-msec interval of time. Each source in both occipitoparietal and occipitotemporal areas evidenced a systematic shift in location associated with changes in stimulus placement parallel to the vertical meridian. These results point to the sensitivity of neuromagnetic techniques. Additional studies using fMRI have also shown general retinotopic organization within visual areas. These methods are able to define the boundaries of different visual areas quickly and effectively (Sereno *et al.*, 1995; Tootell *et al.*, 1995b; 1998; Hadjikhani *et al.*, 1998).

Hari and colleagues examined the occipitoparietal region to determine if it is the homolog of monkey area V6, situated on the anterior bank of the medial parietooccipital sulcus (POS), or if it is an area unique to humans (Portin *et al.*, 1998;

Portin and Hari, 1999; Vanni *et al.*, 2001). Portin and Hari (1999) noted that as they varied the eccentricity of 5.5° semicircles presented in the left and right visual fields (0°–16° eccentricity), the V1 source revealed retinotopic organization whereas the medial parietal source did not. They suggest that both the lack of retinotopic organization and the lack of enhanced foveal representation suggest that the POS area in humans is the homolog of V6 in monkeys (Shipp *et al.*, 1998; Galletti *et al*, 1999). Vanni and colleagues (2001) attempted to examine the temporal dynamics of these two cortical areas, V1 and the anteromedial cuneus (V6 complex). They presented pattern reversal checkerboard stimuli to four quadrants, extending 4–12° from the fixation point. Their results suggested that V1 and the anteromedial cuneus had similar onset times (~56 msec poststimulus) compared to other posterior sources such as temporo-occipital and superior temporal regions.

Previously, Aine and colleagues (1995) noted the simultaneous activation of V1 and occipitoparietal sources [the source locations of POS found by Vanni *et al.* (2001) were quite similar to those found by Aine and colleagues] for peripheral stimulation. Central field stimulation, in contrast, resulted in the sequential activation of V1, occipitoparietal, and occipitotemporal sources. This interesting timing difference noted between central and peripheral field stimulation (centered 0 and 7° in the right visual field, respectively) was investigated further to assess the generality of this effect using stimuli that were not scaled by cortical magnification factor versus those that were scaled. In both cases, V1 and occipitoparietal sources (POS) appeared simultaneous for peripheral stimulation only. Stephen and colleagues (2002) tested this issue further by examining the speed of transmission through dorsal structures such as the POS, versus ventral structures (e.g., area V4), and found equally short onset latencies

throughout the dorsal stream structures compared to the progressive lengthening of onset latencies throughout the ventral stream. Vanni and colleagues (2001) did not compare central versus peripheral field conditions to demonstrate this differential effect, but the fact that several studies found simultaneous activation for V1 and POS for peripheral stimulation speaks to the generality of the effect, because different stimuli, analysis procedures, and recording instruments were used. However, whether POS is or is not retinotopically organized remains to be determined. Supek and colleagues (1999) did reveal retinotopy in this region whereas Portin and Hari (1999) did not. Based on recent results, three to four of the regions identified in the time interval of 60–250 msec appear to reside in parietal cortex, suggesting the possibility that the data may have been undermodeled in the studies of POS mentioned above. [We note that Vanni and Uutela (2000) also resolved three distinct parietal sources and that Supek *et al.* (1999) explicitly noted the possibility of under-modeling their data.] In addition, it is difficult to see small systematic shifts in source location as a function of systematic shifts in field location when large stimuli are utilized.

BASIC VISUAL FUNCTIONS

Spatial Frequency, Temporal Frequency, and Contrast Threshold

Early single-unit studies of feline retinal ganglion cells suggested that the visual system contains two or more classes of neurons that differ in their receptive field (RF) and signal transmission characteristics (Enroth-Cugell and Robson, 1966; Breitmeyer and Ganz, 1976). The RF of a neuron is that area of the retina in which stimulation by light leads to a response of the cell. Y-Type neurons have larger RFs, faster conduction velocities, and respond best to lower spatial frequencies and higher temporal frequencies than do X-Type neurons. X-Type neurons have smaller RFs, slower conduction velocities, and respond best to higher spatial frequencies and lower temporal frequencies. Spatial frequency relates to the amount of detail cells can process and is inversely related to cell size (e.g., Enroth-Cugell and Robson, 1966). Within the feline retina, RF size tends to increase from foveal to peripheral retina, and there is a corresponding shift in the ratio of X to Y cells (Wright and Ikeda, 1974). In other words, the central retina has a higher proportion of X cells and the peripheral retina has more Y cells. As noted above, large-diameter cells generally have faster conduction velocities and prefer lower spatial frequencies. The X and Y cell distinctions in felines are similar to the parvocellular, or P-like, and magnocellular, or M-like, neurons in monkey retina and cortex (Stone and Johnston, 1981). The M and P cells will be discussed in more detail below.

Breitmeyer (1975) examined reaction times (RTs) in humans to gratings of different spatial frequencies and found a correlation; lower spatial frequency gratings yielded shorter reaction times compared to higher spatial frequency gratings. Breitmeyer hypothesized that Y-type cells mediated the responses to the lower spatial frequencies, because their conduction times were fast. Kaufman and Williamson (1980) used MEG to examine this relationship. They measured the phase lag of the evoked neuromagnetic response (i.e., the time from stimulus presentation to response detection) to contrast-reversal gratings when the spatial frequency and reversal rate of these gratings were varied. These data showed that for a grating of a particular spatial frequency, the phase of the response is proportional to the temporal frequency of presentation. Similar to Breitmeyer's RT data, there was an increase in the latency of the neuromagnetic response with an increase in spatial frequency content.

Okada and colleagues (1982) systematically examined peak-to-peak amplitudes (e.g., the amplitude from the maximum positive to the maximum negative peak of the initial response) of the visually evoked magnetic fields (VEFs) to varying spatial frequencies, temporal frequencies, and contrast levels using vertical, contrast-reversal gratings. EEG responses were recorded as well from two active electrode locations and threshold contrasts were determined psychophysically. The peak-to-peak means showed greater amplitude for higher spatial frequencies at low temporal frequencies (see top row of Fig. 1) and, conversely, higher temporal frequencies revealed greater amplitudes to low spatial frequencies (see bottom row). The characteristics of these transfer functions agreed qualitatively with transfer functions obtained with visual evoked potentials (VEPs) (Campbell and Maffei, 1970; Campbell and Kulikowski, 1972; Regan, 1978) and the psychophysical contrast sensitivity function (Kelly, 1966; Robson, 1966). The contrast sensitivity function of the VEF was quite similar in shape to the psychophysical contrast sensitivity function determined in the same experiment and the phase lag increased linearly with temporal frequency of the stimulus, similar to results found by Williamson and colleagues (Williamson et al., 1978; Kaufman and Williamson, 1980). Okada and colleagues also showed that the latency of the VEF increased with higher spatial frequency and decreased when contrast was increased. Although many of these results had been shown previously, this was the first study to document quantitatively the linear relation between the steady-state magnetic field and electrical potential for both phase and amplitude. These data suggested that the VEP and VEF were produced by a common source.

Several studies set out to examine the relationship between MEG response strength and latency as a function of check size and/or contrast of a checkerboard

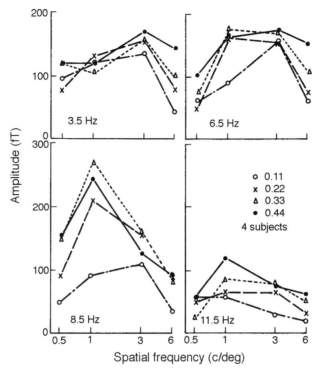

FIGURE 1 Mean peak-to-peak amplitudes of the visually evoked magnetic fields of four subjects are shown as a function of spatial frequency and contrast level. Each subplot shows this relation for four different temporal frequencies (3.5, 6.5, 8.5, and 11.5 Hz). Mean luminance = 10 cpd/m². Reprinted from *Vision Research*, **22**; Y. C. Okada, L. Kaufman, D. Brenner, and S. J. Williamson; Modulation transfer functions of the human visual system revealed by magnetic field measurements; pp. 319–333. Copyright 1982, with permission from Elsevier Science.

stimulus. In addition, the neural origin of the P100 visual response, which was so elusive in the ERP studies, became a focus of MEG studies because MEG was capable of better spatial resolution compared to ERPs (Leahy *et al.*, 1998). Early ERP studies labeled peaks in the evoked responses either as components 1, 2, and 3 (CI, CII, CIII) or as peaks denoted by polarity (negative versus positive) and latency (N70, P100, N200, P200, P300), depending on the type of stimulation (e.g., pattern reversal, pattern onset, flash stimulation) and the country in which the studies were conducted (e.g., United Kingdom versus United States). Considerable effort was expended on attempts at localizing the underlying generators of these peaks either qualitatively (Jeffreys and Axford, 1972a,b; Michael and Halliday, 1971) or quantitatively via

source localization procedures (e.g., Butler *et al.*, 1987; Darcey *et al.*, 1980; Maier *et al.*, 1987; Ossenblok and Spekreijse, 1991), but it eventually became clear that single peaks/components in the wave forms (e.g., P100) do not necessarily reflect activity from a single cortical area (i.e., a peak can reflect activity from a number of different sources). A MEG study by Seki and colleagues (1996) reported very few differences in source locations associated with the MEG correlate of P100 to pattern reversals of full-field (subtending 17° visual angle), half-field, and quadrant-field stimulation. They used a single-dipole model to account for activity occurring in the 90- to 135-msec time window and found that all of the sources localized to the bottom of the calcarine fissure. Other MEG studies focused on localizing the sources of the different components of the VEFs and showed various localizations around the calcarine fissure for the first through third components (Harding *et al.* 1991, 1994; Hashimoto *et al.* 1999; Seki *et al.*, 1996, Shigeto *et al.*, 1998). Unfortunately, the MEG results were quite variable, similar to the ERP results. This was probably because multiple generators were contributing to the peaks in the MEG wave forms but the peaks were analyzed using primarily a single-dipole model.

Armstrong and colleagues (1991) attempted to establish norms for MEG responses to visual stimuli, similar to what had been done with EEG, using a second-order gradiometer in an unshielded environment. They studied 100 subjects aged 18–87 years and found that pattern reversal stimuli evoked a major positive component between 90 and 120 msec, whereas flash stimulation produced a major positive component between 90 and 140 msec. They noted that the latencies were considerably more variable in MEG than in EEG. This is most likely because MEG primarily measures intracellular current flow rather than the return currents, which can cause significant differences from subject to subject in the field patterns at each sensor location, due to the variable orientations of the sources that contribute to these components. Armstrong did find, however, that there was a steep increase in latency after age 55.

Hashimoto and colleagues (1999) used large checkerboard patterns to identify three peaks in the MEG data similar to those found in the ERPs (N75, P100, N145) and attempted to localize the cortical generators of these peaks by applying a single-dipole model around the peak latencies. These investigators noted that the sources for the first and third peaks were adjacent to one another with similar orientations within calcarine fissure, but the generator of the second peak had a different source location in the medial occipital lobe. Furthermore, when different contrast

levels were applied, the first component was quite sensitive to the contrast modulations whereas the third component was not. They concluded that the first and third components had different physiological properties and recalled data from Aine *et al.* (1995) indicating a recurrence of activation in both striate and extrastriate cortices, suggesting that the third component might be a reactivation of primary visual cortex. More recently, Aine and Stephen (2002) have carefully characterized temporal response profiles from several cortical areas and have concluded that response profiles from primary visual and primary auditory areas have initial "spikelike" activity followed by "slow wave" activity. The "spikelike" activity does appear to have different physiological properties, compared to the "slow wave" activity, even though both of these activities are generated from the same cortical region; the former appears to reflect primarily feedforward activity and the latter primarily reflects efferent activity. These data are discussed more fully under the section "Higher Order Processes."

Nakamura and colleagues (2000), aware of the animal studies indicating that the retinal ganglion cells most sensitive to higher spatial frequency stimuli have a predominantly foveal location (Novak *et al.*, 1988), tested whether checkerboard patterns consisting of different check sizes would evoke neuromagnetic activity in slightly different regions of V1, as a function of spatial frequency. These investigators used half-field checkerboard patterns presented to the right field (subtending 12.5° visual angle) with pattern reversal rates at 1 Hz. Similar to many ERP studies, these investigators found that check size significantly affected the latency and amplitude of the 100-msec peak (i.e., longer latencies and reduced amplitude for many of the higher spatial frequencies), but check size did not produce a shift in source location within V1.

Dorsal and Ventral Processing Streams or Object and Spatial Vision

De Monasterio and Gouras (1975) found a division of retinal ganglion cells in monkey retina, similar to those reported previously in the cat retina. Two types prevailed, color-opponent and broadband ganglion cells; color-opponent cells were mostly found in the fovea and broadband cells were more prominent in the periphery (Wiesel and Hubel, 1966; De Monasterio and Gouras, 1975; Leventhal et al., 1981; Perry et al., 1984). The color-opponent cells project to the four dorsal (parvocellular) layers of LGN and the broadband cells project to the two ventral (magnocellular) layers (Wiesel and Hubel, 1966; Schiller and Malpeli, 1978; Leventhal et al., 1981; Perry et al., 1984). These parallel streams of processing continue through primary and higher order visual areas in primate cortex. The large cell types (magnocellular, M cells) predominantly project to posterior parietal cortex, or dorsal stream areas, while the small cell types (parvocellular, P cells) predominantly project to inferior temporal cortex or ventral stream areas (Livingstone and Hubel, 1987; DeYoe and Van Essen, 1988; Shipp and Zeki, 1985; Tootell et al., 1988; Maunsell et al., 1990). In general, "dorsal" stream structures (related to motion processing and spatial vision) are sensitive to luminance differences, relatively insensitive to color, and more sensitive to lower spatial frequencies and higher temporal frequencies. "Ventral" stream structures (related to color processing and object vision), in contrast, are sensitive to chromatic contrast, higher spatial frequencies, and lower temporal frequencies (DeYoe and Van Essen, 1988; Van Essen and Maunsell, 1983; Livingstone and Hubel, 1988; Maunsell and Newsome, 1987; Ungerleider and Mishkin, 1982). The major components of the color/form or object pathway include V1, V2, V4, TEO, and TE (TEO and TE are located within the inferior temporal lobe), and the major components of the motion or spatial pathway include V1, V2, V3, middle temporal area, medial superior temporal area (MST), and area 7A of parietal cortex (Maunsell and Newsome, 1987).

It was Ungerleider and Mishkin (1982) who originally proposed the existence of two cortical streams mediating object and spatial vision, based on lesion studies in monkeys. Livingstone and Hubel (1987, 1988) later suggested that the M and P pathways may be the neural substrates of these processing streams. The goal of several early functional neuroimaging studies in humans was to dissociate the dorsal and ventral processing streams by focusing on color and motion tasks (e.g., Corbetta et al., 1991; Zeki et al., 1991; Kleinschmidt et al., 1996; Shah et al., 1998); they attempted to dissociate M and P pathways in ways similar to those used by Livingstone and Hubel (1987, 1988). It has become very clear, however, that the two streams of processing are not completely segregated, even as early as V1 (e.g., Lachica et al., 1992; Nealy and Maunsell, 1994). Area MT, associated with the parietal/dorsal stream, receives predominantly M cell input from the lateral geniculate nucleus, but area V4, associated with the temporal/ventral stream, receives strong input from both M and P subdivisions of the LGN (Maunsell et al., 1990; Ferrera et al., 1994; Merigan and Maunsell, 1993). Given the controversy that ensued over the separation or lack of separation between the M and P streams, the focus of the neuroimaging studies appeared to turn toward tasks emphasizing object versus spatial vision.

A dissociation between object and spatial pathways was attempted by Haxby and colleagues (1991) and others (Haxby et al., 1994; Kohler et al., 1995), using PET methods. These investigators compared regional cerebral blood flow (rCBF) responses when subjects were engaged in a face-matching task (object processing) versus a dot-location matching task (spatial processing). They concluded that lateral occipital extrastriate cortex is involved in both the face- and dot-matching tasks whereas the face-matching task also activated an occipital temporal region that was anterior and inferior to the lateral occipital region. In addition to activating the lateral occipital region, the dot-matching task also engaged a lateral superior parietal region.

Sato and colleagues (1999), using MEG, attempted to separate out the two processing streams by having subjects discriminate familiar from unfamiliar scenes and faces. They hypothesized that discrimination of familiar versus unfamiliar faces would activate lingual and fusiform gyri, whereas discrimination of familiar versus unfamiliar scenes would invoke activity in the right parahippocampal gyrus and the right POS. In the latter case, they rationalized that both parahippocampal gyrus and parietal cortex are involved in orientation and navigation in space (topographic processing). Using single-dipole modeling methods, they found prominent signals in the MEG response to scenes occurring 200–300 msec after stimulus onset in right parahippocampal and parietooccipital regions. In contrast, prominent MEG signals in response to face processing appeared between 150 and 200 msec in the lingual or bilateral fusiform gyri.

Portin and colleagues (1998) used MEG to study the properties of POS, belonging to the dorsal pathway, by presenting hemifield luminance versus patterned stimuli to the left and right visual fields. Hemifield luminance stimuli were hypothesized to activate dorsal stream structures whereas patterned stimuli were hypothesized to activate ventral stream structures preferentially. The hemifield stimuli, semicircular in shape, subtended either a complete semicircle covering the fovea (a circular radius of 8°; foveal stimuli) or a segment of a circle starting at an eccentricity of 1.5° (nonfoveal stimuli). Source locations were determined by first applying a single-dipole model to various groups of sensor locations (28–32 sensors) over the maximum response area, at various time intervals. The source locations determined from three different cortical regions (bilateral occipital and midline POS sources) were then introduced into a time-varying three-dipole model (fixed locations) to determine the time courses of the three cortical locations. Dipole strengths were allowed to vary as a function of time in order to explain the measured signals in all 122 sensor locations. Patterned stimuli evoked strong contralateral activity in V1 (65–75 msec, maximum peak), followed by sustained activation during the presentation of the stimulus. Weaker activation was localized in the POS. In contrast, the luminance stimulus (also of semicircular shape) evoked bilateral activity in occipital cortex, which occurred 10 msec earlier on average than for patterned stimuli, and caused strong activation of POS. These investigators concluded that they had preferentially activated the parvocellular pathway via the patterned stimulus, and the magnocellular pathway via the luminance stimulus. They also speculated that the stronger bilateral activation of occipital cortex noted for the luminance stimuli was due to the preferential interhemispheric transfer of low spatial frequencies.

As mentioned earlier, Stephen and colleagues (2002) tested the hypothesis that peripheral field stimulation should lead to faster onset latencies in the dorsal stream structures relative to central field stimulation, because (1) peripheral representations of V1 and V2 have been associated with faster conduction velocities [associated with larger cell sizes (Nowak and Bullier, 1997)] and (2) peripheral field representations of V1/V2 have direct projections to MT and parietal cortex (Nowak and Bullier, 1997; Rockland, 1995; Movshon and Newsome, 1996; Ungerleider and Desimone, 1986; Felleman and Van Essen, 1991). Small circular sinusoids with luminance-matched backgrounds were contrast reversed at four alternation rates (0–14 Hz) along the horizontal meridian in central and peripheral visual fields (2.3 and 24°, respectively). A whole-head MEG system (Neuromag 122) was used to acquire the data and new automated analysis methods were applied to the MEG data (Huang *et al.*, 1998; Aine *et al.*, 2000). Multiple starting parameters (e.g., 3000) were randomly chosen from within a head volume for the multidipole, spatiotemporal models applied to the entire sensor array [see Stephen *et al.*, (2002) for details on how the best fits to the data were determined]. Onset latencies for each cortical response (i.e., the time course for a specific cortical area) were calculated for the different visual areas for each subject. The onset latencies in the two representative dorsal stream structures, superior lateral occipital gyrus (S. LOG, putative MT) and intraparietal sulcus (IPS), were significantly shorter for peripheral versus central field stimulation (see tabular data in Fig. 2A), whereas the onset latencies in V1, V2, and inferior lateral occipital gyrus (I. LOG, putative V4) were statistically identical across the field of stimulation. The results indicate that although central and peripheral field stimulation activates similar cortical regions, information from central and peripheral fields arrives in some higher visual areas via different routes. These results are consistent with results from several nonhuman studies (e.g., Breitmeyer and Ganz, 1976; Nowak and Bullier, 1997). Unlike Portin and colleagues (1998), the current results did not find a difference in onset times in V1 when stimulating foveal versus peripheral representations of V1 with the same type of patterned stimulus (circular sinusoids), scaled by the cortical magnification. It is possible that the earlier onset latency noted in V1 by Portin and colleagues, associated with the luminance stimulus, was due to the greater mean luminance of their luminance stimuli compared to their patterned stimuli, as acknowledged by these authors. As noted earlier, higher contrast

stimuli (clearly exhibited by the luminance stimuli) shorten peak latencies and reaction times (Campbell and Kulikowski, 1972; Robson, 1966; Okada *et al.*, 1982).

Color/Form or Object Vision (Ventral Processing Stream)

A brief overview of structures comprising the ventral stream in monkeys is considered next, in order to discuss the wealth of neuroimaging studies that have attempted to separate face-selective areas from object areas within the ventral processing stream of humans. Dorsal stream structures are discussed later under the heading "Motion or Spatial Vision (Dorsal Processing Stream)." Zeki (1973, 1978) originally proposed that area V4 is specifically and selectively involved in color analysis. However, it appears that there are at least four extrastriate visual areas that play a role in color analysis: V2, V3, VP, and V4 (Van Essen and Maunsell, 1983). Recent studies indicate that V4 has a crude retinotopic organization (e.g., Schein and Desimone, 1990) and the RFs in this area contain the central 20–30° of the retina (Zeki, 1980). The major outputs of V4 are to areas TEO and TE in the inferior temporal cortex (ITC) (e.g., Desimone *et al.*, 1980). The RFs of TEO in monkeys are intermediate in size compared to V4 and TE. The neuronal properties in TEO are also intermediate in complexity between V4 and TE, suggesting that the neural coding of visual objects in TEO is based on object features that are more global than those in V4 but not as global as those in TE (Boussaoud *et al.*, 1991). TEO is probably more important for making fine visual discriminations as opposed to memory functions. Area TE is located at the end of the "ventral" stream, in the ITC. The RFs in this area are large and always include the fovea and extend into the ipsilateral visual field (Richmond *et al.*, 1983; Saleem and Tanaka, 1996; Boussaoud *et al.*, 1991). TE RFs have complex selectivities, responding best in

A.

Table 1. Onset latencies of contralateral visual areas					
Visual Field	**V1**	**V2/V3**	**I. LOG**	**S. LOG**	**IPS**
central	78±3 (40)	88±7 (12)	88±7 (14)	98±5 (20)†	100±5 (22)*
peripheral	83±5 (27)	88±5 (17)	86±5 (7)	82±5 (22)†	75±4 (21)*

*p < 0.001; †p < 0.05; mean±SEM (N)

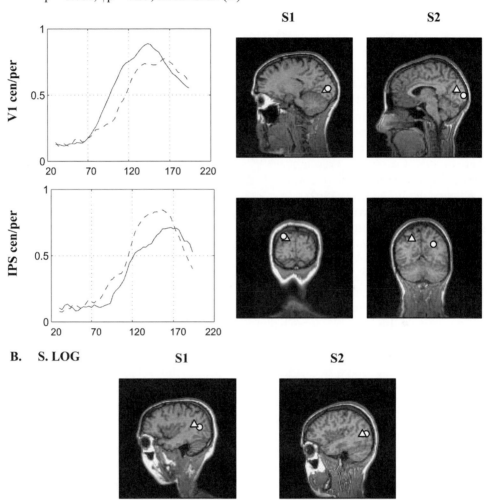

FIGURE 2 (A) The mean onset times across individual time courses (along with the standard error and the number of observations shown in parentheses) for five different cortical regions evoked by stimulating the central versus peripheral visual fields. Onset latencies were computed by an algorithm, where onset time was defined as the time when the activity exceeded two standard deviations of the noise level. The group-averaged cortical response profiles shown for two cortical areas [V1 and intraparietal sulcus (IPS)] display curves associated with central field stimulation (solid lines) and peripheral field stimulation (dashed lines). The IPS is a dorsal stream structure. The MRIs shown at the right reveal the locations of these visual areas for two subjects. The small triangles and circles shown on the MRIs reflect source locations associated with peripheral field and central field stimulation, respectively. (B) Another parietal location (dorsal stream structure), the superior lateral occi-pital gyrus (S. LOG), which revealed earlier onset times for peripheral field stimulation, as well.

the region of the fovea for real objects or faces (Desimone and Gross, 1979, Gross *et al.*, 1974; Perrett *et al.*, 1982; Baylis *et al.*, 1987). Responses to faces are 2–10 times greater than responses to grating stimuli, simple geometrical stimuli, or complex three-dimensional objects (Perrett *et al.*, 1982; Baylis *et al.*, 1987). These cells have some properties of perceptual invariance because they respond well even when the faces are inverted or rotated. TE projects heavily into the perirhinal region, a region important for visual recognition memory of objects, because this region projects to the hippocampus via entorhinal cortex. Ablation of TE produces long lasting deficits in the monkey's ability to learn visual discriminations but leaves intact the ability to learn discriminations in other modalities (e.g., Mishkin, 1982; Cowey and Weiskrantz, 1967; Gross, 1973; Sahgal and Iversen, 1978; Bagshaw *et al.*, 1972; Butter, 1969).

The use of tasks involving face perception or face recognition in functional neuroimaging studies became popular because of the converging lines of evidence crossing nonhuman animal studies, human lesion studies, and noninvasive functional imaging studies in humans, suggesting that a region of the temporal lobe, belonging to the object-processing stream, is selective for face processing. Face-selective neurons in monkeys have been identified in (1) area TE in monkeys (Gross *et al.*, 1972; Rolls *et al.*, 1977), (2) superior temporal sulcus (STS), which receives projections from inferotemporal cortex (Gross *et al.*, 1972; Perrett *et al.*, 1982), and (3) amygdala, parietal cortex, and frontal cortex, all of which receive projections from the fundus of the STS (Sanghera *et al.*, 1979; Aggleton *et al.*, 1980; Leinonen and Nyman, 1979; Seltzer and Pandya, 1978; Pigarev *et al.*, 1979; Jacobsen and Trojanowski, 1977; Rolls, 1984).

Clinical evidence for face-selective regions in humans comes from cases of prosopagnosia, a difficulty in recognizing faces of familiar persons that is associated with damage to the inferior occipitotemporal region (Meadows, 1974; Whiteley and Warrington, 1977; Damasio, 1985; Sergent and Poncet, 1990). Object recognition, in contrast, is not typically impaired in prosopagnosic patients (De Renzi, 1986). As Damasio and colleagues (1982) and Logothetis and Sheinberg (1996) point out, prosopagnosics tend to have difficulties making within-category discriminations. For example, these patients have difficulties differentiating between various cars, or fruits.

Dissociation between face- and object-selective areas within ITC was attempted by Sergent and colleagues (1992) by comparing rCBF measures when subjects were engaged in several tasks (e.g., discriminating the orientation of sine wave gratings, face gender, face identity, object identity). They concluded that face identity caused activation of right extrastriate cortex, fusiform gyrus, and the anterior temporal cortex of both hemispheres. In contrast, object recognition primarily activated left occipitotemporal cortex. Other PET studies (Kim *et al.*, 1999; Kapur *et al.*, 1995; Campanella *et al.*, 2001) and fMRI studies (e.g., Puce *et al.*, 1995; Courtney *et al.*, 1997; Kanwisher *et al.*, 1997; Haxby *et al.*, 1999; Halgren *et al.*, 1999; Jiang *et al.*, 2000; Maguire *et al.*, 2001) attempted to demonstrate the selectivity and locus of face-selective areas. Results from all of these studies generally agree in showing fusiform gyrus involvement (either medial, lateral, or posterior), but some studies revealed additional areas as well, such as inferior temporal cortex, right middle occipital gyrus, right lingual gyrus, superior temporal, inferior occipital sulcus, lateral occipital sulcus, and middle temporal gyrus/STS, in addition to prefrontal regions.

In addition, the fMRI/PET studies generally suggest that object perception activated occipitotemporal regions (fusiform gyrus), an area similar to the area activated by face perception, but more medial

(Malach *et al.*, 1995; Martin *et al.*, 1995; Puce *et al.*, 1995; Halgren *et al.*, 1999; Haxby *et al.*, 1999; Martin and Chao, 2001; Maguire *et al.*, 2001). However, there are clear differences of opinion concerning the exact locations of the object areas. Malach and colleagues (1995), for example, proposed that lateral occipital cortex (LO) near the temporal border was the homolog of monkey TE, because pictures of objects activated this region much more strongly than did scrambled images. Kanwisher and colleagues (1997) also found a region selective to images of objects compared to scrambled images, but this region was just anterior and ventral to Malach's LO. In both cases, the putative object region evoked strong responses to objects and faces, as well as familiar and novel objects.

MEG examinations of face processing primarily focused on deflections seen in MEG-averaged wave forms to face stimuli versus other objects or degraded face stimuli. Lu and colleagues (1991) found that faces evoked greater amplitude deflections than did birds at 150, 260, and 500 msec, which were localized to bilateral occipitotemporal junction, inferior parietal cortex, and middle temporal lobe, respectively. Sams and colleagues (1997) found a face-selective area in four of seven subjects in occipitotemporal cortex peaking at 150–170 msec. They noted, however, that the source locations of the face-specific response varied across subjects and that even nonface stimuli can activate the face area, although with less magnitude. Swithenby and colleagues (1998) also found a significant difference for faces versus other images (i.e., greater normalized regional power) at 140 msec in the sensors over the right occipitotemporal region, and source modeling suggested the ventral occipitotemporal region (see Fig. 3). Each stimulus image subtended a visual angle of 8 × 6° and was luminance matched to the other images. In contrast, Liu and colleagues (1999), using magnetic field tomography (MFT) analysis on single-trial

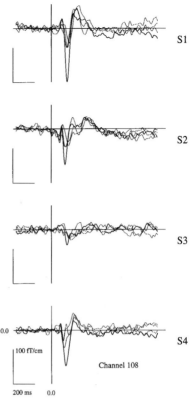

FIGURE 3 Averaged evoked field patterns recorded over right occipitotemporal cortex for four subjects. Responses to faces are depicted by solid tracings; responses to other images are shown as dotted lines. The largest peaks, occurring between 130 and 150 msec for each subject, were evoked by face stimuli. Reprinted with permission from *Experimental Brain Research*; Neural processing of human faces: A magnetoencephalographic study; S. J. Swithenby, A. J. Bailey, S. Bräutigam, O. E. Josephs, V. Jousmäki, and C. D. Tesche; Vol. 118, p. 505, Fig. 3, 1998. Copyright 1998 Springer-Verlag.

data, found no evidence of a face-specific area in the sense that all complex objects appear to activate the fusiform gyrus (at 125–175 msec and 240–265 msec in the left hemisphere and 150–180 msec for the right fusiform), along with many other areas. A previous report from the same laboratory (Streit *et al.*, 1999), using MFT analysis on averaged responses from single subjects, found early activity (~160 msec) related to the emotional content of faces in the posterior sector of superior right temporal cortex and inferior occipito temporal cortex, followed by bilateral activity (right hemisphere leading the left hemisphere) in the middle sector of temporal cortex (~200 msec) and in the amygdala (~220 msec).

In contrast with the Liu *et al.* study (1999), for each condition (faces, pointillized faces, and inverted faces), Linkenkaer-Hansen and colleagues (1998) also localized activity around 170 msec to the fusiform gyrus, but they interpreted these results as evidence for face-selectivity [Halgren *et al.* (2000) found bilateral fusiform activity]. They also suggested that face selectivity may occur as early as 120 msec (although differences in latencies were not statistically significant), because latency differences were evident in the MEG wave forms between faces and pointillized faces (i.e., degraded faces). However, even though these investigators controlled for many of the low-level features such as luminance, contrast, and intensity distribution of the gray-scale levels, such latency differences can occur due to differences in spatial frequency between these stimuli (see Okada *et al.*, 1982). Face stimuli are usually regarded as containing content of low spatial frequency, but pointillized faces have additional high-frequency content. In the face and inverted-face conditions, however, where spatial frequency was held constant, inverted faces resulted in greater amplitude and longer peak latency when compared to upright faces. Liu and colleagues (2000) did not attempt source localization but they found that face stimuli evoked larger responses as compared to nonface stimuli (animal and human hand) at 160 msec after stimulus onset in sensors over both left and right occipitotemporal cortex. Inverted-face stimuli and face stimuli produced similar response magnitudes, but the former occurred 13 msec later than the latter. The latency differences were similar to results noted above in the study by Linkenkaer-Hansen and colleagues (1998)

In conclusion, the MEG studies, along with PET and fMRI studies of face selectiv-

ity, generally suggest that the right fusiform gyrus produces larger response amplitudes to face stimuli as compared with other nonface stimuli. Other regions were also identified (e.g., extrastriate) as being more strongly activated in response to face stimuli. However, most of these studies did not apply appropriate controls to eliminate an alternative interpretation that response strengths or peak latencies and moments may vary between faces and other objects because (1) the area of retinal stimulation was not the same, (2) contrast or luminance was not equated, and (3) spatial frequency content was not equated. The MEG studies presented here indicate that each of these parameters can have a large impact on source amplitude, latency, and location. In this sense, these studies have not demonstrated that a region of the fusiform gyrus is *selective* for faces until all of these lower level features are controlled.

Other functional neuroimaging studies (e.g., Shen *et al.*, 1999; Haxby *et al.*, 1999) also question the selectivity of the face area, because face perception does not appear to be associated with a region or sets of regions that are dedicated solely to face processing. These "face-selective" regions also respond significantly to objects such as houses. Gauthier and colleagues (1999) suggest that results showing a specialized face area in the fusiform gyrus merely reflect the expertise we have at perceiving and remembering faces, rather than being specific to faces. These investigators showed that expertise with nonface objects can also activate the right fusiform gyrus. Recent single-unit studies have also shown that the selectivity of inferotemporal (IT) neurons found for faces could be generated for any novel object (e.g., computer-generated wire and spheroidal objects) as the result of extensive training (reviewed in Logethetis and Sheinberg, 1996; Kobatake *et al.*, 1998). According to Logothetis and Sheinberg (1996), the anterior region of IT is more concerned with object class, whereas the posterior end of IT is concerned with the specifics of an object item (also see review by Tanaka, 1997). Consistent with the suggestion by Gauthier and colleagues, face selectivity is viewed as another form of object recognition. The site of activation within the inferior temporal lobe (i.e., anterior versus posterior) depends on whether object class or object identity is manipulated by the experimental task. Lesion studies also suggest two functional subdivisions of inferotemporal cortex: (1) lesions in posterior TEO lead to simple pattern deficits and (2) lesions in anterior TE lead to associative and visual memory deficits (see review by Logothetis and Sheinberg, 1996).

Cue Invariance

A few studies have tackled the issue of cue invariance of the object-related processing areas. As touched on briefly above, monkey studies indicate both segregation of visual cues into different processing streams such as the M and P streams (e.g., Livingstone and Hubel, 1988) and convergence of several primary cues within single visual areas or even within single neurons. In the latter case, the visual system can be viewed as a series of processing stages that represent a progressive increase in complexity of neuronal representations that are dependent on the output of preceding stages (e.g., Zeki, 1978; Van Essen, 1985; Van Essen and Maunsell, 1983; De Yoe *et al.*, 1994; Sary *et al.*, 1993). As Grill-Spector and colleagues (1998) note, the organizational principles underlying the specialization of visual areas remain a matter of debate (e.g., Ungerleider and Haxby, 1994; Goodale *et al.*, 1994). Grill-Spector and colleagues used fMRI to determine the cue invariance of object-related areas; i.e., does the same preferential activation exist for objects defined solely by luminance, motion, and texture cues? These authors found a region in LO that was preferentially activated by objects defined by all

cues tested. They also found an earlier retinotopic area, V3a, which exhibited convergence of object-related cues as well.

Okusa and colleagues (2000), using MEG, examined cue-invariant shape perception in humans. These investigators presented three different dynamic random-dot patterns (flicker, texture, and luminance), subtending $5 \times 5°$ in the central field. Three different stimulus figures (diamond, noise, and a cross) were presented in the foreground against the background random dots. In the luminance condition, for example, dots comprising the stimulus figure (e.g., diamond) were abruptly reduced in luminance. MEG recordings were made from occipitotemporal cortex using a 37-channel system. By measuring the peak amplitude and peak latency of the first component in the wave forms, they found that the peak latency was different for the cues (250 msec for luminance, 270 msec for flicker, and 360 msec for texture) but not for the figures (diamond, cross, noise). In contrast, the peak amplitude was different for the figures (96–114 fT), but not for the cues. Source locations were determined using a single-dipole model for a time interval of 0–500 msec poststimulus. Source locations evoked by the figures were similar across conditions within subjects but were different across subjects (fusiform gyrus, lateral occipital gyrus, etc.). Reaction times correlated with the peak latency differences noted above for the different cues. They concluded that the shape defined by different visual cues activated the same region in lateral extrastriate cortex regardless of differences between the visual cues. The correspondence between the RTs and peak latencies for the cues suggest that LO is responsible for the perception of shape.

Motion or Spatial Vision (Dorsal Processing Stream)

The magnocellular layers of monkey LGN, associated with motion pathways, project to V1, V2, V3, MT, MST, ventral intraparietal area (VIP), and area 7a in parietal cortex (Van Essen and Maunsell, 1983). In general, the retinotopic specificity decreases progressively in successive levels of the motion pathway and average RF area increases (Maunsell and Newsome, 1987). MT, found on the posterior bank and floor of the superior temporal sulcus, is the lowest order area in which a selective emphasis on motion analysis is apparent (Van Essen and Maunsell, 1983). V1, V2, and MT all have direction-selective cells, but the preferred range of speeds for the overall population of cells is nearly an order of magnitude greater in MT than in V1. In addition, there are pronounced surround interactions in MT permitting the inhibition of responses within the excitatory RF due to motion in other parts of the visual field (signaling relative motion). MST receives strong input from MT, is position invariant, and is sensitive to translational motion, expansion, contraction, and rotation (Geesaman and Andersen, 1996). In general, there is convergence of inputs in the STS from the far peripheral representations of V1 and V2. Inputs to parietal cortex tend to arise either from areas that have been implicated in spatial or motion analysis (e.g., areas within the STS) or from peripheral field representations in the prestriate cortex (Baizer et al., 1991).

Many types of motion have been studied by the functional neuroimaging techniques that have been available over the past 20 years (Watson et al., 1993; Tootell et al., 1995a,b; Cheng et al., 1995; Cornette et al., 1998). Most of this research has focused on trying to identify and characterize the human homolog of monkey area MT. MT in monkeys has been studied extensively by a number of different groups to identify the characteristics of this motion-sensitive area, including identifying cells that are direction selective, speed selective, and orientation selective (Zeki, 1980; Maunsell and Van Essen, 1983;

Albright, 1984; Lagae et al., 1993), as well as defining the receptive field properties (Felleman and Kaas, 1984) and M and P contributions to this area (Maunsell et al., 1990). The overall conclusion of these studies is that the monkey area MT is sensitive to a diverse range of motion stimuli while being fairly insensitive to other visual characteristics such as color. Therefore, functional neuroimaging studies have studied a variety of motion stimuli, including continuous motion using random-dot displays, changes in direction of motion, onset and offset of motion, as well as apparent motion. The functional imaging tools that rely on measuring metabolic or blood flow changes have had reasonable success at locating a region in humans near the parieto-temporo-occipital border that is homologous to monkey area MT/MST (Watson et al., 1993; Tootell et al., 1995a,b; Cheng et al., 1995; Cornette et al., 1998). MEG studies have shown reasonable agreement in the location of the motion-specific activity while adding temporal information about this motion-sensitive area.

The visual MEG studies of motion have attempted to characterize fully the different types of motion, as many VEP (Clarke, 1973a,b), PET, and fMRI studies have done in the past. For example, ffytche et al. (1995a) found that area V5 (or MT) was also activated by the perception of motion defined by hue, rather than luminance cues. In this study, area V4 (typically associated with color processing) was not active, suggesting that although V5 has traditionally been seen as insensitive to color it can apparently use this information to extract the motion information from stimuli. ffytche and colleagues interpreted these results as signifying a parvocellular contribution to area V5, as seen in monkeys. Fylan and colleagues (1997) similarly used isoluminant red/green sinusoidal gratings to demonstrate the presence of chromatic-sensitive units in V1, which play a role in processing motion information. Patzwahl *et al.* (1996) found that the initial response to motion was dipolar and localized to area V5. However, the later activity was much more complex, suggesting multiple areas are necessary to interpret motion stimuli. Holliday *et al.* (1997) found evidence of an additional pathway to V5 based on a case study in which the patient's left hemisphere representation of V1 was absent. The normal hemisphere showed a bimodal response in area V5, but the response was delayed by 25–40 msec compared to controls. The affected side showed a unimodal response that was consistent in time with the second peak from the normal side. This pattern of results suggests that the input for the first peak originated from V1 whereas the second peak had a nongeniculostriate origin.

Anderson and colleagues (1996) performed an extensive set of experiments on area V5 to characterize the spatial and temporal frequency preferences of this area. They found that similar to the monkey literature, area V5 is selective for low spatial frequencies [in cycles per degree (cpd), ≤4 cpd] and a large range of temporal drift frequencies (≤35 Hz). In addition, there was clear response saturation at 10% contrast. Based on psychophysical findings that show that the visual system is sensitive to motion for spatial frequencies ≤35 cpd, and contrary to the ffytche *et al.* (1995a) findings, Anderson *et al.* suggest that the P pathway conveys this information and that this motion information is not processed in area V5. They also suggest that although the M pathway conveys some motion information it is primarily conveying information to the parietal cortex with a more specific goal of identifying motion in the peripheral field.

Although many of the MEG studies on the perception of motion have attempted to localize the motion-specific cortical areas similar to the fMRI and PET studies, they have often extended the analysis to provide additional information about the

temporal characteristics as well. In another study, ffytche *et al.* (1995b) looked at the timing of the V5 response relative to different drift speeds. They found that for speeds greater than 22°/sec, the signals in V5 arrived before the signals in V1, whereas for speeds less than 6°/sec, the signals in V1 arrived before the signals in V5. This timing information is also in agreement with the case study by Holliday *et al.* (1997) that suggested the existence of a separate pathway to area V5.

Lam *et al.* (2000) studied the differences between coherent versus incoherent motion using random-dot stimuli. Although onset latency did not change with speed of the stimuli, there was an inverse relationship between offset latency and speed of the stimuli. They also found that the sources evoked by slower motion stimuli localized more laterally than for faster motion stimuli. Similar results were seen for coherent as well as incoherent motion, suggesting that the same area processed both types of motion. In a study examining changes in the direction of motion (Ahlfors *et al.*, 1999), fMRI locations were used to help guide multidipole analysis of the MEG data (although the MEG locations were not constrained by the fMRI activation areas). These investigators found five different areas responsive to the motion stimuli: MT+, frontal eye field (FEF), posterior STS (pSTS), V3A, and V1/V2. They used the notation MT+ to refer to the collection of motion-sensitive areas, including MT and MST, located along the occipitotemporal border. The onset of the response was first seen in area MT+ around 130 msec, followed by activation of FEF 0–20 msec later. The remaining areas were active later. In general, two types of responses were seen in the five areas, transient (MT, V1/V2) and sustained (pSTS, frontal). They suggest that pSTS is responsible for processing information from a number of different areas due to the long-duration response, consistent with results from monkey studies.

Uusitalo *et al.* (1996) looked at the memory lifetimes in the visual system; that is, how long does it take visual areas to recover from a previous stimulus? They found that the primary and early visual areas with short-onset latencies also had short memory traces (0.2–0.6 sec), whereas the higher order areas (prefrontal, supratemporal gyrus, parieto-occipital-temporal junction), which had later onset times, showed significantly longer memory traces (7–30 sec). A later study examined the memory lifetime of area V5, specifically (Uusitalo *et al.*, 1997). This study showed that area V5 had an activation lifetime of between 0.4 and 1.4 sec across subjects, but the difference between hemispheres, within subjects, was less than 0.1 sec. The activation lifetime of area V5 implies that it is a later stage in the processing hierarchy, as suggested by Felleman and Van Essen (1991).

In addition to testing the different characteristics of continuous motion, there have been a number of studies examining the phenomenon of apparent motion. Apparent motion stimuli are spatially distinct stimuli that are presented sequentially at a sufficiently fast rate for one to perceive the offset of the first stimulus and onset of the second stimulus as a moving stimulus (phi phenomenon). Technically, all motion stimuli created by a computer reflect apparent motion, but the apparent motion stimuli discussed here refer to stimuli that the eye can physically distinguish in a static state but can also be perceived as motion with appropriate timing. Kaneoke and colleagues (1997) have performed the most extensive studies on this type of apparent motion. They initially compared apparent motion with continuous or smooth motion (using random-dot stimuli) to determine if they were perceived in the same way. Although the same area was active in response to these two types of stimuli, the peak latency was significantly shorter for apparent motion (162 and 171 msec) as compared to smooth motion

stimuli (294–320 msec). They suggest that a different pathway is available to the apparent motion stimuli. Based on two additional studies, Kaneoke and colleagues concluded that apparent motion was not a simple summation of on/off responses (Kaneoke *et al.*, 1998; Kawakami *et al.*, 2000). Naito *et al.* (2000) found an interesting field effect in apparent motion. In the lower visual field there were no direction preferences; however in the upper visual field, downward motion produced a significantly stronger response compared to upward motion despite the same location and orientation of the modeled response.

Two additional types of visual motion stimuli that have been studied briefly with significant results are visuomotor integration and action observation. In the first study, Nishitani *et al.* (1999) had the subjects perform three tasks: visual fixation, eye pursuit, and finger–eye pursuit. They found four main areas of activation: V1, anterior intraparietal lobule (aIPL), dorsolateral frontal area (DLF), and superior parietal lobule (SPL). They suggest aIPL is critical for visuomotor integration, whereas SPL played a role in visuospatial attention. They suggested that the lack of V5 activation was due to a weaker response to change in direction, rather than onset/offset of motion in this area. A study by Vanni *et al.* (1999) found enhanced 8- to 15-Hz mu rhythm activity in the postcentral gyrus after a change in perception to a motion stimulus in a binocular rivalry task. This task had a high-contrast stationary horizontal grating stimulus presented to one eye, whereas the other eye was presented with a low-contrast vertical grating. Movement of the weak vertical grating caused perceptual shifts of attention from the high-contrast grating to the low-contrast grating (noted by a verbal response from the subject). The mu enhancement effects were primarily seen during the binocular rivalry task and only very weakly during a separate visual motion task, suggesting that somatosensory cortex plays a role in perception even with no associated movement. They suggest this is possibly related to eye fixation or micro-saccades during the task.

In the remaining studies, the primary task was arm/hand movement with a visual component. In monkeys, it was found that motor cortex was active in response to action observation as well as in response to actually performing the action. There was additional frontal area activation (area F5 in monkeys) that is considered part of the mirror system, i.e., the network of cortical areas employed to mirror someone else's movements or actions (e.g., Gallese *et al.*, 1996; Rizzolatti *et al.*, 1996). Similar MEG studies were performed in humans; the subject was asked to perform hand movements as well as observe another person performing similar hand movements. Salenius (1999) looked initially at the suppression of spontaneous 20-Hz activity in response to hand movement and observation of hand movements. This study showed that viewing the movements significantly diminished the rebound of 20-Hz activity, similar to actual movements. Salenius suggested that the motor cortex is a critical component of the mirror system not only for language but also for inferring someone else's thoughts and actions. Nishitani and Hari (2000) performed a similar study with more extensive localization analysis and found activation of area V5, as well as activation of Brodmann's areas BA44 and BA4 in both the action and the action observation tasks. In addition, BA44 was active much earlier than BA4, suggesting that it plays a critical role in the observation/execution loop. They suggest that BA44, traditionally seen as a language area, is part of the mirror system due to the role hand gestures played in prelingual communication. In addition, these studies show the close link between the different sensory areas in creating a unified percept of the outside world.

OSCILLATORY BEHAVIOR IN THE VISUAL SYSTEM

There are a number of different types of oscillatory behaviors associated with the visual system. First, there is spontaneous oscillatory activity, generally referred to as visual alpha rhythms, which demonstrate oscillatory activity in the 8- to 13-Hz frequency range. Second, one can create oscillatory behavior by driving the system with periodic stimuli. Third, gamma-band oscillatory activity (in the 30- to 45-Hz frequency range) can be induced by various stimuli that do not have any oscillatory characteristics, but evoke an oscillatory response in a particular frequency range.

Alpha rhythms have been studied extensively using EEGs. These studies have ranged from characterizing the normal frequency range of alpha (8–13 Hz) to determining how alpha activity interacts with periodic visual stimulation (e.g., Regan, 1966; Klemm *et al.*, 1982; Mast and Victor, 1991; Pigeau and Frame, 1992). However, due to the lower spatial resolution of EEGs, most of these studies did not focus on the source of the alpha rhythms. Many early MEG studies used the higher spatial resolution of this technique to localize this activity (Ciulla *et al.*, 1999; Chapman *et al.*, 1984; Salmelin and Hari, 1994). Results from these studies primarily agree that the source of the spontaneous activity was located in and around the POS as well as the calcarine fissure. Although results in monkeys suggest that the strongest source of alpha rhythms is found in striate cortex, Salmelin and Hari pointed out that the POS source was probably as strong, if not stronger, in MEG studies due to cancellation of the MEG signal in the calcarine fissure.

A number of different studies have investigated the role of alpha rhythms further by establishing the levels of interaction different stimuli have on the spontaneous alpha activity. Hari *et al.* (1997) used a simple visual stimulus to show that the posterior alpha activity could be dampened within 200 msec of the onset of a visual stimulus. They also saw a rebound of alpha activity beyond baseline levels with the offset of the stimulus. A number of different studies showed differential alpha suppression during different cognitive tasks (Salenius *et al.*, 1995; Tesche *et al.*, 1995; Williamson *et al.*, 1996; Vanni *et al.*, 1997). For example, Salenius and colleagues (1995) and Williamson and colleagues (1996) both found that a visually presented cognitive task and a visual control task caused alpha suppression. However, there was a difference in the degree of alpha suppression between these two studies; Salenius and colleagues found that the alpha suppression was weaker during mental imagery, whereas Williamson and colleagues found equivalent alpha suppression between visual imagery and the visual control task (visual imagery is discussed further under "Higher Order Processes"). Vanni *et al.* (1997) found that alpha suppression was greater for objects than for nonobjects when the objects were the target stimuli, but that there was no difference when the task did not differentiate between these two classes of stimuli. This suggests that the apparent discrepancy in the previous two studies is most likely representing the sensitivity of task relevance, or attention, on the interaction of alpha activity with particular stimuli. In addition to seeing alpha modulation during a mental imagery task, Tesche and colleagues also saw 20-Hz modulation. They suggested that there was probably higher frequency activity in the previous studies that averaged out with the spectral analysis techniques used. As expected, different types of analyses provide different information from a given data set. Given the temporal resolution of MEG, there are a number of different time- and frequency-domain analyses that are appropriate, depending on the tasks and hypotheses of any particular study.

One obvious goal in these studies, besides determining the source of the alpha activity, is to try to determine the purpose of the oscillations. Hari and Salmelin (1997) suggested three possible roles for the spontaneous oscillatory activity seen in many of the sensory modalities while at rest. First, oscillations may reflect a type of idling of the system that allows the system to react more quickly to unexpected incoming stimuli. Second, it may signify the ongoing transfer of information between the peripheral and central nervous system. Third, it might signify periodic stimulation of neuronal groups used to reinforce synaptic connections.

A couple of investigators have suggested clinical applications for the monitoring of alpha activity using MEGs. Parra *et al.* (2000) found that alpha activity and a fixation-off sensitivity-related abnormality (FOS-RA) were separable by applying a cluster analysis to the data. With application of ethosuximide for 1 year, this abnormal activity was reduced. Tesche and Kajola (1993), using a novel time-frequency analysis of the data, found that a spike and slow-wave event found in the time-domain analysis from an epileptic subject localized to a location similar to that of abnormal 2- to 6- Hz activity found in the frequency-domain analysis. They suggested that a time frequency-domain analysis can help with MEG analysis by separating signal and noise, if they are in different frequency bands, as well as by identifying neural activity based on the characteristic that it is spatially correlated, whereas noise often is not.

Driving Oscillatory Activity with Periodic Stimulation

An additional way to interrogate the visual system is not only to observe the spontaneous oscillatory activity but also to drive the system at different frequencies to determine its sensitivity to different temporal characteristics. Narici and colleagues have performed a number of studies looking at the frequency sensitivity of the different sensory systems to stimuli driven at different frequencies (Narici *et al.*, 1990, 1998; Narici and Peresson, 1995). They found that although the different sensory systems can be driven at a number of different frequencies, the preferred frequency is the dominant frequency that is found in the spontaneous activity. That is, when the visual system was driven at the alpha frequency, the driven oscillations lasted considerably longer compared to oscillations at the surrounding frequencies. This is useful in enhancing the signal and improving the stationarity of the oscillations. Although the discussion in the previous section has shown that it is possible to localize and study the alpha activity, the transitory nature of alpha activity seen in short bursts makes the analysis more difficult to perform. In a second study, Narici found that there appeared to be two different components of the occipital alpha, one at 10.5 Hz and one around 12 Hz. The 10.5-Hz component appeared to continue in the background regardless of stimulation, whereas the 12-Hz activity was very stable with periodic stimulation, but it did not continue spontaneously. They suggested the 10.5-Hz activity had an attention component whereas the 12-Hz activity was related to cognitive processing.

In a set of experiments, Tononi *et al.* (1998) and Srinivasan *et al.* (1999) investigated the cortical response to alternating visual stimuli in a binocular rivalry task. That is, different stimuli were presented to the two eyes. These stimuli competed for perceptual dominance similar to a Necker cube that spontaneously changes orientation as the subject maintains fixation. In this set of studies, one eye was presented with a red vertical grating alternating at frequency $f1$, while the other eye was presented with a blue horizontal grating alternating at frequency $f2$. The alternation frequencies presented to the two eyes were chosen from the following set: 7.41, 8.33,

9.5, and 11.12 Hz. The subject activated one of two switches with a right finger movement when the red or blue stimulus was dominant (none if neither was dominant). The stimuli changed dominance every 2–3 sec on average. By collecting a long time interval while the subject performed this task, they were able to obtain a frequency resolution of 0.0032 Hz. They found control values for the power by presenting the two stimuli separately (alternating randomly) for the same length of time as the binocular rivalry task. Tononi and colleagues first found that a signal from both frequency bands was seen during the perceptual dominance of each stimulus. This implies that although only one stimulus was consciously perceived, the visual information from both visual stimuli was registered in cortex at some level. However, there was a significant change in power relative to the consciously perceived stimulus (decreased by 50–85% during the unconscious versus conscious perception). This difference in power was seen in sensors over occipital, temporal, and frontal cortex. Srinivasan *et al.* (1999) extended the work on this task by looking at the coherence at the different frequencies between different cortical areas (compared sensors >12 cm apart). Power at a given channel suggests the level of locally synchronized activity, whereas coherence between channels suggests the level of synchronization in distant brain areas. They found that in addition to an increase in power, the coherence between these widely separated areas was also increased at the stimulus frequency (both intra- and interhemispheric). The most robust change in coherence occurred between interhemispheric sensor pairs between occipital and parietal channels. Other significant coherence pairings included temporal or frontal of one hemisphere with temporal, parietal, and occipital channels of the other hemisphere, and to a lesser extent frontal/temporal pairings with occipital/parietal channels within hemisphere. This study also showed that the coherence information was independent of the change in power, implying that additional information can be gained by looking at coherence results. If one were to extend these methods by performing source analysis of the coherence data, these results suggest one could provide a macroscopic view of network activity and cortical synchrony within the human brain.

Induced Oscillatory Activity

The third type of oscillatory activity that is seen in response to visual stimuli is induced oscillatory activity. That is, the stimulus does not have any oscillatory characteristics, but oscillatory behavior is observed by using a variety of techniques to look at the spectral content of the response. This type of behavior is most commonly seen during cognitive tasks, suggesting that the induced oscillations are part of different cell assemblies that are activated to bind temporally different stimulus characteristics or the activation of a particular system of distributed areas that are necessary to attend or respond to the task. Although most of the original gamma band (30–45 Hz) studies in MEG focused on auditory stimulation, a number of additional studies using visual stimuli in cognitive tasks have shown gamma band activity.

Despite reliable reports of gamma band activation in cats and monkeys, it has been more difficult to see this activity in humans using MEG, as compared to EEG. Eulitz *et al.* (1996) notes that one possible reason why it is difficult to see gamma band activity using MEG relates to the number of neurons in one region that must be active simultaneously (e.g., tens to hundreds of thousands) in order to produce a measurable MEG signal at the surface of the head. If gamma band activity originates from cell assemblies, and at most tens of thousands of neurons make up a particular cell assembly with only a fraction of those cells

active at any one time (Aertsen *et al.*, 1994), then there is an insufficient number of active cells to produce a measurable signal at the surface of the head. An additional difficulty with observing high-frequency oscillations is that if the oscillations are not well phase-locked to the onset of the stimulus, these responses easily average out in the presentation of the 100 stimuli normally needed to achieve an adequate signal-to-noise ratio to obtain a reasonable MEG response. Despite these difficulties, Eulitz and colleagues did see activity in the traditional gamma band using MEG that was reduced during presentation of language stimuli relative to nonlanguage stimuli at 291 and 506 msec. They also observed 60-Hz activity that was specific to language stimuli over language-specific cortex in response to visually presented words and nonword control stimuli. In a related study, Eulitz *et al.* (2000) found that evoked activity and induced activity showed different topographies of activity across the surface of the head. In this case, evoked activity was defined as the normal visual evoked response with its multispectral characteristics and induced activity was defined as specific oscillatory activity that was generated by the non-oscillatory stimulus. Although they confirmed their previous results, only post-hoc analysis showed that the induced 60-Hz activity near the frontotemporal region was specific to automatic word processing.

As suggested by the paucity of studies examining visually induced gamma band activity, novel data analysis techniques are required to provide more information about this type of oscillatory behavior. A large amount of work in this area has been performed by Tallon-Baudry and colleagues (Tallon-Baudry *et al.*, 1997; Tallon-Baudry and Bertrand, 1999). They applied a time–frequency analysis technique that looks for wave packets of gamma band activity using wavelet analysis on unaveraged MEG data. The assumption was that different stimuli would induce gamma band activity at different times. With the wavelet analysis, one can obtain a power value at different time points that can be added together across trials without having to worry about the signal being out of phase and canceling out with averaging. This analysis has provided a significant step forward in using gamma band information to further the understanding of the visual system and cognitive functioning. They have seen both phase-locked gamma band responses (generally early) and non-phase-locked gamma band activity in response to delayed match to sample tasks. Based on a simulation study, they also suggest that the origins of the gamma band activity are the horizontally oriented dendritic fields, which may further explain why MEG has a difficult time detecting this induced activity (Tallon-Baudry and Bertrand, 1999).

Regardless of these difficulties, a number of other studies have reported gamma band activity in a variety of visually presented tasks. Sokolov *et al.* (1999) found that there was an enhancement in gamma band activity in response to coherent motion. In this experiment they presented coherent and incoherent visual and auditory stimuli. The coherent visual stimuli were horizontally oriented bars moving downward (3°/sec) in either the upper or lower half of the screen whereas the coherent auditory stimuli consisted of two alternating tones (300 and 1000 Hz, 60-msec duration). The incoherent visual stimuli consisted of an irregular displacement of the horizontal bars, and the incoherent auditory stimulus was white noise. The auditory and visual coherent stimuli were randomly presented first, always followed by the opposite modality stimulus (unattended condition). The subject had to respond to the offset of the first stimulus and decide if it was auditory or visual (with a choice of finger movements). They found modality-specific attention effects to the coherent stimuli (increased gamma

over visual cortex during the visual stimulus and vice versa), as well as gamma band enhancement for the attended coherent visual stimuli over occipital cortex in 50- to 250-msec time interval (locked to stimulus onset). However, this was only the case when the coherent motion stimulus was attended. If it was not attended, the gamma band activity was the same for coherent and incoherent motion stimuli, suggesting a strong attention rather than a feature-binding component to the gamma band activity.

Braeutigam *et al.* (2001) found a very complex spatio temporal pattern of gamma band responses to visually presented congruent and incongruent words in a sentence completion task. Both congruent and incongruent words showed a typical visual response to the visual word stimuli. However, differences between these two types of stimuli were evident as early as 200 msec poststimulus. The incongruent words showed two different periods of phase-locked responses (230–375 and 570–940 msec). In addition, the incongruent words evoked the well-studied N400 response. The congruent words, on the other hand, showed gamma activity clusters only around the time that the N400 component in the incongruent words was decreasing. This activity was near the traditional Broca's and Wernicke's areas; the authors suggested that this activity was related to a type of syntactic closure. In an interesting, albeit somewhat tangential, study, Amidzic *et al.* (2001) found different patterns of gamma bursts in amateur chess players and in grand masters in the 5 sec following a "move" in chess. The amateur chess players primarily showed gamma activity in the medial temporal lobe, suggesting they were looking at new patterns. In contrast, the grand masters showed no gamma activity in the medial temporal lobe area but revealed activity in the parietal and frontal lobes, suggesting they were searching the data base for known patterns.

Although most of the induced oscillatory studies have focused on gamma band activity, other regions of cortex reveal induced oscillatory behavior in other frequency bands. For example, the hippocampus has been shown in rats to exhibit induced oscillatory activity in the theta frequency band (4–12 Hz) (Vanderwolf, 1969). In another study, Tesche and Karhu (2000) used MEG to determine if this technique could detect stimulus-induced theta activity in the human hippocampus. By engaging their subjects in a working memory task (using a variant of the Sternberg paradigm), they were able to demonstrate stimulus-locked theta activity. Unlike most MEG studies that randomize the timing of the presentation of the stimuli to reduce habituation effects, the stimuli in this task were presented with a constant temporal spacing. They found stimulus-locked theta activity in both left and right hippocampus; however, the left hippocampus theta activity was evident at ~120 msec poststimulus, whereas the right hippocampus theta activity was evident at ~80 msec prestimulus. The duration of the stimulus-locked theta activity was dependent on memory load, suggesting that the duration of theta activity was related to the cognitive process of monitoring incoming sensory stimuli. The memory-load theta was also found to last at most 600 msec, despite a systematic increase in memory load. Tesche and Karhu suggest that the timing of this stimulus-locked theta might be a physiological correlate of the generally accepted memory-load limit of 7 ± 2 items. The prestimulus phase-locking is most likely associated with internal timing mechanisms of the cortex, which are linked to both right hemisphere and cerebellar activity.

HIGHER ORDER PROCESSES

Selective Attention

For the past three decades, behavioral and neurophysiological investigations of selective attention have attempted to specify the functional level at which information is selected for or rejected from further processing (Johnston and Dark, 1986; Kahneman and Treisman, 1984). "Early selection" theories (e.g., Broadbent, 1958; Treisman and Geffen, 1967) have proposed that irrelevant information can be rejected before the semantic analysis of the stimulus, i.e., attention operates at the sensory or perceptual level. "Late selection" theories, in contrast, propose that selection occurs after both the physical and semantic analysis of all stimuli impinging on an organism (e.g., Deutsch and Deutsch, 1963). According to this view, stimuli automatically activate nodes in long-term memory; attention in this case operates at the level of decision or response processes (Deutsch and Deutsch, 1963; Shiffrin and Schneider, 1984; Hoffman, 1978; Posner et al., 1980).

Early event-related potential studies of visual selective attention in humans attempted indirectly to address the question of *when* and *where* stimulus information is selected for further processing. These studies examined peak latencies in the wave forms, peak amplitudes, and scalp distributions, evoked by selective-attention tasks (e.g., Eason et al., 1969; Van Voorhis and Hillyard, 1977; Harter et al., 1982; Hillyard, 1985; Rugg et al., 1987; Neville and Lawson, 1987). The question of "early" versus "late" selection in cognitive studies of selective attention translated into the question of how early in the ERP wave forms the effects of selective attention occur, and more specifically, if selective attention can influence very early levels of the visual system such as primary visual cortex (V1) (e.g., Eason, 1981; Harter and Aine, 1984; Hillyard and Munte, 1984; Hillyard, 1985). Although it is generally assumed that ERP effects at increasing latencies reflect the differential activation of populations of neurons at successive levels in the nervous system, little information is available about the neural structures responsible for attention-related ERP effects in humans.

Early invasive studies of attention, using single-unit recordings in monkeys, were initially unsuccessful in finding any modulation of primary visual cortex as a function of selective attention, at any point in time (e.g., Wurtz and Mohler, 1976; Moran and Desimone, 1985; Haenny and Schiller, 1988; Motter, 1993). However, recent invasive studies in monkeys (e.g., Ito and Gilbert, 1999; Roelfsema *et al.*, 1998; Vidyasagar, 1998; Mehta *et al.*, 2000a,b) and noninvasive fMRI studies in humans (e.g., Tootell *et al.*, 1998; Worden *et al.*, 1996; Brefczynski and De Yoe, 1999; Ghandi *et al.*, 1999; Huk and Heeger, 2000; Shulman *et al.*, 1997, Somers *et al.*, 1999; Watanabe *et al.*, 1998) routinely demonstrate such modulation of activity. Investigators using invasive methods generally agree that attention acts to enhance the mean firing rate of individual neurons (Bushnell *et al.*, 1981; Haenny *et al.*, 1988; Roelfsema *et al.*, 1998; McAdams and Maunsell, 1999; Spitzer *et al.*, 1988; Connor *et al.*, 1997; Motter, 1994; Seidemann and Newsome, 1999). Although effects of attention have been demonstrated at many levels within the visual system of monkeys (Desimone and Duncan, 1995; Ito and Gilbert, 1999; Reynolds and Desimone, 1999; Mehta *et al.*, 2000a,b; Schroeder *et al.*, 2001; Maunsell, 1995; Treue and Martinez-Trujillo, 1999; Moran and Desimone, 1985; Motter, 1993; Treue and Maunsell, 1996), there is still some debate concerning how early effects of attention may be evidenced. Some studies indicate that attention can influence the initial visual response (e.g., Luck *et al.*, 1997; Ito and Gilbert, 1999), but others suggest that attention-related modulations clearly lag the earliest response (~250–300 msec) (Lamme *et al.*, 1998; Haenny and Schiller, 1988; Mehta *et al.*, 2000a; Seidemann and Newsome, 1999; Roelfsema *et al.*, 1998; Motter, 1994).

Spatial location appears to be an especially effective visual cue for guiding selective attention. A number of studies have shown that ERPs recorded over the posterior regions of the head are significantly modulated when subjects are required to focus attention on a sequence of visual stimuli at a particular spatial location while ignoring a concurrent sequence of flashes in the opposite visual field. Stimuli presented at the attended location, compared to stimuli presented at the same location while attention was directed toward stimuli in the opposite visual field, elicit an enhanced sequence of ERP components over the occipital scalp that typically include P1 and N1 components (peak latencies of 80–140 and 140–170 msec, respectively), as well as longer latency deflections (Eason *et al.*, 1969; Van Voorhis and Hillyard, 1977; Harter *et al.*, 1982; Hillyard and Munte, 1984; Mangun and Hillyard, 1988; Neville and Lawson, 1987; Rugg *et al.*, 1987). These early attention-sensitive ERP effects are thought to arise in one or more regions of visual cortex, although direct evidence for this conclusion is lacking. Modulation of even earlier stages of the afferent pathway has been reported by Eason and colleagues (Eason *et al.*, 1983). Taken together, these data suggest that selective attention to spatial location may involve modulation of the earliest stages of the cortical visual system and possibly subcortical structures.

Luber *et al.* (1989) examined spatial attention using MEG by presenting 1° square gratings 5° to the left or right of central fixation (above the horizontal meridian) and instructing subjects to attend to either the right or the left field for a block of trials, while maintaining central fixation. They noted an enhancement of source strengths occurring around 200–360 msec, "well after at least the first component of the cortical response has occurred." This is unlike the earlier ERP studies (e.g., Van Voorhis and Hillyard, 1977; Harter *et al.*, 1982), wherein attention-related effects were noted around 100 msec poststimulus. Effects of attention were not accompanied by changes in the location or orientation of the equivalent current dipoles, suggesting that attention modulates sensory areas that normally process visual stimuli.

Aine and colleagues (1995) examined effects of attending a conjunction of location and spatial frequency. Gratings of 1 and 5 cpd were randomly presented to two locations along the horizontal meridian: the central visual field and 7° in the right visual field. Subjects were instructed to attend to one of the four combinations of field location and spatial frequency (e.g., attend to the 1-cpd stimulus presented to the right visual field). During the nonattend condition in this specific example, striate and occipito temporal regions did not remain active for long; by 130 msec, an occipitoparietal source dominated. A difference field was constructed by subtracting the non-attend wave form the attend wave form and a single-dipole model was applied to this difference wave. The difference wave revealed a strong effect of attention around 150 msec, which localized to striate cortex. When striate sources were compared for the nonattend condition (90 msec) and the attend condition (150 msec), the source locations were adjacent to one another with opposing orientations. The apparent differences in orientation and in the temporal dynamics of the response were interpreted as reflecting feedback into striate cortex, causing a reactivation of this region as a function of attention.

Vanni and Uutela (2000) examined the frontoparietal attentional network using MEG [e.g., frontal eye fields and lateral intraparietal area; Corbetta et al., (1991)], which has been reported to be active when shifts of attention occur between objects or locations and shifts of gaze. Precentral (putative FEF) and parietal responses to peripheral stimuli were compared when subjects were instructed to fixate centrally on a small square while attending versus not attending to peripheral stimuli, versus when subjects were engaged in detecting

auditory tones (i.e., they were not attending to the central fixation point). Regions of interest (ROIs) were selected based on the average of three conditions representing steadily active areas within 400 msec from stimulus onset. Minimum current estimates were calculated for these ROIs. The most systematic difference between experimental conditions was noted in the right precentral region (frontal eye fields). These authors concluded that the focusing of attention on a fixation point enhances right precentral cortical responses (putative FEF) to stimuli in all parts of the visual field, whether attended or not. They suggest that visually evoked right FEF responses, evident around 100 msec in their study, depend on visual attention (e.g., attention to the fixation point), instead of being dependent on making overt responses to target stimuli, as suggested by Corbetta and colleagues (1993). We also note FEF activity (e.g., Stephen et al., 2002) when subjects are required to maintain central fixation but are not required to attend/respond to the visual stimuli. This issue is discussed in more detail under "Final Comments."

Visual Mental Imagery

As mentioned previously, many investigators currently believe that information concerning the attributes of stimuli is not stored as a unified percept in a single cortical location; but rather, it appears to be stored in a distributed cortical system in which information about specific features is stored close to the regions of cortex that mediate the perception of those features (e.g., Ungerleider, 1995; Mesulam, 1998; Goldman-Rakic, 1988). Perception occurs when information is registered directly from the senses. Mental imagery occurs when perceptual information is accessed from memory; perhaps previously perceived objects or events are recalled or mental images may result from a new combination or modification of stored perceptual information. Mental imagery draws on much of the same neural machinery as perception in the same modality, and can engage mechanisms in memory, emotion, and motor control (see Kosslyn *et al.*, 2001). However, although visual mental imagery and visual perception share many mechanisms, they do not draw on identical processes. For example, imagery, unlike perception, does not require low-level organizational processing. On the other hand, perception, unlike imagery, does not require the activation of information in memory when the stimulus is not present. Kosslyn and colleagues report results from a functional neuroimaging study suggesting that, of the brain areas active during visual perception and visual imagery, approximately two-thirds were activated in both cases (Kosslyn *et al.*, 1997). An invasive study conducted in humans examined the neuronal substrates of visual perception and visual imagery by recording from single neurons in the human medial temporal lobe of patients with pharmacologically intractable epilepsy (Kreiman *et al.*, 2000). Neurons in the hippocampus, amygdala, entorhinal cortex, and parahippocampal gyrus altered their firing rates during mental imagery. In addition, of the neurons that fired selectively during both visual stimulation and imagery, 88% had identical selectivity. In general, careful selection of task instruction and stimuli for an imagery task can produce preferential activation of different processing streams. For example, the fusiform face area may be activated by having subjects image faces while parahippocampal regions may become active by instructing subjects to visualize indoor or outdoor scenes (O'Craven and Kanwisher, 2000).

As was noted in the section on oscillatory behavior, many functional neuroimaging studies investigated whether visual imagery could alter activity of the primary visual area (V1). Two studies with results that replicate each other are noted here, indicating that visual mental imagery can alter activity in primary visual cortex just as visual selective attention can alter activity in primary visual cortex. Both PET and fMRI results examined responses evoked by having subjects image different sizes of objects. When the object was imaged as a larger size, activation in the calcarine fissure shifted to more anterior locations, whereas activation shifted to more posterior locations when the object was imaged as a smaller size (i.e., retinotopic organization) (Kosslyn *et al.*, 1995; Tootell *et al.*, 1998).

Several studies examining visual mental imagery utilized a visual mental rotation task similar to one described by Cooper and Shepard (1973). Michel and colleagues (1994) used MEG to test whether the temporal duration of alpha suppression over visual cortex correlates with behavioral reaction time measures, as the time required for completing the mental rotation task increases. In a previous study, Kaufman *et al.* (1990) showed that recognition of previously presented polygon shapes was accompanied by suppression of alpha activity, which correlated with reaction time. In addition, the source of the alpha suppression appeared to reside in visual cortex, similar to earlier blood flow studies (reviewed by Roland and Gulyas, 1994). In the study by Michel and colleagues, subjects were asked to discriminate normal from mirror-reflected versions of alphanumeric characters when the characters were tilted at different angles relative to the upright position. The reaction times paralleled results from Cooper and Shepard (1973), showing increased reaction time with increased rotation of the target figure from the normal orientation. Responses to mirror-reflected letters appeared to be 50 msec longer than responses to letters with the correct orientation. In addition, there was a clear relationship between the increase in duration of suppression of parietooccipital alpha band neuronal activity and reaction time; i.e., both increased by about 200 msec for the largest (most difficult) angles of rotation. This result indicates that the POS region was involved in the mental rotation task. Furthermore, small changes in the spatial pattern during alpha suppression were observed to be dependent on task demands. These authors concluded that alpha suppression directly reflected the cognitive functions that were involved in mental rotation.

Iwaki and colleagues (1999) and Kawamichi and colleagues (1998) also examined cortical processes related to mental rotation using source localization methods. In the study by Iwaki and colleagues, line-drawn objects were presented simultaneously and subjects were instructed to discriminate rotationally symmetrical pairs from mirror-reversed pairs via a finger lift response. A control task consisted of having subjects view the same visual stimuli without making judgments and to respond alternately with their right or left index finger. These investigators report initial activity in occipital cortex (120–180 msec) for both target and control tasks, followed by activation in the posterior part of the inferotemporal or temporal cortex for the target condition around 170–230 msec. Finally, activity was evident in parietal or inferior parietal regions for the target condition around 200–270 msec. Kawamichi and colleagues (1998) found similar regions of activity and temporal sequence when subjects were engaged in making judgments of hand orientation in a mental rotation task. These studies provide information concerning the dynamic properties of distributed cortical activity related to mental rotation processes.

Raij (1999) examined imagery-related activity in visual cortex produced by auditory phonemes. Subjects were instructed to imagine visually the letter (Roman alphabet) corresponding to the auditory phoneme and to examine its visuospatial properties. This activity was compared to responses to the same stimuli when subjects detected tone pips. Imagery-related responses were de-

tected over multiple cortical areas, including left lateral occipital cortex in 2 of 10 subjects and in the calcarine fissure of 1 subject. Posterior parietal cortex, close to the midline (precuneus), was active around 390 msec after voice onset. Aine and colleagues (2002) similarly demonstrated activation of visual cortex (around 200 msec after word onset) during a size categorization task using auditory word stimuli that represent common objects. Mellet and colleagues (2000), using fMRI methods, have also demonstrated that auditory verbal descriptions can produce blood oxygenation changes in visual cortex.

An additional MEG and EEG study that falls somewhere between the categories of selective attention and mental imagery, reported by Gaetz and colleagues (1998), examined the spontaneous reversals of the Necker cube. The subjects were instructed to close their eyes after reversals to mark trigger points in the data. A neural network classification analysis on the MEG data revealed that the individual epochs related to the control stimulus (a square) and the Necker cube conditions were classified appropriately (10/10), showing significant differences between the conditions. The EEG data showed somewhat less specific results, with correct classifications in 6/8 conditions. Both the MEG and EEG data showed that there was a significant increase in correlation across the channels during the Necker cube reversals relative to the control condition. Gaetz and colleagues conclude that there is increased synchrony in a distributed network of cortical areas (including occipital, parietal, and temporal areas) during the perception of Necker cube reversals.

Working Memory

Wang and colleagues (2001) showed MEG results from a Wisconsin Card Sorting Task (WCST). This task has been routinely used as a neuropsychological test of frontal lobe dysfunction (Milner, 1963). Subjects are asked to match a "target" card to a "reference" card, each of which contain colored symbols varying in terms of color, shape, and number of symbols. The correct sorting principle (i.e., sort based on color, sort based on number of symbols, sort based on shape of symbols) is never explicitly described; subjects must determine for themselves, based on the feedback signals received, whether or not they are sorting according to the correct category. Patients suffering from frontal lobe dysfunction have difficulties in switching to a new, correct category. Wang and colleagues were interested in comparing MEG responses to (1) card sorting when subjects were sorting to the appropriate card category versus after they were first notified that they needed to switch their attention to another card category and (2) feedback for correct versus incorrect responses. In general, a frontal–parietal network was identified across subjects (BA9, BA44/45, and BA40) common to both continuous sorting and feedback responses (see Fig. 4). After subjects were first notified that they needed to switch categories, strong activity in middle and inferior prefrontal cortex was evident at 200 msec (primarily BA44/45); at 370 msec, strong activity was evident again in prefrontal cortex (primarily BA9). Differences in response to the wrong versus correct feedback signals were evident around 460–640 msec in the dorsolateral prefrontal and middle frontal gyrus (primarily BA9). These authors concluded that the same general brain areas (frontal–parietal network) were involved in (1) shifting attention after receiving feedback indicating the wrong sorting category was being used and (2) visual

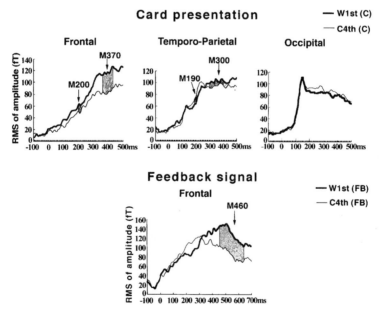

FIGURE 4 Group-averaged RMS from frontal, temporoparietal, and occipital regions are shown across subjects for the card presentation and feedback signal conditions. For card presentation, differences in the frontal and temporoparietal regions can be seen when subjects needed to shift to another category (solid lines) versus when subjects were sorting based on the correct category (thin lines). Note that occipital regions did not reveal such differences. Differences associated with the feedback signal can be seen in frontal regions when the first incorrect feedback signal was delivered (solid lines) versus when the correct feedback signal was delivered (thin line). Shaded regions represent periods when the differences between the two conditions were statistically significant as determined by paired *t*-tests. Frontal regions revealed different patterns of effects—same regions but at different points in time. Reprinted from *Cognitive Brain Research* **12**; L. Wang, R. Kakigi, and M. Hoshiyama; Neural activities during Wisconsin Card Sorting Test-MEG observation; pp. 19–31. Copyright 2001, with permission from Elsevier Science.

working memory associated with correct performance. The timing between these structures differed according to task condition. Numerous studies ranging from single-unit studies in monkeys to noninvasive fMRI studies in humans have shown enhanced activity in prefrontal regions that is maintained throughout working memory tasks (e.g., Jiang *et al.*, 2000). The current MEG study (Wang *et al.*, 2001), however, emphasizes the importance of the temporal dynamics of brain activity. Different functions are not only represented by networks of different brain structures, but different functions may also be represented as different timing patterns within the same network of brain structures. This latter aspect of brain organization has hardly been explored.

Aine and Stephen (2002) explored the mechanisms underlying the enhancement of brain areas (or saliency), as a function of selective-attention/working-memory tasks. Several MEG articles alluded either to the recurrence of activity within a visual area or to the variability in the duration of activity (i.e., lifetimes of activation traces) across visual areas. In the former case, Hari

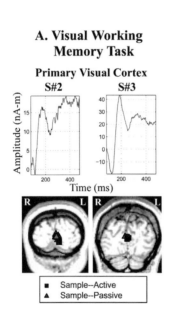

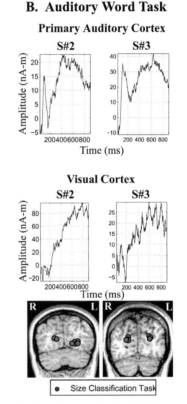

FIGURE 5 "Spikes" and "slow waves" evoked by visual and auditory stimuli. (A) Response profiles for primary visual cortex in two subjects (left and right columns, respectively) evoked by visual stimuli while engaged in a working-memory task (Active Condition). These responses were acquired to the sample stimulus of the delayed nonmatch to sample task. Each tracing represents an average of ~250 individual neuromagnetic responses. MRIs for each subject are shown below, with primary visual cortex highlighted by the symbols representing the best-fitting solutions. (B) Cortical response profiles evoked by the auditory classification task for the same two subjects. The top row shows response profiles from primary auditory cortex and the bottom row shows response profiles from visual cortex when subjects were classifying whether the common nouns they heard represented items larger than a television set. The MRIs below reveal that bilateral lower level visual areas were engaged in this auditory task.

and colleagues (1980) noted that both the N100 and P180 components of the auditory MEG localized to primary auditory cortex. Aine and colleagues (1995) had noted a similar finding in the visual MEG, i.e., there appeared to be a recurrence of activation within primary visual cortex. Williamson and colleagues (Lu *et al.*, 1992; Uusitalo *et al.*, 1996), on the other hand, studied the decay times of neural activity in primary and secondary auditory and visual cortex. They noted that the decay time of the sensory traces in primary areas corresponded to psychophysical memory experiments examining iconic memory (initial representation of visual stimuli) and echoic memory (initial representation of auditory stimuli). As mentioned earlier, Uusitalo and colleagues (1996) suggested that there are two forms of memory representation in each sensory modality. In the visual system, occipital lobes revealed short lifetimes (e.g., 200–300 msec), whereas higher order visual structures revealed lifetimes lasting from 7 to 30 sec.

Our recent memory studies in both auditory and visual modalities, using our newer automated analysis procedures (Huang *et al.*, 1998; Aine *et al.*, 2000), have shown that activity in the primary visual and auditory cortices can be characterized as having an early "spikelike" component followed by later "slow-wave" activity (see rows, A and B, Fig. 5). The early "spikelike" activity in the visual response was experimentally separated from the later "slow-wave" activity by conducting an auditory size classification task which evoked activity in visual cortex, presumably due to imagery (see bottom row of Fig. 5B). Visual cortical activity was evoked when subjects were asked if the auditory words, representing common objects, were larger than a television set. These results were interpreted as reflecting early feedforward activity (similar to Uusitalo's brief lifetime traces from occipital activity) (Uusitalo *et al.*, 1996) and later feedback activity, which was of longer duration and

was particularly sensitive to attention (similar to Uusitalo's long lifetime traces evident in higher order visual areas). The difference between these studies is that primary and secondary areas reflect both types of activity, which can account for the results by Hari *et al.* (1980) and Aine *et al.* (1995) that suggest a recurrence of activation, even in primary areas. Aine and Stephen (2002) link these results to recent studies examining feedforward and feedback components in monkeys when they were engaged in selective attention tasks and studies examining temporal binding.

In the visual working-memory task (a modified version of a delayed nonmatch to sample task), conducted by Aine and Stephen (2002), stimuli were constructed of black and white squares (Walsh functions) with the characteristics that (1) each member had an equal amount of black and white, allowing for equal luminance across the stimulus sets, and (2) they were difficult to label verbally. Subjects were presented with a "Sample" stimulus for 1 sec duration in the central visual field (visual angle 2°) followed by two distractor stimuli in the lower left and right quadrants. A second Walsh stimulus ("Target" of 1 sec duration) was presented approximately 2.5 sec after the offset of the "Sample" stimulus and subjects were instructed to respond with a button press to the "Target" stimulus if it did not match the "Sample" stimulus. Results from the "Sample" stimuli (no behavioral responses were made to these stimuli) showed that selective attention or working memory can sustain activity over quite a number of different cortical areas (thereby increasing the lifetimes of traces in these regions), compared to a passive control task (see Fig. 6A), and acts to increase the synchronicity of the activity (see Fig. 6B) across widespread cortical areas (temporal binding?). Both of these effects were most pronounced for the later "slow-wave" activity.

The topic of temporal binding (i.e., how features and attributes of stimuli become

A. MEG Cortical Response Profiles -- Working Memory

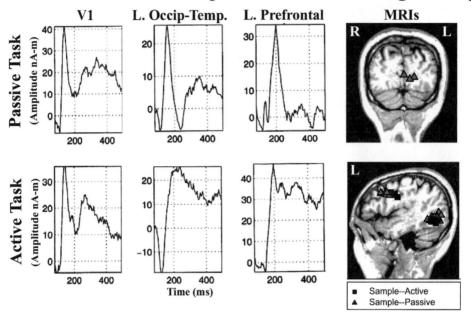

B. Cross-Correlations -- Working Memory

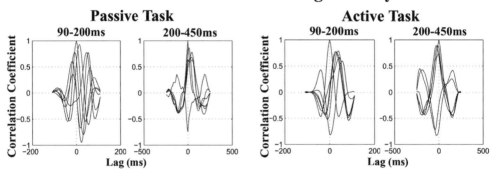

FIGURE 6 (A) MEG cortical response profiles to "Sample" stimuli when the subject was not engaged (first row—Passive Task) versus engaged (second row—Active Task) in the working-memory task. Note that activity localized to left occipital–temporal and prefrontal regions reveal elevated and sustained activity in the later portion of the responses for the "Active" versus "Passive" profiles (bottom vs. top rows, respectively). The clusters of triangles and squares on the MRIs to the right indicate the cortical regions of activity localized for the "Passive" versus "Active" tasks, respectively. The right hemisphere is displayed on the left side of the MRIs, according to radiological convention. (B) Cross-covariance plots of different cortical areas relative to V1. The autocorrelation of V1 with itself is included as a reference. The left and right columns in A show cross-covariance plots of the time-courses for the best solution relative to V1 during the passive and active portions, respectively. Both early (90–200 msec) and late (200–450 msec) time intervals for each "Passive" and "Active" task are shown. Notice that during the early time interval for the "Passive" task there is a large dispersion of the lag at the maximum correlation (peak), whereas during the late time interval of the "Active" task, the maximum correlation of most of the sources is almost synchronous with the V1 slow-wave response. It is also interesting to note that the time-courses appear more synchronous even in the early time interval during the "Active" task, although there is no evidence of an enhancement of the early response (compare initial time courses for "Passive" and "Active" tasks in A).

integrated across widespread cortical regions) has been one of intense interest and debate lately. Singer (1999), along with many others, suggest that synchronous neuronal firing provides one mechanism for *binding* the different features/attributes of stimuli across these widespread cortical areas. Recent results from nonhuman studies support the idea that cortical neurons form networks by synchronizing their activity with other neurons that process similar information (Singer, 1995; 1999; Engel *et al.*, 1991, 1992; Gray, 1999; Roelfsema *et al.*, 1997; Towle *et al.*, 1999). Temporal binding could be postulated if in-phase oscillatory behavior was observed across different cortical areas. One type of activity that has been suggested to mediate temporal binding in this case is the gamma band activity discussed in the previous section. A second situation in which temporal binding could be postulated is if different cortical areas exhibited low-frequency synchronous activity. Our MEG results are consistent with the second notion of temporal binding in that we find that selective attention helps synchronize the late activity across brain regions, similar to a study conducted in monkeys by Fries and colleagues (2001). Our results and results of others reviewed in this paper suggest that by capitalizing on the temporal resolution of neuromagnetic measures, insights into the connectivity patterns of the different cortical regions (i.e., functional systems or networks) can be obtained.

FINAL COMMENTS

A review of MEG visual studies conducted over the past 30 years leads one to note the variety of methods applied to the analysis of MEG data as well as differences in the designs of the studies. A few issues mentioned below capture differences in investigator opinions, both implicit and explicit, which deserve some attention.

Source Modeling Issues

The most frequently used source model in MEG assumes that the observed field pattern at any instant in time can be approximated by using a single equivalent current dipole (ECD). For multiple-dipole modeling, the surface distribution can be approximated by a set of ECDs with fixed locations, the moments of which vary with time. In the ECD approach, the fitting procedure is generally overdetermined because the number of dipole parameters is less than the number of independent MEG measurements. Several investigators have tested the accuracy of source localization using this approach on computer-simulated data and by using physical models, for which the source and head models are known (e.g., Weinberg *et al.*, 1986; Barth *et al.*, 1989; Achim *et al.*, 1991; Supek and Aine, 1993).

Another type of source model divides the entire brain or just the cortex into a large number of grid sites (e.g., distributed source model). Because the number of unknown parameters for the distributed source model is greater than the number of MEG measurements (10,000–1,000,000 unknowns versus 100–200 measurements), the problem is highly underdetermined, thus requiring additional mathematical constraints. The current distribution is obtained at these sites by fitting the data using mathematical constraints such as minimum norm (e.g., Ioannides *et al.*, 1994; Wang *et al.*, 1992; Dale and Sereno, 1993; Hämäläinen and Ilmoniemi, 1994; Pascual-Marqui *et al.*, 1994; Grave de Peralta-Menendez and Gonzalez-Andino, 1998; Uutela *et al.*, 1999).

Analysis methods in the early days of MEG were clearly dominated by use of a single-dipole model applied to instants in time. Currently, single-dipole modeling techniques are still commonly used, as well as multidipole, spatiotemporal models, but variants of minimum norm methods are beginning to gain ground [e.g., minimum current estimates (Uutela *et al.*, 1999)]. Regardless of the method of choice for the investigator, it is important for investigators to apply modeling procedures that are objective and easily described. Current methods that do not require investigators to provide starting parameters and are relatively easy to describe are as follows: (1) variants of multidipole, spatiotemporal modeling (e.g., Scherg, 1990) using R- or RAP-MUSIC algorithms (Mosher and Leahy, 1998; Ermer *et al.*, 2000); (2) variants of multidipole, spatiotemporal modeling using multistart methods (Huang *et al.*, 1998; Aine *et al.*, 2000); (3) variants of minimum norm methods (e.g., Hämäläinen and Ilmoniemi, 1994) using magnetic field tomography (Ioannides *et al.*, 1990, 1993); (4) variants of minimum norm methods using minimum current estimates (Uutela *et al.*, 1999); and (5) bayesian inference (Schmidt *et al.*, 1999).

One criticism of the spatiotemporal, multidipole methods focuses on the assumption that cognitive processes are represented as extended regions of tissue (rather than focal). Indeed, older hierarchical models of cortical organization, which view sensory signals as being elaborated on at successive stages in sensory association cortices with information flow in one basic direction, implied that cognitions might be represented in brain as extended in nature. However, current anatomical and physiological data depict cortical organization of cognitive functions as distributed module-mosaics that are reciprocally interconnected by a finite number of dedicated networks (e.g., Goldman-Rakic, 1988). Ojemann and colleagues (1989), for example, show that even language is highly localized in most patients, using electrical stimulation mapping techniques; it is composed of several mosaics of 1 to 2 cm^2, usually one in the frontal region and one or more in the temporoparietal lobe. Numerous invasive studies in monkeys point to similar conclusions, even for higher order functions such as memory.

Fahy *et al.* (1993), for example, found evidence for clustering of neurons with recognition memory-related activity as if such neurons may occur in cortical columns.

Central Fixation: Attention or Eye Movement?

Many visual functional neuroimaging studies are reporting bilateral activity in the lateral frontal gyri, medial frontal gyrus, and bilateral parietal cortical activity (e.g., intraparietal sulcus) across a number of different tasks (e.g., Kim *et al.*, 1999; Nobre *et al.*, 1997; Kosslyn *et al.*, 1997; Courtney *et al.*, 1997; Campanella *et al.*, 2001; Aine and Stephen, 2002). These cortical regions correspond well with the frontal eye fields, supplementary eye fields, and the parietal eye fields, as discussed by several authors (e.g., Anderson *et al.*, 1994; Berman *et al*, 1999; Petit and Haxby, 1999; Petit *et al.*, 1999; Paus, 1996; Paus *et al.*, 1991; Ploner *et al.*, 1999; Morrow and Sharpe, 1995). Are these regions unique to the specific task instructions at hand (e.g., mental figure rotation or spatial attention), are they related to eye movements, or are they a result of attending to the fixation point? Corbetta (1998) suggests that the attention and eye movement systems share the same neural network, i.e., attention is covert eye movements. To make things even more confusing, eye movements can be as subtle as maintaining fixation, as noted in results reported by Petit and colleagues (1999) and Leinonen and Nyman (1979). This pattern of results has become a hallmark of visual studies, including those that do not require cognitive processing at all, other than maintaining central fixation (e.g., Stephen *et al.*, 2002). Vanni and Uutela (2000) attempted to examine this complex issue and noted large differences in the putative right FEF activity between conditions in which subjects were required to fixate centrally versus a control condition in which subjects were detecting tones. In the latter case, the FEF is not likely to be as active because subjects were not as concerned about maintaining central fixation while engaged in an auditory task. Unfortunately, the details of this control experiment, which was conducted on only 2 of the 11 subjects, is lacking (e.g., how do we know these subjects were fixating centrally during the auditory task?). It is clear that additional studies will be required in order to understand the complex relationship between eye movements, maintaining central fixation, and attention on this frontal-parietal system.

Multimodality Imaging

Most investigators would agree that multimodality imaging is a reasonable direction to pursue because different techniques provide complementary information (e.g., George et al., 1995; Heinze et al., 1994; Ahlfors et al., 1999; Liu et al., 1998; Dale et al., 2000; Dale and Halgren, 2001). However, initial simplistic notions suggesting the use of fMRI locations to constrain multidipole, spatiotemporal models in order to obtain the time courses for fMRI locations can be misleading. Because we do not understand the exact relationship between changes in membrane potentials and changes in blood oxygenation levels, it seems prudent to compare and contrast MEG and fMRI measures initially and to use fMRI location information to "guide," as opposed to "constrain," MEG analyses (e.g., Ahlfors et al., 1999). MEG computer simulations indicate that undermodeling the data, or even having the correct model order (i.e., number of dipoles) but a poor set of starting parameters for an error surface containing many local minima (i.e., many sources and/or low signal-to-noise ratio), can provide erroneous time courses (Supek and Aine, 1997).

There are several reasons why one would not expect to find a one-to-one correspondence between active source regions localized from MEG versus fMRI. First, the optical imaging experiments find that many of the largest signals corresponding with blood volume changes originated from the larger elements of the microvasculature, which were outside of the activated area (Frostig et al., 1990); i.e., the later phase of the vascular response is less localized (Malonek and Grinvald, 1996). Second, fMRI results represent activity averaged across seconds of time whereas most MEG results focus on millisecond windows in time. It may be the case that later slow-wave activity noted in many cognitive MEG studies correlates best with fMRI, because it is sustained for >1 second. This issue needs further investigation. We have also noted that when long time intervals are modeled in the MEG studies (e.g., 500–1000 msec), some of the early activity is not modeled, as if the later and longer duration activity dominates longer time intervals. This problem often prompts one to examine more than one window of time. Third, MEG can detect subtle changes in stimulus parameters (e.g., spatial frequency content, contrast, temporal frequency, and area of retinal stimulation), whereas fMRI requires strong stimulus parameters (larger and brighter stimuli) in order to evoke a noticeable change in blood oxygenation.

In conclusion, the past 30 years has produced very exciting changes in MEG hardware, providing dense, whole-head coverage. Although a significant amount of work has also been devoted toward developing more automated multisource modeling techniques and global minimizers, many of these analysis tools have not been sufficiently evaluated nor widely distributed throughout the MEG community, as evidenced by the number of studies using a single-dipole model for analysis of sensory and cognitive data. However, we are likely to witness significant improvements in this regard during the next decade, because at this point in time, noninvasive MEG and EEG methods provide our best hope for understanding the temporal dynamics of the different functional networks mediating sensory and cognitive processes. A complete understanding of the functional organization of human visual system must incorporate *when* and *how long* events are occurring, in addition to *where* they are occurring.

Okada's group recently demonstrated in swine that MEG is capable of monitoring the synchronized population spikes of the thalamocortical axonal terminals and cortical neurons from outside the skull (Ikeda *et al.*, 2002), thereby providing the most compelling evidence yet that MEG is capable of directly examining population spike activity. Our own personal experiences indicate that MEG is capable of showing much more detail about brain functions than originally imagined, and MEG has much better spatial resolution than originally postulated, given that appropriate models are applied to the data. Once appropriate head models become available to EEG studies, many of the MEG analysis tools can be applied to EEG data as well, which will enable us to examine the complementary nature of these two methods. We look forward to a meaningful integration of MEG, EEG, fMRI, and PET results to help elucidate the functional organization of the human brain.

Acknowledgments

This work was supported by the NIH (NEI, 5R01-EY08610-10; and NCRR, 1-P20-RR-15636; the MIND Institute (#2006); the VA Merit Review ("Functional Neuroimaging of Normal Aging"); the Research Service, Department of Veterans Affairs; and the Department of Radiology, UNM School of Medicine. We wish to thank Selma Supek, David Hudson, Sanja Kovacevic, and Chad Woodruff for their helpful comments on the manuscript.

References

Achim, A., Richer, F., and Saint-Hilaire, J. M. (1991). Methodological considerations for the evaluation of spatiotemporal source models. *Electroencephalogr. Clin. Neurophysiol.* **79**, 227–240.

Aersten, A., Erb, M., Palm, G., and Schütz, A. (1994). Coherent assembly dynamics in the cortex: Multineuron recordings, network simulations and anatomical considerations. *In* "Oscillatory Event Related Brain Dynamics" (C. Pantev *et al.*, eds.), pp. 59–83. Plenum, New York.

Aggleton, J. P., Burton, M. J., and Passingham, R. E. (1980). Cortical and subcortical afferents to the amygdala in the rhesus monkey (*Macaca mulatta*). *Brain Res.* **190**, 347–368.

Ahlfors, S. P., Ilmoniemi, R. J., Hämäläinen, M. S. (1992). Estimates of visually evoked cortical currents. *Electroencephalogr. Clin. Neurophysiol.* **82**, 225–236.

Ahlfors, S. P., Simpson, G. V., Dale, A. M., Belliveau, J. W., Liu, A. K., Korvenoja, A., Virtanen, J., Huotilainen, M., Tootell, R. B., Aronen, H. J., and Ilmoniemi, R. J. (1999). Spatiotemporal activity of a cortical network for processing visual motion revealed by MEG and fMRI. *J. Neurophysiol.* **82**, 2545–2555.

Aine, C. J., and Stephen, J. M. (2002). Task relevance enhances and synchronizes late slow-wave activity of distributed cortical sources (submitted).

Aine, C. J., Supek, S., and George, J.S. (1995). Temporal dynamics of visual-evoked neuromagnetic sources: Effects of stimulus parameters and selective attention. *Int. J Neurosci.* **80**, 79–104.

Aine, C. J., Supek, S., George J. S., Ranken, D., Lewine, J., Sanders, J., Best, E., Tiee, W., Flynn, E., and R.R., Wood, C. C. (1996). Retinotopic organization of human visual cortex: Departures from the classical model. *Cereb. Cortex* **6**, 354–361.

Aine, C. J., Huang, M., Stephen, J., and Christner, R. (2000). Multistart algorithms for MEG empirical data analysis reliably characterize locations and time courses of multiple sources. *NeuroImage* **12**, 159–172.

Albright, T. D. (1984). Direction and orientation selectivity of neurons in visual area MT of the macaque. *J. Neurophysiol.* **52**, 1106–1130.

Amidzic, O., Riehle, H. J., Fehr, T., Wienbruch, C., and Elbert, T. (2001). Pattern of focal gamma-bursts in chess players. *Nature* **412**, 603.

Anderson, S. J., Holliday, I. E., Singh, K. D., and Harding, G. F. (1996). Localization and functional analysis of human cortical area V5 using magnetoencephalography. *Proc. R. Soc. Lond. B. Biol. Sci.* **263**, 423–431.

Anderson, L. J., Jenkins, I. H., Brooks, D. J., Hawken, M. B., Frackowiak, R. S. J., and Kennard, C. (1994). Cortical control of saccades and fixation in man: A PET study. *Brain* **117**, 1073–1084.

Armstrong, R. A., Slaven, A., and Harding, G. F. (1991). Visual evoked magnetic fields to flash and pattern in 100 normal subjects. *Vis. Res.* **31**, 1859–1864.

Bagshaw, M.H., Mackworth, N. H., and Pribram, K. H. (1972). The effect of resections of the inferotemporal cortex or the amygdala on visual orienting and habituation. *Neuropsychologia.* **10**, 153–162.

Baizer, J. S., Ungerleider, L. G., and Desimone, R. (1991). Organization of visual inputs to the inferior temporal and posterior parietal cortex in macaques. *J. Neurosci.* **11**, 168–190.

Barth, D. S., Baumgartner, C., and Sutherling, W. W. (1989). Neuromagnetic field modeling of multiple brain regions producing interictal spikes in human epilepsy. *Electroencephalogr. Clin. Neurophysiol.* **73**, 389–402.

Barth, D. S., Sutherling, W., Broffman, J., and Beatty, J. (1986). Magnetic localization of a dipolar current source implanted in a sphere and a human cranium. *Electroencephalogr. Clin. Neurophysiol.* **63**, 260–273.

Baylis, G. C., Rolls, E. T., and Leonard, C. M. (1987). Functional subdivisions of the temporal lobe neocortex. *J. Neurosci.* **7**, 330–342.

Berman, R. A., Colby, C. L., Genovese, C. R., Voyvodic, J. T., Luna, B., Thulborn, K. R., and Sweeney, J. A. (1999). Cortical networks subserving pursuit and saccadic eye movements in humans: an fMRI study. *Human Brain Mapping* **8**, 209–225.

Boussaoud, D., Desimone, R., and Ungerleider, L. G. (1991). Visual topography of area TEO in the macaque. *J. Comp. Neurol.* **306**, 554–575.

Braeutigam, S., Bailey, A. J., and Swithenby, S. J. (2001). Phase–locked gamma band responses to semantic violation stimuli. *Brain. Res. Cogn. Res.* **10**, 365–377.

Brefczynski, J. A., and De Yoe, E. A. (1999). A physiological correlate of the 'spotlight' of visual attention. *Nature Neurosci.* **2**, 370–374.

Breitmeyer, B. (1975). Simple reaction time as a measure of the temporal response properties of transient and sustained channels. *Vis. Res.* **15**, 1411–1412.

Breitmeyer, B. G., and Ganz, L. (1976). Implications of sustained and transient channels for theories of visual pattern masking saccadic suppression, and information processing. *Psychol. Rev.* **83**, 1–36.

Brenner, D., Williamson, S. J., and Kaufman, L. (1975). Visually evoked magnetic field of the human brain. *Science* **190**, 480–482.

Broadbent, D. E. (1958). "Perception and Communication." Pergamon, London.

Bushnell, M. C., Goldberg, M. E., and Robinson, D. L. (1981). Behavioral enhancement of visual responses in monkey cerebral cortex. I. Modulation in posterior parietal cortex related to selective visual attention. *J. Neurophysiol.* **46**, 755–772.

Butler, S. R., Georgiou, G. A., Glass, A., Hancox, R. J., Hopper, J. M., and Smith, K. R. H. (1987). Cortical generators of the CI component of the pattern-onset visual evoked potential. *Electroencephalogr. Clin. Neurophysiol.* **68**, 256–267.

Butter, C. M. (1969). Impairments in selective attention to visual stimuli in monkeys with inferotemporal and lateral striate lesions. *Brain Res.* **12**, 374–383.

Campanella, S., Joassin, F., Rossion, B., De Volder, A., Bruyer, R., and Crommelinck, M. (2001). Association of the distinct visual representations of faces and names: A PET activation study. *NeuroImage* **14**, 873–882.

Campbell, F. W., and Kulikowski, J. J. (1972). The visual evoked potential as a function of contrast of a grating pattern. *J. Physiol.* **222**, 345–356.

Campbell, F. W., and Maffei, L. (1970). Electrophysiological evidence for the existence of orientation and size detectors in the human visual system. *J. Physiol.* **207**, 534–652.

Chapman, R. M., Ilmoniemi, R. J., Barbanera, S., and Romani, G. L. (1984). Selective localization of alpha brain activity with neuromagnetic measurements. *Electroencephalogr. Clin. Neurophysiol.* **58**, 569–572.

Cheng, K., Fujita, H., Kanno, I., Miura, S., and Tanaka, K. (1995). Human cortical regions activated by wide-field visual motion: An H2 (15)O PET study. *J. Neurophysiol.* **74**, 413–427.

Ciulla, C., Takeda, T., and Endo, H. (1999). MEG characterization of spontaneous alpha rhythm in the human brain. *Brain Topogr.* **11**, 211–222.

Clarke, P. G. (1973a). Visual evoked potentials to changes in the motion of patterned field. *Exp. Brain Res.* **18**, 145–155.

Clarke, P. G. (1973b). Comparison of visual evoked potentials to stationary and to moving patterns. *Exp. Brain Res.* **18**, 156–164.

Clarke, S., and Miklossy, J. (1990). Occipital cortex in man: Organization of callosal connections, related myelo- and cytoarchitecture, and putative boundaries of functional visual areas. *J. Comp. Neurol.* **298**, 188–214.

Cohen, D. (1968). Magnetoencephalography: evidence of magnetic fields produced by alpha-rhythm currents. *Science* **161**, 784–786.

Cohen, D. (1972). Magnetoencephalography: Detection of the brain's electrical activity with a superconducting magnetometer. *Science* **175**, 664–666.

Connor, C. E., Preddie, D. C., Gallant, J. L., and Van Essen, D. C. (1997). Spatial attention effects in Macaque Area V4. *J. Neurosci.* **17**, 3201–3214.

Cooper, L. A., and Shepard, R. N. (1973). The time required to prepare for a rotated stimulus. *Memory Cogn.* **1**, 246–250.

Corbetta, M. (1998). Frontoparietal cortical networks for directing attention and the eye to visual locations: identical, independent, or overlapping neural systems? *Proc. Natl. Acad. Sci. U.S.A.* **95**, 831–838.

Corbetta, M., Miezin, F. M., Dobmeyer, S., Shulman, G. L., and Petersen, S. E. (1991). Selective and divided attention during visual discriminations of shape, color, and speed: functional anatomy by positron emission tomography. *J. Neurosci.* **11**, 2383–2402.

Corbetta, M., Miezin, F. M., Shulman, G. L., and Petersen, S. E. (1993). A PET study of visuospatial attention. *J. Neurosci.* **13**, 1202–1226.

Cornette, L., Dupont, P., Spileers, W., Sunaert, S., Michiels, J., Van Hecke, P., Mortelmans, L., and Orban, G. A. (1998). Human cerebral activity evoked by motion reversal and motion onset. A PET study. *Brain* **121**, 143–157.

Courtney, S. M., Ungerleider, L. G., Kell, K., and Haxby, J. V. (1997). Transient and sustained activity in a distributed neural system for human working memory. *Nature* **386**, 608–611.

Cowey, A., and Weiskrantz, L. (1967). A comparison of the effects of inferotemporal and striate cortical lesions on visual behavior of rhesus monkeys. *Q. J. Exp. Psychol.* **19**, 246–253.

Cragg, B. G. (1969). The topography of the afferent projections in the circumstriate visual cortex of the monkey studied by the Nauta method. *Vis. Res.* **9**, 733–747.

Cuffin, B. N. (1990). Effects of head shape on EEG's and MEG's. *IEEE BME* **32**, 905–910.

Dale, A. M., and Halgren, E. (2001). Spatiotemporal mapping of brain activity by integration of multiple imaging modalities. *Curr. Opin. Neurobiol.* **11**, 202–208.

Dale, A. M., and Sereno M. I. (1993). Improved localization of cortical activity by combining EEG and MEG with MRI cortical surface reconstruction: a linear approach. *J. Cogn. Neurosci.* **5**, 162–176.

Dale, A. M., Liu, A. K., Fischl, B. R., Buckner, R. L., Belliveau, J. W., Lewine, J. D., and Halgren, E. (2000). Dynamic statistical paramagnetic mapping: Combining fMRI and MEG for high-resolution imaging of cortical activity. *Neuron* **26**, 55–67.

Damasio, A. R. (1985). Prosopagnosia. *Trends Neurosci.* **8**, 132–135.

Damasio, A. R. Damasio, H., and Van Hoesen, G. W. (1982). Prosopagnosia: Anatomic basis and behavioral mechanisms. *Neurology* **32**, 331–334.

Darcey, T. M., Ary, J. P., and Fender, D. H. (1980). Spatiotemporal visually evoked scalp potentials in response to partial-field patterned stimulation. *Electroencephalogr. Clin. Neurophysiol.* **50**, 348–355.

De Monasterio, F. M., and Gouras, P. (1975). Functional properties of ganglion cells of the Rhesus monkey retina. *J. Physiol.* **251**, 167–195.

De Renzi, E. (1986). Current issues in prosopagnosia. *In* "Aspects of Face Processing" (H. D. Ellis, M. A. Jeeves, F. Newcombe, and A. Young, eds), pp. 153–252. Marinus Nijhoff, Dordrecht.

Desimone, R., and Duncan, J. (1995). Neural mechanisms of selective visual attention. *Annu. Rev. Neurosci.* **18**, 193–222.

Desimone, R., Fleming, J., and Gross, C. G. (1980). Prestriate afferents to inferior temporal cortex: an HRP study. *Brain Res.* **184**, 41–55.

Desimone, R., and Gross, C. G. (1979). Visual areas in the temporal cortex of the macaque. *Brain Res.* **178**, 363–380.

Deutsch, J. A., and Deutsch, D. (1963). Attention: Some theoretical considerations. *Psychol. Rev.* **70**, 80–90.

De Yoe, E. A., and Van Essen, D. C. (1988). Concurrent processing streams in monkey visual cortex. *Trends Neurosci.* **11**, 219–226.

De Yoe, E. A., Felleman, D. J., Van Essen, D. V., and McClendon, E. (1994). Multiple processing streams in occipitotemporal cortex. *Nature* **371**, 151–154.

Drasdo, N. (1980). Cortical potentials evoked by pattern presentation in the foveal region. *In* "Evoked Potentials" (C. Barber ed.), pp. 167–174 MTP Press, Lancaster.

Eason, R. G. (1981). Visual evoked potential correlates of early neural filtering during selective attention. *Bull. Psychonom. Soc.* **18**, 203–206.

Eason, R. G., Harter, M. R., and White, C. T. (1969). Effects of attention and arousal on visually evoked cortical potentials and reaction time in man. *Physiol. Behavior.* **4**, 283–289.

Eason, R. G., Oakley, M., and Flowers, L. (1983). Central neural influences on the human retina during selective attention. *Physiol. Psychol.* **11**, 18–28.

Engel, A. K., König, P., Kreiter, A. K., Schillen, T. B., and Singer, W. (1992). Temporal coding in the visual cortex: new vistas on integration in the nervous system. *Trends Neurosci.* **15**, 218–226.

Engel, A. K., König, P., Kreiter, A. K., and Singer, W. (1991). Interhemispheric synchronization of oscillatory neuronal responses in cat visual cortex. *Science* **252**, 1177–1179.

Enroth-Cugell, C., and Robson, J. G. (1966). The contrast sensitivity of retinal ganglion cells of the cat. *J. Physiol.* **187**, 517–551.

Ermer, J. J., Mosher, J. C., Huang, M., and Leahy, R. M. (2000). Paired MEG data set source localization using recursively applied and projected (RAP) MUSIC. *IEEE Trans. Biomed. Eng.* **47**, 1248–1260.

Eulitz, C., Maess, B., Pantev, C., Friederici, A. D., Feige, B., and Elbert, T. (1996). Oscillatory neuromagnetic activity induced by language and nonlanguage stimuli. *Cogn. Brain Res.* **4**, 121–132.

Eulitz, C., Eulitz, H., Maess, B., Cohen, R., Pantev, C., and Elbert, T. (2000). Magnetic brain activity evoked and induced by visually presented words and nonverbal stimuli. *Psychophysiology.* **37**, 447–455.

Fahy, F. L., Riches, I. P., and Brown, M. W. (1993). Neuronal activity related to visual recognition memory: Long-term memory and the encoding of recency and familiarity information in the primate anterior and medial inferior temporal and rhinal cortex. *Exp. Brain Res.* **96**, 457–472.

Felleman, D. J., and Kaas, J. H. (1984). Receptive-field properties of neurons in middle temporal visual area (MT) of owl monkeys. *J. Neurophysiol* **52**, 488–513.

Felleman, D. J., and Van Essen, D. C. (1991). Distributed hierarchical processing in the primate cerebral cortex. *Cereb. Cortex.* **1**, 1–47.

Ferrera, V. P., Nealey, T. A., and Maunsell, J. H. R. (1994). Responses in Macaque visual area V4 following inactivation of the parvocellular and magnocellular LGN pathways. *J. Neurosci.* **14**, 2080–2088.

ffytche, D. H., Skidmore, B. D., and Zeki, S. (1995a). Motion-from-hue activates area V5 of human visual cortex. *Proc. R. Soc. Lond. B Biol. Sci.* **260**, 353–358.

ffytche, D. H., Guy, C. N., and Zeki, S. (1995b). The parallel visual motion inputs into areas V1 and V5 of human cerebral cortex. *Brain* **118**, 1375–1394.

Fries, P., Reynolds, J. H., Rorie, A. E., and Desimone, R. (2001). Modulation of oscillatory neuronal synchronization by selective visual attention. *Science* **291**, 1560–1563.

Frostig, R., Lieke, E., Ts'o, D., and Grinvald, A. (1990). Cortical functional architecture and local coupling between neuronal activity and the microcirculation revealed by in vivo high-resolution optical imaging of intrinsic signals. *Proc. Natl. Acad. Sci. U.S.A.* **87**, 6082.

Fylan, F., Holliday, I. E., Singh, K. D., Anderson, S. J., and Harding, G. F. A. (1997). Magnetoencephalographic investigation of human cortical area V1 using color stimuli. *NeuroImage* **6**, 47–57.

Gaetz, M., Weinberg, H., Rzempoluck, E., and Jantzen, K. J. (1998). Neural network classifications and correlation analysis of EEG and MEG activity accompanying spontaneous reversals of the Necker cube. *Cogn. Brain Res.* **6**, 335–346.

Gallese, V., Fadiga, L., Fogassi, L., and Rizzolatti, G. (1996). Action recognition in the premotor cortex. *Brain* **119**, 593–609.

Galletti, C., Fattori, P., Kutz, D. F., and Gamberini, M., (1999). Brain location and visual topography of cortical area V6A in the Macaque monkey. *Euro. J. Neurosci.* **11**, 575–582.

Gauthier, I., Tarr, M. J., Anderson, A. W., Skudlarski, P., and Gore, J. C. (1999). Activation of the middle fusiform 'face area' increases with expertise in recognizing novel objects. *Nat. Neurosci.* **2**, 568–573.

Geesaman, B. J., and Andersen, R. A. (1996). The analysis of complex motion patterns by form/cue invariant MSTd neurons. *J. Neurosci.* **16**, 4716–4732.

George, J. S., Aine, C. J., Mosher, J. C., Schmidt, D. M., Ranken, D. M., Schlitt, H. A., Wood, C. C., Lewine,

J. D., Sanders, J. A., and Belliveau, J. W. (1995). Mapping function in the human brain with magnetoencephalography, anatomical magnetic resonance imaging and functional magnetic resonance imaging. *J. Clin. Neurophysiol.* **12**, 406–431.

Ghandi, S. P., Heeger, D. J., and Boynton, G. M. (1999). Spatial attention affects cortical activity in human primary visual cortex. *Proc. Natl. Acad. Sci. U.S.A.* **96**, 3314–3319.

Goldman-Rakic, P. S. (1988). Topography of cognition: Parallel distributed networks in primate association cortex. *Annu. Rev. Neurosci.* **11**, 137–156.

Goodale, M. A., Meenan, J. P., Bulthoff, H. H., Nicolle, D. A., Murphy, K. J., and Racicot, C. I. (1994). Separate neural pathways for the visual analysis of object shape in perception and prehension. *Curr. Biol.* **4**, 604–610.

Grave de Paralta-Menendez, R., and Gonzalez-Andino, S. L. (1998). A critical analysis of linear inverse solutions to the neuroelectromagnetic inverse problem. *IEEE Trans. Biomed. Eng.* **45**, 440–8.

Gray, C. M. (1999). The temporal correlation hypothesis of visual feature integration: Still alive and well. *Neuron* **24**, 31–47.

Grill-Spector, K., Kushnir, T., Edelman, S., Itzchak, Y., and Malach, R. (1998). Cue-invariant activation in object-related areas of the human occipital lobe. *Neuron* **21**, 191–202.

Gross, C. G. (1973). Visual functions of inferotemporal cortex. *In* "Handbook of Sensory Physiology" (R. Jung, ed), Vol. 7, pp. 451–482. Springer-Verlag, Berlin.

Gross, C. G., Rocha-Miranda, C. E., and Bender, D. B. (1972). Visual properties of neurons in inferotemporal cortex of the macaque. *J. Neurophysiol.* **35**, 96–111.

Gross, C. G., Bender, D. B., and Rocha-Miranda, C. E. (1974). Inferotemporal cortex: a single-unit analysis. *In* "The Neurosciences (Third Study Program)" (F. O. Schmitt and F. G. Worden, eds.), pp. 229–238, MIT Press, Cambridge.

Hadjikhani, N., Liu, A. K., Dale, A. M., Cavanagh, P., and Tootell, R. B. H. (1998). Retinotopy and color sensitivity in human visual cortical area V8. *Nat. Neurosci.* **1**, 235–241.

Haenny, P. E., and Schiller, P. H. (1988). State dependent activity in monkey visual cortex. I. Single cell activity in V1 and V4 on visual tasks. *Exp. Brain Res.* **69**, 225–244.

Haenny, P. E., Maunsell, J. H. R., and Schiller, P. H. (1988). State dependent activity in monkey visual cortex. II. Extraretinal factors in V4. *Exp. Brain Res.* **69**, 245–259.

Halgren, E., Dale, A. M., Sereno, M. I., Tootell, R. B. H., Marinkovic, K., and Rosen, B. R. (1999). Location of human face-selective cortex with respect to retinotopic areas. *Human Brain Mapping.* **7**, 29–37.

Halgren, E., Raij, T., Marinkovic, K., Jousmäki, V., and Hari, R. (2000). Cognitive response profile of the human fusiform face area as determined by MEG. *Cereb. Cortex.* **10**, 69–81.

Hämäläinen, M. S., and Ilmoniemi, R. J. (1994). Interpreting magnetic fields of the brain: Minimum norm estimates. *Med. Biol. Eng. Comput.* **32**, 35–42.

Hämäläinen, M. S., and Sarvas, J. (1987). Feasibility of the homogeneous head model in the interpretation of neuromagnetic fields. *Phys. Med. Biol.* **32**, 91–97.

Hämäläinen, M. S., and Sarvas, J. (1989). Realistic conductivity geometry model of the human head for interpretation of neuromagnetic data. *IEEE BME* **36**, 165–171.

Harding, G. F. A., Janday, B., and Armstrong, R. A. (1991). Topographic mapping and source localization of the pattern reversal visual evoked magnetic response. *Brain Topogr.* **4**, 47–55.

Harding, G. F. A., Degg, C., Anderson, S. J. , Holliday, I., Fylan, F., Barnes, G., and Bedford, J. (1994). Topographic mapping of the pattern onset evoked magnetic response to stimulation of different portions of the visual field. *Int. J. Psychophysiol.* **16**, 175–183.

Hari, R., and Salmelin, R. (1997). Human cortical oscillations: a neuromagnetic view through the skull. *Trends Neurosci.* **20**, 44–49.

Hari, R., Salmelin, R., Makela, J. P., Salenius, S., and Helle, M. (1997). Magnetoencephalographic cortical rhythms. *Int. J. Psychophysiol.* **26**, 51–62.

Hari, R., Aittoniemi, L., Järvinen, M. L., Katila, T., and Varpula, T. (1980). Auditory evoked transient and sustained magnetic fields of the human brain. *Exp. Brain Res.* **40**, 237–240.

Harrison, R. R., Aine, C. J., Chen, H.-W., and Flynn, E. R. (1996). Comparison of minimization methods for spatio-temporal electromagnetic source localization using temporal constraints. *NeuroImage* **3**, S64.

Harter, M. R., and Aine, C. J. (1984). Brain mechanisms of visual selective attention. *In* (R. Parasuraman and D. R. Davies, (eds.), "Varieties of Attention" pp. 293–321. Academic Press, New York.

Harter, M. R., Aine, C. J., and Schroeder, C. (1982). Hemispheric differences in the neural processing of stimulus location and type: Effects of selective attention on visual evoked potentials. *Neuropsychologia* **20**, 421–438.

Hashimoto, I., Kashii, S., Kikuchi, M., Honda, Y., Nagamine, T., and Shibasaki, H. (1999). Temporal profile of visual evoked responses to pattern-reversal stimulation analyzed with a whole-head magnetometer. Exp. Brain. Res. 125, 375–382.

Haxby, J. V., Grady, C. L., Horwitz, B., Ungerleider, L. G., Mishkin, M., Carson, R. E., Herscovitch, P., Schapiro, M. B., and Rapoport, S. I. (1991). Dissociation of object and spatial visual processing pathways in human extrastriate cortex. *Proc. Natl. Acad. Sci. U.S.A.* **88**, 1621–1625.

Haxby, J. V., Horwitz, B., Ungerleider, L. G., Maisog, J. M., Pietrini, P., and Grady, C. L. (1994). The functional organization of human extrastriate cortex: A PET-rCBF study of selective attention to faces and locations. *J. Neurosci.* **14**, 6336–6353.

Haxby, J. V., Ungerleider, L. G., Clark, V. P., Schouten, J. L., Hoffman, E. A., and Martin, A. (1999). The effect of face inversion on activity in human neural systems for face and object perception. *Neuron* **22**, 189-199.

Heinze, H. J., Mangun, G. R., Burchert, W., Hinrichs, H., Scholz, M., Munte, T. F., Gos, A., Scherg, M., Johannes, S., and Hundeshagen, H. (1994). Combined spatial and temporal imaging of the brain activity during visual selective attention in humans. *Nature* **372**, 543-546.

Hillyard, S. A. (1985). Electrophysiology of human selective attention. *Trends Neurosci.* **8**, 400–405.

Hillyard, S. A., and Munte, T. F. (1984). Selective attention to color and locational cues: An analysis with event-related brain potentials. *Percept. Psychophys.* **36**, 185–198.

Hoffman, J. E. (1978). Search through a sequentially presented visual display. *Percept. Psychophys.* **23**, 1–11.

Holliday, I. E., Anderson, S. J., and Harding, G. F. (1997). Magnetoencephalographic evidence for non-geniculostriate visual input to human cortical area V5. *Neuropsychologia* **35**, 1139–1146.

Huang, M., Aine, C. J., Supek, S., Best, E., Ranken, and Flynn, E. R. (1998). Multi-start downhill simplex method for spatiotemporal source localization in magnetoencephalography. *Electroencephalogr. Clin. Neurophysiol.* **108**, 32–44.

Huk, A. C., and Heeger, D. J. (2000). Task-related modulation of visual cortex. *J. Neurophysiol.* **83**, 3525–3536.

Ikeda, H., Leyba, L., Bartolo, A., Wang, Y., and Okada, Y. C. (2002). Synchronized spikes of thalamocortical axonal terminals and cortical neurons are detectable outside the brain of piglet with high-resolution of MEG. *J. Neurophysiol.* **87**, 626–630.

Ioannides, A. A., Bolton, J. P., and Clarke, C. J. (1990). Continuous probabilistic solutions to the biomagnetic inverse problem. *Inverse Problem* **6**, 523–542.

Ioannides, A. A., Muratore, R., Balish, M., and Sato, S. (1993). *In vivo* validation of distributed source solutions for the biomagnetic inverse problem. *Brain Topogr.* **5**, 263–273.

Ioannides, A. A., Fenwick, P. B., Lumsden, J., Liu, M. J., Bamidis, P. D., Squires, K. C., Lawson, D., and Fenton, G. W. (1994). Activation sequence of discrete brain areas during cognitive processes: results from magnetic field tomography. *Electroencephalogr. Clin. Neurophysiol.* **91**, 399–402.

Ito, M., and Gilbert, C. D. (1999). Attention modulates contextual influences in the primary visual cortex of alert monkeys. *Neuron* **22**, 593–604.

Iwaki, S., Ueno, S., Imada, T., and Tonoike, M. (1999). Dynamic cortical activation in mental image processing revealed by biomagnetic measurement. *NeuroReport* **10**, 1793–1797.

Jacobsen, S., and Trojanowski, J. Q. (1977). Prefrontal granular cortex of the rhesus monkey. I. Intrahemispheric cortical afferents. *Brain Res.* **132**, 209–233.

Jeffreys, D. A., and Axford, J. G. (1972a). Source locations of pattern-specific components of human visual evoked potentials. I. Component of striate cortical origin. *Exp. Brain. Res.* **16**, 1–21.

Jeffreys, D. A., and Axford, J. G. (1972b). Source locations of pattern-specific components of human visual evoked potentials. II. Component of extrastriate cortical origin. *Exp. Brain. Res.* **16**, 22–40.

Jiang, Y., Haxby, J. V., Martin, A., Ungerleider, L. G., and Parasuraman, R. (2000). Complementary neural mechanisms for tracking items in human working memory. *Science* **287**, 643–646.

Johnston, W. A., and Dark, V. J. (1986). Selective attention. *Annu. Rev. Psychol.* **37**, 43–75.

Kahneman, D., and Treisman, A. (1984). Changing views of attention and automaticity. *In* "Varieties of Attention" (R. Parasuraman and D. R. Davies, eds.), pp. 29–61. Academic Press, London.

Kaneoke, Y., Bundou, M., Koyama, S., Suzuki, H., and Kakigi, R. (1997). Human cortical area responding to stimuli in apparent motion. *NeuroReport* **8**, 677–682.

Kaneoke, Y., Bundou, M., and Kakigi, R. (1998). Timing of motion representation in the human visual system. *Brain Res.* **790**, 195–201.

Kanwisher, N., McDermott, J., and Chun, M. M. (1997). The fusiform face area: A module in human extrastriate cortex specialized for face perception. *J. Neurosci.* **17**, 4302–4311.

Kapur, N., Friston, K. J., Young, A., Frith, C. D., and Frackowiak, R. S. J. (1995). Activation of human hippocampal formation during memory for faces: A PET study. *Cortex* **31**, 99–108.

Kaufman, L., and Williamson, S. J. (1980). The evoked magnetic field of the human brain. *Ann. N.Y. Acad. Sci.* **340**, 45–65.

Kaufman, L., Schwartz, B., Salustri, C., and Williamson, S. J. (1990). Modulation of spontaneous brain activity during mental imagery. *J. Cogn. Neurosci.* **2**, 124–132.

Kawakami, O., Kaneoke, Y., and Kakigi, R. (2000). Perception of apparent motion is related to the neural activity in the human extrastriate cortex as measured by magnetoencephalography. *Neurosci. Lett.* **285**, 135–138.

Kawamichi, H., Kikuchi, Y., Endo, H., Takeda, T., and Yoshizawa, S. (1998). Temporal structure of implicit motor imagery in visual hand-shape discrimination as revealed by MEG. *NeuroReport* **9**, 1127–1132.

Kelly, D. H. (1966). Frequency doubling in visual responses. *J. Opt. Soc. Am.* **56**, 1628–1633.

Kim, J. J., Andreasen, N. C., O'Leary, D. S., Wiser, A. K., Boles Ponto, L. L., Watkins, G. L., and Hichwa, R. D. (1999). Direct comparison of the neural substrates of recognition memory for words and faces. Brain **122**, 1069–1083.

Kleinschmidt, A., Lee, B. B., Requardt, M., and Frahm, J. (1996). Functional mapping of color processing by magnetic resonance imaging of responses to selective P- and M-pathway stimulation. *Exp. Brain. Res.* **110**, 279–288.

Klemm, W. R., Gibbons, W. D., Allen, R. G., and Harrison, J. M. (1982). Differences among humans in steady-state evoked potentials: evaluation of alpha activity, attentiveness and cognitive awareness of perceptual effectiveness. *Neuropsychologia* **20**, 317–325.

Kobatake, E., Wang, G., and Tanaka, K. (1998). Effects of shape-discrimination training on the selectivity of inferotemporal cells in adult monkeys. *J. Neurophysiol.* **80**, 324–330.

Kohler, S., Kapur, S., Moscovitch, M., Winocur, G., and Houle, S. (1995). Dissociation of pathways for object and spatial vision: a PET study in humans. *NeuroReport* **6**, 1865–1868.

Kosslyn, S. M. (1988). Aspects of a cognitive neuroscience of mental imagery. *Science* **240**, 1621–1626.

Kosslyn, S. M., Ganis, G., and Thompson, W. L. (2001). Neural foundations of imagery. *Nat. Rev.* **2**, 635–642.

Kosslyn, S. M., Thompson, W. L., and Alpert N. M. (1997). Neural systems shared by visual imagery and visual perception: A positron emission tomography study. *NeuroImage* **6**, 320–334.

Kosslyn, S. M., Thompson, W. L., Kim, I. J., and Alpert, N. M. (1995). Topographical representations of mental images in primary visual cortex. *Nature* **378**, 496–498.

Koyama, S., Kakigi, R., Hoshiyama, M., and Kitamura, Y. (1998). Reading of Japanese Kanji (morphograms) and Kana (syllabograms): A magnetoencephalographic study. *Neuropsychologia* **36**, 83–98.

Kreiman, G., Koch, C., and Fried, I. (2000). Imagery neurons in the human brain. *Nature* **408**, 357–361.

Kuriki, S., Hirata, Y., Fujimaki, N., and Kobayashi, T. (1996). Magnetoencephalographic study on the cerebral neural activities related to the processing of visually presented characters. *Cogn. Brain Res.* **4**, 185–199.

Lachica, E. A., Beck, P. D., and Casagrande, V. A. (1992). Parallel pathways in macaque monkey striate cortex: Anatomically defined columns in layer III. *Proc. Natl. Sci. U.S.A.* **89**, 3566–3570.

Lagae, L., Raiguel, S., and Orban, G. A. (1993). Speed and direction selectivity of macaque middle temporal neurons. *J. Neurophysiol.* **69**, 19–39.

Lam, K., Kaneoki, Y., Gunji, A., Yamasaki, H., Matsumoto, E., Naito, T., and Kakigi, R. (2000). Magnetic response of human extrastriate cortex in the detection of coherent and incoherent motion. *Neuroscience* **97**, 1–10.

Lamme, V. A. F., Zipser, K., and Spekreijse, H. (1998). Figure–ground activity in primary visual cortex is suppressed by anesthesia. *Proc. Natl. Acad. Sci. U.S.A.* **95**, 3263–3268.

Leahy, R. M., Mosher, J. C., Spencer, M. E., Huang, M. X., and Lewine, J. D. (1998). A study of dipole localization accuracy for MEG and EEG using a human skull phantom. *Electroencephalogr. Clin. Neurophysiol.* **107**, 159–173.

Leinonen, L., and Nyman, G. (1979). Functional properties of cells in antero-lateral part of area 7 associative face area of awake monkeys. *Exp. Brain. Res.* **34**, 321–333.

Lesevre, N., and Joseph, J. P. (1979). Modifications of the pattern-evoked potentials (PEP) in relation to the stimulated part of the visual field (clues for the most probable origin of each component). *Electroencephalogr. Clin. Neurophysiol.* **47**, 183–203.

Leventhal, A. G., Rodieck, R. W., and Dreher, B. (1981). Retinal ganglion cell classes in the Old World Monkey: morphology and central projections. *Science* **213**, 1139–1142.

Linkenkaer-Hansen, K., Palva, J. M., Sams, M., Hietanen, J. K., Aronen, H., and Ilmoniemi, R. (1998). Face-selective processing in human extrastriate cortex around 120 msec after stimulus onset revealed by magnetoencephalography and electroencephalography. *Neurosci. Lett.* **253**, 147–150.

Liu, A. K., Belliveau, J. W., and Dale, A. M. (1998). Spatiotemporal imaging of human brain activity using functional MRI constrained magnetoencephalography data: Monte Carlo simulations. *Proc. Natl. Acad. Sci. U.S.A.* **95**, 8945–50.

Liu, L., Ioannides, A. A., and Streit, M. (1999). Single trial analysis of neurophysiological correlates of the recognition of complex objects and facial expressions of emotion. *Brain Topogr.* **11**, 291–303.

Liu, J., Higuchi, M., Marantz, A., and Kanwisher, N. (2000). The selectivity of the occipitotemporal M170 for faces. *NeuroReport* **11**, 337–341.

Livingstone, M. S., and Hubel, D. H. (1987). Psychophysical evidence for separate channels for the perception of form, color, movement, and depth. *J. Neurosci.* **7**, 3416–3468.

Livingstone, M. S., and Hubel, D. H. (1988). Segregation of form, color, movement, and depth: Anatomy, physiology, and perception. *Science* **240**, 740–749.

Logothetis, N. K., and Sheinberg, D. L. (1996). Visual object recognition. *Annu. Rev. Neurosci.* **19**, 577–621.

Lu, S. T., Hämäläinen, M. S., Hari, R., Ilmoniemi, R. J., Lounasmaa, O. V., Sams, M., and Vilkman, V. (1991). Seeing faces activates three separate areas outside the occipital visual cortex in man. *Neuroscience* **43**, 287–290.

Lu, Z. L., Williamson, S. J., and Kaufman, L. (1992). Behavioral lifetime of human auditory sensory memory predicted by physiological measures. *Science* **258**, 1668–1670.

Luber, B., Kaufman, L., and Williamson, S. J. (1989). Brain activity related to spatial visual attention. *In* "Advances in Biomagnetism" (S. J. Williamson, M. Hoke, G. Stroink, and M. Kotani, eds.), pp. 213–216. Plenum, New York.

Luck, S. J., Chelazzi, L., Hillyard, S. A., and Desimone, R. (1997). Neural mechanisms of spatial selective attention in areas V1, V2, and V4 of macaque visual cortex. *J. Neurophysiol.* **77**, 24–42.

Maclin, E., Okada, Y. C., Kaufman, L., and Williamson, S. J. (1983). Retinotopic map on the visual cortex for eccentrically placed patterns: First noninvasive measurement. *Nuovo Cimento* **2**, 410–419.

Maguire, E. A., Frith, C. D., and Cipolotti, L. (2001). Distinct neural systems for the encoding and recognition of topography and faces. *NeuroImage* **13**, 743–750.

Maier, J., Dagnelie, G., Spekreijse, H., and Van Dijk, B. W. (1987). Principal components analysis for source localization of VEPs in man. *Vis. Res.* **27**, 165–177.

Malach, R., Reppas, J. B., Benson, R. R., Kwong, K. K., Jiang, H., Kennedy, W. A., Ledden, P. J., Brady, T. J., Rosen, B. R., and Tootell, R. B. H. (1995). Object-related activity revealed by functional magnetic resonance imaging in human occipital cortex. *Proc. Natl. Acad. Sci. U.S.A.* **92**, 8135–8139.

Malonek, D., and Grinvald, A. (1996). Interactions between electrical activity and cortical microcirculation revealed by imaging spectroscopy: Implications for functional brain mapping. *Science* **272**, 551–554.

Mangun, G. R., and Hillyard, S. A. (1988). Spatial gradients of visual attention: behavioral and electrophysiological evidence. *Electroencephalogr. Clin. Neurophysiol.* **70**, 417–428.

Martin, A., and Chao, L. L. (2001). Semantic memory and the brain: Structure and processes. *Curr. Opin. Neurobiol.* **11**, 194–201.

Martin, A., Haxby, J. V., Lalonde, F. M. Wiggs, C. L., and Ungerleider, L. G. (1995). Discrete cortical regions associated with knowledge of color and knowledge of action. *Science* **270**, 102–105.

Mast, J., and Victor, J. D. (1991). A new statistic for steady-state evoked potentials. *Electroencephalogr. Clin. Neurophysiol.* **78**, 389–401.

Maunsell, J. H. R. (1995). The brain's visual world: Representation of visual targets in cerebral cortex. *Science* **270**, 764–768.

Maunsell, J. H. R., and Newsome, W. T. (1987). Visual processing in monkey extrastriate cortex. *Annu. Rev. Neurosci.* **10**, 363–401.

Maunsell, J. H. R., and Van Essen, D. C. (1983). Anatomical connections of the middle temporal visual area in the macaque monkey and their relationship to a hierarchy of cortical areas. *J. Neurosci.* **3**, 2563–2586.

Maunsell, J. H. R., Nealey, T. A., and DePriest D. D. (1990). Magnocellular and parvocellular contributions to responses in the middle temporal visual area (MT) of the Macaque monkey. *J. Neurosci.* **10**, 3323–3334.

McAdams, C. J., and Maunsell, J. H. R. (1999). Effects of attention on the reliability of individual neurons in monkey visual cortex. *Neuron* **23**, 765–773.

Meadows, J. C (1974). The anatomical basis of prosopagnosia. *J. Neurol. Neurosurg. Psychiatr.* **37**, 489–501.

Mehta, A. D., Ulbert, I., and Schroeder, C. E. (2000a). Intermodal selective attention in monkeys. I. Distribution and timing of effects across visual areas. *Cereb. Cortex* **10**, 343–358.

Mehta, A. D., Ulbert, I., and Schroeder, C. E. (2000b). Intermodal selective attention in monkeys. II. Physiological mechanisms of modulation. *Cereb. Cortex* **10**, 359–370.

Mellet, E., Tzourio-Mazoyer, N., Bricogne, S., Mazoyer, B., Kosslyn, S. M., and Denis, M. (2000). Functional anatomy of high-resolution visual mental imagery. *J. Cogn. Neurosci.* **12**, 98–109.

Merigan, W. H., and Maunsell J. H. R. (1993). How parallel are the primate visual pathways? *Annu. Rev. Neurosci.* **16**, 369–402.

Mesulam, M.-M. (1998). From sensation to cognition. *Brain* **121**: 1013–1052.

Michael, W. F., and Halliday, A. M. (1971). Differences between the occipital distribution of upper and lower field pattern evoked responses in man. *Brain Res.* **32**, 311–324.

Michel, C. M., Kaufman, L., and Williamson, S. J. (1994). Duration of EEG and MEG α suppression increases with angle in a mental rotation task. *J. Cogn. Neurosci.* **6**, 139–150.

Milner, B. (1963). Effects of different brain lesions on card sorting: The role of the frontal lobes. *Arch. Neurol.* **9**, 100–110.

Mishkin, M. (1982). A memory system in the monkey. *Philos. Trans. R. Soc. Lond.* **298**, 85–95.

Moran, J., Desimone, R. (1985). Selective attention gates visual processing in the extrastriate cortex. *Science* **229**, 782–784.

Morrow, M. J., and Sharpe, J. A. (1995). Deficits of smooth-pursuit eye movement after unilateral frontal lobe lesions. *Ann. Neurol.* **37**, 443–451.

Mosher, J. C., and Leahy, R. M. (1998). Recursive MUSIC: A framework for EEG and MEG source localization. *IEEE Trans. Biomed. Eng.* **45**, 1342–1354.

Motter, B. C. (1993). Focal attention produces spatially selective processing in visual cortical areas V1, V2, and V4 in the presence of competing stimuli. *J. Neurophysiol.* **70**, 909–919.

Motter, B. C. (1994). Neural correlates of feature selective memory and pop-out in extrastriate Area V4. *J. Neurosci.* **14**, 2190–2199.

Movshon, J. A., and Newsome, W. T. (1996). Visual response properties of striate cortical neurons projecting to area MT in macaque monkeys. *J. Neurosci.* **16**(23), 7733–7741.

Naito, T., Kaneoke, Y., Osaka, N., and Kakigi, R. (2000). Asymmetry of the human visual field in magnetic response to apparent motion. *Brain Res.* **865**, 221–226.

Nakamura, M., Kakigi, R., Okusa, T., Hoshiyama, M., and Watanabe, K. (2000). Effects of check size on pattern reversal visual evoked magnetic field and potential. *Brain Res.* **872**, 77–86.

Narici, L., and Peresson, M. (1995). Discrimination and study of rhythmical brain activities in the alpha band: A neuromagnetic frequency responsiveness test. *Brain Res.* **703**, 31–44.

Narici, L., Pizzella, V., Romani, G. L., Torrioli, G., Traversa, R., and Rossini, P. M. (1990). Evoked alpha- and mu-rhythm in humans: A neuromagnetic study. *Brain Res.* **520**, 222–231.

Narici, L., Portin, K., Salmelin, R., and Hari, R. (1998). Responsiveness of human cortical activity to rhythmical stimulation: A three-modality, whole-cortex neuromagnetic investigation. *NeuroImage* **7**, 209–223.

Nealey, T. A., and Maunsell, J. H. R. (1994). Magnocellular and parvocellular contributions to the responses of neurons in macaque striate cortex. *J. Neurosci.* **14**, 2069–2079.

Neville, H. J., and Lawson, D. (1987). Attention to central and peripheral visual space in a movement detection task: An event-related potential and behavioral study. I. Normal hearing adults. *Brain Res.* **405**, 253–267.

Nishitani, N., and Hari, R. (2000). Temporal dynamics of cortical representation for action. *Proc. Natl. Acad. Sci.* **97**, 913–918.

Nishitani, N., Uutela, K., Shibasaki, H., and Hari, R. (1999). Cortical visuomotor integration during eye pursuit and eye-finger pursuit. *J. Neurosci.* **19**, 2647–2657.

Nobre, A. C., Sebestyn, G. N., Gitelman, D. R., Mesulam, M. M., Frackowiak, R. S. J., and Frith, C. D. (1997). Functional localization of the system for visuospatial attention using positron emission tomography. *Brain* **120**, 515–533.

Novak, G. P., Wiznitzer, M., Kurtzberg, D., Giesser, B. S., and Vaughan, Jr., H. G. (1988). The utility of visual evoked potentials using hemifield stimulation and several check sizes in the evaluation of suspected multiple sclerosis. *Electroencephalogr. Clin. Neurophysiol.* **71**, 1–9.

Nowak, L. G., and Bullier, J. (1997). The timing of information transfer in the visual system. *Cereb. Cortex.* **12**, 205–232.

O'Craven, K. M., and Kanwisher, N. (2000). Mental imagery of faces and places activates corresponding stimulus-specific brain regions. *J. Cogn. Neurosci.* **12**, 1013–1023.

Ojemann, G., Ojemann, J., Lettich, E., and Berger, M. (1989). Cortical language localization in left, dominant hemisphere. *J. Neurosurg.* **71**, 316–326.

Okada, Y. C., Kaufman, L., Brenner, D., and Williamson, S. J. (1982). Modulation transfer functions of the human visual system revealed by magnetic field measurements. *Vis. Res.* **22**, 319–333.

Okada, Y., Wu, J., and Kyuhou, S. (1997). Genesis of MEG signals in a mammalian CNS structure. *Electroencephalogr. Clin. Neurophysiol.* **103**, 474–485.

Okada, Y., Lähteenmäki, A., and Xu, C. (1999a). Comparison of MEG and EEG on the basis of somatic evoked responses elicited by stimulation of the snout in the juvenile swine. *Clin. Neurophysiol.* **110**, 214–229.

Okada, Y., Lahteenmäki, A., and Xu, C. (1999b). Experimental analysis of distortion of magnetoencephalography signals by the skull. *Clin. Neurophysiol.* **110**, 230–238.

Okusa, T., Kakigi, R., and Osaka, N. (2000). Cortical activity related to cue-invariant shape perception in humans. *Neuroscience.* **98**, 615–624.

Ossenblok, P., and Spekreijse, H. (1991). The extrastriate generators of the EP to checkerboard onset. A source localization approach. *Electroencephalogr. Clin. Neurophysiol.* **80**, 181–193.

Parra, J., Meeren, H. K., Kalitzin, S., Suffczynski, P., de Munck, J. C., Harding, G. F., Trenite, D. G., and Lopes da Silva, F. H. (2000). Magnetic source imaging in fixation-off sensitivity: Relationship with alpha rhythm. *J. Clin. Neurophysiol.* **17**, 212–223.

Pascual-Marqui, R. D., Michel, C. M., and Lehmann, D. (1994). Low resolution electromagnetic tomography: A new method for localizing electrical activity of the brain. *Int. J. Psychophysiol.* **18**, 49–65.

Patzwahl, D. R., Elbert, T., Zanker, J. M., and Altenmuller, E. O. (1996). The cortical representation of object motion in man is interindividually variable. *NeuroReport* **7**, 469–472.

Paus, T. (1996). Location and function of the human frontal eye-field: A selective review. *Neuropsychologia* **34**, 475–483.

Paus, T., Kalina, M., Patockova, L., Angerova, Y., Cerny, R., Mecir, P., Bauer, J., and Krabec, P. (1991). Medial vs lateral frontal lobe lesions and differential impairment of central-gaze fixation maintenance in man. *Brain* **114**, 2051–2067.

Perrett, D. I., Rolls, E. T., and Caan, W. (1982). Visual neurons responsive to faces in the monkey temporal cortex. *Exp. Brain. Res.* **47**, 329–342.

Perry, V. H., and Cowey, A. (1985). The ganglion cell and cone distributions in the monkey's retina: Implication for central magnification factors. *Vis. Res.* **25**, 1795–1810.

Perry, V. H., Oehler, R., and Cowey, A. (1984). Retinal ganglion cells that project to the dorsal lateral geniculate nucleus in the Macaque monkey. *Neuroscience* **12**, 1101–1123.

Petit, L., and Haxby, J. V. (1999). Functional anatomy of pursuit eye movements in humans as revealed by fMRI. *J. Neurophysiol.* **81**, 463–471.

Petit, L., Dubois, S., Tzourio, N., Dejardin, S., Crivello, F., Michel, C., Etard, O., Denise, P., Roucoux, A., and Mazoyer, B. (1999). PET study of the human foveal fixation system. *Human Brain Mapping* **8**, 28–43.

Pigarev, I. N., Rizzolatti, G., and Scandolara, C. (1979). Neurones responding to visual stimuli in the frontal lobe of macaque monkeys. *Neurosci. Lett.* **12**, 207–212.

Pigeau, R. A., and Frame, A. M. (1992). Steady-state visual evoked responses in high and low alpha subjects. *Electroencephalogr. Clin. Neurophysiol.* **84**, 101–109.

Ploner, C. J., Rivaud-Pechous, S., Gaymard, B. M., Agid, Y., and Pierrot-Deseilligny, C. (1999). Errors of memory-guided saccades in humans with lesions of the frontal eye field and the dorsolateral prefrontal cortex. *J. Neurophysiol.* **82**, 1086–1090.

Polyak, S. I. (1957). The Vertebrate Visual system. University of Chicago Press, Chicago.

Portin, K., and Hari, R. (1999). Human parieto-occipital visual cortex: Lack of retinotopy and foveal magnification. *Proc. R. Soc. Lond. B* **266**, 981–985.

Portin, K., Salenius, S., Salmelin, R., and Hari, R. (1998). Activation of the human occipital and parietal cortex by pattern and luminance stimuli: neuromagnetic measurements. *Cereb. Cortex.* **8**, 253–260.

Posner, M. I., Snyder, C. R., and Davidson, B. J. (1980). Attention and the detection of signals. *J. Exp. Psychol.* **109**, 160–174.

Puce, A., Allison, T., Gore, J. C., and McCarthy, G. (1995). Face-sensitive regions in human extrastriate cortex studied by functional MRI. *J. Neurophysiol.* **74**, 1192–1199.

Raij, T. (1999). Patterns of brain activity during visual imagery of letters. *J. Cogn. Neurosci.* **11**, 282–299.

Regan, D. (1966). Some characteristics of average steady-state and transient responses evoked by modulated light. *Electroencephalogr. Clin. Neurophysiol.* **20**, 238–248.

Regan, D. (1978). Assessment of visual acuity by evoked potential recording: Ambiguity caused by temporal dependence of spatial frequency selectivity. *Vis. Res.* **18**, 439–443.

Regan, D. (1989). "Human Brain Electrophysiology: Evoked Potentials and Evoked Magnetic Fields in Science and Medicine." Elsevier, New York.

Reynolds, J. H., and Desimone, R. (1999). The role of neural mechanisms of attention in solving the binding problem. *Neuron* **24**, 19–29.

Richmond, B. J., Wurtz, R. H., and Sato T. (1983). Visual responses of inferior temporal neurons in awake Rhesus monkey. *J. Neurophysiol.* **50**, 1415–1432.

Rizzolatti, G., Fadiga, L., Gallese, V., and Fogassi, L. (1996). Premotor cortex and the recognition of motor actions. *Cog. Brain Res.* **3**, 131–141.

Robson, J. G. (1966). Spatial and temporal contrast-sensitivity functions of the visual system. *J. Opt. Soc. Am.* **56**, 1141–1142.

Rockland, K. S. (1995). Morphology of individual axons projecting from area V2 to MT in the macaque. *J. Comp. Neurol.* **355**, 15–26.

Rodieck, R. W. (1979). Visual Pathways. *Annu. Rev. Neurosci.* **2**, 193–225.

Roelfsema, P. R., Engel, A. K., König, P., and Singer, W. (1997). Visuomotor integration is associated with zero time-lag synchronization among cortical areas. *Nature* **385**, 157–161.

Roelfsema, P. R., Lamme, V. A. F., and Spekreijse, H. (1998). Object-based attention in the primary visual cortex of the Macaque monkey. *Nature* **395**, 376–381.

Roland, P. E., and Gulyas, B. (1994). Visual imagery and visual representation. *Trends Neurosci.* **17**, 281–296.

Rolls, E. T. (1984). Neurons in the cortex of the temporal lobe and in the amygdala of the monkey with responses selective for faces. *Hum. Neurobiol.* **3**, 209–222.

Rolls, E. T., Judge, S. J., and Sanghera, M. K. (1977). Activity of neurons in the inferotemporal cortex of alert monkey. *Brain Res.* **130**, 229–238.

Rovamo, J., and Virsu, V. (1979). An estimation and application of the human cortical magnification factor. *Exp Brain Res.* **37**, 495–510.

Rugg, M. D., Milner, A. D., Lines, C. R., and Phalp, R. (1987). Modulation of visual event-related potentials by spatial and non-spatial visual selective attention. *Neuropsychologia* **25**, 85–96.

Saghal, A., and Iversen, S. D. (1978). The effects of foveal prestriate and inferotemporal lesions on matching to sample behavior in monkeys. *Neuropsychologia.* **16**, 391–406.

Saleem, K. S., and Tanaka, K. (1996). Divergent projections from the anterior inferotemporal area TE to the perirhinal and entorhinal cortices in the macaque monkey. *J. Neurosci.* **16**, 4757–4775.

Salenius, S. (1999). 'Human see, human do' cortex. *Mol. Psychiatr.* **4**, 307–309.

Salenius, S., Kajola, M., Thompson W. L., Kosslyn, S., and Hari, R. (1995). Reactivity of magnetic parieto-occipital alpha rhythm during visual imagery. *Electroencephalogr. Clin. Neurophysiol.* **95**, 453–462.

Salmelin, R., and Hari, R. (1994). Characterization of spontaneous MEG rhythms in healthy adults. *Electroencephalogr. Clin. Neurophysiol.* **91**, 237–248.

Salmelin, R., Hari, R., Lounasmaa, O. V., and Sams, M. (1994). Dynamics of brain activation during picture naming. *Nature* **368**, 463–465.

Sams, M., Hietanen, J. K., Hari, R., Ilmoniemi, R. J., and Lounasmaa, O. V. (1997). Face-specific responses from the human inferior occipito-temporal cortex. *Neuroscience* **77**, 49–55.

Sanghera, M. K., Rolls, E. T., and Roper-Hall, A. (1979). Visual responses of neurons in the dorso-lateral amygdale of the alert monkey. *Exp. Neuro.* **163**, 610–626.

Sary, G., Vogels, R., and Orban, G. A. (1993). Cue-invariant shape selectivity of macaque inferior temporal neurons. *Science* **260**, 995–997.

Sato, N., Nakamura, K., Nakamura, A., Sugiura, M., Ito, K., Fukuda, H., and Kawashima, R. (1999). Different time course between scene processing and face processing: a MEG study. *NeuroReport* **10**, 3633–3637.

Schein, S. J., and Desimone, R., (1990). Spectral properties of V4 neurons in the macaque. *J. Neurosci.* **10**, 3369–3389.

Scherg, M. (1990). Fundamentals of dipole source potential analysis. *In* "Advances in Audiology, Vol. 6, Auditory Evoked Magnetic Fields and Electric Potentials" (F. Grandori, M. Hoke, and G. L. Romani, eds.), pp. 40–69 Karger, Basel.

Schiller, P. H., and Malpeli, J. G. (1978). Functional specificity of lateral geniculate nucleus laminae of the Rhesus monkey. *J. Neurophysiol.* **41**, 788–797.

Schmidt, D. M., George, J. S., and Wood, C. C. (1999). Bayesian inference applied to the electromagnetic inverse problem. *Human Brain Mapping* **7P**, 195–212.

Schneider, G. E. (1969). Two visual systems. *Science* **163**, 895–902.

Schroeder, C. E., Mehta, A. D., and Foxe, J. J. (2001). Determinants and mechanisms of attentional modulation of neural processing. *Front. Biosci.* **6**, D672–684.

Seidemann, E., and Newsome, W. T. (1999). Effect of spatial attention on the responses of Area MT neurons. *J. Neurophysiol.* **81**, 1783–1794.

Seki, K., Nakasato, N., Fujita, S., Hatanaka, K., Kawamura, T., Kanno, A., and Yoshimoto, T. (1996). Neuromagnetic evidence that the P100 component of the pattern reversal visual evoked response originates in the bottom of the calcarine fissure. *Electroencephalogr. Clin. Neurophysiol.* **100**, 436–442.

Seltzer, B., and Pandya, D. N. (1978). Afferent cortical connections and architectonics of the superior temporal sulcus and surrounding cortex in rhesus monkey. *Brain Res.* **149**, 1–24.

Sereno, M. I., Dale, A. M., Reppas, J. B., Kwong, K. K., Belliveau, J. W., Brady, T. J., Rosen, B. R., and Tootell, R. B. H. (1995). Borders of multiple visual areas in humans revealed by functional magnetic resonance imaging. *Science* **268**, 889–893.

Sergent, J., and Poncet, M. (1990). From covert to overt recognition of faces in a prosopagnosic patient. *Brain* **113**, 989–1004.

Sergent, J., Ohta, S., and MacDonald, B. (1992). Functional neuroanatomy of face and object processing. *Brain* **115**, 15–36.

Shah, N. J., Aine, C. J., Schlitt, H., Krause, B. J., Ranken, D., George, J., and Müller-Gärtner, H.-W. (1998). Activation of the visual ventral stream in humans: An fMRI study. *In* "Positron Emission Tomography: A Critical Assessment of Recent Trends" (B. Gulya and H. W. Müller, eds). Kluwer Academic Publishers, Dordrecht.

Shen, L., Hu, X., Yacoub, E., and Ugurbil, K. (1999). Neural correlates of visual form and visual spatial processing. *Human Brain Mapping.* **8**, 60–71.

Shiffrin, R. M., and Schneider, W. (1984). Automatic and controlled processing revisited. *Psychol. Rev.* **91**: 269–276.

Shigeto, H., Tobimatsu, S., Yamamoto, T., and Kobayashi, M. (1998) Visual evoked cortical magnetic responses to checkerboard reversal stimulation: A study on the neural generators of N75 and N145. *J. Neurol. Sci.* **156**, 186–194.

Shipp, S., and Zeki, S. (1985). Segregation of pathways leading from area V2 to areas V4 and V5 of macaque monkey visual cortex. *Nature* **315**, 322–325.

Shipp, S., Blanton, M., and Zeki, S. (1998). A visuo-somatomotor pathway through superior parietal cortex in the Macaque monkey: Cortical connections of areas V6 and V6A. *Euro. J. Neurosci.* **10**, 3171–3193.

Shulman, G. H. M., Corbetta, M., Buckner, R. L., Raichle, M. E., Fiez, J. A., Miezen, F. M., and Peterson, S. E. (1997). Top-down modulation of early sensory cortex. *Cereb. Cortex* **7**, 193–206.

Singer, W. (1995). Visual feature integration and the temporal correlation hypothesis. *Annu. Rev. Neurosci.* **18**, 555–586.

Singer, W. (1999). Neuronal synchrony: A versatile code for the definition of relations? *Neuron* **24**, 49–65.

Sokolov, A., Lutzenberger, W., Pavlova, M., Preissl, H., Braun, C., and Birbaumer, N. (1999). Gamma-band MEG activity to coherent motion depends on task-driven attention. *NeuroReport* **10**, 1997–2000.

Somers, D. C., Dale, A. M., Seiffert, A. E., and Tootell, R. B. (1999). Functional MRI reveals spatially specific attentional modulation in human primary visual cortex. *Proc. Natl. Acad. Sci. U.S.A.* **96**, 1663–1668.

Spitzer, H., Desimone, R., and Moran, J. (1988). Increased attention enhances both behavioral and neuronal performance. *Science* **240**, 338–340.

Squire, L. R., (1986). Mechanisms of memory. *Science* **232**, 1612–1619.

Srinivasan, R., Russell, D. P., Edelman, G. M., and Tononi, G. (1999). Increased synchronization of neuromagnetic responses during conscious perception. *J. Neurosci.* **19**(13), 5435–5448.

Stensaas, S. S., Eddington, D. K., and Dobelle, W. H. (1974). The topography and variability of the primary visual cortex in man. *J. Neurosurg.* **40**, 747–755.

Stephen, J. M., Aine, C. J., Christner, R. F., Ranken, D., Huang, M., and Best, E. (2002). Temporal frequency sensitivity of the human visual system measured with MEG: I. Central versus peripheral field stimulation (submitted).

Stone, J., and Johnston, E. (1981). The topography of primate retina: A study of the human, bushbaby, and new and old-world monkeys. *J. Comp. Neurol.* **196**, 205–223.

Streit, M., Ioannides, A. A., Liu, L., Wölwer, W., Dammers, J., Gross, J., Gaebel, W., and Müller-Gärtner, H.-W. (1999). Neurophysiological correlates of the recognition of facial expressions of emotion as revealed by magnetoencephalography. *Cogn. Brain Res.* **7**, 481–491.

Supek, S., and Aine, C. J. (1993). Simulation studies of multiple dipole neuromagnetic source localization: Model order and limits of source resolution. *IEEE Trans. Biomed. Eng.* **40**, 529–540.

Supek, S., and Aine, C. J. (1997). Spatio-temporal modeling of neuromagnetic data: I. Multi-source location versus time-course estimation accuracy. *Human Brain Mapping* **5**, 139–153.

Supek, S., Aine, C. J., Ranken, D., Best, E., Flynn, E. R., and Wood, C. C. (1999). Single vs. paired visual stimulation: Superposition of early neuromagnetic responses and retinotopy in extrastriate cortex in humans. *Brain Res.* **830**, 43–55.

Swithenby, S. J., Bailey, A. J., Bräutigam, S., Josephs, O. E., Jousmäki, V., and Tesche, C. D. (1998). Neural processing of human faces: A magnetoencephalographic study. *Exp. Brain Res.* **118**, 501–510.

Tallon-Baudry, C., and Bertrand, O. (1999). Oscillatory gamma activity in humans and its role in object representation. *Trends Cogn. Sci.* **3**, 151–162.

Tallon-Baudry, C., Bertrand, O., Wienbruch, C., Ross, B., and Pantev, C. (1997). Combined EEG and MEG recordings of visual 40 Hz responses to illusory triangles in human. *NeuroReport* **8**, 1103–1107.

Tanaka, K. (1997). Mechanisms of visual object recognition: Monkey and human studies. *Curr. Opin. Neurobiol.* **7**, 523–529.

Tesche, C. D., and Kajola, M. (1993). A comparison of the localization of spontaneous neuromagnetic activity in the frequency and time domains. *Electroencephalogr. Clin. Neurophysiol.* **87**, 408–416.

Tesche, C. D., and Karhu, J. (2000). Theta oscillations index human hippocampal activation during a working memory task. *Proc. Natl. Acad. Sci. U.S.A.* **97**(2), 919–924.

Tesche, C. D., Krusin-Elbaum, L., and Knowles, W. D. (1988). Simultaneous measurement of magnetic and electrical responses of *in vitro* hippocampal slices. *Brain Res.* **462**, 190–193.

Tesche, C. D., Uusitalo, M. A., Ilmoniemi, R. J., and Kajola, M. J. (1995). Characterizing the local oscillatory content of spontaneous cortical activity during mental imagery. *Brain Res. Cogn. Brain Res.* **2**, 243–249.

Teyler, T. J., Cuffin, B. N., and Cohen, D. (1975). The visual evoked magnetoencephalogram. *Life Sci.* **17**, 683–692.

Tononi, G., Srinivasan, R., Russell, D. P., and Edelman, G. M. (1998). Investigating neural correlates of conscious perception by frequency-tagged neuromagnetic responses. *Proc. Natl. Acad. Sci. U.S.A.* **95**, 3198–3203.

Tootell, R. B. H., Hamilton, S. L., and Switkes, E. (1988). Functional anatomy of macaque striate cortex. IV. Contrast and magno-parvo streams. *J. Neurosci.* **8**, 1594–1609.

Tootell, R. B., Reppas, J. B., Dale, A. M., Look, R. B., Sereno, M. I., Malach, R., Brady, T. J., and Rosen, B. R. (1995a). Visual motion aftereffect in human cortical area MT revealed by functional magnetic resonance imaging. *Nature* **375**, 139–141.

Tootell, R. B., Reppas, J. B., Kwong, K. K., Malach, R., Bom, R. T., Brady, T. J., Rosen, B. R., and Belliveau, J. W. (1995b). Functional analysis of human MT and related visual cortical areas using magnetic resonance imaging. *J. Neurosci.* **15**, 3215–3230.

Tootell, R. B. H., Hadjikani, N. K., Mendola, J. D., Marrett, S., and Dale, A. M. (1998). From retinotopy to recognition: fMRI in human visual cortex. *Trends Cogn. Sci.* **2**, 174–183.

Towle, V. L., Carder, R. K., Khorasani, L., and Lindberg, D. (1999). Electrocorticographic coherence patterns. *J. Clin. Neurophysiol.* **16**, 528–547.

Treisman, A., and Geffen, G. (1967). Selective attention: Perception or response? *Q. J. Exp. Psychol.* **19**, 1–17.

Treue, S., and Maunsell, J. H. R. (1996). Attentional modulation of visual motion processing in areas MT and MST. *Nature* **382**, 538–541.

Treue, S., and Martinez-Trujillo, J. C. (1999). Feature-based attention influences motion processing gain in macaque visual cortex. *Nature* **399**, 575–579.

Ungerleider, L. G. (1995). Functional brain imaging studies of cortical mechanisms for memory. *Science* **270**, 769–775.

Ungerleider, L. G., and Desimone, R. (1986). Projections to the superior temporal sulcus from the central and peripheral field representations of V1 and V2. *J. Comp. Neurol.* **248**, 147–163.

Ungerleider, L. G., and Haxby, J. V. (1994). "What" and "where" in the human brain. *Curr. Opin. Neurobiol.* **4**, 157–165.

Ungerleider, L. G., and Mishkin, M. (1982). Two cortical visual systems. *In* "Analysis of Visual Behavior" (D. J. Ingle, M. A. Goodale, and R. J. W. Mansfield, eds.), pp. 549–586 MIT Press, Cambridge.

Uusitalo, M. A., Williamson, S. J., and Seppa, M. T. (1996). Dynamical organization of the human visual system revealed by lifetimes of activation traces. *Neurosci. Lett.* **213**, 149–152.

Uusitalo, M. A., Jousmaki, V., and Hari, R. (1997). Activation of trace lifetime of human cortical responses evoked by apparent motion. *Neurosci. Lett.* **224**, 45–48.

Uutela, K., Hämäläinen, M., and Somersalo, E. (1999). Visualization of magnetoencephalographic data using minimum current estimates. *NeuroImage* **10**, 173–180.

Vanderwolf, C. H. (1969). Hippocampal electrical activity and voluntary movement in the rat. *Electroencephalogr. Clin. Neurophysiol.* **26**(4), 407–18.

Van Essen, D. C. (1979). Visual areas of the mammalian cerebral cortex. *Annu. Rev. Neurosci.* **2**, 227–263.

Van Essen, D. C. (1985). Functional organization of primate visual cortex. *In* "In Cerebral Cortex" A. Peters and E. G. Jones (eds.), Vol. 3, pp. 259–329. Plenum, New York.

Van Essen, D. C., and Maunsell, J. H. R. (1983). Hierarchical organization and functional streams in the visual cortex. *Trends Neurosci.* **6**, 370–375.

Van Essen, D. C., Newsome, W. T. N., and Bixby, J. L. (1982). The pattern of interhemispheric connections and its relationship to extrastriate visual areas in the macaque monkey. *J. Neurosci.* **2**, 265–283.

Vanni, S., and Uutela, K. (2000). Foveal attention modulates responses to peripheral stimuli. *J. Neurophysiol.* **83**, 2443–2452.

Vanni, S., Revonsuo, A., and Hari, R. (1997). Modulation of the parieto-occipital alpha rhythm during object detection. *J. Neurosci.* **17**, 7141–7147.

Vanni, S., Portin, K., Virsu, V., and Hari, R. (1999). Mu rhythm modulation during changes of visual percepts. *Neuroscience.* **91**, 21–31.

Vanni, S., Tanskanen, T., Seppä, M., Uutela, K., and Hari, R. (2001). Coinciding early activation of the human primary visual cortex and anteromedial cuneus. *Proc. Natl. Acad. Sci. U.S.A.* **98**, 2776–2780.

Van Voorhis, S., and Hillyard, S. A. (1977). Visual evoked potentials and selective attention to points in space. *Percept. Psychophys.* **22**, 54–62.

Vidyasagar, T. R. (1998). Gating of neuronal responses in macaque primary visual cortex by an attentional spotlight. *NeuroReport* **9**, 1947–1952.

Walla, P., Hufnagl, B., Lindinger, G., Imhof, H., Deecke, L., and Lang, W. (2001). Left temporal and temporoparietal brain activity depends on depth of word encoding: A magnetoencephalographic study in healthy young subjects. *NeuroImage* **13**, 402–409.

Wang, J. Z., Williamson, S. J., and Kaufman, L. (1992). Magnetic source images determined by a lead-field analysis: The unique minimum-norm. *IEEE Trans. Biomed. Eng.* **39**, 665–675.

Wang, L., Kakigi, R., and Hoshiyama, M. (2001). Neural activities during Wisconsin Card Sorting Test-MEG observation. *Cogn. Brain Res.* **12**, 19–31.

Watanabe, T., Sasaki, Y., Miyauchi, S., Putz, B., Fujimaki, N., Nielsen, M., Takino, R., and Miyakawa, S. (1998). Attention-regulated activity in human primate visual cortex. *J. Neurophysiol.* **79**, 2218–2221.

Watson, J. D., Myers, R., Frackowiak, R. S., Hajnal, J. V., Woods, R. P., Mazziotta, J. C., Shipp, S., and Zeki, S. (1993). Area V5 of the human brain: Evidence from a combined study using positron emission tomography and magnetic resonance imaging. *Cereb. Cortex* **3**, 79–94.

Weinberg, H., Brickett, P., Coolsma, F., and Baff, M. (1986). Magnetic localization of intracranial dipoles: Simulation with a physical model. *Electroencephalogr. Clin. Neurophysiol.* **64**, 159–170.

Whiteley, A. M., and Warrington, E. K. (1977). Prosopagnosia: A clinical, psychological, and anatomical study of three patients. *J. Neurol. Neurosurg. Psychiatr.* **40**, 394–430.

Wiesel, T. N., and Hubel, D. H. (1966). Spatial and chromatic interactions in the lateral geniculate body of the rhesus monkey. *J. Neurophysiol.* **29**, 1115–1156.

Williamson, S. J., Kaufman, L., and Brenner, D. (1978). Latency of the neuromagnetic response of the human visual cortex. *Vis. Res.* **18**, 107–110.

Williamson, S. J., Kaufman, L., Curtis, S., Lu, Z. L., Michel, C. M., and Wang, J. Z. (1996). Neural substrates of working memories are revealed magnetically by the local suppression of alpha rhythm.

Electroencephalogr. Clin. Neurophysiol. (Suppl.) **47**, 163–180.

Wilson, M. (1978). Visual system: Pulvinar-extrastriate cortex. In R. B. Masterton (ed) "Handbook of Behavioral Neurobiology" (R. B. Masterton, ed.), Vol. 1, pp. 209–247. Plenum, New York.

Worden, M. S., Wellington, R., and Schneider, W. (1996). Determining the locus of attentional selection with functional magnetic resonance imaging. *NeuroImage* **3**, 244.

Wright, M. J., and Ikeda, H. (1974). Processing of spatial and temporal information in the visual system. *In* "The Neurosciences (Third Study Program)" (F. O. Schmitt and F. G. Worden, eds.), pp. 115–122. MIT Press, Cambridge.

Wu, J., and Okada, Y. C. (1998). Physiological bases of the synchronized population spikes and slow wave of the magnetic field generated by a guinea-pig longitudinal CA3 slice preparation. *Electroencephalogr. Clin. Neurophysiol.* **107**, 361–373.

Wurtz, R. H., and Mohler, C. W. (1976). Enhancement of visual responses in monkey striate cortex and frontal eye fields. *J. Neurophysiol.* **39**, 766–772.

Zeki, S. M. (1969). Representation of central visual fields in prestriate cortex of monkey. *Brain Res.* **14**, 271–291.

Zeki, S. M. (1973). Colour coding in rhesus monkey prestriate cortex. *Brain Res.* **53**, 422–427.

Zeki, S. (1978). Functional specialisation in the visual cortex of the rhesus monkey. *Nature* **274**, 423–428.

Zeki, S. M. (1980). A direct projection from area V1 to area V3A of rhesus monkey visual cortex. *Proc. R. Soc. Lond.* **207**, 499–506.

Zeki, S., Watson, J. D. G., Lueck, C. J., Friston, K. J., Kennard, C., and Frackowiak, R. S. J. (1991). A direct demonstration of functional specialization in human visual cortex. *J. Neurosci.* **11**, 641–649.

Zouridakis, G., Simos, P. G., Breier, J. I., and Papanicolaou, A. C. (1998). Functional hemispheric asymmetry assessment in a visual language task using MEG. *Brain Topogr.* **11**, 57–65.

6

Aligning Linguistic and Brain Views on Language Comprehension

Kara D. Federmeier, Robert Kluender, and Marta Kutas

INTRODUCTION

Language affords human beings an incredible degree of representational flexibility within the limits of highly restrictive constraints. For example, despite the remarkable ability of the human vocal tract to produce all kinds of sounds, only a limited subset of these is actually used in the world's languages. A native speaker of any of the world's languages will have an intuitive sense for what kinds of sounds can and cannot (e.g., coughs and raspberry noises) figure as possible sounds in a human language, even if none of the sounds in question occurs in his or her own particular language. Individual languages exhibit an even more restricted inventory of speech sounds, the lowest attested number being eleven. However, this small repertoire of sounds is grouped and ordered to create a very much larger set of words in a language, termed its lexicon. Likewise, the entries in this lexicon, although large in number—typically consisting of many thousands of entries—can be combined to form literally an infinite number of sentences describing real, imaginary, and impossible objects and events, not to mention emotional states and abstract concepts.

Especially striking is that almost all humans learn this complicated coding system early in life and use it throughout their life span with ease. Every day, humans produce and comprehend completely new strings of words, at a rate of about 150 words per minute (Maclay and Osgood, 1959). No other species is capable of this tremendous versatility, either naturally in the wild or when trained in humanlike communication systems for experimental purposes in the laboratory. Our linguistic ability is one of the many salient characteristics that distinguish humans from other species. Another is the relative size and complexity of our brains, and surely these two features are not unrelated or logically independent. In fact, we can say that the degree of flexibility and efficiency we exhibit in this cognitive domain is a consequence of the structure of language, together with the structure of the entity that represents it and mediates its processing, the human brain. In this chapter we examine how these come together in neural imaging studies of language comprehension relying on physiological measures, with an emphasis on electrical brain activity (an equally compelling story could be told for language production, but that tale will not be told here).

LANGUAGE STRUCTURE: THE LINGUIST'S VIEW AND THE BRAIN'S VIEW

The language system is structured at multiple levels, ranging from its physical form to its referential meaning in context. Phonetics and phonology are the study of language sounds. Phonetics describes how the speech sounds utilized by all human languages are produced, transmitted, and perceived. Within any given language, sounds (and hand shapes in signed languages) come to be systematically organized and categorized (into "phonemes"). For example, various combinations of different actual sound patterns (mediated by measurably different vocal tract configurations) may all yield something that an English speaker interprets as a "t"—the (different) sounds in the words "top," "stop," "pot," and "button," for example. Phonology is the study of such sound systems and the kind of knowledge that people have about the sound patterns of their particular language.

"Morphemes" are combinations of phonemes that have come to have their own meaning. Some are whole words (e.g., "cat"), whereas others are affixes that modulate the meaning of whole words (e.g., the /s/, which, when added to the end of an English word, makes that word plural). Morphology, then, is the study of the patterns that govern word formation, including both how morphemes combine to yield new meanings or parts of speech (derivational morphology), and how they combine to create different forms of the same word (inflectional morphology). Just as morphemes are combined to create new words and new forms of words, whole words are combined to make larger units of language—phrases, clauses, sentences, and discourses. Within and across languages, the way in which certain words and types of words come to be put together to create these larger language units is patterned. Phrases, for example, are built around particular types of words. Noun phrases may contain several different types of words but must contain at least one noun and must not contain a verb. Phrases act as units that can be found in multiple places in a sentence—for instance, noun phrases may be subjects, objects, or parts of prepositional phrases. The study of language grammars—of how words (and affixes) pattern across phrases, sentences and discourses—is known as syntax.

Ultimately, humans use language to transmit information—meaning—that depends not just on the general pattern of sounds or words, but on the specific words used, their specific pattern, and the specific context (linguistic, social, environmental) in which they occur. The study of language meaning in general, known as semantics, and of meaning in its larger context, known as pragmatics, asks how language is used to transmit and, in some cases, affect or even distort reality.

From a linguist's perspective, then, language is a highly structured system, and this structure is important for understanding how language can be used so readily and efficiently. However, it cannot be the structure of language *alone* that makes it such a useful tool, for if that were the case it would be difficult to understand why humans alone come to have fully developed language skills. Rather, it must be the structure of language in combination with that of the human brain that explains how humans acquire, use, and create language. A question then arises: Does the human brain "see" language the way that linguists see language?

As just discussed, linguists have uncovered language patterns at various levels—phonological, morphological, syntactic, semantic, pragmatic. Cognitive neuroscientists and psycholinguists have long sought to determine whether these regularities arise from some aspect of sensory and cognitive processing. It seems likely that at least some of these distinctions are also important to the brain. At some level, for example, the brain probably does process phonological patterns differently from semantic or syntactic ones, and there is likely to be some difference between the brain's processing of two different sounds that are ultimately treated alike and two that are ultimately distinguished. However, linguists have typically focused on general principles of language organization and function that cut across individual languages, across individual language speakers, and even across individual instances of language performance. In other words, they are generally not concerned with processing issues and thus often examine patterns collapsed across time and space. However, the brain's processing of language necessarily takes place in time and space, and brain scientists are dedicated to delineating the importance of both. For example, linguistic inputs that are separated by different stretches of time (e.g., different numbers of words) or that require different numbers/sizes of saccadic eye movements are liable to be treated differently by the brain, though not, perhaps, by linguists. At the same time, not all differences noted by linguists are likely to be meaningful to all brain areas at all times. Early in visual processing, for instance, the brain responds similarly to letter strings that can be pronounced (i.e., are phonologically legal) and those that cannot.

Clearly then, any processing account of language must reconcile the categories that linguists have inferred from analysis of the world's languages (competence) with the processes that brain scientists have inferred from various neurobiological measures of brain activity during language performance; thus cognitive neuroscientists and psycholinguists have long been interested in the brain's "view." However, the issue of whether the brain sees language as linguists do (and why the answer should matter) has been of some debate among linguists. To a large extent, the debate has

played out along the lines of functionalist versus reductionist views of the study of mind (Churchland, 1984; Fodor, 1981). The strongest functionalist stance on this issue came from Noam Chomsky. With a pronounced emphasis on mental phenomena over and above mere observable linguistic behavior, Chomsky firmly established modern linguistic science as practiced in the latter half of the twentieth century as a functionalist enterprise par excellence:

> Mentalistic linguistics is simply theoretical linguistics that uses performance as data (along with other data, for example, the data provided by introspection) for the determination of competence, the latter being taken as the primary object of its investigation. The mentalist, in this traditional sense, need make no assumptions about the possible physiological basis for the mental reality that he studies. In particular, he need not deny that there is such a basis. One would guess, rather, that it is the mentalistic studies that will ultimately be of greatest value for the investigation of neurophysiological mechanisms, since they alone are concerned with determining abstractly the properties that such mechanisms must exhibit and the functions they must perform. [Chomsky, 1965, p. 193, fn. 1]

> From this point of view we can proceed to approach the study of the human mind much in the way that we study the physical structure of the body. In fact, we may think of the study of mental faculties as actually being a study of the body—specifically the brain—conducted at a certain level of abstraction. [Chomsky, 1980, p. 2]

In essence, Chomsky's original answer to this question was that ultimately, the brain would indeed have to see language the way the linguist does, because only the linguist is in a position to determine the primitives and operations in need of neural implementation. Chomsky later modified this position by acknowledging that primary linguistic data provided by introspection were no longer able to decide among competing linguistic theories, and that linguists would therefore need to take into consideration other sources of evidence derived from performance measures, including neural imaging data.

At the opposite extreme, perhaps the strongest reductionist answer to the question of the appropriate characterization of the brain–language relationship came from a structural linguist, Charles Hockett:

> The essential difference between the [analytical] process in the child and the procedure of the linguist is this: the linguist has to make his analysis overtly, in communicable form, in the shape of a set of statements which can be understood by any properly trained person, who in turn can predict utterances not yet observed with the same degree of accuracy as can the original analyst. The child's 'analysis' consists, on the other hand, of a mass of varying synaptic potentials in his central nervous system. The child in time comes to **behave** the language; the linguist must come to **state** it.... . [The linguistic scientist's] purpose in analyzing a language is not to create structure, but to determine the structure actually created by the speakers of the language. For the scientist, then, 'linguistic structure' refers to something existing quite independently of the activities of the analyst: a language is what it is, it has the structure it has, whether studied and analyzed by a linguist or not. [Hockett, 1963, p. 280]

Although this was originally published in 1948 and reflects the behaviorism of the time, it nonetheless seems not all that far removed from a present-day neoempirist position on this issue.

Nowadays, both psychological functionalists and reductionists are interested in how the brain "sees" language. For example, one of the characteristics that Fodor (1983) assigns to mental modules is association with fixed neural architecture. In part because of this, much of the current interest in neural imaging techniques among linguists and psycholinguists comes from those with functionalist leanings. Thus, taking the brain's perspective on language will likely yield useful data for scientists of any theoretical persuasion, and that is what we will attempt to do here.

METHODS FOR EXAMINING BRAIN FUNCTION

The brain not only represents language but also is involved in its creation and its real-time use. To understand how requires knowing something about the brain and about what regularities in language the brain notices and under what circumstances. Thus, cognitive neuroscientists interested in language processing have turned to a number of noninvasive brain imaging techniques in order to get various mutually constraining pictures of the brain in action as it processes language. These include direct measures of brain electrical activity and measures of metabolic processes that support such activity.

Comprehending and producing language are brain functions that require the coordinated activity of large groups of neurons. This neural communication is electrochemical in nature, involving the movement of electrically charged elements known as ions. Under normal (nonstimulated) conditions, each neuron has a "resting" electrical potential that arises due to the distribution of ions inside and outside it. Stimulation of the neuron changes the permeability of the neural membrane to these charged elements, thereby altering the electrical potential. A transient increase in potential (depolarization) at the cell body can cause an all-or-none wave of depolarization that moves along the cell's axon, known as an "action potential." The action potential then spreads to other neurons via the release of neurotransmitters from the axon terminals; these neurotransmitters diffuse across extracellular space (synaptic cleft) and cause permeability changes in the dendrites of nearby neurons. These permeability changes may cause an action potential in the receiving cell as well, or may simply alter the electrical potential of that cell such that it will be more or less sensitive to ensuing stimulation.

Neural communication thus involves wavelike changes in the electrical potential along neurons and their processes. These current flows are the basis for electrophysiological recordings in the brain and at the scalp surface, because changes in electrical potential can be monitored by placing at least two electrodes somewhere on the head (or in the brain) and measuring the voltage difference between them. The resulting electroencephalogram (EEG) observed at the scalp is due to the summed potentials of multiple neurons acting in concert. In fact, much of the observed activity at the scalp likely arises from cortical pyramidal cells whose organization and firing satisfy the constraints for an observable signal (for details, see, e.g., Allison, et al., 1986; Kutas and Dale, 1997; Nunez and Katznelson, 1981).

The EEG measures spontaneous, rhythmic brain activity occurring in multiple frequency bands. For the purposes of understanding the neural basis of language processing, however, cognitive neuroscientists are often interested in the brain's response to a particular event or kind of event, such as the appearance of a word on a computer screen. To examine event-related activity in particular, one can average the EEG signal time-locked to the stimuli of interest to create an "event-related potential" or ERP. The ERP is a wave form consisting of voltage fluctuations in time, one wave form for each recording site. This wave form consists of a series of positive- and negative-going voltage deflections (relative to some base line activity prior to event onset). Under different experimental conditions, one can observe changes in wave form morphology (e.g., presence or absence of certain peaks), the latency, duration, or amplitude (size) of one or more peaks, or their distribution over the scalp. Until recently, electrophysiological investigations of language have focused on relatively fast (high-frequency), transient ERP responses; more recently, however, slower potentials that develop over the course of clauses and sentences have also been monitored.

ERPs are informative indices of language-related processes because they are a continuous, multidimensional signal. Specifically, ERPs provide a direct estimate of what a significant part of the brain is doing just before, during, and after an event of interest, even if it is extended in time. And, they do so with millisecond resolution. ERPs can indicate not only that two conditions are different, but also how—whether, for example, there is a quantitative change in the timing or size of a process or a qualitative change in the nature of processing or involvement of different brain generators as reflected in a different morphology or scalp distribution. To a limited extent, ERPs can also be used to infer where in the brain processes take place [via source modeling techniques and in combination with other neuroimaging techniques; for more information see Dale and Halgren (2001) and Kutas et al., (1999)].

Because it is difficult to localize precisely the neural source of electrical signals recorded at the scalp from the electrical recordings alone, other types of brain imaging methods have been brought to bear on attempts to link specific brain areas with cognitive processes. The brain requires a constant supply of blood to meet its metabolic demands, which in turn change with neural activity. With increased neuronal activity, glucose consumption goes up and there are concomitant local increases in blood flow and changes in oxygen extraction from the blood. These hemodynamic (and metabolic) changes can be monitored with techniques such as positron emission tomography (PET) and functional magnetic resonance imaging (fMRI). Local changes in blood flow during a cognitive task, for example, can be followed with PET using ^{15}O-labeled water. Because these increases in blood flow exceed increases in local oxygen extraction, blood near regions of neural activity eventually has higher concentrations of oxygenated hemoglobin compared to blood near inactive regions. Such differences can be measured with fMRI, because as hemoglobin becomes deoxygenated it becomes more paramagnetic than the surrounding tissue, thereby creating a magnetically inhomogeneous environment. Under the right circumstances, these hemodynamic imaging methods can localize regions of neural activity with high spatial resolution. Their temporal resolution, however, is poorer, because hemodynamic responses typically lag the electrical signal by 1–2 sec and do not track activity on a millisecond-by-millisecond basis. Combinations of these measures of brain activity thus seem to offer the most complete picture of where, when, and how language is processed in the brain.

Using neuroimaging techniques, researchers have looked at language processing from early stages of word recognition through the processing of multisentence discourses, from the planning of a speech act to its articulation (e.g., Kutas and Van Petten, 1994; Osterhout, 1994; Osterhout and Holcomb, 1995). So doing reveals that the brain's processing of language involves many different kinds of operations taking place at different times and different temporal scales and in multiple brain areas. These operations differ in the extent to which they are general purpose versus language specific, in the extent to which they are affected by context (and to what types of contexts they are sensitive), and in the extent to which they interact with one another in space and time.

LANGUAGE COMPREHENSION

Initially, the brain cannot know whether an incoming stimulus is linguistic or not. Thus, its first task when confronted with a written, spoken, or signed word—as with any external, perceptual stimulus—is to determine what it is, or at least to what categories it might belong. This (unconscious)

decision is crucial and difficult; in order to process a stimulus effectively, attention must be distributed over the stimulus appropriately, certain kinds of feature information must be extracted and possibly stored in memory, information needed to interpret the stimulus must be accessed from long-term memory, and so on. Because the brain cannot always know what kind of stimulus it will encounter at any given moment, some aspects of (especially early) perceptual processing are likely to be similar regardless of the nature of the stimulus. At times, processing decisions may also be guided by guesses—based on frequency, recency, and other predictive regularities gained from experience with the sensory world—about what the stimulus is likely to be. When it can, it seems that the brain makes use of both top-down (expectancy or context-based) and bottom-up (stimulus-based) information to guide its analysis of input. Thus, if someone has been reading or listening to a stream of linguistic stimuli, their brain might be biased to treat incoming input as linguistic; in other contexts, the same input may initially be interpreted as nonlinguistic (e.g., Johnston and Chesney, 1974). To the extent that the context allows, the brain might also form expectations about the physical nature of the stimulus—color, size, font, loudness, voice, etc. Modulation of attention to such stimulus parameters is reflected in variations in the amplitude of early sensory ERP components that originate from primary and secondary sensory-processing areas in the brain (e.g., P1, N1, mismatch negativity, Nd, processing negativity; see relevant chapters in this book). Depending on the task demands, there may also be various kinds of effects on later ERP components such as N2, P3, RP, etc., shown to vary systematically with cognitive variables.

From Perception to Language

Regardless of the nature or degree of available top-down information, however, the first task for successful language comprehension involves early sensory classification of the input. In the visual modality, for example, this might include differentiating single objectlike stimuli from strings, orthographically legal words from illegal words, or pseudowords from nonwords. Schendan and colleagues (1998) examined the time course of this type of classification by comparing the ERP responses to object like (real objects, pseudoobjects), wordlike (words, letter strings, pseudofont strings), and intermediate (icon strings) stimuli. Around 95 msec a negativity (N100) over midline occipital sites distinguished single objectlike stimuli from strings (see Fig. 1). This differentiation is important because, as supported by the neuropsychological literature, different attentional resources are required to process sets of spatially distinct objects as opposed to a single, spatially contiguous form, and these processes are mediated by different brain areas (e.g., Farah, 1990). This classification was followed shortly by a distinction between strings made from real letters (words and pseudowords) and those made from other characters (icon strings, pseudofont), suggesting that the visual system of experienced readers has developed the ability rapidly to detect physical stimuli with the properties of real letters. Results from intracranial recording and fMRI studies suggest that such differentiations may be occurring in areas in the posterior fusiform gyrus (Allison et al., 1994) and the occipitotemporal and inferior occipital sulci (Puce et al., 1996). Finally, the ERPs showed a distinction between words and pseudowords, beginning approximately 200 msec poststimulus onset. Similar time courses of analyses and categorizations seem to hold for auditory inputs as well; for example, the ERPs to meaningful and nonsense words are very similar within the first 150 msec of processing and begin to be distinguishable by 200–250 msec (Novick et al., 1985).

Although ERPs provide a very temporally precise means of determining an upper limit on the time by which the brain must have appreciated the difference between two conditions or stimuli, they do not explicitly tell us either what that differ-

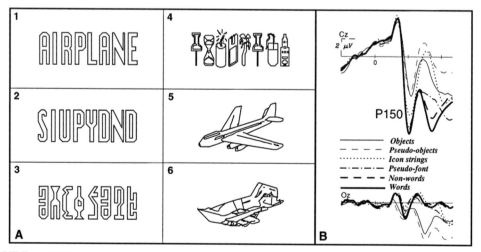

FIGURE 1 ERPs to visual stimuli. Sample stimuli (A) including (1) words, (2) nonwords, (3) pseudofont, (4) icon strings, (5) objects, (6) and pseudoobjects and the associated grand average ERPs (B) from a midline central (Cz) and occipital (Oz) electrode site. The P150 is large for stringlike stimuli (words, nonwords, and pseudofont), small for objectlike stimuli (objects and pseudoobjects), and intermediate for icon strings. From Schendan et al. (1998); reprinted with the permission of Cambridge University Press.

ence means or the extent to which information about that difference will be available for or actually used in further processing. So, the fact that the processing of real words and pseudowords is differentiated at some level by 200–250 msec does not necessarily mean that the brain has identified one type of stimulus as a word and the other as not a word (in the same way that a linguist or psycholinguist might). It may just reflect the brain's greater exposure to one class of stimuli than the other or its sensitivity to unusual (infrequent) letter combinations that characterize one class of stimuli more than the other. In fact, pronounceable pseudowords continue to be processed much like real words (in terms of the components elicited, though not necessarily in their size and latency) for several hundred milliseconds more. Unlike nonwords, but like stimuli bearing meaning, including real words, pronounceable pseudowords elicit a negativity peaking approximately 400 msec poststimulus onset (N400). Thus, it would seem that at least some of the processing circuits of the brain deal with pseudowords, which have no particular learned meaning, no differently than these circuits do with real words for some time after an initial differentiation. Perhaps the early differentiation has less to do with whether

any item is or is not a word and more to do with the extent of prior exposure. ERP research with children just acquiring language and/or reading skills as well as with adults learning a second language may provide a means for examining this hypothesis (Mills *et al.*, 1997; Neville *et al.*, 1997; Weber-Fox and Neville, 1996). Indeed, answering such questions poses one of the major challenges in cognitive neurolinguistics.

It is around the time that the brain's response to words seems to first diverge from that to pseudowords that the ERP also first shows a sensitivity to a word's frequency of occurrence in a given language (Francis and Kucera, 1982)—or, from the brain's point of view, the context-independent probability of encountering a particular word. King and Kutas (1998b) found that the latency of a left anterior negativity (which they labeled the lexical processing negativity, or LPN) occurring between 200 and 400 msec poststimulus onset is strongly correlated with a word's frequency of occurrence in the language (see Fig. 2). In short, the brain seems to process more rapidly words that it has had more experience processing. This kind of early difference in the speed with which words are processed can have large consequences later in the processing stream.

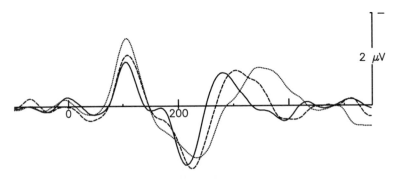

FIGURE 2   The lexical processing negativity is sensitive to word frequency. Grand average ERPs in response to words presented one at a time in sentences read for comprehension. Overlapped are the ERPs (digitally high-pass filtered at 4 Hz) to words sorted as a function of their frequency of occurrence in the English language. The latency of the negative peak is longest (~340 msec) for low-frequency (·····) and shortest (~280 msec) for high-frequency (——) words. Medium-frequency (----) words peak at ~300 msec. Data from King and Kutas (1998b).

King and Kutas (1998b) suggested that at least some of the reported differences between the processing of "open class" (nouns, verbs, adjectives, adverbs) and "closed class" (determiners, articles, prepositions) words were due to differences in their average frequency and the consequences this had on their early neural processing (also see Brown *et al.*, 1999; Münte *et al.*, 2001; Osterhout *et al.*, 1997a).

It is important to point out, however, that there is no single time or place where "word frequency" is processed and/or stored. Rather, word frequency affects multiple stages of processing, including word identification, access of associated phonological or semantic information from long-term memory, maintenance of word form or associated information in working memory, etc. In fact, ERP results clearly demonstrate that word frequency has different effects later in a word's processing. For example, with all other factors held constant (especially in the absence of semantic context), N400 amplitude is an inverse function of word frequency (Van Petten and Kutas, 1991). As will be discussed later, the N400 seems to be related to the access of semantic information from long-term memory and/or the integration of this information into a larger context. This aspect of processing is also affected by more "immediate" or local frequency information—namely, repetition in the experimental context (e.g., Rugg, 1985). Similar to the effects of global frequency information, repetition reduces the amplitude of the N400 activity, among the effects it has on other components (Van Petten *et al.*, 1991).

Processing Patterns

The fact that a word is encountered frequently or was just encountered thus affects the way it is processed by the brain. Moreover, it affects the processing at different times and most likely in different ways: the time interval since the last repetition, the number of repetitions, and the context within which the repetition occurs all seem to matter, albeit differently as a function of the individual's age (Besson and Kutas, 1993; Besson *et al.*, 1992; Kazmerski and Friedman, 1997; Nagy and Rugg, 1989; Rugg *et al.*, 1997; Young and Rugg, 1992). More specifically, words repeated in the context of a word list are typically characterized by an enhanced positivity; the effects of repetition overlap but are not limited to the region of the N400 and are thought to comprise multiple components. Repetition effects are large on immediate repetition (with no delay lag) in young and older adults. At longer lags, the pattern of effects is more variable in general and apparently smaller, if present at all, in older individuals. Although multiple repetitions of a word progressively diminish the amplitude of the N400 component, this reduction is modulated by the nature of the context in which the word reappears; a word repeated in an altered context seems to show little signs of N400 reduction (Besson and Kutas, 1993). However, when a word is repeated in the same context, its N400 amplitude is progressively reduced by repetition, even if it is semantically anomalous within its context, such that by a third presentation, the N400 region is characterized by a large posterior positive component. In fact, the repetition effect is more pronounced for semantically anomalous than for semantically congruous sentence endings.

Effects like these are likely to hold for language units larger than words as well—e.g., frequent and infrequent word combinations and frequent or infrequent syntactic structures. Indeed, ERPs reveal the importance of probability in the brain's processing of syntactic aspects of a sentence. A late positivity, variously called the P600 or "syntactic positive shift" (SPS), has most commonly been elicited in response to dispreferred, low-frequency, but possible continuations of sentences, as well as to outright syntactic violations (e.g., Coulson *et al.*, 1998b; Hagoort *et al.*, 1993; Neville

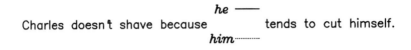

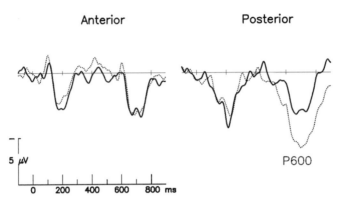

FIGURE 3   The P600. Grand average ERPs to target words in grammatical (solid) and ungrammatical (dotted) sentences at one anterior (left) and one posterior (right) electrode site. Compared to grammatical controls, ERPs to ungrammatical stimuli (here, case violations) are associated with enhanced positivity between 600 and 800 msec over posterior scalp sites.

et al., 1991; Osterhout and Holcomb, 1992). This positivity has a variable onset latency (generally late, but sometimes as early as 200 msec, depending on stimulus onset asynchrony) and a midpoint around 600 msec—though this may vary with the complexity of the linguistic structure involved (Münte *et al.*, 1997b). Its scalp distribution is most often posterior, though anterior effects have also been reported (see Fig. 3).

The P600 is typically observed when some aspect of a sentence violates structural (as opposed to semantic) expectations. For example, the P600 is reliably elicited when low-level morphosyntactic violations occur in a sentence, as when a subject does not agree in number with its verb ("Every Monday he mow the lawn"), when a noun phrase is incorrectly marked for case ("Ray fell down and skinned he knee") or number ("It has a nasty tempers and bites"), or when the second verb of a compound form is incorrectly inflected ("Dew does not fell like rain does"). In addition, late positivity is also seen in the

ERP response when the expected canonical word order of a phrase is disrupted ("Max's of proof the theorem") or when a verb's argument structure requirements are not met ("The broker persuaded to sell the stock"). It is important to note, however, that the P600 is not contingent on the presence of a grammatical violation; it is also elicited by points of processing difficulty, when the difficulty stems from processing at a grammatical or structural level (Kaan *et al.*, 2000; Osterhout and Holcomb, 1992). Although these manipulations are all "syntactic" to linguists, they differ significantly from one another in ways that are likely to matter to the brain. For example, some, such as word order violations, depend almost exclusively on position in the linear string, whereas others, such as morphosyntactic violations, depend instead on the relationship between words in a sentence, relatively independent of their linear sentence position. Still others, such as verb argument structure violations, depend not only on the relationship between sentence elements, but also on the relationship of those sentence elements to requirements specified in the lexical entry of the verb.

So what might the P600 be indexing? A clue comes from work by Coulson and colleagues (1998b), who examined the response to morphosyntactic violations of subject–verb agreement and case marking when these violations were either frequent or infrequent in an experimental run. They observed a P600 response to ungrammatical as compared with grammatical trials, although infrequent ungrammatical events elicited larger P600s than did frequently occurring ungrammatical events. Moreover, even grammatical events elicited some P600 activity when they occurred infrequently among many ungrammatical sentences (for further discussion see Coulson et al., 1998a; Gunter et al., 1997; Münte et al., 1998a; Osterhout and Hagoort, 1999; Osterhout et al., 1996).

It seems, then, that the part of the brain that is sensitive to syntactic violations is also sensitive to the subjective probability of those violations. Although the P600 is not typically elicited by semantically improbable events, it can be elicited subsequent to N400 effects in such contexts, and can even be elicited in response to nonstandard but orthographically and phonologically licit spellings of words (Münte et al., 1997b). This may suggest that, at least at some point, the processing of syntax takes place by reference to the relative (perceived?) frequency and reliability of various expected regularities in the language, a frequency that is continuously updated with experience. However, much work still remains to be done detailing the sensitivity of P600 amplitude to nonlinguistic variables, and understanding the nature of its relationship (identity, overlap, independence) from the group of positivities variously called the P3, P3b, P300, and late positive component, which likely encompass several distinct subcomponents.

The nature of early, sometimes left-lateralized frontal negativities that frequently precede the P600 in the ERPs to syntactic violations is somewhat less well understood. These negativities have been reported in two latency ranges: about 100 to 300 msec postword onset, the early left anterior negativity (ELAN), and, more commonly, about 300 to 500 or 600 msec postword onset, the left anterior negativity (LAN). These negativities have thus far eluded definitive identification as to their eliciting conditions, presumably because the experimental designs across studies have manipulated different variables and because, within individual studies, the manipulations undertaken have often been subject to more than one interpretation.

The left anterior negativity elicited between 300 and 600 msec has basically been interpreted in one of two different ways. One is as a direct and immediate response to syntactic or morphosyntactic ill-formedness (e.g., Münte et al., 1993; Neville et al., 1991; Osterhout and Holcomb, 1992), and the other is as an index of working memory processes during sentence comprehension (Coulson et al., 1998b; King and Kutas, 1995; Kluender and Kutas, 1993). The problem in deciding between these two alternatives is that manipulations of syntactic well-formedness have often occurred in sentences that incorporate long-distance relationships, which tax working memory resources, and working memory manipulations of long-distance sentence relationships have often resulted in—or been confounded with—less than complete well-formedness, as measured by either grammaticality or acceptability. Moreover, there is additional evidence in support of both interpretations. In the case of morphosyntactic and word order violations, LAN effects have been dissociated from P600 effects when such violations occur in jabberwocky sentences containing pseudowords: in these cases, the P600 effects can be suppressed but the LAN effect persists (Canseco-Gonzalez et al., 1997; Münte et al., 1997a; but see also Hahne and Jescheniak,

2001). This dissociation has been taken to mean that the LAN is the true marker of ill-formedness, whereas the P600 is merely an index of attempts on the part of the brain to recompute the sentence and make sense of the faulty input it is getting; this attempt at recomputation purportedly does not occur in jabberwocky sentences because no sense is to made of them in the first place. On the other hand, in support of the working memory interpretation, LAN effects have also been observed in tandem with P600 effects in response to long-distance, purely semantic violations of hyponymy that crucially range across two separate clauses (Shao and Neville, 1996). It may well be the case that both interpretations of the LAN are correct, i.e., that it is influenced both by syntactic ill-formedness and by working memory load (Kluender *et al.*, 1998; Vos *et al.*, 2001). Because both syntactic processing and verbal working memory are known functions of left frontal cortex, and because both tend to activate Broca's area in neural imaging studies (e.g., Dapretto and

Bookheimer, 1999; Embick *et al.*, 2000; Kang *et al.*, 1999; Ni *et al.*, 2000), this could be one clear instance in which the brain is not strictly respecting linguistic analysis (see Fig. 4).

The early left anterior negativity elicited between 100 and 300 msec postword onset is of slightly more recent vintage. The ELAN has most reliably been elicited in response to word category violations using auditory presentation (Friederici *et al.*, 1993; Hahne and Friederici, 1999) and has been interpreted as an index of a first-stage syntactic parser sensitive only to word category (i.e., part of speech) information in building an initial phrase structure tree. Because of its early latency and variability, it has been highly controversial. The morphology of the component varies from study to study in an as yet unpredictable manner: sometimes it is part of a broad negativity extending throughout the entire epoch (Friederici *et al.*, 1993, 1996), whereas at other times it is a phasic component with a clear peak (Hahne and Jescheniak, 2001). The relation of the ELAN to the

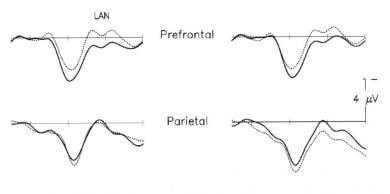

—— Inanimate(Animate): *The poetry that the editor recognized* **depressed**
········ Animate(Inanimate): *The editor that the poetry depressed* **recognized**

FIGURE 4   The left anterior negativity (LAN). Grand average ERPs to target sentence intermediate words (shown in bold type in the sentences) at left and right prefrontal (top) and left and right parietal (bottom) electrode sites. Responses at the main clause verb of object-relative sentences with an inanimate subject (solid lines) are compared with object-relative sentences with an animate subject (dotted lines). Animate subjects are harder to process in this construction because, although they tend to be subjects, they are here being used as objects of the relative-clause verb. In response to this increased ambiguity in syntactic processing, one observes increased negativity between 300 and 500 msec over frontal sites, with a left-lateralized distribution (LAN). Over parietal sites, the beginning of a P600 response can also be observed. Data from Weckerly and Kutas (1999).

LAN is also unclear. With low-contrast visual input, the latency of the component falls within that of the LAN (Gunter *et al.*, 1999); in jabberwocky studies, very similar manipulations have resulted in ELAN effects in one case (Hahne and Jescheniak, 2001) and in LAN effects in another (Münte *et al.*, 1997a); sometimes the ELAN is followed by a LAN, usually as a continuing negativity (Friederici *et al.*, 1993, 1996; Hahne and Friederici, 1999), and sometimes it is not (Hahne and Friederici, 1999; Hahne and Jescheniak, 2001).

More generally, the relation of the anterior phasic negativities to the P600 is unclear—at times they precede it, at other times they do not. Is this due to an interaction with verbal working memory, activated in some cases more than others? Moreover, the relation of the anterior phasic negativities to the slow anterior negative potentials indexing verbal working memory load (as discussed in the next section) is equally unclear. These are issues that will need to be sorted out in future research. What such results do make clear, however, is that the brain is sensitive to the frequency and recency of exposure to particular patterns. Its sensitivities range from the probability of encountering a particular physical stimulus to the probability of those stimuli patterning in a particular way with respect to one another in a phrase or sentence.

Working Memory

The brain's sensitivity to linguistic patterns of various types highlights another important aspect of language, namely, the need to process relations between items, at different levels of abstraction. Many linguistic patterns emerge over the course of multiple words separated by time and/or space, depending on the modality of presentation. Processing relations between these items necessitates that the brain maintain them in some kind of temporary store or "working memory." Even simple,

declarative sentences (e.g., "John really likes his pet dog") require working memory resources. At minimum, "John" must be held in memory so that the reader/listener knows who is being referred to when the pronoun "his" is encountered. Indeed, ERP data show that the brain is sensitive to the relationship between a pronoun and its antecedent. When an occupational title (e.g., "secretary") is paired with the more "probable" pronoun "she" (based on United States census data), less negativity is observed around 200 msec over left anterior sites than when the same occupation is paired with the less probable pronoun "he" (King and Kutas, 1998a). In the latter case, the brain may assume that the "he" refers to a new participant because the pronoun–antecedent pair seems less likely; the increased negativity may then reflect the working memory load associated with storing and/or holding onto information about two participants as opposed to only one. In a somewhat similar design with reflexive pronouns, Osterhout and co-workers (1997b) found that pronouns that disagreed with the gender definition or gender stereotype of an antecedent noun elicited a large positivity (i.e., the P600 typically associated with syntactic violations). The important point, however, is that pronouns elicit reliable ERP effects that can be used to investigate the link between them and the nouns to which they refer—a link that clearly relies on working memory.

Although all sentences tap into working memory, some clearly absorb more working memory resources than others (see Fig. 5). For instance, a sentence containing a relative clause (e.g., "The reporter who followed the senator admitted the error") typically requires more working memory resources than a simple declarative sentence, in part because a participant ("the reporter") is involved in two clauses/actions ("following" and "admitting"). These "subject-relative clauses," however, are presumed to require fewer

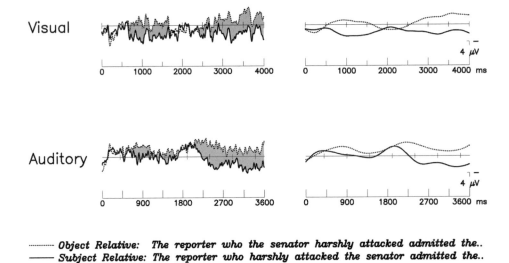

Visual

Auditory

·········· **Object Relative:** *The reporter who the senator harshly attacked admitted the..*
———— **Subject Relative:** *The reporter who harshly attacked the senator admitted the..*

FIGURE 5 Working memory and sentence processing. Comparison of grand average ERPs to subject-relative (solid lines) and object-relative (dotted lines) sentences from a left anterior site. On the left are the unfiltered data and on the right are the same data after they have been low-pass filtered to highlight slowly developing responses. The visual sentences were presented one word at a time, whereas the auditory sentences were presented as natural speech. The shading represents the area where object-relative sentences are reliably more negative than are subject-relative sentences. Visual data from Kutas and King (1996) and auditory data from Muller *et al.* (1997).

working memory resources than are object-relative clauses, such as "The reporter who the senator followed admitted the error". In object-relative clauses, the subject of the main clause ("the reporter") must be kept distinct from the subject of the relative clause ("the senator"). By examining sentences that vary in the extent to which they require working memory resources, one can examine the nature of the brain's response to working memory load (e.g., Friederici *et al.*, 1998; King and Kutas, 1995; Kutas and King, 1996; Mecklinger *et al.*, 1995; Muller *et al.*, 1997). In addition, one can assess individual variation in the brain's response to sentences of varying structural complexity as a function of the amount of working memory resources available (e.g., comparing individuals with high working memory "spans" with those who have fewer working memory resources). For example, King and Kutas (1995) compared ERP responses to subject- and object-relative sentences read one

word at a time. As soon as the sentence structures varied, good comprehenders elicited greater left, frontal negativities in the object-relative as compared with the subject-relative clauses. This is the point in the sentence where, in the case of object relatives, a second participant ("the senator") must be stored in working memory (along with "the reporter"). In contrast, the response of poor comprehenders (with fewer working memory resources) was quite negative to both types of sentences; thus, both types of sentences seemed to tax working memory resources for poorer comprehenders. Similar effects were observed for these same sentences presented as natural speech (Muller *et al.*, 1997). These results led to the hypothesis that the left anterior effect reflects general, as opposed to modality-specific, working memory operations. A similar left anterior negativity effect has also been observed for wh-questions (Kluender and Kutas, 1993). In English wh-questions (e.g., "Who did the doctor cure __?"), the wh-element (the "filler," in this case the word "who") appears at the beginning of the sentence, leaving a "gap" in the canonical word order (which in English is subject–verb–object). Another example comes from uncommon (and therefore difficult) word orders in German (Roesler *et al.*, 1998). The role of working memory operations in sentence processing can also be examined by simply adding an irrelevant or elaborative clause to a simple transitive sentence (Gunter *et al.*, 1995).

The extended nature of various working memory operations is also manifest in less transient, slow potential effects (long-lasting potentials on the order of seconds). For example, in response to the subject versus object-relative clauses discussed above, good comprehenders show a slow positive shift to the subject-relative sentences over frontal sites that lasts for the duration of the relative clause and beyond; poor comprehenders do not show either this slow positivity or this difference (Kutas and King, 1996). This comprehension-related ERP difference shows up even for simple transitive sentences, with good comprehenders generating much more of a frontal positive shift compared to poorer comprehenders. At the same time, poorer comprehenders show enhanced early sensory visual components such as the P1–N1–P2 relative to the better comprehenders. This suggests that poorer comprehenders (as compared to good comprehenders) may have devoted more resources to lower level perceptual processing, thereby having fewer resources to devote to higher order (possibly working-memory demanding) language processes. The potentials in normal elderly individuals for both simple transitive and object-relative sentences most resemble those of the poorer comprehending younger individuals (Kutas and King, 1996).

A number of PET and fMRI studies also have compared subject-relative and object-relative clauses, in the interest of localizing verbal working memory processes within the human brain. Because the left inferior frontal gyrus is a well-established language area commonly implicated in aspects of syntactic processing and production (i.e., Broca's area), it is perhaps not surprising that in all such studies to date, the left inferior frontal gyrus has emerged as a reliable locus of activation when the hemodynamic response to object-relative clauses has been compared to that for subject-relative clauses. This is also consistent with the finding that the neural circuitry for visuospatial working memory in the rhesus monkey involves extensive networks in prefrontal cortex (e.g., Goldman-Rakic, 1990). Thus in an fMRI study, Just *et al.* (1996) compared center-embedded subject- and object-relative clauses like those above with active conjoined clauses (e.g., "The reporter followed the senator and admitted the error"), and found increased activation in both Broca's and Wernicke's areas for object-relative clauses compared to subject-relative clauses and for subject-relative clauses as compared to active conjoined clauses. On the other hand, a series of PET studies of center-embedded object relatives (e.g., "The juice [that the child spilled] stained the rug") vs. right-branching subject relatives (e.g., "The child spilled the juice [that stained the rug]") by Caplan and colleagues has consistently shown increased activation only in Broca's area, though the exact locus of activation *within* Broca's area has shifted slightly from study to study: the pars opercularis (Brodmann's area 44) in Stromswold *et al.* (1996) and Caplan *et al.* (1998), and the pars triangularis (Brodmann's area 45) in Caplan *et al.* (1999, 2000).

However, a Japanese fMRI study that manipulated center-embedded vs. left-branching structures using only subject-relative clauses in Japanese, a verb-final language, yielded a widespread increase in activation in response to the center-embedded subject relatives (Inui *et al.*, 1998). This increase in activation appeared in both BA 44 and BA 45 of the left inferior frontal gyrus (i.e., Broca's area), as well as in the posterior portion of the left superior temporal gyrus (BA 22, i.e., Wernicke's area), and in left dorsolateral prefrontal cortex (the posterior part of BA 9). What is interesting about this comparison is that in order to maintain strict left branching in Japanese, the canonical subject–object–verb (SOV) word order of Japanese, preserved in the center-embedded condition, must be disrupted: the object noun plus its (preceding) relative clause must be moved to the front of the sentence, resulting in relatively rare OSV word order (corpus studies of both spoken and written Japanese text show that the OSV pattern occurs less than 1% of the time) (Yamashita, 2002). Note that this emulates the word order of object relatives in English ("…who the senator followed," "…that the child spilled," etc.). Thus at least in Japanese, center embedding with canonical word order seems to present a greater load for working memory than fronting an object in noncanonical word order. Naturally, more cross-linguistic studies of this nature are needed to tease apart conclusively the effects of center embedding, object fronting, basic word order, and neural imaging technique (PET vs. fMRI) in these working memory studies.

In general, neuroimaging results support claims originally made in the behavioral literature that successful language comprehension involves the storage and retrieval of information in working memory (e.g., Carpenter and Just, 1989; Daneman and Carpenter, 1980; Daneman and Merikle, 1996). Only through the use of working memory can the brain process critical relationships between sensory stimuli distributed over time and space. In addition, these results suggest that successful relational processing may call for more general, attentional resources. If more attention must be paid to lower level perceptual processes necessary for language comprehension, less attentional resources are available for the working memory operations especially critical for the processing of complex language structures.

Long-Term Memory

Although the processing of relations between items is crucial for successful language comprehension, at its heart language involves the processing of a different kind of relation—the relation between language elements and real-world knowledge stored in long-term memory (see McKoon and Ratcliff, 1998). Words are symbols—that is, they are associated with information that is not contained in the physical form of the word. It has been suggested that the human ability to remember, transform, and flexibly combine thousands of symbols is what especially sets us apart from other species (e.g., Deacon, 1997). Early in their processing, words are but perceptual objects with visual or acoustic properties that must be processed sufficiently to allow categorization and identification. Eventually, however, words serve as entry points into vast amounts of information stored in long-term memory. This associated information has been derived from many modalities (e.g., the shape and color of a carrot, its smell, its taste, its firmness, and smoothness; the crunching sound made when eating it) and has come to be associated with the word form through experience. The nature of the organization of long-term memory, the types of information that are stored, and the extent to which different information types are accessed under various conditions are all highly controversial issues.

Mirroring the concerns of psycholinguistics in general, many ERP investigations have been aimed at determining what kinds of information about words are typically retrieved during reading and listening and the time courses with which this information is retrieved. Moreover, given its unique ability to track word, sentence, and discourse-level processing with equal resolution, the ERP technique has also been directed at determining how information retrieved from the various words in a sentence is ultimately combined into a single message. ERP data suggest that the brain is clearly sensitive to some aspects of meaning by at least 250–300 msec post stimulus onset. In this time window, the brain's response to words (and pronounceable pseudowords) in all modalities (spoken, printed, signed) (e.g., Holcomb and Neville, 1990; Kutas and Hillyard, 1980a, b; Kutas *et al.*, 1987), to pictures (Ganis *et al.*, 1996; Nigam *et al.*, 1992) and faces (Barrett and Rugg, 1989; Bobes *et al.*, 1994; Debruille *et al.*, 1996), and to meaningful environmental sounds (Chao *et al.*, 1995; Van Petten and Rheinfelder, 1995) contains a negativity with a posterior, slightly right hemisphere distribution at the scalp. Potentials at the same latency and sensitive to these same semantic variables are observed in the fusiform gyrus of patients with electrodes implanted for localizing seizure activity (e.g., McCarthy *et al.*, 1995; Nobre and McCarthy, 1995); note that the polarity of a recorded potential depends on the location of the active electrode and reference, such that the intracranially recorded "N400s" are not always negative. This so-called N400 component was mentioned previously in the discussion of frequency and repetition effects, because its amplitude varies with both. In children and intact adults, the N400 seems to be the normal response to stimuli that are potentially meaningful. Some have suggested that the N400 reflects some kind of search through long-term, semantic memory; indeed N400 amplitude does vary with factors that also influence memory, such as the number of items to be remembered (Stuss *et al.*, 1986) and the length of the delay between presentations of an item (e.g., Chao *et al.*, 1995). Its amplitude is diminished and its latency is prolonged with normal aging, and even more

so with various dementias (e.g., Iragui *et al.*, 1993, 1996).

We have suggested that the N400 indexes some aspect of meaning because its amplitude is modulated by semantic aspects of a preceding context, be it a single word, a sentence, or a multisentence discourse. For instance, the amplitude of the N400 to a word in a list is reduced if that word is preceded by one with a similar meaning (e.g., N400 amplitude to "dog" is reduced when preceded by "cat" compared to "cup") (Brown and Hagoort, 1993; Holcomb and Neville, 1990; Van Petten *et al.*, 1995). Brain activity in the same time region is also sensitive to phonological and orthographic relations between words (Barrett and Rugg, 1990; Polich *et al.*, 1983; Praamstra *et al.*, 1994; Rugg, 1984a; Rugg and Barrett, 1987). Similarly, the amplitude of the N400 to a word in a sentence is reduced to the extent that the word is compatible with the ongoing semantic context. An anomaly (e.g., "He takes his coffee with cream and dog") elicits the largest N400 response. Nonanomalous but less probable words (e.g., "He takes his coffee with cream and honey") generate less N400 activity than do anomalies but N400s of greater amplitude than more probable completions (e.g., "He takes his coffee with cream and sugar") (Kutas and Donchin, 1980; Kutas and Hillyard, 1980ab, 1984; Kutas *et al.*, 1984). Discourse-level factors may also affect the magnitude of the N400 response. As single sentences, both "the mouse quickly went into its hole" and "the mouse slowly went into its hole" are congruous. However, in a larger discourse context (e.g., "Prowling under the kitchen table, the cat surprised a mouse eating crumbs. The mouse ... "), the two adverbs (quickly and slowly) are no longer equally expected; in fact, the N400 response to "slowly" in this type of context is larger than the response to "quickly" (van Berkum *et al.*, 1999). Thus, at least around 400 msec, lexical, sentential, and discourse factors seem to converge to influence language comprehension and do so in a fairly similar manner. When both lexical and sentential factors are present, they seem to influence the N400 amplitude independently (Kutas, 1993; Van Petten, 1993, 1995; see also Fischler *et al.*, 1985, for a similar conclusion). The relation of the N400 to semantic integrative processes is further supported by the observation that its amplitude is greatly attenuated and its latency is delayed in aphasic patients with moderate to severe comprehension problems, but not in patients with equivalent

amounts of damage to the right hemisphere (Swaab *et al.*, 1997).

The N400 is thus sensitive to the relationship between a word and its immediate sentential context and to that between a word and other words in the lexicon (see Fig. 6). Insofar as N400 indexes some aspect of search through memory, it seems then that the brain uses all the information it can as soon as it can to constrain its search. How does context serve to guide this search? We can think of information about word meaning as existing in a kind of space, structured by experience. The nature of this structure is often inferred

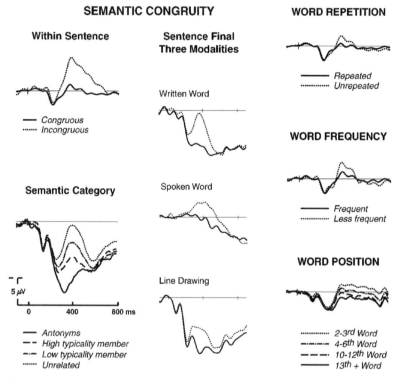

FIGURE 6 The N400 responses to various experimental manipulations, all shown here at a representative right posterior site. Incongruous words elicit large N400 amplitudes relative to congruous words, whether these items are in midsentence position (top left of figure) or in sentence final position. As shown in the center, this effect can be observed in all modalities, including written words, spoken words, and line drawings (here, all using the same experimental materials). As seen at bottom left, the N400 is similarly sensitive to varying degrees and types of semantic relations in more minimal contexts, including highly constrained antonyms (e.g., "The opposite of black … white"; solid line), and category membership relations (e.g., "A type of bird …") with high (e.g., "robin"; dashed line) or low (e.g., "turkey"; dot–dash line) typicality, as compared with unrelated items (dotted line). N400 amplitudes also vary with factors such as repetition, word frequency, and word position (see right side of figure).

from the outcome of various categorization or sentence verification tasks (e.g., Kounios, 1996; Kounios and Holcomb, 1992; Kounios *et al.*, 1994). Context (as well as the other factors known to influence N400 amplitude such as frequency or repetition) may serve to direct processing into different parts of this space—usually parts that render subsequent searches easier by bringing the processor into a state "closer" to the meaning of upcoming words. We have examined this hypothesis in a study in which participants were asked to read the following types of pairs of sentences:

> Ann wanted to treat her foreign
> guests to an all-American dessert.
> She went out in the back yard and
> picked some apples.

These sentence pairs were terminated with either the contextually expected item ("apples"), a contextually unexpected item that came from the same semantic category as the expected item (e.g., "oranges," another fruit), or an unexpected item from a different semantic category (e.g., "carrots"). Both types of unexpected endings elicited an N400 relative to congruent endings. However, even though both kinds of unexpected endings were equally inappropriate and implausible in the context, the unexpected item from the expected category elicited a smaller N400 than did the one from a different category. Moreover, the N400 reduction to such "within-category" violations was largest in highly constraining sentence contexts, where these violations were most implausible. The N400 does more than simply index the semantic fit between an item and its local context, therefore. Rather, this data pattern shows that the organization of sensory, motor, and higher order features in the brain built up of years of experience with the world (the fact that apples and oranges share more features in common than apples and carrots) has an inevitable impact on the neural processes (here seen in the N400 response) by which brains

make sense of language in real time (Federmeier and Kutas, 1999b; Kutas and Federmeier, 2001).

An integral part of language comprehension, therefore, involves retrieving world knowledge associated with words and groups of words from long-term semantic memory. ERP data in conjunction with neuropsychological data and data from other neuroimaging techniques suggest that this meaning-related information resides in featural mosaics distributed across multiple brain areas, including higher order perceptual and motor-processing areas. fMRI studies (in accord with neuropsychological findings), for example, have shown that different brain areas become active in response to words (and/or pictures) representing different kinds of information (e.g., actions vs. colors) (Martin *et al.*, 1995) and that patterns of activation within general brain areas, such as the ventral temporal cortex, vary as a function of semantic category as well (e.g., tools, animals) (see reviews by Humphreys *et al.*, 1999; Martin and Chao, 2001). N400 data also reveal that the nature of the meaning information retrieved from long-term memory differs—even within the same linguistic context—for different types of stimuli (e.g., a picture vs. word representing the same concept) (Federmeier and Kutas, 2001) and as a function of which cerebral hemisphere preferentially (based on location of presentation) processes that information (Federmeier and Kutas, 1999a, 2002). The ERP data further suggest that meaning emerges from these distributed systems by virtue of temporally coincident and functionally similar activity within a number of brain areas [see also intracranial recording studies by Halgren *et al.* (1994a,b), McCarthy *et al.* (1995), and Nobre and McCarthy (1995)].

Language meaning thus emerges from an interaction between structure in the brain, built out of experience, and structure in the language stream. Context serves to shape not only the ease with which information can be found but also the nature of the information that is retrieved. Conceptual information also serves to shape language processing by providing a structure ("frame" or "schema") within which details beyond the level of individual words can be fit and related to one another. These "schemas" can be thought of as the brain's general expectations about the nature of information that will be retrieved and the order in which it will come. These schemas might well influence the extent to which various aspects of information are attended, how they are stored in working memory, and the ease with which they are comprehended. A study by Münte *et al.* (1998b) examined how people's schemas about time (built of daily experience) may affect the brain's processing of sentences and thus interact with working memory variables. People read sentences describing the temporal order of two events; the sentences differed only in whether their initial word was "before" or "after" (e.g., "Before/after the students took the exam the teacher called the parents"). Although these sentence types are otherwise identical in lexical content and syntactic structure, they differ in the extent to which they fit with our schema of time as a dimension moving from past to future. In "after" sentences, the two events are mentioned in accordance with this conception—the temporally earlier event coming first and the temporally later event coming second. By contrast, "before" sentences reverse this natural order. Münte *et al.* found that starting within 300 msec of the initial word (the temporal term), "after" sentences showed a larger sustained positivity than did "before" sentences; this positivity was similar to that described for the relative-clause (object vs subject) contrast. This difference was, again, most pronounced for individuals with high working memory spans. The data suggest that our knowledge of the world (in this case, about time)

has an immediate, lasting effect on processing, and that this impact is modulated by working memory capacity and/or availability. Words such as "before" and "after" serve as cues about the relationship between elements to come. These relations, in turn, are easier to process if they conform to general conceptual patterns derived from experience.

CONCLUSIONS

Comprehending language thus entails a number of different kinds of brain processes, including perceptual analysis, attention allocation, retrieval of information from long-term memory, storage of information in working memory, and comparisons between/transformations of information contained in working memory. These processes take place at multiple levels for different types of information (orthographic/phonological word form information, morphological/syntactic information, conceptual/semantic information) and unfold with different time courses; they are thus reflected in different electrophysiological processes with different time-courses, mediated by different brain areas.

Understanding language processing, therefore, demands that we apprehend how the multiple subprocesses involved interact over time and space. This, in turn, compels us to appreciate how the brain's processing of language interacts with more general processing demands. For example, both N400 and P600 amplitudes are responsive to attentional manipulations. The N400, for instance, is not observed when the priming context is masked (Brown and Hagoort, 1993), and N400 effects in word pair tasks are larger when the prime target interval is short and the proportion of related word pairs is high (Chwilla *et al.*, 1995; Holcomb, 1988). Similarly, the P600 to verb inflection errors is greatly attenuated if not absent when people are asked to scan sentences merely to determine whether a word in a sentence is printed in upper case (Gunter and Friederici, 1999). Orthographic, phonological, morphological, syntactic, and pragmatic priming and context ERP effects seem to overlap temporally between 200 and 400 msec. Various and sundry memory-related and some attention-related ERP effects are observed in this very same interval. Moreover, the transient ERPs elicited during the analysis of a visual stimulus as a word are superimposed on the slower potentials that seem to be elicited during the processing of sentences and during various tasks requiring that information be retrieved from longer term memory. Indeed, the language specificity of any of these processes remains unknown to date.

What we do know is that language processing is a complex skill engaging the whole brain. The goal of electrophysiological investigations of language, as well as the goal of research exploring language processing with other tools, is to fashion an understanding of how the various processes involved in language comprehension and production are coordinated to yield the message-level apprehension we attain from reading or listening to speech. Linguists, psycholinguists, and neurolinguists alike strive to understand how the brain "sees" language—because, in turn, language is such an important facet of how humans "see" their world.

References

Allison, T., Wood, C. C., and McCarthy, G. (1986). The central nervous system. *In* "Psychophysiology: Systems, Processes, and Applications" (M. G. Coles, E. Donchin, and S. W. Porges, eds.), pp. 5–25. Guilford Press, New York.

Allison, T., McCarthy, G., Nobre, A., Puce, A., and Belger, A. (1994). Human extrastriate visual cortex and the perception of faces, words, numbers, and colors. *Cereb. Cortex* **4**(5), 544–554.

Barrett, S. E., and Rugg, M. D. (1989). Event-related potentials and the semantic matching of faces. *Neuropsychologia* **27**(7), 913–922.

Barrett, S. E., and Rugg, M. D. (1990). Event-related potentials and the phonological matching of picture names. *Brain Lang.* **38**(3), 424–437.

Besson, M., and Kutas, M. (1993). The many facets of repetition: A cued-recall and event-related potential analysis of repeating words in same versus different sentence contexts. *J. Exp. Psycho.: Learning Memory Cogn.* **19**(5), 1115–1133.

Besson, M., Kutas, M., and Van Petten, C. (1992). An event-related potential (ERP) analysis of semantic congruity and repetition effects in sentences. *J. Cogn. Neurosci.* **4**(2), 132–149.

Bobes, M. A., Valdes-Sosa, M., and Olivares, E. (1994). An ERP study of expectancy violation in face perception. *Brain Cogn.* **26**(1), 1–22.

Brown, C., and Hagoort, P. (1993). The processing nature of the N400: Evidence from masked priming. *J. Cogn. Neurosci.* **5**(1), 34–44.

Brown, C. M., Hagoort, P., and ter Keurs, M. (1999). Electrophysiological signatures of visual lexical processing: Open- and closed-class words. *J. Cogn. Neurosci.* **11**(3), 261–281.

Canseco-Gonzalez, E., Love, T., Ahrens, K., Walenski, M., Swinney, D., and Neville, H. (1997). Processing of grammatical information in Jabberwocky sentences: An ERP study. Paper presented at the Cognitive Neuroscience Society, Fourth Annual Meeting, Boston, Massachusetts.

Caplan, D., Alpert, N., and Waters, G. (1998). Effects of syntactic structure and propositional number on patterns of regional cerebral blood flow. *J. Cogn. Neurosci.* **10**(4), 541–552.

Caplan, D., Alpert, N., and Waters, G. (1999). PET studies of syntactic processing with auditory sentence presentation. *Neuroimage* **9**(3), 343–351.

Caplan, D., Alpert, N., Waters, G., and Olivieri, A. (2000). Activation of Broca's area by syntactic processing under conditions of concurrent articulation. *Human Brain Mapping* **9**(2), 65–71.

Carpenter, P. A., and Just, M. A. (1989). The role of working memory in language comprehension. *In* "Complex Information Processing: The Impact of Herbert A. Simon" D. Klahr and K. Kotovsky, eds.), pp. 31–68. Lawrence Erlbaum Assoc., Hillsdale, New Jersey.

Chao, L. L., Nielsen-Bohlman, L., and Knight, R. T. (1995). Auditory event-related potentials dissociate early and late memory processes. *Electroencephalogr. Clin. Neurophysiol.*, **96**(2), 157–168.

Chomsky, N. (1965). "Aspects of the Theory of Syntax." MIT Press, Cambridge, Massachusetts.

Chomsky, N. (1980). "*Rules and representations*. B. Blackwell, London.

Churchland, P. M. (1984). "Matter and Consciousness: A Contemporary Introduction to the Philosophy of Mind." MIT Press, Cambridge, Massachusetts.

Chwilla, D. J., Brown, C. M., and Hagoort, P. (1995). The N400 as a function of the level of processing. *Psychophysiology* 32(3), 274–285.

Coulson, S., King, J. W., and Kutas, M. (1998a). ERPs and domain specificity: Beating a straw horse. *Lang. Cogn. Processes* 13, 653–672.

Coulson, S., King, J. W., and Kutas, M. (1998b). Expect the unexpected: Event-related brain response to morphosyntactic violations. *Lang. Cogn. Processes* 13(1), 21–58.

Dale, A. M., and Halgren, E. (2001). Spatiotemporal mapping of brain activity by integration of multiple imaging modalities. *Curr. Opin. Neurobiol.* 11(2), 202–208.

Daneman, M., and Carpenter, P. A. (1980). Individual differences in working memory and reading. *J. Verbal Learn. Verbal Behav.* 19(4), 450–466.

Daneman, M., and Merikle, P. M. (1996). Working memory and language comprehension: A meta-analysis. *Psychonom. Bull. Rev.* 3(4), 422–433.

Dapretto, M., and Bookheimer, S. Y. (1999). Form and content: Dissociating syntax and semantics in sentence comprehension. *Neuron* 24(2), 427–432.

Deacon, T. W. (1997). "The Symbolic Species." W. W. Norton, New York.

Debruille, J. B., Pineda, J., and Renault, B. (1996). N400-like potentials elicited by faces and knowledge inhibition. *Cogn. Brain Res.* 4(2), 133–144.

Embick, D., Marantz, A., Miyashita, Y., O'Neil, W., and Sakai, K. L. (2000). A syntactic specialization for Broca's area. *Proc. Natl. Acad. Sci. U.S.A.* 97(11), 6150–6154.

Farah, M. J. (1990). "Visual Agnosia: Disorders of Object Recognition and What They Tell Us about Normal Vision." MIT Press, Cambridge.

Federmeier, K. D., and Kutas, M. (1999a). Right words and left words: Electrophysiological evidence for hemispheric differences in meaning processing. *Cogn. Brain Res.* 8(3), 373–392.

Federmeier, K. D., and Kutas, M. (1999b). A rose by any other name: Long-term memory structure and sentence processing. *J. Mem. Lang.* 41(4), 469–495.

Federmeier, K. D., and Kutas, M. (2001). Meaning and modality: Influences of context, semantic memory organization, and perceptual predictability on picture processing. *J. Exp. Psychol.: Learning Mem. Cogn.* 27(1), 202–224.

Federmeier, K. D., and Kutas, M. (2002). Picture the difference: Electrophysiological investigations of picture processing in the cerebral hemispheres. *Neuropsychologia* 40, 730–747.

Fischler, I., Childers, D. G., Achariyapaopan, T., and Perry, N. W. (1985). Brain potentials during sentence verification: Automatic aspects of comprehension. *Biol. Psychol.* 21(2), 83–105.

Fodor, J. A. (1981). The mind–body problem. *Sci. Am.* 244(1), 114–123.

Fodor, J. A. (1983). "The Modularity of Mind: An Essay on Faculty Psychology." MIT Press, Cambridge, Massachusetts.

Francis, W. N., and Kucera, H. (1982). "*Frequency Analysis of English Usage.*" Houghton Mifflin Company, Boston.

Friederici, A. D., Pfeifer, E., and Hahne, A. (1993). Event-related brain potentials during natural speech processing: Effects of semantic, morphological and syntactic violations. *Cogn. Brain Res.* 1(3), 183–192.

Friederici, A. D., Hahne, A., and Mecklinger, A. (1996). Temporal structure of syntactic parsing: Early and late event-related brain potential effects. *J. Exp. Psychol.: Learning Memory Cogn.* 22(5), 1219–1248.

Friederici, A. D., Steinhauer, K., Mecklinger, A., and Meyer, M. (1998). Working memory constraints on syntactic ambiguity resolution as revealed by electrical brain responses. *Biol. Psychol.* 47(3), 193–221.

Ganis, G., Kutas, M., and Sereno, M. I. (1996). The search for 'common sense': An electrophysiological study of the comprehension of words and pictures in reading. *J. Cogn. Neurosci.* 8, 89–106.

Goldman-Rakic, P. S. (1990). Cortical localization of working memory. *In* "Brain Organization and Memory: Cells, Systems, and Circuits" J. L. McGaugh and N. M. Weinberger *et al.*, (eds.), pp. 285–298. Oxford University Press, New York.

Gunter, T. C., and Friederici, A. D. (1999). Concerning the automaticity of syntactic processing. *Psychophysiology* 36, 126–137.

Gunter, T. C., Jackson, J. L., and Mulder, G. (1995). Language, memory, and aging: An electrophysiological exploration of the N400 during reading of memory-demanding sentences. *Psychophysiology* 32(3), 215–229.

Gunter, T. C., Stowe, L. A., and Mulder, G. (1997). When syntax meets semantics. *Psychophysiology* 34(6), 660–676.

Gunter, T. C., Friederici, A. D., and Hahne, A. (1999). Brain responses during sentence reading: Visual input affects central processes. *Neurorep.: Rapid Commun. Neurosci. Res.* 10(15), 3175–3178.

Hagoort, P., Brown, C., and Groothusen, J. (1993). The syntactic positive shift (SPS) as an ERP measure of syntactic processing. Special Issue: Event-related brain potentials in the study of language. *Lang. Cogn. Processes* 8(4), 439–483.

Hahne, A., and Friederici, A. D. (1999). Electrophysiological evidence for two steps in syntactic analysis: Early automatic and late controlled processes. *J. Cogn. Neurosci.* 11(2), 194–205.

Hahne, A., and Jescheniak, J. D. (2001). What's left if the Jabberwock gets the semantics? An ERP investigation into semantic and syntactic processes during auditory sentence comprehension. *Cogn. Brain Res.* 11(2), 199–212.

Halgren, E., Baudena, P., Heit, G., Clarke, J. M., Marinkovic, K., Chauvel, P., and Clarke, M. (1994a). Spatio-temporal stages in face and word processing. 2. Depth-recorded potentials in the human frontal and Rolandic cortices [published erratum appears in *J. Physiol. Paris* **88**(2) (1994), following p. 151]. *J. Physiol.* **88**(1), 51–80.

Halgren, E., Baudena, P., Heit, G., Clarke, J. M., Marinkovic, K., and Clarke, M. (1994b). Spatio-temporal stages in face and word processing. I. Depth-recorded potentials in the human occipital, temporal and parietal lobes [corrected] [published erratum appears in *J. Physiol. Paris* **88**(2) (1994), following p. 151]. *J. Physiol.* **88**(1), 1–50.

Hockett, C. F. (1963). A note on structure. In "Readings in Linguistics" (M. Joos, ed.), pp. 279–280. American Council of Learned Societies, New York.

Holcomb, P. J. (1988). Automatic and attentional processing: An event-related brain potential analysis of semantic priming. *Brain Lang.* **35**(1), 66–85.

Holcomb, P. J., and Neville, H. J. (1990). Auditory and visual semantic priming in lexical decision: A comparison using event-related brain potentials. *Lang. Cogn. Processes* **5**(4), 281–312.

Humphreys, G. W., Price, C. J., and Riddoch, M. J. (1999). From objects to names: A cognitive neuroscience approach. *Psychol. Res./Psychol. Forsch.* **62**(2-3), 118–130.

Inui, T., Otsu, Y., Tanaka, S., Okada, T., Nishizawa, S., and Konishi, J. (1998). A functional MRI analysis of comprehension processes of Japanese sentences. *Neurorep.: Int. J. Rapid Commun. Res. Neurosci.* **9**(14), 3325–3328.

Iragui, V. J., Kutas, M., Mitchiner, M. R., and Hillyard, S. A. (1993). Effects of aging on event-related brain potentials and reaction times in an auditory oddball task. *Psychophysiology* **30**(1), 10–22.

Iragui, V., Kutas, M., and Salmon, D. P. (1996). Event-related potentials during semantic categorization in normal aging and senile dementia of the Alzheimer's type. *Electroencephalogr. Clin. Neurophysiol.* **100**, 392–406.

Johnston, V. S., and Chesney, G. L. (1974). Electrophysiological correlates of meaning. *Science* **186**(4167), 944–946.

Just, M. A., Carpenter, P. A., Keller, T. A., Eddy, W. F., and Thulborn, K. R. (1996). Brain activation modulated by sentence comprehension. *Science* **274**(5284), 114–116.

Kaan, E., Harris, A., Gibson, E., and Holcomb, P. (2000). The P600 as an index of syntactic integration difficulty. *Lang. Cogn. Processes* **15**(2), 159–201.

Kang, A. M., Constable, R. T., Gore, J. C., and Avrutin, S. (1999). An event-related fMRI study of implicit phrase-level syntactic and semantic processing. *Neuroimage* **10**(5), 555–561.

Kazmerski, V. A., and Friedman, D. (1997). Old/new differences in direct and indirect memory tests using pictures and words in within- and cross-form conditions: Event-related potential and behavioral measures. *Cogn. Brain Res.* **5**(4), 255–272.

King, J. W., and Kutas, M. (1995). Who did what and when? Using word- and clause-level ERPs to monitor working memory usage in reading. *J. Cogn. Neurosci.* **7**(3), 376–395.

King, J. W., and Kutas, M. (1998a). He really is a nurse: ERPs and anaphoric coreference. *Psychophysiology* **35**(Suppl. 1), S47.

King, J. W., and Kutas, M. (1998b). Neural plasticity in the dynamics of human visual word recognition. *Neurosci. Lett.* **244**(2), 61–64.

Kluender, R., and Kutas, M. (1993). Bridging the gap: Evidence from ERPs on the processing of unbounded dependencies. *J. Cogn. Neurosci.* **5**(2), 196–214.

Kluender, R., Münte, T., Cowles, H. W., Szentkuti, A., Walenski, M., and Wieringa, B. (1998). Brain potentials to English and German questions. *J. Cogn. Neurosci. (Suppl.)* **1**, 24.

Kounios, J. (1996). On the continuity of thought and the representation of knowledge: Electrophysiological and behavioral time-course measures reveal levels of structure in semantic memory. *Psychonom. Bull. Rev.* **3**(3), 265–286.

Kounios, J., and Holcomb, P. J. (1992). Structure and process in semantic memory: Evidence from event-related brain potentials and reaction times. *J. Exp. Psychol. Gen.* **121**(4), 459–479.

Kounios, J., Montgomery, E. C., and Smith, R. W. (1994). Semantic memory and the granularity of semantic relations: Evidence from speed-accuracy decomposition. *Memory Cogn.* **22**(6), 729–741.

Kutas, M. (1993). In the company of other words: Electrophysiological evidence for single-word and sentence context effects. Special Issue: Event-related brain potentials in the study of language. *Lang. Cogn. Processes* **8**(4), 533–572.

Kutas, M., and Dale, A. (1997). Electrical and magnetic readings of mental functions. In "Cognitive Neuroscience" (M. D. Rugg, ed.), pp. 197–242. Psychology Press, Hove, East Sussex.

Kutas, M., and Donchin, E. (1980). Preparation to respond as manifested by movement-related brain potentials. *Brain Res.* **202**(1), 95–115.

Kutas, M., and Federmeier, K. D. (2001). Electrophysiology reveals semantic memory use in language comprehension. *Trends Cogn. Sci.* **4**(12), 463–470.

Kutas, M., and Hillyard, S. A. (1980a). Event-related brain potentials to semantically inappropriate and surprisingly large words. *Biol. Psychol.* **11**(2), 99–116.

Kutas, M., and Hillyard, S. A. (1980b). Reading senseless sentences: Brain potentials reflect semantic incongruity. *Science* **207**(4427), 203–205.

Kutas, M., and Hillyard, S. A. (1984). Brain potentials during reading reflect word expectancy and semantic association. *Nature* **307**(5947), 161–163.

Kutas, M., and King, J. W. (1996). The potentials for basic sentence processing: Differentiating integrative processes. *In* "Attention and Performance 16: Information Integration in Perception and Communication" (T. Inui and J. L. McClelland, eds.), pp. 501–546. MIT Press, Cambridge, Massachusetts.

Kutas, M., and Van Petten, C. K. (1994). Psycholinguistics electrified: Event-related brain potential investigations. *In* "Handbook of Psycholinguistics" (M. A. Gernsbacher, ed.), pp. 83–143. Academic Press, San Diego.

Kutas, M., Lindamood, T. E., and Hillyard, S. A. (1984). Word expectancy and event-related brain potentials during sentence processing. *In* "Preparatory States and Processes" (S. Kornblum and J. Requin, eds.), pp. 217–237. Lawrence Erlbaum Assoc., Hillsdale, New Jersey.

Kutas, M., Neville, H. J., and Holcomb, P. J. (1987). A preliminary comparison of the N400 response to semantic anomalies during reading, listening, and signing. *Electroencephalogr. Clin. Neurophysiol. (Suppl.)* **39**, 325–330.

Kutas, M., Federmeier, K. D., and Sereno, M. I. (1999). Current approaches to mapping language in electromagnetic space. *In* "The Neurocognition of Language" (C. M. Brown and P. Hagoort, eds.), pp. 359–392. Oxford University Press, Oxford.

Maclay, H., and Osgood, C. E. (1959). Hesitation phenomena in spontaneous English speech. *Word* **15**, 19–44.

Martin, A., and Chao, L. L. (2001). Semantic memory and the brain: Structure and processes. *Curr. Opin. Neurobiol.* **11**(2), 194–201.

Martin, A., Haxby, J. V., Lalonde, F. M., and Wiggs, C. L. (1995). Discrete cortical regions associated with knowledge of color and knowledge of action. *Science* **270**(5233), 102–105.

McCarthy, G., Nobre, A. C., Bentin, S., and Spencer, D. D. (1995). Language-related field potentials in the anterior-medial temporal lobe: I. Intracranial distribution and neural generators. *J. Neurosci.* **15**(2), 1080–1089.

McKoon, G., and Ratcliff, R. (1998). Memory-based language processing: Psycholinguistic research in the 1990s. *Annu. Rev. Psychol.* **49**, 25–42.

Mecklinger, A., Schriefers, H., Steinhauer, K., and Friederici, A. D. (1995). Processing relative clauses varying on syntactic and semantic dimensions: An analysis with event-related potentials. *Memory Cogn.* **23**(4), 477–494.

Mills, D. L., Coffey-Corina, S., and Neville, H. J. (1997). Language comprehension and cerebral specialization from 13 to 20 months. *Dev. Neuropsychol.* **13**(3), 397–445.

Muller, H. M., King, J. W., and Kutas, M. (1997). Event-related potentials elicited by spoken relative clauses. *Cogn. Brain Res.* **5**(3), 193–203.

Münte, T. F., Heinze, H.-J., and Mangun, G. R. (1993). Dissociation of brain activity related to syntactic and semantic aspects of language. *J. Cogn. Neurosci.* **5**(3), 335–344.

Münte, T. F., Matzke, M., and Johannes, S. (1997a). Brain activity associated with syntactic incongruencies in words and pseudo-words. *J. Cogn. Neurosci.* **9**(3), 318–329.

Münte, T. F., Szentkuti, A., Wieringa, B. M., Matzke, M., and Johannes, S. (1997b). Human brain potentials to reading syntactic errors in sentences of different complexity. *Neurosci. Lett.* **235**(3), 105–108.

Münte, T. F., Heinze, H. J., Matzke, M., Wieringa, B. M., and Johannes, S. (1998a). Brain potentials and syntactic violations revisited: No evidence for specificity of the syntactic positive shift. *Neuropsychologia* **36**(3), 217–226.

Münte, T. F., Schiltz, K., and Kutas, M. (1998b). When temporal terms belie conceptual order: An electrophysiological analysis. *Nature* **395**, 71–73.

Münte, T. F., Wieringa, B. M., Weyerts, H., Szentkuti, A., Matzke, M., and Johannes, S. (2001). Differences in brain potentials to open and closed class words: Class and frequency effects. *Neuropsychologia* **39**(1), 91–102.

Nagy, M. E., and Rugg, M. D. (1989). Modulation of event-related potentials by word repetition: The effects of inter-item lag. *Psychophysiology* **26**(4), 431–436.

Neville, H. J., Coffey, S. A., Lawson, D. S., Fischer, A., Emmorey, K., and Bellugi, U. (1997). Neural systems mediating American Sign Language: Effects of sensory experience and age of acquisition. *Brain Lang.* **57**(3), 285–308.

Neville, H. J., Nicol, J. L., Barss, A., Forster, K. I., and Garrett, M. F. (1991). Syntactically based sentence processing classes: Evidence from event-related brain potentials. *J. Cogn. Neurosci.* **3**(2), 151–165.

Ni, W., Constable, R. T., Mencl, W. E., Pugh, K. R., Fulbright, R. K., Shaywitz, S. E., Shaywitz, B. A., Gore, J. C., and Shankweiler, D. (2000). An event-related neuroimaging study distinguishing form and content in sentence processing. *J. Cogn. Neurosci.* **12**(1), 120–133.

Nigam, A., Hoffman, J. E., and Simons, R. F. (1992). N400 to semantically anomalous pictures and words. *J. Cogn. Neurosci.* **4**(1), 15–22.

Nobre, A. C., and McCarthy, G. (1995). Language-related field potentials in the anterior-medial temporal lobe: II. Effects of word type and semantic priming. *J. Neurosci.* **15**(2), 1090–1098.

Novick, B., Lovrich, D., and Vaughan, H. G. (1985). Event-related potentials associated with the discrimination of acoustic and semantic aspects of speech. *Neuropsychologia* **23**(1), 87–101.

Nunez, P. L., and Katznelson, R. D. (1981). "Electric Fields of the Brain: The Neurophysics of EEG." Oxford University Press, New York.

Osterhout, L. (1994). Event-related brain potentials as tools for comprehending language comprehension. In "Perspectives on sentence processing" (J. Charles Clifton, L. Frazier and K. Rayner, eds.), . pp. 15–44. Lawrence Erlbaum Assoc., Hillsdale, New Jersey.

Osterhout, L., and Hagoort, P. (1999). A superficial resemblance doesn't necessarily mean you're part of the family: Counterarguments to Coulson, King, and Kutas (1998) in the P600/SPS-P300 debate. *Lang. Cogn. Processes* **14**, 1–14.

Osterhout, L., and Holcomb, P. J. (1992). Event-related brain potentials elicited by syntactic anomaly. *J. Memory Lang.* **31**(6), 785–806.

Osterhout, L., and Holcomb, P. J. (1995). Event related potentials and language comprehension. In "Electrophysiology of Mind: Event-Related Brain Potentials and Cognition" (M. D. Rugg and M. G. H. Coles, eds.), Vol. 25, pp. 171–215. Oxford University Press, Oxford.

Osterhout, L., McKinnon, R., Bersick, M., and Corey, V. (1996). On the language specificity of the brain response to syntactic anomalies: Is the syntactic *J. Cogn. Neurosci.* **8**(6), 507–526.

Osterhout, L., Bersick, M., and McKinnon, R. (1997a). Brain potentials elicited by words: Word length and frequency predict the latency of an early negativity. *Biol. Psychol.* **46**(2), 143–168.

Osterhout, L., Bersick, M., and McLaughlin, J. (1997b). Brain potentials reflect violations of gender stereotypes. *Memory Cogn.* **25**(3), 273–285.

Polich, J., McCarthy, G., Wang, W. S., and Donchin, E. (1983). When words collide: Orthographic and phonological interference during word processing. *Biol. Psychol.* **16**(3-4), 155–180.

Praamstra, P., Meyer, A. S., and Levelt, W. J. M. (1994). Neurophysiological manifestations of phonological processing: Latency variations of a negative ERP component time-locked to phonological mismatch. *J. Cogn. Neurosci.* **6**(3), 204–219.

Puce, A., Allison, T., Asgari, M., Gore, J. C., and McCarthy, G. (1996). Differential sensitivity of human visual cortex to faces, letterstrings, and textures: A functional magnetic resonance imaging study. *J. Neurosci.* **16**(16), 5205–5215.

Roesler, F., Pechmann, T., Streb, J., Roeder, B., and Hennighausen, E. (1998). Parsing of sentences in a language with varying word order: Word-by-word variations of processing demands are revealed by event-related brain potentials. *J. Memory Lang.* **38**(2), 150–176.

Rugg, M. D. (1984a). Event-related potentials and the phonological processing of words and nonwords. *Neuropsychologia* **22**(4), 435–443.

Rugg, M. D. (1984b). Event-related potentials in phonological matching tasks. *Brain Lang.* **23**(2), 225–240.

Rugg, M. D. (1985). The effects of semantic priming and word repetition on event-related potentials. *Psychophysiology* **22**(6), 642–647.

Rugg, M. D., and Barrett, S. E. (1987). Event-related potentials and the interaction between orthographic and phonological information in a rhyme-judgment task. *Brain Lang.* **32**(2), 336–361.

Rugg, M. D., Mark, R. E., Gilchrist, J., and Roberts, R. C. (1997). ERP repetition effects in indirect and direct tasks: Effects of age and interitem lag. *Psychophysiology* **34**(5), 572–586.

Schendan, H. E., Ganis, G., and Kutas, M. (1998). Neurophysiological evidence for visual perceptual categorization of words and faces within 150 ms. *Psychophysiology* **35**(3), 240–251.

Shao, J., and Neville, H. (1996). *ERPs elicited by semantic anomalies: Beyond the N400*. Paper presented at the Cognitive Neuroscience Society, Third Annual Meeting, San Francisco, California.

Stromswold, K., Caplan, D., Alpert, N., and Rauch, S. (1996). Localization of syntactic comprehension by positron emission tomography. *Brain Lang.* **52**(3), 452–473.

Stuss, D. T., Picton, T. W., and Cerri, A. M. (1986). Searching for the names of pictures: An event-related potential study. *Psychophysiology* **23**(2), 215–223.

Swaab, T., Brown, C., and Hagoort, P. (1997). Spoken sentence comprehension in aphasia: Event-related potential evidence for a lexical integration deficit. *J. Cogn. Neurosci.* **9**(1), 39–66.

van Berkum, J. J. A., Hagoort, P., and Brown, C. M. (1999). Semantic integration in sentences and discourse: Evidence from the N400. *J. Cogn. Neurosci.* **11**(6), 657–671.

Van Petten, C. (1993). A comparison of lexical and sentence-level context effects in event-related potentials. Special Issue: Event-related brain potentials in the study of language. *Lang. Cogn. Processes* **8**(4), 485–531.

Van Petten, C. (1995). Words and sentences: Event-related brain potential measures. *Psychophysiology* **32**(6), 511–525.

Van Petten, C., and Kutas, M. (1991). Influences of semantic and syntactic context in open- and closed-class words. *Memory Cogn.* **19**(1), 95–112.

Van Petten, C., and Rheinfelder, H. (1995). Conceptual relationships between spoken words and environmental sounds: Event-related brain potential measures. *Neuropsychologia* **33**(4), 485–508.

Van Petten, C., Kutas, M., Kluender, R., Mitchiner, M., and McIsaac, H. (1991). Fractionating the word repetition effect with event-related potentials. *J. Cogn. Neurosci.* **3**(2), 131–150.

Van Petten, C., Reiman, E., and Senkfor, A. (1995). PET and ERP measures of semantic and repetition priming. Poster, *Soc. Psychophysiol. Res.*

Vos, S. H., Gunter, T. C., Kolk, H. H. J., and Mulder, G. (2001). Working memory constraints on syntactic processing: An electrophysiological investigation. *Psychophysiology* **38**(1), 41–63.

Weber-Fox, C., and Neville, H. J. (1996). Maturational constraints on functional specializations for language processing: ERP and behavioral evidence in bilingual speakers. *J. Cogn. Neurosci.* **8**(3), 231–256.

Weckerly, J., and Kutas, M. (1999). An electrophysiological analysis of animacy effects in the processing of objective relative sentences. *Psychophysiology* **36**(5), 559–570.

Yamashita, H. (2002). Scrambled sentences in Japanese. Linguistic properties and motivations for production (In press).

Young, M. P., and Rugg, M. D. (1992). Word frequency and multiple repetition as determinants of the modulation of event-related potentials in a semantic classification task. *Psychophysiology* **29**(6), 664–676.

Episodic Memory Encoding and Retrieval: Recent Insights from Event-Related Potentials

Edward L. Wilding and Helen Sharpe

INTRODUCTION

Episodic memory is memory of personally experienced events in which the "rememberer" was involved as a participant, an observer, or both. Successful episodic retrieval can—and frequently does—involve memory for the context in which an event or events occurred. The term *recollection* is often employed to refer to this kind of episodic retrieval. The processes that are engaged when an episode was experienced (Craik and Lockhart, 1972), as well as those that are engaged during an attempt to retrieve the episode influence conjointly the likelihood of remembering. An additional influential factor is the degree of correspondence between those processes that are active at encoding and those that are active at retrieval (Tulving and Thomson, 1973; Morris *et al.*, 1977). The focus of this chapter is on episodic memory retrieval processing, and is concerned primarily with insights into the neural and functional bases of episodic memory encoding and retrieval that have been garnered from studies in which event-related potentials (ERPs) have been acquired.

The view that neurally and functionally distinct processes underpin episodic memory is supported by the findings in studies of patients with circumscribed brain damage, wherein the memory impairment varies according to the location as well as to the extent of the lesion (for review, see Gabrieli, 1993). Although this form of evidence is important for identifying neural structures that are necessary for the normal operation of episodic memory, delineation of the functional roles played by such structures is less straightforward. This observation is especially relevant with respect to encoding and retrieval operations, because on the basis of behavioral manipulations alone it is difficult to determine whether a memory impairment results from a processing deficit that is restricted to encoding or to retrieval, or is in fact due to deficits that occur at both stages (Mayes and Roberts, 2001).

Measures that permit neural activity to be recorded during the encoding and retrieval phases of episodic memory tasks are less subject to these concerns, and are thus well suited to questions about the processes and brain regions that may be engaged only at encoding or retrieval, or at both stages. In this context, there are three principal ways in which electrophysiological measures can inform about the neural (hence cognitive) processes that support episodic memory operations. They can provide information about (1) the time course of cognitive processes, (2) the extent (or degree) to which such processes are engaged as a result of experimental manipulations, and (3) whether qualitatively distinct processes are engaged within and/or across experimental conditions of interest. With respect to this final observation, it should be emphasized that inferences about the engagement of distinct processes need not include specification of the neural structures that support those processes. The limited spatial resolution of ERPs means that inferences about the neural generators responsible for indices of memory-related processes acquired via electrodes placed on the scalp can be made only when supported by converging forms of evidence, a point addressed in greater depth elsewhere in this volume (also see Rugg, 1998; Wilding, 2001). In keeping with this observation, discussion of the likely neural basis of scalp-recorded neuroelectric activity in this chapter relies heavily on related findings taken from neuropsychological studies, intracranial recordings, and functional neuroimaging, which is the term used here to refer to studies in which blood-flow correlates of neural activity have been obtained using either positron emission tomography (PET) or functional magnetic resonance imaging (fMRI).

The bulk of this review is concerned with ERP studies of retrieval from episodic memory. The review of effects obtained by recording ERPs evoked by items at retrieval is preceded by a brief commentary on ERP studies of encoding. The emphasis on ERP studies of episodic retrieval reflects the greater proportion of research that has been devoted to this aspect of memory retrieval processing—at least insofar as this can be gauged from the published literature. Recent developments in ERP studies of memory encoding warrant some comment, however, because they mark an important shift in the field.

This is due in part to the impetus toward understanding memory-encoding operations that has been provided by the application of event-related fMRI to the study of memory encoding. The ability to separate and classify the blood-flow correlates of neural activity on a trial-by-trial basis became available in the past decade (Dale and Buckner, 1997; Josephs et al., 1997), and in a short space of time has been applied widely to questions concerning the neural and functional basis of episodic memory encoding as well as episodic retrieval (Wagner, et al. 1999; Rugg and Henson, 2002).

EPISODIC ENCODING

Not everything that we encounter is remembered. Although we know that manipulations such as levels of processing and full versus divided attention influence the likelihood of subsequent remembering (e.g., Richardson-Klavehn and Bjork, 1988), we know less about the time course of effective encoding into episodic memory, and about the neural substrates responsible for effective encoding of different kinds of information. Event-related potential studies of memory encoding have focused on modulations of the electrical record that are referred to as *subsequent memory* or *Dm* effects (Paller et al., 1987). Subsequent memory effects are differences between event-related potentials evoked by items presented during memory-encoding tasks, and separated afterward according to whether the items were remembered or forgotten on a subsequent memory test. The logic underpinning this approach is that reliable differences between ERPs separated according to this criterion may reflect processes that are influential in the effective encoding of information into memory.

The likelihood that ERP subsequent memory effects will be observed depends on at least two factors. First, among the set of ERPs recorded at encoding there must be sufficient variability to support two (or more) reliably different subsets. Second, performance on the subsequent memory test must depend on or be correlated with at least some of the processes that are responsible for that variability. Consequently, if a given encoding task results in little intertrial variability, there will be no subsequent memory effects, irrespective of the form of the following memory test or the level of memory performance. Furthermore, even if there is sufficient variability at encoding to support a subsequent memory effect, such an effect will not be observed if the memory test can be completed on the basis of processes that do not contribute to that variability. This characterization of ERP subsequent memory effects—and the implications that it has for null results—underlies a number of discussions of the likely functional significance of the effects (for example, see Paller et al., 1988; Van Petten and Senkfor, 1996), although the assumptions are stated explicitly only rarely.

Excellent and comprehensive reviews of ERP studies of subsequent memory effects are provided by Johnson (1995), Friedman and Johnson (2000), and Wagner and colleagues (1999). Our purpose here is to highlight a small number of recent findings that we believe to be of particular importance. They relate to two key questions concerning the nature of encoding of information into episodic memory: first, whether the neural correlates of successful retrieval vary qualitatively according to the type of retrieval task that is completed, and second, whether the correlates vary qualitatively according to the operations to which items are subjected at the time of encoding.

Although visual inspection of the ERP subsequent memory effects obtained in studies of episodic encoding up to the mid-1990s is suggestive of differences in the distribution of the effects according to encoding task and retrieval task, there is

little statistical support for this impression (Johnson, 1995). There is some evidence that for verbal stimuli the scalp distribution of subsequent memory effects changes with time (Fernandez et al., 1998), although in this study there was no evidence that these electrophysiologically separable effects had distinct functional correlates. Other findings, however, speak to the issues raised by both of the aforementioned questions. For the latter—whether subsequent memory effects differ qualitatively according to encoding operations— an important study is due to Sommer and colleagues (Sommer et al., 1997), who reported that the subsequent memory effect for unfamiliar faces has a scalp distribution that differs reliably from the distribution of the effect for words [for precursors and related findings, see Sommer et al. (1991, 1995)]. In the 1997 study by Sommer et al., participants were exposed to study stimuli comprising words (unfamiliar names) and unfamiliar faces. In separate test blocks they were represented with words or faces and required to rate the items on a 4-point scale from "not at all familiar" to "very familiar." For both stimulus types the scalp distributions of the ERP subsequent memory effects were obtained by subtracting the study ERPs attracting "not at all familiar" ratings at test from those attracting "very familiar" ratings.

The effect for words was in line with previous findings, with the effect being largest at frontocentral electrode sites, and displaying a slight tendency to be larger at right- than at left-hemisphere sites (Johnson, 1995). The effect for faces, by contrast, was relatively more symmetric, and was largest at central scalp sites. This is one of the first studies to demonstrate that the scalp distribution of subsequent memory effects varies according to stimulus type. An important caveat, however, follows from the observation that the names-versus-faces contrast involved manipulations at encoding as well as at retrieval. As a consequence, it is not straightforward to determine whether the operations engaged at one or both of these phases contribute to the different scalp distributions that were observed. It may be that successful encoding of faces versus names came about because different brain regions are important for the successful encoding of these two stimulus types. An alternative interpretation is that the distinct ERP subsequent memory distributions arose because at the time of retrieval participants interrogated their memories for different attributes of the memory trace. To cast this in terms of the earlier abstract characterization, due to the fact that separate "face" and "name" blocks were employed at test, participants may have exploited different sources of variation in ostensibly the same set of evoked potentials that were recorded during the two study tasks.

This criticism cannot be leveled at a study by Otten and Rugg (2001a), who recorded ERPs during an encoding task in which participants were cued on a trial-by-trial basis as to whether they should make an animacy (living/nonliving) or an alphabetic (order of first and last letter) judgment to each study word. In a subsequent test phase, participants were presented with an equal number of old (previously studied) words from the alphabetic and animacy conditions, alongside the same number of new words. A modified recognition memory procedure was employed in which participants were asked to make old/new judgments to test items and to indicate whether the judgment was made with high or low confidence. The subsequent memory effects obtained by subtracting the ERPs evoked by subsequently forgotten items from those evoked by items that were remembered confidently differed qualitatively according to the encoding operations to which they were subjected (see Fig. 1). These findings indicate that successful episodic encoding depends on neural systems and cognitive

operations that vary according to the nature of the processing to which words are subjected. Interesting questions for future research include whether the same or different subsequent memory effects are observed when encoding (but not retrieval) tasks are blocked rather than interleaved, and whether the effects are also influenced by the form of the subsequent retrieval task.

Finally, on a methodological point Sommer et al. (1997) as well as Otten and Rugg (2001a) employed variants on standard recognition tasks in which it was possible to select classes of responses such that the ERPs contributing to subsequent memory effects did not include what could be classed as nonconfident or "unsure" responses. In subsequent memory studies in which only a binary distinction is required—as has been the case in most ERP subsequent memory studies that employ recognition as the retrieval task—these omitted responses would have been distributed in some ratio between the ERPs evoked by the remembered and the forgotten (or missed) items. The likely outcome of this is a reduction in the magnitude of any modulations that distinguish remembered from forgotten items. These observations have two implications. First, they may go some way to explaining the fact that the number of reports failing to reveal reliable ERP subsequent memory effects for recognition outweighs the number in which reliable effects have been obtained (Johnson, 1995; Wagner et al., 1999). Second, they suggest that in future ERP studies employing variants on recognition memory tasks it may be beneficial to incorporate as part of the procedure a test manipulation that enables more than a binary separation between remembered and forgotten items [for related comments and findings in the context of event-related fMRI studies, see Otten and Rugg, 2001b)].

The second question outlined at the start of this section concerned whether mani-

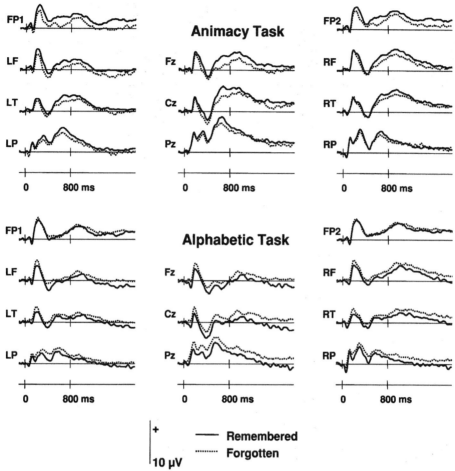

FIGURE 1 Group-average ERPs elicited by remembered and forgotten words in the study of Otten and Rugg (2001a), separated according to encoding task. The data are shown for three midline sites and four paired left- and right-hemisphere sites. Reprinted from *Cognitive Brain Research*, **12**; L. J. Otten and M. D. Rugg; Electrophysiological correlates of memory encoding are task-dependent, pp. 11–18. Copyright, 2001, with permission from Elsevier Science.

pulations at test influenced the scalp distribution of ERP subsequent memory effects. To our knowledge, there have been no studies to date in which this has been demonstrated. One reason for this may be that the focus in some studies has been on paired contrasts in which recognition was one of the retrieval tasks (e.g., Paller *et al.*, 1988). As noted previously, standard recognition memory tasks have not yielded subsequent memory effects in a number of studies, and in those in which they have been obtained the effects have not been particularly robust (Johnson, 1995).

An issue somewhat related to this point, however, is the question of the brain regions that are responsible for supporting different classes of phenomenal experience that may accompany recognition judgments. According to dual-process accounts of recognition memory, correct "old" judgments can be made on the basis of two dissociable processes—recollection and familiarity (Mandler, 1980; Jacoby and Dallas, 1981). Operationally, the distinction between the two is that although both can support the ability to determine whether a test item is old or new, only the former is accompanied by memory for contextual details of a prior encounter with the item. One procedure that may capture to some degree the recollection/familiarity distinction was introduced by Tulving (1985) and has since been developed and explored extensively by Gardiner and colleagues (for reviews, see Gardiner and Java, 1993; Gardiner, 2001). In this procedure, participants are asked at test to denote whether their "old" judgment on a recognition task was accompanied by memory for any aspects of the context of the previous presentation of the item. If it was, they are asked to assign a "remember" (R) response to the item, and otherwise to assign a "know" (K) response.

The fact that the probabilities of R and K responses can be manipulated independently is consistent with the view that distinct processes underlie these two classes of response (Gardiner, 2001) [for some caveats, see Donaldson (1996)]. Furthermore, a number of variables that affect R or K responses selectively have also been found to affect recollection or familiarity selectively (Gardiner, 1988; Gardiner and Java, 1990; Jacoby and Kelley, 1992; Gardiner and Java, 1993), suggesting that, as long as appropriate transformations of the data are performed (Yonelinas and Jacoby, 1995), there is a relatively direct mapping between the two kinds of subjective reports and the processes proposed by dual-process theorists.

What are the implications of these accounts for ERP studies of subsequent memory? To the extent that dissociable cognitive (hence neural) processes support R and K responses, then one prediction would be that the subsequent memory effect accompanying R responses should different qualitatively from that which accompanies K responses. If this was not the case, then the findings would be consistent with the view that K responses are essentially weak R responses. That is, the two kinds of phenomenal experience are not dissociable (see Donaldson, 1996;

Hirshman and Master, 1997; Hirshman and Henzler, 1998). Given this perspective, it might be regarded as surprising that in at least two studies there has been no evidence for qualitative differences between the ERP subsequent memory effects that accompanied R and K judgments at test (Smith, 1993; Friedman and Trott, 2000). In the earlier of these, Smith (1993) reported that the subsequent memory effects for R and K responses were equivalent, whereas Friedman and Trott (2000) observed the same pattern for elderly participants but evidence for a reliable subsequent memory effect for R responses only for a young participant group. The reasons for the disparity across studies are not clear, but in neither case was there evidence consistent the view that the neural activity promoting subsequent R and K judgments differed qualitatively.

These findings contrast, however, with those obtained in a study by Mangels and colleagues (2001). They identified reliable subsequent memory effects for "remember" and "know" responses, with the latter being a subset of the former. These findings indicate that there are encoding processes common to items that will subsequently attract R or K judgments, as well as additional processes that are correlated only with the likelihood of a subsequent R judgment. Mangels et al. (2001) went on to suggest that the subsequent memory effect common to R and K responses is an index of processes that would support subsequent judgments based on familiarity, whereas the anteriorly distributed modulations restricted to predicting R responses reflect study processing necessary for subsequent recollection.

An important first step in substantiating these claims will be identifying the reasons for the disparities between the findings in this study and those of Smith (1993) and Friedman and Trott (2000). This is unlikely to be a straightforward exercise because the three studies differed in a number of ways, including the electrode montage that was used, the manipulations employed at encoding, the precise instructions given at test, and the specific test requirements. These comments notwithstanding, the findings of Mangels and colleagues are consistent with those obtained in an fMRI study of memory encoding in which the R/K procedure was employed (Henson et al., 1999). As in the electrophysiological study, the findings of Henson and colleagues are consistent with the view that the brain regions engaged at encoding are not equivalent for items attracting an R or a K response at test. It will be interesting to know whether findings permitting the same conclusion will be obtained when forced-choice context judgments are used instead of the remember/know procedure.

To summarize, recent findings in ERP studies of subsequent memory have provided data that speak to the two questions identified at the outset of this section: namely, do the neural correlates of successful episodic encoding vary according to study and/or test tasks? The answer to the first question is in the affirmative, and the studies of Sommer et al. (1997) and Otten and Rugg (2001a) provide some indications as to the kinds of paradigms that might be employed fruitfully in order to determine the classes of encoding manipulations that yield distinct subsequent memory effects. The answer to the second question is not clear, but there is some evidence to suggest that R and K responses are associated with distinct subsequent memory effects (Mangels et al., 2001).

It is worthwhile considering the findings of Mangels et al. (2001) alongside two other observations. The first is the suggestion that robust ERP subsequent memory effects for recognition memory may be obtained if confidence judgments (Otten and Rugg, 2001a) or some variant thereon (Sommer et al., 1997) are employed to identify low-confidence (or midrange familiarity) test judgments. The ERPs recorded at study with respect to those items can then be discarded in order to permit a cleaner separation between remembered and forgotten items. The second observation is that recall is presumably less dependent on familiarity than is recognition. In combination these observations suggest that one direction for future work is to revisit, in the light of current knowledge, a question that was prevalent in the ERP subsequent memory literature more than a decade ago—namely, whether the brain regions that support subsequent recall are isomorphic with those that support recognition memory (Paller et al., 1988; Johnson, 1995).

EPISODIC RETRIEVAL

Event-related potential studies of retrieval from episodic memory have gained prominence largely over the past 20–25 years. Prior to this, the primary focus of ERP memory studies was on the Sternberg memory-scanning paradigm, in which participants were asked to remember a small set of items (Sternberg, 1966; for a review see Kutas, 1988). Much of the contemporary focus in ERP studies of retrieval from long-term memory has been on differences between the ERPs that are evoked by old (previously studied) items—most commonly words—and an appropriate base line. In recognition memory tasks and variants the common base line is the electrical activity evoked by correctly identified new (unstudied) items, and the differences between these classes of ERPs are hereafter referred to as ERP old/new effects. The logic behind this contrast is straightforward: reliable differences between the ERPs evoked by these two classes of test item are candidate electrophysiological indices of processes that reflect or are contingent on successful memory retrieval.

It is now accepted that there is a family of old/new effects (Donaldson et al., 2002), which are distinguishable on the basis of their time courses, scalp distributions, and sensitivity to experimental variables. Some of the old/new effects have a longer history than do others, and the effects also vary considerably according to the degree of consensus that exists concerning their likely functional significance. Here we review old/new effects that have been observed in recognition memory tasks and in tasks in which retrieval of contextual information is required. We make no claims about completeness [for example, see Friedman and Johnson (2000)]. Rather, we have selected these effects on the grounds that there is sufficient evidence to support the view that they index functionally distinct processes, and recent developments provide good reason to comment. In this review we restrict ourselves to effects that have been observed in direct memory tasks, meaning tasks in which participants are asked explicitly to retrieve information that was encoded in a prior study phase. Indirect memory tasks, by contrast, are those in which no reference to a prior study phase is made. The findings from studies in which indirect tasks were employed are referred to only when they relate to the old/new effects that have been obtained using direct tasks [for reviews of the ERP findings in indirect tasks, see Rugg and Doyle (1994) and Rugg and Allan (2000)]. At this point it is also worth noting a comment concerning terminology. The term *repetition effects* will be employed to refer to differences between ERPs evoked by old and new words in indirect tasks. The term *old/new effects* will be used only to refer to differences between ERPs evoked by old and new items to which accurate old/new judgments have been made.

The Left-Parietal ERP Old/New Effect

Sanquist and colleagues (1980) were the first to report that ERPs differentiated old and new words to which correct judgments were made on a test of recognition memory. It is instructive to read the original report of Sanquist and colleagues for a number of reasons. One striking aspect is that the majority of the paper is concerned with the ERPs that were recorded during an encoding task that involved participants making judgments about the orthographic, phonemic, or semantic similarities between pairs of stimuli that were presented sequentially. The relatively small proportion of the paper that is devoted to the ERPs recorded at test is perhaps surprising given that contrasts between the ERPs evoked by classes of old and new test stimuli are now probably the most widely reported data type in ERP studies of episodic memory.

The principal finding for the ERPs recorded at test was that the amplitude of a positive-going wave form was greater for *hits* (studied words identified correctly) than it was for three other classes of ERPs: *correct rejections* (unstudied words identified correctly), as well as *misses* and *false alarms* (incorrectly identified old and new words, respectively). The amplitude differences between correct rejections, misses, and false alarms were markedly smaller than the differences that separated these three measures from the corresponding mean amplitude measure for hits. These findings were important, because they suggested that the relative positivity elicited by hits was not due simply to repetition of a studied item, to processes that are related to the act of making an "old" response, or simply to the belief that an item was "old."

The relative positivity elicited by hits in the study of Sanquist and colleagues (1980) is likely the first report of what is now termed the *left-parietal ERP old/new effect*. Subsequent studies have revealed that the effect onsets 400–500 msec poststimulus is often larger at left than at right parietal scalp sites, and typically has a duration of 500–800 msec (Karis *et al.*, 1984; Johnson *et al.*, 1985; Friedman and Sutton, 1987; Rugg and Nagy, 1989; Smith and Halgren, 1989; Friedman, 1990a,b; Noldy *et al.*, 1990; Bentin *et al.*, 1992; Potter *et al.*, 1992; Rugg *et al.*, 1992; Smith and Guster, 1993). The link between this effect and memory retrieval operations is strengthened by the fact that the absence of the effect for misses and false alarms reported initially by Sanquist and colleagues (1980) has been replicated in a number of studies (Neville *et al.*, 1986; Rugg and Doyle, 1992; Wilding *et al.*, 1995; Van Petten and Senkfor, 1996; Wilding and Rugg, 1996). In combination, these findings are consistent with the view that the effect is an electrophysiological index of veridical retrieval of information from memory.

Mnemonic functional interpretations of the parietal old/new effect can be divided into those that have linked the effect to recollection (e.g., Smith and Halgren, 1989; Van Petten *et al.*, 1991; Paller and Kutas, 1992; Smith, 1993; Paller *et al.*, 1995; Rugg *et al.*, 1995), and those that have linked it with fluency-based recognition or familiarity (Johnson *et al.*, 1985; Friedman, 1990b; Potter *et al.*, 1992; Rugg and Doyle, 1992, 1994). The distinction between recognition and familiarity has been introduced already in the discussion of subsequent memory effects, and it is now generally accepted that the parietal old/new effect indexes processes that are related more closely to recollection than to familiarity (Allan *et al.*, 1998).

Arguably the strongest evidence in support of this view has come from studies in which recollection has been operationalized as the ability to retrieve contextual (or *source*) details of the prior occurrence of a test item—such as where on the study list it occurred, or what associations were evoked by the stimulus at study. For example, Smith (1993) used the remember/know paradigm in order to distinguish recollected from familiar test items (Tulving, 1985; Gardiner and Java, 1993). In the study of Smith (1993), a larger parietal old/new effect was associated with R than with K responses that were made to old test words (also see Düzel *et al.*, 1997). Complementary findings stem from two studies by Wilding and colleagues (Wilding *et al.*, 1995; Wilding and Rugg, 1996), who used a forced-choice paradigm in which participants made an initial old/new judgment to test words, and, for those judged to be old, a second judgment denoting in which of two contexts the words had been presented at study. In the first report, the context manipulation was modality (auditory versus visual) (Wilding *et al.*, 1995). In the second, it was speaker voice (male versus female) (Wilding and Rugg, 1996). In a total of four experiments, the parietal old/new effect was larger when participants made correct source judgments compared to when they made incorrect source judgments following a correct "old" judgment. In combination, these findings argue strongly for the link between the parietal effect and recollection, because the magnitude of any ERP old/new effect that reflected familiarity should not vary with the success or otherwise of retrieval of contextual information.

On the basis of these and similar findings, it has been proposed that the amplitude of the left-parietal old/new effect is correlated positively with either the quality or the amount of information of information that is retrieved from memory (Rugg, 1995; Wilding and Rugg, 1996). How to distinguish between these two possibilities is unclear; nonetheless, common to them both is the prediction that the effect should be of greater amplitude when evoked by test items that are associated with accurate rather than inaccurate source judgments, or R rather than K judgments. This is, of course, the pattern of data that has been reviewed in the previous paragraph. Further consideration of the findings in these studies, however, suggests an alternative interpretation.

The starting point for this argument is the observation that the use of forced-choice measures for source judgments means that when ERPs are separated according to the accuracy of the source judgment, both resulting categories will contain a proportion of trials on which recollection did not occur. In more detail, the old/new effect for words associated with incorrect source judgments may have arisen as a result of averaging two types of trials: those not associated with recollection (which do not evoke parietal old/new effects), and those associated with recollection of information that was not diagnostic for the source judgment that was required in the task [e.g., voice in the study of Wilding and Rugg (1996)]. Second, the larger old/new effect for words associated with correct source judgments may have arisen because, in addition to containing trials of the two types described above, on some trials recollection of voice information would have occurred. A consequence of this is that the findings in the studies reviewed above cannot rule out the possibility that the parietal old/new effect indexes recollection in an "all-or-none" fashion. According to this account, the differences between the two critical response categories (correct vs. incorrect source judgments) in the studies of Wilding and colleagues (1995; Wilding and Rugg, 1996) arose because the category associated with incorrect source judgments contained higher proportions of trials on which recollection did not occur. Broadly similar arguments can be applied to comparable findings in other ERP studies of memory that have required source memory judgments (Smith, 1993; Senkfor and Van Petten, 1998). Furthermore, the results in studies in which there is a positive correlation between recognition memory performance and the magnitude of the left-parietal ERP old/new effect (e.g., Paller and Kutas, 1992; Johnson et al., 1998) are consistent with an all-or-none account, because the level of recognition performance may well vary inversely with the proportion of trials in which recollection does not occur.

In order to disentangle the graded and all-or-none accounts of the parietal old/new effect, Wilding (2000) designed an experiment in which the larger proportion of trials not associated with recollection would be associated with the response category that should, according to the graded account, evoke the largest left-parietal old/new effect. The experiment consisted of study phases in which each word was associated with two aspects of source information. These were followed by test phases in which two forced-choice source decisions were required for items judged to be old. This design permitted a contrast between the old/new effects evoked by items that attracted either *one* or *two* correct source judgments. In this design the probability of one correct source judgment necessarily exceeds the probability of two correct judgments (the actual probabilities in the experiment, collapsed across study task were as follows: 1 correct, 0.75; 2 correct, 0.57). Assuming that trials in which recollection did not occur are distributed equally between the 2-correct and 1-correct response categories, then the relative attenuating influence exerted by these trials should be greater in the 2-correct case, due to the fact that this category contains less trials. The experiment thus constitutes a strong test of the graded hypothesis because the likely influence of guesses would be to reduce the amplitude of the 2-correct parietal effect to a greater degree than the amplitude of the 1-correct category.

The results shown in Fig. 2 provide strong support for the graded hypothesis, because the magnitude of the left-parietal old/new effect was correlated positively with the number of correct source judgments. At first pass this finding may seem to run counter to at least one dual-process account of recognition memory, according to which recollection is modeled as an all-or-none process, where the success or failure of recollection is defined relative to a fixed threshold (Yonelinas, 1994; Yonelinas et al., 1996; Jacoby, 1998). This disparity is more apparent than real, however, because threshold accounts make

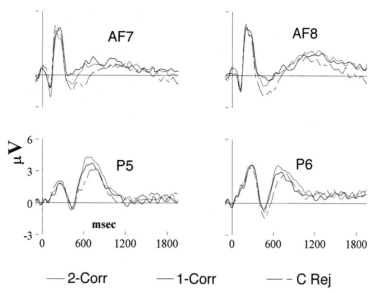

FIGURE 2 Grand-average ERPs elicited by words attracting either one (1-Corr) or two correct (2-Corr) source judgments (collapsed across material retrieved), contrasted with the ERPs evoked by correct rejections (C Rej). Data from Wilding (2000) for left- and right-hemisphere frontal (AF7/AF8) and parietal (P5/P6) electrode sites.

no predictions as to how far above or below threshold the signal strength for a given item will be.

In summary, the link between the left-parietal ERP old/new effects and recollection is well established, and recent findings have contributed to a more detailed understanding of the way in which recollection is indexed. A final comment is that the left-parietal effect has been evoked in studies in which numerous different kinds of source material have been retrieved (Donaldson *et al.*, 2002). The fact that the effect is observed consistently, irrespective of the contents of retrieval, suggests that it indexes what might be considered "central" or "core" aspects of recollection that are shared across content domains (Allan *et al.*, 2000; Donaldson *et al.*, 2002).

A Putative Electrophysiological Correlate of Familiarity

An important aspect of the studies reviewed in the previous section is that they provide little or no evidence that the ERP old/new effects evoked by correct versus incorrect source judgments, or R versus K judgments,[1] are associated with scalp distributions that differ reliably. To the extent that any ERP index of familiarity would be relatively more prominent in the ERPs evoked by incorrect source or K judgments, these findings provide little support for dual-process accounts of recognition memory (Mandler, 1980; Jacoby and Dallas, 1981). That is, the ERP findings are consistent with the view that the difference between recognition with or without retrieval of source is one of degree rather than one of kind (Wilding and Rugg, 1996). There are two (not mutually exclusive) reasons for treating this conclusion somewhat cautiously. The first is the domain-general conclusion that null results in cognitive electrophysiological

---

[1]Düzel and colleagues (1997) reported differential scalp distributions of the neural activity associated with correct R and K responses. Because their claims were not based on analyses of appropriately rescaled data (McCarthy and Wood, 1985), their results must be treated cautiously at present.

studies must be interpreted with a good degree of circumspection, by virtue of the fact that ERPs provide only a partial measure of the neural activity that is evoked by stimuli in cognitive tasks (Rugg and Coles, 1995; Rugg, 1998; Wilding, 2001). The second observation is that we concur with the authors of an earlier review, who, the aforementioned findings notwithstanding, find compelling the evidence from behavioral studies that recollection and familiarity are indeed independent bases for recognition-memory judgments (Allan *et al.*, 1998). These observations are particularly apposite in light of the fact that the question of whether ERPs are in fact sensitive to familiarity as well as to recollection has been addressed in recent studies. These studies suggest that the reasons for the absence of putative indices of familiarity in the electrical record in previous studies of recognition memory was that the paradigms employed were not optimal for revealing a correlate of this process, although other results, described below, qualify this statement.

In an influential study, Rugg and colleagues (1998) identified putative correlates of recollection and familiarity in a single experiment. In their study, the authors compared old/new effects following deep (semantic) and shallow (orthographic) encoding tasks. Over the time window of 500–800 msec, the parietal old/new effect was larger for deeply than for shallowly studied words, in keeping with previous findings (e.g., Paller and Kutas, 1992). At frontocentral sites over the 300- to 500-msec time period, both categories of old item were more positive-going than correct rejections, and of equal amplitude. Rugg and colleagues proposed that this earlier modulation indexes familiarity, a proposal supported by two aspects of their data. First, the fact that the putative index of familiarity precedes the index of recollection is consistent with findings that the time after stimulus presentation at which familiarity is most influential for recognition judgments is earlier than the comparable time point for recollection (Yonelinas and Jacoby, 1994). Second, the frontocentral effect was of equivalent size in the deep and shallow conditions, which concurs with findings that depth of processing manipulations using the R/K paradigm has little influence on the probability of a K response, whereas the proportion of R responses increases with depth of encoding (Gardiner, 1988; Gardiner *et al.*, 1996; although see Toth, 1996; Yonelinas, 1998).

The possible link between this frontocentrally distributed old/new effect and familiarity has been pursued by Curran (1999, 2000). In the earlier of these two studies a frontocentral repetition effect analogous to the old/new effect reported by Rugg and colleagues was evident for both words and pronounceable nonwords (pseudowords) when the task was either lexical decision or recognition memory.[2] A repetition effect analogous to the left-parietal ERP old/new effect was also evident and this effect varied according to lexical status, being larger for words than for pseudowords. Drawing on findings that words are more likely to be associated with recollection than are pseudowords, Curran proposed, in keeping with the proposal of Rugg *et al.* (1998), that the frontocentral and left-parietal old/new effects index familiarity and recollection, respectively. His findings in a subsequent study revealed the same one-way dissociation between the two effects. In this case, the manipulation involved presentation of singular and plural words and the ERPs were separated according to response accuracy at test. In two experiments the left-parietal ERP old/new effect was larger when plurality matched across study and test phases, whereas the frontocentral effect

---

[2] Old and new words were not separated according to response accuracy in the recognition task so as to avoid biasing the contrast between the repetition effects obtained in lexical decision and old/new recognition.

was insensitive to changes in plurality between study and test. To the extent that re-presentation of words in the same plurality is associated with a greater likelihood of rec-ollection than is re-presentation of words in the opposite plurality, these findings are also consistent with the view that the frontocen-tral modulation indexes familiarity.

A similar between-groups dissociation was reported by Tendolkar and colleagues (1999), who contrasted the ERPs evoked by correctly identified old and new stimuli in patients with Alzheimer disease (AD) with those evoked by matched controls. The AD patients were impaired on judgments requiring recollection relative to their con-trols, and a parietal old/new effect was evident for controls only, whereas a fronto-central effect was evident for both groups (see Fig. 3). Finally, Mecklinger (2000) reports patient data as well as data from studies in which participants had no neurological disorder that are consistent with the view that a frontocentral effect indexes familiarity, but the left-parietal ERP old/new effect indexes recollection (also see Mecklinger, 1998; Mecklinger and Meins-hausen, 1998). In combination, the findings reviewed to this point in this section are thus consistent with dual-process accounts of recognition memory (Rugg *et al.*, 1998; Curran, 1999, 2000).

The findings in an additional study, however, suggest that the frontocentral effect does not index familiarity directly. In the study of Tsivilis *et al.* (2001) partici-pants saw stimuli that comprised pictures of everyday objects set against background scenes. The experiment was designed such that during old/new recognition for the

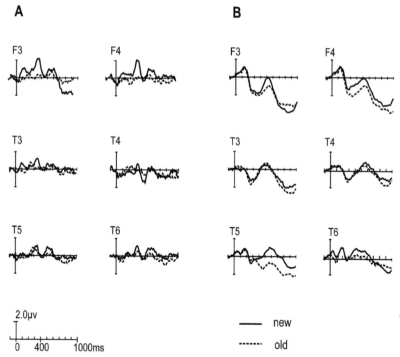

FIGURE 3 Group-average ERPs elicited by old and new words attracting correct recognition judgments for Alzheimer disease patients (A) and matched controls (B). ERPs are shown for left- and right-hemisphere frontal (F3/F4), central (T3/T4), and parietal (T5/T6) electrode sites. Note that negative is plotted upward on this figure. Reprinted from *Neuroscience Letters*, **263**; I. Tendolkar, A. Schoenfeld, G. Golz, G. Fernandez, K.-P. Kuhl, R. Ferszt, and H.-J. Heinze; Neural correlates of recognition memory with and without recollection in patients with Alzheimer's disease and healthy controls, pp. 45–48. Copyright 1999, with permission from Elsevier Science.

objects the object/background pairings could be one of five types: studied objects against the same background or against a different background (which could be previously seen or novel), and novel objects against a novel background or one that had been seen at study. The putative index of familiarity was evident only when both object and background were old (relative to a novel object/novel background base line), leading Tsivilis and colleagues to suggest that the putative correlate of familiarity is in fact a negative-going index of novelty, whereby the modulation will be evident when any aspect of task-relevant information is new to the experiment. Were the effect to be considered an index of familiarity, then the relative positivity seen for object/background conjunctions when both elements were old should also have been observed when an old object was seen against a new background.

The findings of Tsivilis and colleagues suggest that ERPs are not sensitive to familiarity directly, but remain consistent with the view that ERPs index multiple distinct processes during recognition memory and variants thereon. Tsivilis *et al.* (2001) also observed a left-parietal old/new effect that was dissociable from the putative index of novelty, as well as an earlier anteriorly distributed component that was sensitive to any pairing that involved at least one component (object or background) that was encountered at study. A commentary on the likely functional significance of this early frontal component is deferred until more is known about its antecedents. In combination, however, the findings in this study extend those in previous studies. Common to the majority of findings reviewed in this section is that they support dual-process accounts of recognition memory to the extent that they indicate there are at least two neurally and functionally dissociable processes engaged during recognition tasks. The findings of Tsivilis *et al.*, however, suggest that the mapping

between the memory-related processes evident in the electrical record and the processes postulated in dual-process accounts is not a direct one.

Electrophysiological Indices of Implicit Memory

Another important result from the study of Rugg and colleagues (1998), reviewed above, stemmed from the fact that, for shallowly studied words, it was possible to form ERPs evoked by old words that were judged incorrectly to be new (*misses*). At frontal sites over the time window of 300–500 msec, these ERPs did not differ from those for correct rejections, whereas at parietal sites during the same time period the misses were associated with a positive-going modulation of magnitude equivalent to those observed for correct old judgments to deeply and shallowly studied words. This early parietal effect is therefore functionally dissociable from the fronto-central effect, which was evident for both classes of old words, and the left- parietal old/new effect, which was evident principally for old words studied in the deep encoding task. On the basis of the facts that this modulation discriminates old from new items, but does not vary in amplitude according to the accuracy of old judgments, Rugg and colleagues proposed that it is an electrophysiological index of implicit memory (Rugg *et al.*, 1998).

The fact that ERPs differentiate old from new words over this early time period at parietal scalp sites has been documented in a number of indirect memory tasks (e.g., Rugg, 1987; Bentin and Peled, 1990), as well as in continuous recognition memory (e.g., Friedman, 1990a,b) and study-test recognition tasks (see especially Smith and Halgren, 1989). In addition, the link between this effect and processes related to implicit memory has been noted in some previous studies (e.g., Bentin *et al.*, 1992; Friedman *et al.*, 1992), and is suggested by visual inspection of ERPs elicited by misses and correct rejections in other reports (for example, see Johnson *et al.*, 1998). Nonetheless, the combination of functional dissociations reported by Rugg and colleagues represents the first convincing demonstration that ERPs index implicit memory, and perhaps more importantly the first demonstration, in normal participants, that implicit and explicit memory are associated with distinct neural substrates. These findings provide a potentially important springboard to investigate issues that include, but are not restricted to, the sensitivity of ERPs to different forms of implicit memory (e.g., conceptual versus perceptual priming) and the question of the degree to which implicit and explicit memory are independent processes. Strong evidence in support of independence would accrue from findings that the putative electrophysiological correlates of implicit and explicit memory processes can be manipulated such that across experimental conditions both occur in the absence of the other (Rugg *et al.*, 2000).

Old/New Effects at Frontal Scalp Sites

Neuropsychological findings indicate that the functional integrity of both the medial temporal lobes and the prefrontal cortex is necessary for veridical source memory. Patients with extensive damage to medial temporal lobe structures commonly exhibit a marked inability to acquire and/or bring to mind new information (Scoville and Milner, 1957; Mayes, 1988). By contrast, patients with damage restricted to prefrontal cortex exhibit a more selective impairment. While often able to make simple judgments of prior occurrence, impairments are commonly observed on tasks that require more complex judgments that involve using contextual details from a prior episode (Schacter *et al.*, 1984; Shimamura and Squire, 1987; Janowsky *et al.*, 1989; Glisky *et al.*, 1995).

On the basis of these findings it has been proposed that the medial temporal lobes

and prefrontal cortex have distinct functional roles in recollection. According to one class of accounts, the former is responsible for information retrieval, whereas the latter is involved in postretrieval processes that operate on the products of retrieval (Moscovitch, 1992, 1994; Squire *et al.*, 1993). For example, Moscovitch (1992) has referred to the prefrontal cortex as a "working-with-memory" structure, which incorporates the idea that this structure is involved in coordinating information necessary for veridical recollection, as well as being influential in the ways in which memories are used to guide behavior.

The starting point for this discussion of ERP studies that are relevant to the multicomponent nature of recollection is the study of Wilding and Rugg (1996), which was introduced earlier. To recap, in that study participants completed an initial lexical decision task, in which equal numbers of word and pronounceable nonword stimuli were spoken in a male or a female voice. In a subsequent test phase, participants made initial old/new judgments to old and new words. For those words judged old, participants made a second judgment, denoting whether the old words had been spoken in a male or female voice at study. This allowed the comparison of three classes of ERPs: those to correct rejections, and those to words judged old correctly that were assigned either correctly or incorrectly to study voice.

As discussed previously, the left-parietal old/new effect was larger following a correct source judgment than it was following an incorrect source judgment. In addition, this study revealed a second old/new effect that differentiated correctly identified old and new words. The effect was largest over frontal scalp sites, and larger over the right hemisphere than over the left. The effect onset was at around the same time as the parietal effect but had a duration that extended until at least 1400

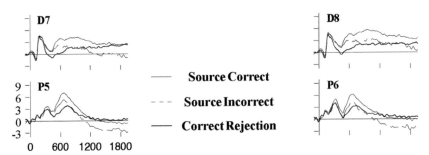

FIGURE 4 Grand-average ERPs elicited by old and new words to which either correct or incorrect source judgments were made (collapsed across retrieval task), contrasted with those evoked by correct rejections. Data are shown
for left- and right-hemisphere frontal (D7/D8) and parietal (P5/P6) electrode sites. Data from Wilding (1999).

msec poststimulus. This right-frontal
old/new effect was dissociable from the
left-parietal effect in terms of time course
and scalp distribution, thereby allowing
the conclusion that two distinct neural
populations are engaged during retrieval
of source information. An example of the
right-frontal old/new effects is shown in
Fig. 4, which also provides an illustration
of amplitude differences between ERPs
evoked by words attracting correct or
incorrect source judgments.

Like the parietal old/new effect, the
right-frontal effect was larger for correct
than for incorrect source judgments,
leading Wilding and Rugg to suggest that
the effect played a functional role in source
memory judgments—a conclusion supported by the fact that equivalent effects
over frontal scalp were not observed for
false alarms or for misses (Wilding and
Rugg, 1996, 1997b). Consequently, following the neurologically inspired models of
Moscovitch and Squire (also see Stuss et al.,
1994), Wilding and Rugg proposed that the
left-parietal effect reflected information
retrieval, whereas the right-frontal effect
reflected processes necessary for integrating retrieved information into a coherent
representation of a prior episode. Johnson
and colleagues (Johnson et al., 1996) came
to a similar conclusion on the basis of
findings that activity at right-frontal electrode sights was greater in tasks requiring
source judgments than in tasks requiring

recognition memory judgments (also see
Senkfor and Van Petten, 1998).

Although Wilding and Rugg made this
proposal in the absence of direct electrophysiological evidence to support the view
that the left-parietal and right-frontal
old/new effects index distinct processes,
subsequent findings support the claim
(e.g., Wilding and Rugg, 1997a,b). These
subsequent findings also, however, indicated that the initial functional interpretation of the right-frontal effect required
modification. The effect does not always
vary in magnitude according to the accuracy of source judgments (Trott et al., 1997;
Senkfor and Van Petten, 1998; Van Petten
et al., 2000; Cycowicz et al., 2001), it is
on occasions evident in recognition tasks
in which there is no overt source
retrieval requirement (Allan and Rugg,
1997; Donaldson and Rugg, 1998; Rugg
et al., 2000), it is not an obligatory correlate
of successful source retrieval (Rugg et al.,
1996; Wilding and Rugg, 1997b), it varies in
magnitude according to the type of source
information that is retrieved (Wilding,
1999; Donaldson et al., 2002), and it has
been statistically indistinguishable for R
and K judgments to old items (Düzel et al.,
1997). In addition, it is not always evident
that the same effects are in fact being
observed across studies (in particular, see
Tendolkar and Rugg, 1998). Visual inspection suggests that under certain retrieval
conditions frontal old/new effects vary

with respect to the degree of laterality as well as with the relative anterior/central distribution of the effects (Trott et al., 1997; Tendolkar and Rugg, 1998; Cycowicz et al., 2001). Furthermore, under some circumstances the effect can be dissociated into an early bilateral component (600–900 msec) and a longer duration right-frontal component (Wilding and Rugg, 1997a; Donaldson and Rugg, 1998). The conditions under which these two components are evident, either separately or in conjunction, are not well established. A general rule of thumb is that the earlier of the two effects tends to be more prominent in tasks in which an old/new judgment precedes the source judgment than in studies in which item and source judgments are combined (cf. Wilding and Rugg, 1996, 1997b), as is the case in the recognition memory exclusion task procedure (Jacoby, 1998).

Rather than reassessing ground that has been reviewed in detail elsewhere (Friedman and Johnson, 2000; Rugg and Allan, 2000; Van Petten et al., 2000), we restrict discussion here to a couple of broad observations. First, the weight of evidence supports the view that these frontal effects are likely an index of processes that operate in some way on retrieved information in pursuit of task-specific goals. A more precise characterization is elusive at present [for related comments, see Van Petten et al. (2000)]. Second, a number of related points stem from the view that the frontal old/new effects described above are likely to be generated in the frontal cortex. This claim is supported by the neuropsychological evidence mentioned previously (Stuss et al., 1994), and the consistent findings from functional neuroimaging studies that frontal brain regions are engaged during episodic encoding and retrieval (Cabeza and Nyberg, 2000). In a review of the functional neuroimaging literature relevant to the question of the functional roles played by frontal cortex in episodic memory, Fletcher and Henson (2001) proposed that three separate regions

of lateral frontal cortex—anterior, dorsolateral and ventrolateral—support distinct cognitive operations. The specification of these operations was derived in part from protocols reported by participants in effortful episodic retrieval tasks, as well as consideration of the more domain-general roles that frontal cortex plays in cognition (Burgess and Shallice, 1996; Shallice and Burgess, 1998). Fletcher and Henson (2001) proposed that anterior frontal cortex supports processes involved in the selection of goals and subgoals, whereas the integrity of ventrolateral and dorsolateral frontal cortex is necessary for updating working memory and monitoring as well as selecting among the contents of working memory, respectively.

As the authors acknowledge, this tripartite division is unlikely, ultimately, to have sufficient anatomical or cognitive resolution. Models of this type, however (also see Wagner, 1999), emphasize that subtle differences between retrieval tasks are likely to result in engagement of some combination of the control processes that can in principle be required during episodic retrieval. The differential engagement of these processes across different retrieval tasks may go some way to explaining the disparities across studies in the ERP episodic memory literature. A detailed examination of this possibility is beyond the scope of this review. In closing, though, it is perhaps worth noting what may turn out to be a more fundamental concern. Although the existing data permit some conclusions about the relative engagement of right- versus left-frontal cortex, more fine-grained delineation within each hemisphere is speculative at this stage. It may be the case, that it will not be possible to separate reliably the contributions of distinct frontal cortical regions with scalp-recorded event-related potentials. If this turns out to be the case, then event-related potentials may not be particularly influential in developing either cognitive or functional neuroanatomical accounts of the control processes that are engaged during episodic retrieval. This conclusion is premature at present, however, and a resolution to this issue will stem at least in part from studies that incorporate two improvements on the majority of studies to date. The first is the use of electrode montages that have better spatial resolution than those that have been employed to date. The second is a tighter specification of the cognitive processes that are engaged during retrieval tasks.

ELECTROPHYSIOLOGICAL INDICES OF RETRIEVAL ATTEMPTS

In this final section, we review recent studies in which contrasts have not been restricted to those between the ERPs evoked by correct rejections and those evoked by various classes of responses to old items. Rather, they have been extended to include contrasts between classes of new (unstudied) test items that have been obtained in different retrieval tasks. The logic for this contrast is that unstudied items on a given direct memory task will presumably be subject to processes that can broadly be defined as constituting a retrieval attempt (Wilding, 1999). Of course, old items will also be subject to this class of retrieval processes, but these may be confounded in the electrical record with activity that reflects retrieval success, or the postretrieval processing of retrieved information (Rugg and Wilding, 2000). The activity elicited by unstudied test items is assumed to be less subject to this confound due to the fact that these items were not presented in the relevant prior study phase.

Rugg and Wilding (2000; Rugg et al., 2000) distinguished two classes of process that might be considered to form part of a retrieval attempt. The first is retrieval effort, defined as the recruitment of

resources in pursuit of retrieval. The second is retrieval orientation, which determines the task-specific processes that may be engaged in pursuit of retrieval of specific mnemonic contents. Rugg and Wilding argued that separating these two classes of retrieval process requires them to be manipulated independently. This has been achieved in some studies but not in others.

To our knowledge, the initial report of a contrast between ERPs evoked by classes of new items is due to Johnson and colleagues (1996). In that study, two groups of participants completed incidental encoding tasks on an equal number of words and pictures. One group was asked to think of uses for each object designated by the word or picture. The other was asked to rate how easy it would be to draw each stimulus (either the picture or the image evoked by each word). In the retrieval task participants were shown an equal number of old and new words. They were asked to distinguish old from new words, and for the old words, to indicate whether they had been encountered as a word or as a picture at study. Distinct modulations over frontal and posterior scalp sites differentiated the ERPs that were evoked by correct rejections for the two groups. The same modulations were evident in the ERPs that were evoked by old words associated with a correct picture/word designation. Johnson and colleagues (1996) proposed that the differences reflected shifts in evaluative operations that were engaged in the two cases, depending on the emphasis at study. They argued that new items would be subject to the same evaluative operations as old items and it was these processes that were indexed by the modulations differentiating the ERPs evoked by new items from the two groups.

A similar line of enquiry was pursued by Wilding (1999) using a within-participants design. Whereas Johnson and colleagues manipulated the processes engaged at retrieval indirectly via an encoding manipulation, in the study of Wilding (1999) all participants completed the same encoding task and then different retrieval tasks in separate blocks. ERPs were recorded to visual presentations of old and new words in separate test blocks that required source judgments based either on voice or task information. The voice and task information had been encoded in a task in which participants heard words, an equal number of which were spoken by a male/female voice. To each word participants made one of two judgments—an active/passive judgment (action task) or a pleasant/unpleasant judgment (liking task). The type of judgment varied across trials, and was determined by a cue that preceded each spoken word. In one test condition, participants made a three-way distinction between new words and old words spoken at study by the male or female voice. In the second condition, participants distinguished new words from old words, to which either an active/passive or a pleasant/unpleasant judgment had been made at study. There was no systematic relationship at study between task and voice, thereby precluding successful retrieval task performance being accomplished by focusing on one aspect of context information only. Participants were informed of the retrieval orientation for each test block only after completion of the immediately preceding study phase.

The likelihood of a correct rejection was equivalent in both retrieval tasks, as were the reaction times for these items. The ERPs evoked by correct rejections in the two retrieval tasks were distinguished by a polarity reversal at left- and right-hemisphere frontal sites, with the differences extending to central scalp locations. In light of the behavioral data, Wilding proposed that the effects were unlikely to reflect processes tied closely to task difficulty, hence retrieval effort, and in keeping with the interpretation offered by

Johnson *et al.* (1996) proposed that the processes reflected differential monitoring or evaluation of the mnemonic information that was activated by new test items.

Contrasts between classes of correct rejections were also reported in two studies by Ranganath and Paller (1999, 2000). In the earlier of these two studies (Ranganath and Paller, 1999), each participant completed the same picture-encoding task followed by two different retrieval tasks. At test each picture took one of three forms: old, new, or new but perceptually similar to old pictures (previously presented pictures were rescaled, resulting in small changes to their height and width). In one test condition (general retrieval), participants made old/new recognition judgments to pictures, responding *old* to previously studied pictures as well as to perceptually similar pictures. In the other test condition (specific retrieval), participants responded *old* only to previously studied pictures. These two conditions were designed to differ in the degree to which participants were required to process perceptual details of the test items.

The differences between the ERPs that were evoked by the two classes of new items were most evident over left-frontal scalp, where those from the specific retrieval condition (respond old only to studied pictures) were more positive-going from approximately 400 to 1200 msec poststimulus. The authors reasoned that, in contrast to the general retrieval test condition, the specific retrieval condition required participants to attend more closely to perceptual features of the stimuli, and to engage in more evaluative operations before making an old/new judgment. They proposed that the differences over left-frontal scalp reflected the greater demands that these information-processing operations imposed on attention and working memory in pursuit of retrieval. This amounts to a retrieval effort interpretation of the findings, which might be considered to run counter to the behavioral findings: there were no reliable differences between reaction times for the two classes of new items, and no differences between the probabilities for correct "new" responses.

The probability of a correct judgment to an old item was, however, lower in the specific than in the general retrieval task. This raises an interesting question, because in this experiment, as well as that of Wilding (1999), task difficulty can be considered constant across the retrieval tasks of interest only if the data supporting the claim for parity are restricted to responses attracted by new items. If task difficulty is assessed in relation to the likelihood of correct responses to old items, or perhaps in terms of the discrimination measure *p(hit) minus p(false alarm)* (Snodgrass and Corwin, 1988), then the specific task in the study of Ranganath and Paller and the voice retrieval task in the study of Wilding are more difficult. Which aspects of the behavioral data to include when determining task difficulty is not at all clear.

Two studies in which there is little argument with the claim that effort and orientation are confounded are due to Rugg *et al.* (2000) and Wilding and Nobre (2001). Rugg and colleagues also revealed differences at left-frontal scalp locations between the ERPs that were evoked by classes of unstudied test items. In this case, however, the differences were related to an encoding manipulation rather than to different instructions at test. Participants completed encoding tasks in which visually presented low-frequency words were processed with respect to either their semantic or their orthographic characteristics (hereafter the *deep* and *shallow* encoding tasks, respectively). In subsequent old/new recognition blocks, each block contained words that had been processed in only one of the two encoding tasks. For unstudied items the ERPs at left-frontal scalp locations were more positive-going for the blocks that contained shallowly encoded old words. Because memory was poorer in the

shallow than in the deep retrieval task, it is reasonable to assume that greater demands were placed on attention and working memory in pursuit of recognition decisions in this task. The findings are, therefore, consistent with the interpretation offered by Ranganath and Paller (1999, 2000).

The findings of Rugg *et al.* for written words also indicate that the left-frontal modulation is not a consequence of using picture stimuli at test, and that the differences observed by Ranganath and Paller (1999, 2000) likely do not reflect processes related to differential inspection of the surface features of test stimuli. While noting that their results were consistent with a working memory-load interpretation, however, Rugg *et al.* (2000) also discussed an alternative account of the left-frontal effect that can be defined broadly as an "effort" interpretation. They observed that participants adopted different response criteria in the deep and shallow retrieval blocks, and that a difference in response criterion across conditions was also evident in the behavioral data from the study of Ranganath and Paller (1999). In both cases, a more stringent (conservative) criterion was adopted in the more demanding task. The left-frontal effect could therefore reflect processes related to criterion setting rather than to the differential demands placed on working memory and/or attention (Rugg *et al.*, 2000).

In addition to this left-frontal modulation, Rugg *et al.* (2000) also observed a second modulation that differentiated the ERPs elicited by unstudied items in the deep and shallow retrieval conditions. This effect was largest at right-hemisphere centroparietal scalp locations, and comprised a greater negativity in the ERPs evoked by unstudied items from the deep retrieval condition. The authors suggested that this modulation likely indexes processes that are distinct from those indexed by the left-frontal effect. The principal support for this proposal was drawn from the similarity between this modulation and the N400 ERP component. This negative-going component was identified initially in studies of language processing (Kutas and Hillyard, 1980) and is larger in tasks that require semantic rather than nonsemantic processing of stimuli (Rugg *et al.*, 1988; Chwilla *et al.*, 1995). On the basis of this similarity, Rugg *et al.* (2000) proposed that participants employed retrieval strategies at test that varied according to their experiences at the time of encoding, with the N400-like modulation reflecting the greater emphasis on semantic retrieval processing in the easier of the two retrieval tasks. Whether the N400-like modulation indexes processes that are in fact distinct from those indexed by the left-frontal modulation was not clear, however, because there was no statistical evidence to support the view that the two effects were either neurally or functionally dissociable.

Their claims for functionally separable processes draw support from a study in which participants were directed at test to retrieve either semantically or phonologically encoded material (Wilding and Nobre, 2001). Participants initially completed two different encoding tasks. The first involved generating a word and saying aloud a word that rhymed with it. The second involved generating a mental image of a concept denoted by a word and saying aloud a word denoting a concept with a similar mental image. These encoding tasks were blocked and each block was followed by a corresponding retrieval phase in which participants made R/K/new judgments to old and new words. They were asked to make an R response only to those words for which they could remember the associate (either image based or phonological) that was generated at study. In keeping with the findings of Rugg and colleagues (Rugg *et al.*, 2000), memory performance was superior following image-based encoding (Craik and Lockhart, 1972). The ERPs evoked by correct rejections in this task

were also associated with a larger N400-like effect than those evoked in the phonological retrieval task. To the extent that the image-based retrieval task is likely to encourage greater emphasis on semantic processing, compared to the phonological task, these findings are consistent with those of Rugg *et al.* (2000).

Wilding and Nobre (2001) included a second experiment in their study, again incorporating the image-based/phonological manipulation. The principal difference between this experiment and the one described already was that at test participants were cued on a trial-by-trial basis as to which retrieval task to complete, and frequent switches between tasks were required. Memory accuracy was no worse in this experiment than when the two retrieval tasks were blocked. By contrast, the modulations that differentiated the ERPs evoked by the two classes of correct rejections in the blocked design were attenuated in the mixed-trial design, as is shown in Fig. 5.

Wilding and Nobre argued that the reason for this attenuation was that participants in the mixed-trial design were not provided with sufficient opportunity to engage in task-specific processing [and/or to disengage from processing relevant on previous trials: see Rogers and Monsell (1995) and Allport and Wylie (2000)]. Furthermore, they observed that the correspondence across studies at the level of the behavioral data was consistent with the view that the processes reflected in the differences between the ERPs evoked by correct rejections in the blocked design were not influential in determining the success or failure of memory retrieval. Rather, they argued that the differences likely reflected processes that optimized the evaluation of task-relevant aspects of a memory trace. Although this interpretation may turn out to be correct, it presumes that the differences observed in the blocked design reflect orientation rather than effort. The behavioral data indicate

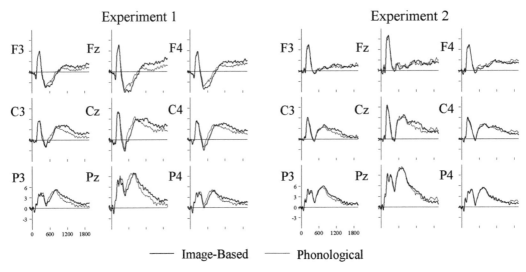

FIGURE 5 Group-average ERPs elicited by new words attracting correct judgments in the blocked (Experiment 1) and mixed-trial (Experiment 2) designs for frontal (F3, Fz, F4), central (C3, Cz, C4), and parietal (P3, Pz, P4) electrode sites. The ERPs elicited by new items are separated according to the retrieval task (image based or phonological) in which they were presented. Data from Wilding and Nobre (2001).

that memory accuracy was superior in the image-based tasks, and it remains to be determined whether effort and orientation are influenced equivalently by the requirement to switch frequently between retrieval tasks.

To our knowledge, retrieval effort and orientation have been manipulated independently in only one study. Robb and Rugg (2002) recorded ERPs while participants completed four separate recognition memory tasks. Old/new judgments to visually presented words were made in each. In two of the blocks words were presented at study; in the remainder, pictures were presented. One block in each pair comprised an easy recognition task, and the other a difficult one. This was accomplished by manipulating study-list length and the study–test interval. The design therefore enabled identification of neural activity predictive of effort and activity predictive of orientation.

Indices of both classes of processes were evident in the electrical record, although the authors encourage caution concerning the putative index of processes related to

difficulty, given the size of the effect and its level of significance. The effect of orientation, by contrast, was robust, extending from 300 to 1900 msec poststimulus with a broad scalp distribution. Whatever the eventual status of the putative correlate of difficulty, these findings are important because they are consistent with the view that effort, at least as operationalized in terms of task difficulty, is not simply manifest as changes in activity in the same brain regions that support retrieval orientations (Rugg and Wilding, 2000).

In summary, the deployment of ERPs in order to index processes that are engaged in pursuit of retrieval is a relatively recent endeavour. The findings to date provide some support for the distinction between orientation and effort, but require generalization. This will involve the use of a wider range of stimuli and task types, as well as implementation in designs when electrophysiological correlates of these two classes of process can be disentangled. To date, attention to processes that form part of a retrieval attempt has been somewhat lacking in ERP studies in comparison to studies in which other functional neuroimaging modalities have been employed (Rugg and Wilding, 2000). It is to be hoped that this situation will change in the near future.

CONCLUDING REMARKS

In this review we have focused on recent developments in electrophysiological studies of episodic memory processes. In the case of both episodic encoding and episodic retrieval there are good grounds to believe that important advances and insights are being—and will continue to be—made. Although this review has focused on processes that are time locked to the presentation of discrete task stimuli, it may turn out that in future studies it will be important to supplement these approaches with designs that permit the monitoring of activity that is engaged before stimuli are presented. There are two ways in which this could be achieved. The first is to employ designs in which participants are cued as to which encoding or retrieval task to complete on a trial-by-trial basis (e.g., Otten and Rugg, 2001a; Wilding, 2001; Morcom and Rugg, 2002), and to record the activity that is evoked by the cues. Such activity will presumably reflect preparatory processes that are set in train by the cue and may well influence the accuracy and/or time course of successful episodic encoding and retrieval.

A second approach is to record direct current (DC) potentials during encoding and retrieval tasks. These recordings can be employed to monitor slow (low-frequency) changes in neural activity that can be sustained for several seconds and may reflect the adoption and maintenance of a cognitive set. A set is a preparatory state that determines the processing to which task stimuli will be subjected (Gibson, 1941). The extent to which the success or otherwise of episodic encoding and retrieval are influenced by the adoption of a set or

mode (Tulving, 1983) remains to be determined, but it is an issue that ERPs are well suited to address. This is due to the fact that by adopting a suitably broad frequency range at acquisition it is in principle possible to index two classes of process. The first is state-related activity that is time locked to task onset, may be maintained for the duration of the task, and is likely reflected in low-frequency modulations of the electrical record. The second is item-related activity that is set in train by stimuli that are presented during the task. The activity engaged by these stimuli is assumed to have a time course that is shorter than the interstimulus interval, and will be indexed by higher frequency components of the electrical record than those indexing state-related activity. The results of one study in which state- and item-related measures of episodic retrieval operations were obtained (Düzel et al., 1999) suggest strongly that the use of this approach will provide a valuable adjunct to the methods that are employed most often at present in event-related potential studies of episodic memory encoding and retrieval.

References

Allan, K., and Rugg, M. D. (1997). An event-related potential study of explicit memory on tests of cued recall and recognition. *Neuropsychologia* **35**, 387–397.

Allan, K. A., Wilding, E. L., and Rugg, M. D. (1998). Electrophysiological evidence for dissociable processes contributing to recollection. *Acta Psychol.* **98**, 231–252.

Allan, K., Robb, W. G. K., and Rugg, M. D. (2000). The effect of encoding manipulations on neural correlates of episodic retrieval. *Neuropsychologia* **38**, 1188–1205.

Allport, A., and Wylie, G. (2000). Task-switching: Positive and negative priming of task-set. *In* "Attention, Space and Action: Studies in Cognitive Neuroscience" (G. W. Humphreys, J. Duncan, and A. M. Treisman, eds.), pp. 273–296. Oxford University Press, Oxford.

Bentin, S., and Peled, B. S. (1990). The contribution of task-related factors to ERP repetition effects at short and long lags. *Mem. Cogn.* **18**, 359–366.

Bentin, S., Moscovitch, M., and Heth, I. (1992). Memory with and without awareness: Performance and electrophysiological evidence of savings. *J. Exp. Psychol. Learn. Mem. Cogn.* **18**, 1270–1283.

Burgess, P. W., and Shallice, T. (1996). Confabulation and the control of recollection. *Memory* **4**, 359–411.

Cabeza, R., and Nyberg, L. (2000). Imaging cognition II: An empirical review of 275 PET and fMRI studies. *J. Cogn. Neurosci.* **12**, 1–47.

Chwilla, D. J., Brown, C. M., and Hagoort, P. (1995). The N400 as a function of the level of processing. *Psychophysiology* **32**, 274–285.

Craik, F. I. M., and Lockhart, R. S. (1972). Levels of processing: A framework for memory research. *J.Verbal Learn. Verbal Behav.* **16**, 519–533.

Curran, T. (1999). The electrophysiology of incidental and intentional retrieval: ERP old/new effects in lexical decision and recognition memory. *Neuropsychologia* **37**, 771–785.

Curran, T. (2000). Brain potentials of recollection and familiarity. *Mem. Cogn.* **28**, 923–938.

Cycowicz, Y. M., Friedman, D., and Snodgrass, J. G. (2001). Remembering the colour of objects: An ERP investigation of source memory. *Cereb. Cortex* **11**, 322–334.

Dale, A. M., and Buckner, R. L. (1997). Selective averaging of rapidly presented trials using fMRI. *Hum. Brain Mapping* **5**, 329–340.

Donaldson, W. (1996). The role of decision processes in remembering and knowing. *Mem. Cogn.* **24**, 523–533.

Donaldson, D. I., and Rugg, M. D. (1998). Recognition memory for new associations: Electrophysiological evidence for the role of recollection. *Neuropsychologia* **36**, 377–395.

Donaldson, D. I., Wilding, E. L., and Allan, K. (2002). Fractionating retrieval from episodic memory using event-related potentials. *In* "The Cognitive Neuroscience of Memory: Episodic Encoding and Retrieval" (A. E. Parker, E. L. Wilding, and T. J. Bussey, eds.). Psychology Press, Hove.

Düzel, E., Yonelinas, A.P., Mangun, G.R., Heinze, H.J., and Tulving, E. (1997). Event-related brain potential correlates of two states of conscious awareness in memory. *Proc. Natl. Acad. Sci. U.S.A* **94**, 5973–5978.

Düzel, E., Cabeza, R., Picton, T. W., Yonelinas, A. P., Scheich, H., Heinze, H. J., and Tulving, E. (1999). Task-related and item-related brain processes of memory retrieval. *Proc. Natl. Acad. Sci. U.S.A.* **96**, 1794–1799.

Fernandez, G., Weyerts, H., Tendolkar, I., Smid, H. G., Scholz, M., and Heinze, H. J. (1998). Event-related potentials of verbal encoding into episodic memory: Dissociation between the effects of subsequent memory performance and distinctiveness. *Psychophysiology* **35**, 709–720.

Fletcher, P. C., and Henson, R. N. A. (2001). Frontal lobes and human memory: Insights from functional neuroimaging. *Brain* **124**, 849–881.

Friedman, D. (1990a). Cognitive event-related potential components during continuous recognition memory for pictures. *Psychophysiology* **27**, 136–148.

Friedman, D. (1990b). Endogenous event-related brain potentials during continuous recognition memory for words. *Biol. Psychol.* **30**, 61–87.

Friedman, D., and Johnson, R. J. (2000). Event-related potential (ERP) studies of episodic memory encoding and retrieval: A selective review. *Micros. Res. Techniq.* **51**, 6–28.

Friedman, D., and Sutton, S. (1987). Event-related potentials during continuous recognition memory. *In* "Current Trends in Event-Related Potential Research" (Supplement 40 to "Electroencephalography and Clinical Neurophysiology") (R. Johnson, J. W. Rohrbaugh, and R. Parasuraman, eds.), pp. 316–321. Elsevier, Amsterdam.

Friedman, D., and Trott, C. (2000). An event-related potential study of encoding in young and older adults. *Neuropsychologia* **38**, 542–557.

Friedman, D., Hamberger, M., Stern, Y., and Marder, K. (1992). Event-related potentials during repetition priming in Alzheimer's patients and young and older controls. *J. Clin. Exp. Neuropsychol.* **14**, 448–462.

Gabrieli, J. D. E. (1993). Disorders of memory in humans. *Curr. Opin. Neurol. Neurosurg.* **6**, 93–97.

Gardiner, J. M. (1988). Functional aspects of recollective experience. *Mem. Cogn.* **16**, 309–313.

Gardiner, J. M. (2001). Episodic memory and autonoetic consciousness: A first-person approach. *Philos. Trans. Roy. Soc. (Lond.)* **356**, 1351–1361.

Gardiner, J. M., and Java, R.I. (1990). Recollective experience in word and non-word recognition. *Mem. Cogn.* **18**, 23–30.

Gardiner, J. M., and Java, R. I. (1993). Recognising and remembering. *In* "Theories of Memory" (A. Collins, M. A. Conway, S. E. Gathercole, and P. E. Morris, eds.), pp. 163–188. Erlbaum, Assoc. Hillsdale, New Jersey.

Gardiner, J. M., Java, R. I., and Richardson-Klavehn, A. (1996). How level of processing really influences awareness in recognition memory. *Can. J. Exp. Psychol.* **50**, 114–122.

Gibson, J. J. (1941). A critical review of the concept of set in contemporary experimental psychology. *Psychol. Bull.* **38**, 781–817.

Glisky, E. L., Polster, M. L., and Routhieaux, B. C. (1995). Double dissociation between item and source memory. *Neuropsychology* **9**, 229–235.

Henson, R. N. A., Rugg, M. D., Shallice, T., Josephs, O., and Dolan, R. J. (1999). Recollection and familiarity in recognition memory: An event-related functional magnetic resonance imaging study. *J. Neurosci.* **19**, 3962–3972.

Hirshman, E., and Henzler, A. (1998). The role of decision processes in conscious recollection. *Psychol. Sci.* **9**, 61–65.

Hirshman, E., and Master, S. (1997). Modelling the conscious correlates of recognition memory: Reflections on the remember–know paradigm. *Mem. Cogn.* **25**, 345–351.

Jacoby, L. L. (1998). Invariance in automatic influences of memory: Toward a user's guide for the process–dissociation procedure. *J. Exp. Psychol. Learn. Mem. Cogn.* **24**, 3–26.

Jacoby, L. L., and Dallas, M. (1981). On the relationship between autobiographical memory and perceptual learning. *J. Exp. Psychol. Gen.* **3**, 306–340.

Jacoby, L. L., and Kelley, C. (1992). Unconscious influences of memory: Dissociations and automaticity. *In* "The Neuropsychology of Consciousness" (A. D. Milner and M. D. Rugg, eds.), pp. 201–233. Academic Press, London.

Janowsky, J. S., Shimamura, A. P., and Squire, L. R. (1989). Source memory impairment in patients with frontal lobe lesions. *Neuropsychologia* **27**, 1043–1056.

Johnson, R. (1995). Event-related potential insights into the neurobiology of memory systems. *In* "Handbook of Neuropsychology" (F. Boller and J. Grafman, eds.), pp. 135–164. Elsevier, Amsterdam.

Johnson, R., Pfefferbaum, A., and Kopell, B. S. (1985). P300 and long-term memory: Latency predicts recognition performance. *Psychophysiology* **22**, 497–507.

Johnson, M. K., Kounios, J., and Nolde, S. F. (1996). Electrophysiological brain activity and memory source monitoring. *NeuroReport* **8**, 1317–1320.

Johnson, Jr., R., Kreiter, K., Russo, B., and Zhu, J. (1998). A spatio-temporal analysis of recognition-related event-related brain potentials. *Int. J. Psychophysiol.* **29**, 83–104.

Josephs, O., Turner, R., and Friston, K. J. (1997). Event-related fMRI. *Hum. Brain Mapping* **5**, 243–248.

Karis, D., Fabiani, M., and Donchin, E. (1984). P300 and memory: Individual differences in the Von Restorff effect. *Cogn. Psychol.* **16**, 177–216.

Kutas, M. (1988). Review of event-related potential studies of memory. *In* "Perspectives in Memory Research" (M.S. Gazzaniga, ed.), pp. 182–217. MIT Press, Cambridge, Massachusetts.

Kutas, M., and Hillyard, S. A. (1980). Reading senseless sentences: Brain potentials reflect semantic incongruity. *Science* **207**, 203–205.

Mandler, G. (1980). Recognising: The judgment of previous occurrence. *Psychol. Rev.* **87**, 252–271.

Mangels, J. A., Picton, T. W., and Craik, F. I. M. (2001). Attention and successful episodic encoding: an event-related potential study. *Cogn. Brain Res.* **11**, 77–95.

Mayes, A. R. (1988). "Human Organic Memory Disorders." Cambridge University Press, Cambridge.

Mayes, A. R., and Roberts, N. (2001). Theories of episodic memory. *Philos. Trans. Roy. Soc. (Lond.)* **356**, 1395–1408.

McCarthy, G., and Wood, C. C. (1985). Scalp distributions of event-related potentials: An ambiguity associated with analysis of variance models. *Electroencephalogr. Clin. Neurophysiol.* **62**, 203–208.

Mecklinger, A. (1998). On the modularity of recognition memory for object form and spatial location: A topographic ERP analysis. *Neuropsychologia* **36**, 441–460.

Mecklinger, A. (2000). Interfacing mind and brain: A neurocognitive model of recognition memory. *Psychophysiology* **37**, 565–582.

Mecklinger, A., and Meinshausen, R. (1998). Recognition memory for object forms and spatial locations: An event-related potential study. *Mem. Cogn.* **26**, 1068–1088.

Morcom, A., and Rugg, M. D. (2002). Getting ready to remember: The neural correlates of task set during recognition memory. *Neuroreport* **13**, 149–152.

Morris, C. D., Bransford, J. D., and Franks, J. J. (1977). Levels of processing versus transfer appropriate processing. *J. Verbal Learn. Verbal Behav.* **16**, 519–533.

Moscovitch, M. (1992). Memory and working-with-memory: A component process model based on modules and central systems. *J. Cogn. Neurosci.* **4**, 257–267.

Moscovitch, M. (1994). Models of consciousness and memory. *In* "The Cognitive Neurosciences" (M.S. Gazzaniga, ed.), pp. 1341–1356. MIT Press, Cambridge, Massachusetts.

Neville, H. J., Kutas, M., Chesney, G., and Schmidt, A. L. (1986). Event-related brain potentials during initial encoding and recognition memory of congruous and incongruous words. *J. Mem. Lang.* **25**, 75–92.

Noldy, N. E., Stelmack, R. M., and Campbell, K. B. (1990). Event-related potentials and recognition memory for pictures and words: The effects of intentional and incidental learning. *Psychophysiology* **27**, 417–428.

Otten, L. J., and Rugg, M. D. (2001a). Electrophysiological correlates of memory encoding are task-dependent. *Cogn. Brain Res.* **12**, 11–18.

Otten, L. J., and Rugg, M. D. (2001b). Task-dependency of the neural correlates of episodic encoding as measured by fMRI. *Cereb. Cortex* **11**, 1150–1160.

Paller, K. A., and Kutas, M. (1992). Brain potentials during retrieval provide neurophysiological support for the distinction between conscious recollection and priming. *J. Cogn. Neurosci.* **4**, 375–391.

Paller, K. A., Kutas, M., and Mayes, A. R. (1987). Neural correlates of encoding in an incidental learning paradigm. *Electroencephalogr. Clin. Neurophysiol.* **67**, 360–371.

Paller, K. A., McCarthy, G., and Wood, C. C. (1988). ERPs predictive of subsequent recall and recognition performance. *Biol. Psychol.* **26**, 269–276.

Paller, K. A., Kutas, M., and McIsaac, H. K. (1995). Monitoring conscious recollection via the electrical activity of the brain. *Psychol. Sci.* **6**, 107–111.

Potter, D. D., Pickles, C. D., Roberts, R. C., and Rugg, M. D. (1992). The effects of scopolamine on event-related potentials in a continuous recognition memory task. *Psychophysiology* **29**, 29–37.

Ranganath, C., and Paller, K. A. (1999). Frontal brain potentials during recognition are modulated by requirements to retrieve perceptual details. *Neuron* **22**, 605–613.

Ranganath, C., and Paller, K. A. (2000). Neural correlates of memory retrieval and evaluation. *Cogn. Brain Res.* **9**, 209–222.

Richardson-Klavehn, A., and Bjork, R. A. (1988). Measures of memory. *Annu. Rev. Psychol.* **39**, 475–543.

Robb, W. G. K., and Rugg, M. D. (2002). Electrophysiological dissociation of retrieval orientation and retrieval effort. *Psychonom. Bull. Rev.* (in press).

Rogers, R. D., and Monsell, S. (1995). Costs of a predictable switch between simple cognitive tasks. *J. Exp. Psychol. Gen.* **124**, 207–231.

Rugg, M. D. (1987). Dissociation of semantic priming, word and non-word repetition by event-related potentials. *Q. J. Exp. Psychol.* **39A**, 123–148.

Rugg, M. D. (1995). ERP studies of memory. *In* "Electrophysiology of Mind: Event-Related Brain Potentials and Cognition" (M. D. Rugg and M. G. H. Coles, eds.), pp. 132–170. Oxford Univ. Press, Oxford.

Rugg, M. D. (1998). Functional neuroimaging in cognitive neuroscience. *In* "The Neurocognition of Language" (C.M. Brown and P. Hagoort, eds.), pp. 15–36. Oxford University Press, Oxford.

Rugg, M. D., and Allan, K. (2000). Event-related potential studies of Memory. *In* "The Oxford Handbook of memory" (E. Tulving and F. I. M. Craik, eds.), pp. 521–537. Oxford University Press, Oxford.

Rugg, M. D., and Coles, M. G. H. (1995). The ERP and cognitive psychology: Conceptual issues. *In* "Electrophysiology of Mind: Event-Related Brain Potentials and Cognition" (M. D. Rugg and M. G. H. Coles, eds.), pp. 27–39. Oxford University Press, Oxford.

Rugg, M. D., and Doyle, M. C. (1992). Event-related potentials and recognition memory for low- and high-frequency words. *J. Cogn. Neurosci.* **4**, 69–79.

Rugg, M. D., and Doyle, M. C. (1994). Event-related potentials and stimulus repetition in direct and indirect tests of memory. *In* "Cognitive Electrophysiology" (H. J. Heinze, T. Munte, and G. R. Mangun, eds.), pp. 124–148. Birkhauser, Boston.

Rugg, M. D., and Henson, R. N. A. (2002). Episodic memory retrieval: An (event-related) functional neuroimaging perspective. *In* "The Cognitive Neuroscience of Memory: Episodic Encoding and Retrieval" (A. E. Parker, E. L. Wilding, and T. J. Bussey, eds.). Psychology Press, Hove.

Rugg, M. D., and Nagy, M. E. (1989). Event-related potentials and recognition memory for words. *Electroencephalogr. Clin. Neurophysiol.* **72**, 395–406.

Rugg, M. D., and Wilding, E. L. (2000). Retrieval processing and episodic memory. *Trends Cogn. Sci.* **4**, 108–115.

Rugg, M. D., Furda, J., and Lorist, M. (1988). The effects of task on the modulation of event-related potentials by word repetition. *Psychophysiology* **25**, 55–63.

Rugg, M. D., Brovedani, P., and Doyle, M. C. (1992). Modulation of event-related potentials by word repetition in a task with inconsistent mapping between repetition and response. *Electroencephalogr. Clin. Neurophysiol.* **84**, 521–531.

Rugg, M. D., Cox, C. J. C., Doyle, M. C., and Wells, T. (1995). Event-related potentials and the recollection of low and high frequency words. *Neuropsychologia* **33**, 471–484.

Rugg, M. D., Schloerscheidt, A. M., Doyle, M. C., Cox, C. J. C., and Patching, G. R. (1996). Event-related potentials and the recollection of associative information. *Cogn. Brain Res.* **4**, 297–304.

Rugg, M. D., Mark, R. E., Walla, P., Schloerscheidt, A. M., Birch, C. S., and Allan, K. (1998). Dissociation of the neural correlates of implicit and explicit memory. *Nature* **392**, 595–598.

Rugg, M. D., Allan, K., and Birch, C. S. (2000). Electrophysiological evidence for the modulation of retrieval orientation by depth of study processing. *J. Cogn. Neurosci.* **12**, 664–678.

Sanquist, T. F., Rohrbaugh, J. W., Syndulko, K., and Lindsley, D. B. (1980). Electrocortical signs of levels of processing: Perceptual analysis and recognition memory. *Psychophysiology* **17**, 568–576.

Schacter, D. L., Harbluk, J. L., and McLachlan, D. R. (1984). Retrieval without recollection: An experimental analysis of source amnesia. *J. Verbal Learn. Verbal Behav.* **23**, 593–611.

Scoville, W. B., and Milner, B. (1957). Loss of recent memory after bilateral hippocampal lesions. *J. Neurol. Neurosurg. Psychiatr.* **20**, 11–21.

Senkfor, A. J., and Van Petten, C., V. P. (1998). Who said what: An event-related potential investigation of source and item memory. *J. Exp. Psychol. Learn. Mem. Cogn.* **24**, 1005–1025.

Shallice, T., and Burgess, P. (1998). The domain of supervisory processes and the temporal organisation of behaviour. *In* "The Prefrontal Cortex: Executive and Cognitive Functions" (A. C. Roberts,

T. W. Robbins, and L. Weiskrantz, eds.), pp. 22–35. Oxford University Press, Oxford.

Shimamura, A. P., and Squire, L. R. (1987). A neuropsychological study of fact memory and source amnesia. *J. Exp. Psychol. Learn. Mem. Cogn.* **13**, 464–473.

Smith, M. E. (1993). Neurophysiological manifestations of recollective experience during recognition memory judgements. *J. Cogn. Neurosci.* **5**, 1–13.

Smith, M. E., and Guster, K. (1993). Decomposition of recognition memory event-related potentials yields target, repetition, and retrieval effects. *Electroencephalogr. Clin. Neurophysiol.* **86**, 335–343.

Smith, M. E., and Halgren, E. (1989). Dissociation of recognition memory components following temporal lobe lesions. *J. Exp. Psychol. Learn. Mem. Cogn.* **15**, 50–60.

Snodgrass, J. G., and Corwin, J. (1988). Pragmatics of measuring recognition memory: Applications to dementia and amnesia. *J. Exp. Psychol. Gen.* **117**, 34–50.

Sommer, W., Schweinberger, S. R., and Matt, J. (1991). Human brain potential correlates of face encoding into memory. *Electroencephalogr. Clin. Neurophysiol.* **79 (6)**, 457–463.

Sommer, W., Heinz, A., Leuthold, H., Matt, J., and Schweinberger, S. R. (1995). Metamemory, distinctiveness, and event-related potentials in recognition memory for faces. *Mem. Cogn.* **23**, 1–11.

Sommer, W., Komoss, E., and Schweinberger, S. R. (1997). Differential localisation of brain systems subserving memory for names and faces in normal subjects with event-related potentials. *Electroencephalogr. Clin. Neurophysiol.* **102**, 192–199.

Squire, L. R., Knowlton, B., and Musen, G. (1993). The structure and organization of memory. *Annu. Rev. Psychol.* **44**, 453–495.

Sternberg, S. (1966). High-speed scanning in human memory. *Science* **153**, 652–654.

Stuss, D. T., Eskes, G. A., and Foster, J. K. (1994). Experimental neuropsychological studies of frontal lobe functions. *In* "Handbook of Neuropsychology, Volume 10" (F. Boller and J. Grafman, eds.), pp. 149–183. Elsevier, New York.

Tendolkar, I., and Rugg, M. D. (1998). Electrophysiological dissociation of recency and recognition memory. *Neuropsychologia* **36**, 477–490.

Tendolkar, I., Schoenfeld, A., Golz, G., Fernandez, G., Kuhl, K.-P., Ferszt, R., and Heinze, H.-J. (1999). Neural correlates of recognition memory with and without recollection in patients with Alzheimer's disease and healthy controls. *Neurosci. Lett.* **263**, 45–48.

Toth, J. P. (1996). Conceptual automaticity in recognition memory: Levels of processing effects on familiarity. *Can. J. Exp. Psychol.* **50**, 123–128.

Trott, C. T., Friedman, D., Ritter, W., and Fabiani, M. (1997). Item and source memory: Differential age

effects revealed by event-related potentials. *NeuroReport* **8**, 3373–3378.

Tsivilis, D., Otten, J., and Rugg, M. D. (2001). Context effects on the neural correlates of recognition memory: An electrophysiological study. *Neuron* **31**, 1–20.

Tulving, E. (1983). "Elements of Episodic Memory." Oxford University Press, Oxford.

Tulving, E. (1985). Memory and Consciousness. *Can. Psychol.* **26**, 1–12.

Tulving, E., and Thomson, D.M. (1973). Encoding specificity and retrieval processes in episodic memory. *Psychol. Rev.* **80**, 353–373.

Van Petten, C., and Senkfor, A. J. (1996). Memory for words and novel visual patterns: Repetition, recognition, and encoding effects in the event-related brain potential. *Psychophysiology* **33**, 491–506.

Van Petten, C., Kutas, M., Kluender, R., Mitchiner, M., and McIsaac, H. (1991). Fractionating the word repetition effect with event-related potentials. *J. Cogn. Neurosci.* **3**, 129–150.

Van Petten, C., Senkfor, A. J., and Newberg, W. M. (2000). Memory for drawings in locations: Spatial source memory and event-related potentials. *Psychophysiology* **4**, 551–564.

Wagner, A. D. (1999). Working memory contributions to human learning and remembering [Review]. *Neuron* **22**, 19–22.

Wagner, A. D., Koutstaal, W., and Schachter, D. L. (1999). When encoding yields remembering: insights from event-related neuroimaging. *Philos. Trans. Roy. Soc. (Lond.)* **354**, 1307–1324.

Wilding, E. L. (1999). Separating retrieval strategies from retrieval success: An event-related potential study of source memory. *Neuropsychologia* **37**, 441–454.

Wilding, E. L. (2000). In what way does the parietal ERP old/new effect index recollection? *Int. J. Psychophysiol.* **35**, 81–87.

Wilding, E. L. (2001). Event-related functional imaging and episodic memory. *Neurosci. Biobehav. Rev.* **25**, 545–554.

Wilding, E. L., and Nobre, A. C. (2001). Task-switching and memory-retrieval processing: Electrophysiological evidence. *NeuroReport* **12**, 3613–3617.

Wilding, E. L., and Rugg, M. D. (1996). An event-related potential study of recognition memory with and without retrieval of source. *Brain* **119**, 889–905.

Wilding, E. L., and Rugg, M. D. (1997a). An event-related potential study of memory for spoken and heard words. *Neuropsychologia* **35**, 1185–1195.

Wilding, E. L., and Rugg, M. D. (1997b). Event-related potentials and the recognition memory exclusion task. *Neuropsychologia* **35**, 119–128.

Wilding, E. L., Doyle, M. C., and Rugg, M. D. (1995). Recognition memory with and without retrieval of study context: An event-related potential study. *Neuropsychologia* **33**, 743–767.

Yonelinas, A. P. (1994). Receiver-operating characteristics in recognition memory: Evidence for a dual-process model. *J. Exp. Psychol. Learn. Mem. Cogn.* **20**, 1341–1354.

Yonelinas, A. P. (1998). Recollection and familiarity in recognition memory: Convergence of remember/know, process dissociation and ROC data. *Neuropsychology* **12**, 323–329.

Yonelinas, A. P., and Jacoby, L. L. (1994). Dissociations of processes in recognition memory: Effects of interference and of response speed. *Can. J. Exp. Psychol.* **48**, 516–534.

Yonelinas, A. P., and Jacoby, L. L. (1995). The relationship between remembering and knowing as bases for recognition: Effects of size congruency. *J. Mem. Lang.* **34**, 622–643.

Yonelinas, A. P., Dobbins, I., Szymanski, M. D., Dhaliwal, H. S., and King, L. (1996). Signal-detection, threshold, and dual-process models of recognition memory: ROCs and conscious recollection. *Conscious. Cogn.* **5**, 418–441.

COGNITIVE AND AFFECTIVE PROCESSING OF THE BRAIN

B. AFFECTIVE AND DEVELOPMENTAL PERSPECTIVES OF NEURAL COGNITION

Self-Regulation and the Executive Functions: Electrophysiological Clues

Phan Luu and Don M. Tucker

INTRODUCTION

Cognitive models typically describe executive functions as higher level processes that exert control over elementary mental operations (Norman and Shallice, 1986). Executive control includes supervisory functions that must be engaged in situations in which well-learned behavior is inadequate. These situations include demands for planning, error correction, execution of novel actions, inhibition of routinized behavior, and alerting to danger. When executive functions are impaired, such as by frontal lobe lesions, the patient's actions may be guided by demand characteristics of the environment without regard for social or practical appropriateness (Eslinger and Damasio, 1985; Lehrmitte, 1986; Lehrmitte *et al.*, 1986).

As recognized in the cognitive analysis of attention, concepts of executive functions run the risk of invoking a homunculus (Posner, 1978). The requirement for an external or supervisory control of information processing naturally leads to the assumption of an external agent that must direct the cognitive traffic. Because executive deficits are particularly apparent with frontal lesions, it has been natural for clini-

cians and researchers to assume, tacitly of course, that the homunculus resides in the frontal lobe.

A more attractive scientific model would explain how executive psychological operations might emerge from more elementary adaptive mechanisms. Since the middle of the twentieth century, neuroanatomical studies have provided important clues to such mechanisms, showing dense connections of the primate frontal lobe with the visceral and emotional functions of limbic cortex (MacLean and Pribram, 1953; Pribram and MacLean, 1953). Developing the anatomical evidence further, Nauta (1971) emphasized that the frontal lobe's connectivity with limbic circuits implies primary roles for emotion and motivation in self-regulation. For Nauta, the frontal lobe lesion syndromes reflect the lack of control by affective, subjective evaluation in action planning. Even though a patient with a prefrontal lobe lesion can accurately describe the environmental situation, behavior occurs as if there is no evaluative control (Nauta's limbic "set points"). In addition to the evaluation of action plans, the limbic set points provide ongoing monitoring in order for the plan to be maintained in relation to adaptive goals. Nauta's reasoning has been influential on modern concepts, and it remains consistent

199

with the more recent emphasis on affective cues in frontal self-regulation by Damasio *et al.* (1990).

In this chapter, we begin with the assumption that an adequate scientific theory of human self-regulation must explain how higher executive functions emerge from more elementary mechanisms of learning. These mechanisms must achieve the adaptive control of actions in contexts. We review both hemodynamic and electrophysiological evidence suggesting that activity in regions of limbic cortex, particularly the cingulate gyrus, may be integral to the frontal executive functions. Neurophysiological studies of learning and memory in animals have provided important models of the corticolimbic and corticothalamic mechanisms of self-regulation. Findings of basal ganglia mechanisms are also instructive for understanding motivational control of action, and we attempt to point out how these might be relevant to corticolimbic and corticothalamic mechanisms. We review several interesting clues that scalp electrophysiological measures in humans could be related to the essential limbic, striatal, and thalamic circuits. One of the clues is the oscillatory nature of corticolimbic activity that appears to underlie conventional electrophysiological measures (such as the error-related negativity, N2, and P300). By considering current electrophysiological findings in humans in relation to neurophysiological findings in animal research, we propose that there are important new perspectives to be gained on the intrinsic mechanisms of human self-regulation.

ANTERIOR CINGULATE CORTEX AND THE EXECUTIVE FUNCTIONS

Broca identified the limbic lobe at the core of the cerebral hemisphere. In addition to the medial temporal cortex, the limbic lobe is composed of the cingulate gyri, bordering the corpus callosum on the medial surface of each hemisphere and set off from the callosum by the callosal sulcus. Historically, the cingulate cortex was also referred to as the gyrus fornicatus, emphasizing its anatomical relation with the fornix. From its initial identification, the cingulate's relation to the primitive limbic regions was a subject of debate, with a number of early workers suggesting that it belonged to the olfactory system. With the advent of more precise methods for studying anatomical connectivity and cytoarchitecture, it is now clear that the entire cingulate gyrus was derived from the archicortex (i.e., the hippocampus) and not the olfactory cortex (Pandya *et al.*, 1988; Sanides, 1970). This relation with the hippocampus explains the dense connections of the cingulate with the hippocampus and other dorsal cortical structures derived from archicortex.

Prior to functional studies, little was known about the functional significance of the cingulate cortex. However, there were many speculations based on its anatomical connections and its comparatively old anatomical position. As a result of its inclusion with olfactory structures, it was believed to be involved in olfactory function, which was considered to be unimportant in humans (MacLean, 1993). But studies by Ward (1948a,b) demonstrated that the anterior cingulate cortex (ACC) was important to autonomic and motor functions. This is clearly demonstrated in patients with lesions to the ACC, who show a host of symptoms, including apathy, inattention, dysregulation of autonomic functions, akinetic mutism, and emotional instability (Barris and Schuman, 1953).

Modern cognitive neuroimaging methods have allowed researchers to study the relation between executive functions and the ACC. Hemodynamic studies identified ACC activation in tasks that required subjects to make responses that are either novel or that required them to overcome competing responses (George *et al.*, 1994; Pardo, *et al.*, 1990; Posner *et al.*, 1988). These results were interpreted to reflect the role of the ACC in attention, particularly attention for action (Posner and Dehaene, 1994). According to this view, the ACC provides top-down control to resolve competing neural activations (Posner and DiGirolamo, 1998). More recent theories of the ACC state that rather than strategically implementing attention allocation-like functions, the ACC is involved in evaluating conflicting demands (i.e., competing neural activation) (Carter *et al.*, 1998, 1999). According to this theory, the ACC signals when executive control, i.e., functions controlled by the dorsolateral prefrontal cortex (MacDonald *et al.*, 2000), is required.

It is well known that the ACC is not a homogeneous structure, both in terms of cytoarchitectonics and function (Devinsky *et al.*, 1995; Vogt *et al.*, 1993a). A review by Bush *et al.* (2000) noted that cognitive tasks tend to activate the dorsal ACC and deactivate the rostroventral ACC. Conversely, emotional tasks activate the rostroventral ACC and deactivate the dorsal ACC. These two subdivisions of the ACC appear to be warranted on neuroanatomical grounds as well (Pandya *et al.*, 1981; Vogt *et al.*, 1987). The findings that both cognitive and emotional tasks activate different regions of the ACC have proved to be difficult to reconcile for pure cognitive theories of executive functions and the ACC. However, they are consistent with theories that emphasize the central role of affect in self-regulation (Nauta, 1971), and this integration of emotions with cognition in the ACC is now recognized to be important (Allman *et al.*, 2001; Paus, 2001).

Executive Control and Action Monitoring

Another aspect of executive function is the ability to integrate negative feedback, that is, to monitor for the occurrence of errors and to adjust behavior accordingly.

This self-regulatory function is so important to adaptive behavior that failure to appreciate the significance of mistakes often leads to the inability to manage one's life, as is often observed in frontal lobe patients (Eslinger and Damasio, 1985; Rylander, 1947). Frontal lobe patients are often capable of recognizing errors. However, as described in classic studies (Rylander, 1947), they are often remarkably untroubled by their mistakes.

Using scalp electrophysiological methods in normals, two research groups identified an event-related potential (ERP) that appears to index the recognition of erroneous responses (Falkenstein *et al.*, 1991; Gehring *et al.*, 1993). This ERP component, termed the *error negativity* (Ne) or the *error-related negativity* (ERN), has a negative distribution over mediofrontal scalp sites and it peaks approximately 100 msec after response onset (see Fig. 1). The scalp distribution of the ERN suggests a mediofrontal neural generator. Dehaene *et al.* (1994) source analyzed the ERN with dense-array electroencephalogram (EEG) data and found a generator that lies in the region of the ACC. This result has been corroborated in subsequent studies (Holroyd *et al.*, 1998; Luu *et al.*, 2000a; Miltner *et al.*, 1997) and is consistent with results of error-related activity recorded in the ACC in monkeys (Gemba *et al.*, 1986; Niki and Watanabe, 1979).

The ERN is seen after hand (Falkenstein *et al.*, 1991), feet (Holroyd *et al.*, 1998), vocal (Masaki *et al.*, 2001), and saccadic eye movement errors (Van't Ent and Apkarian, 1999), findings that are consistent with an output-independent system of action monitoring. The ERN was originally thought to index the activity of an error detection system that compared the actual response with an internal representation of the correct response (Falkenstein *et al.*, 1991; Gehring *et al.*, 1993; Scheffers *et al.*, 1996). According to this proposal, ERN amplitude should be largest when the error response is substantially different

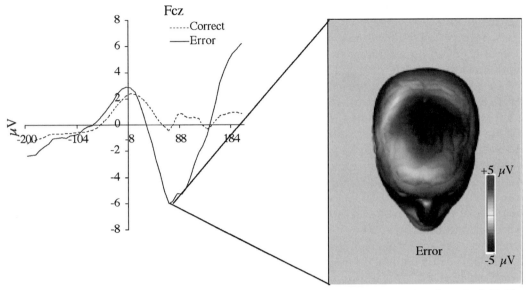

FIGURE 1 Response-locked ERP wave form for correct and error responses at the Fcz electrode (left). The scalp distribution of the ERN at its maximum is shown on the right.

from the correct response, and this was confirmed in a study by Bernstein *et al.* (1995). Although some have proposed that conscious awareness of having made an error is required for the manifestation of the ERN (Dehaene *et al.*, 1994; Luu *et al.*, 2000b), a study using an antisaccade test indicates that this may not be the case (Nieuwenhuis *et al.*, 2001). That is, the comparison of an error response with the expected response need not reach the level of awareness to elicit an ERN.

Recordings of error potentials in the ACC of the monkey support the error detection view of the ERN. Gemba *et al.* (1986) found that error-related potentials are not observed in the ACC prior to the animal evincing behavioral evidence that indicates that insight into the nature of the task (i.e., what constitutes a correct response) has been grasped. It should be noted that the ERN appears to be unrelated to other error-related processes, such as inhibiting or correcting the erroneous response. For example, the ERN still occurs in situations in which errors cannot be corrected, such as pushing a button when a

response is not required (Scheffers *et al.*, 1996) or when the response is erroneous by a speed criterion (Luu *et al.*, 2000b).

This error detection view of the ERN has been questioned because of several findings. First, mediofrontal negativities can be found after correct responses. The smaller negativity associated with correct responses has been labeled the correct-related negativity (CRN) by Ford (1999). Ford noted that the ERN and CRN differed in their topographic distribution, but this is in contrast to what was found by Vidal *et al.*(2000) and Luu *et al.* (2000b), who used dense-array EEGs to compare the scalp distribution of the CRN and ERN. Scheffers and Coles (2000) have found that the ERN can be observed after correct responses if subjects believe that a response is in error. This finding is consistent with an error detection view of the ERN and has been used by Coles *et al.* (2001) to explain why ERN-like negativities are observed after correct responses. Another hypothesis put forth is that the CRN reflects the monitoring process and that the ERN reflects an additional signal, in response to errors, that is overlaid on top of the CRN (Falkenstein *et al.*, 2000).

Second, it has been suggested that the ERN, rather than indexing the output of an error detection system, reflects the conflict-monitoring responses of the ACC (Carter *et al.*, 1998). According to this theory, errors are instances in which response conflict is high. The conflict-monitoring hypothesis is attractive in that it also explains ACC activity in a host of other tasks that require executive control. Using functional magnetic resonance imaging (fMRI) methods, Carter *et al.* found the ACC to be active for error responses and for correct responses that had high response competition demands. This proposal has stimulated a number of studies because it is clear and testable. Falkenstein *et al.* (2000) found the ERN amplitude to be of equivalent size for tasks that have strong response conflict and those that have no response conflict. Similarly, when responses are sorted according to degree of response conflict, as measured by activation of motor cortices, the ERN was largest for errors with the wrong response hand, which had little or no response conflict (Luu *et al.*, 2000b). In contrast, Gehring and Fencsik (2001) conducted a study in which they found errors that were similar to the correct response in terms of motor output produced larger ERN amplitudes than those that were dissimilar. They interpreted these findings to be consistent with the conflicting monitoring theory of the ACC. Other fMRI studies have found activity in the rostroventral ACC to be specific to errors and the dorsal ACC to be common to both errors and response conflict manipulation (Kiehl *et al.*, 2000; Menon *et al.*, 1997). Thus, ERN responses may be influenced by conflicting response demands in some experiments and not others, and there may be regional differentiation within the ACC in the conflict-monitoring function.

One intriguing property of the ERN is that it can be elicited by a feedback informing subjects of the accuracy of their response. In time-interval tasks, subjects are required to produce a response within a certain time interval. In these tasks, a correct response cannot immediately be determined because a correct response is not defined *a priori* by an internal representation of the action. Therefore, the ERN is not observed until a feedback is presented to the subject (Badgaiyan and Posner, 1998; Miltner *et al.*, 1997). This observation has proved difficult for the conflict-monitoring theory to reconcile, but it suggests interesting relations to affective reactions in response to errors (Tucker *et al.*, 1999). Tucker *et al.* observed that during the time window of the late-positive complex (LPC, approximately 472 msec) to targets, a medial prefrontal negativity differentiated between good and bad targets; bad targets elicited a larger negativity than did good targets. This "evaluative negativity" effect was found to be superposed over the topography of the LPC. The time course of this effect and its superposition with the LPC is very reminiscent of the stimulus-locked error-related negativity (Falkenstein *et al.*, 1991). Moreover, this effect was again observed when a feedback was presented to subjects informing them of their performance; a negative feedback elicited larger mediofrontal negativity than did a positive feedback. The results from this study suggest that the observed evaluative negativity is separable from the response because the effect was observed in response to the target and the feedback.

Luu *et al.* (2000a) proposed that evaluation of action occurs along the affective dimension of distress. These authors found that subjects who are high on the dimension of personality known as negative emotionality (Tellegen and Waller, 1996), which describes the tendency to experience subjective distress, should show exaggerated ERN responses because of their affective reactions to errors. Indeed, early in the experiment subjects with high negative emotionality subjects displayed larger

ERN amplitudes compared to subjects with low negative emotionality. Anxiety disorders, such as obsessive–compulsive disorder (OCD), are related to negative emotionality through the dimension of subjective distress. Gehring *et al.* (2000) found that ERN amplitudes were larger for OCD subjects in comparison to controls. Moreover, the ERN amplitude was correlated with symptom severity. In a similar study, Johannes *et al.* (2001b) confirmed these findings. In addition, these researchers found latency and topographic differences of the ERN for OCD subjects when compared to controls. At the low end of the distress dimension are those people who are not prone to feeling anxious. Dikman and Allen (2000) found that subjects who are low on a scale measuring sociability (which indicates low levels of anxiety) exhibited small ERN amplitudes when their error responses were punished. A more direct test of the relation between distress and ERN amplitude was demonstrated by Johannes *et al.* (2001a). These researchers administered oxazepam and found that the amplitude of the ERN was reduced in those subjects who received this anxiolytic drug compared to those subjects who received a placebo. This reduction of the ERN with an anxiolytic is thus consistent with increased ERNs in subjects high in negative affect (Luu *et al.*, 2000a).

Theta Dynamics and the ERN

Examining the morphology of the ERN wave form, researchers have noted that the ERN is often preceded and followed by other negative deflections. Taking this as a clue that the ERN is actually part of an ongoing oscillatory process, Luu and Tucker (2001) found that the ERN emerges as one component of a midline oscillation whose activity is at the theta frequency. Moreover, this midline theta oscillation was interposed with sensorimotor oscillations, which are also at the theta frequency. Figure 2 shows the series of events recorded in a typical (Eriksen flanker task) ERN paradigm (Luu and Tucker, 2001). At approximately 80 msec prior to the button press, there is a negative potential along the midline that occurs again after a response (at approximately 88 msec). When this negativity occurs after an erroneous button press, it is much larger compared to a correct button press and is recognized as the ERN. Prior to the button press (at approximately –32 msec), a negative potential is observed over the contralateral sensorimotor recording sites and it is observed again at approximately 136 msec after the button press. When an error is committed, the ERN becomes correlated with these sensorimotor potentials.

Applying independent components analysis (ICA) (Makeig *et al.*, 1997) to data from individual subjects, Makeig *et al.* (2002a) discovered that the ERN is actually composed of multiple independent components with maximal power at the theta frequency. The trial-by-trial phase resettings of the ongoing theta oscillation sum up to provide the averaged deflection recognized as the ERN. The independent components demonstrate interesting relations to the different events that occur in the task. Figure 3 shows the ERP of two independent vertex and frontal components scaled to microvolt

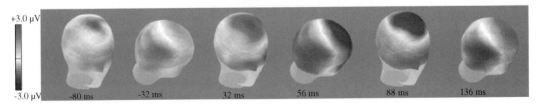

FIGURE 2 Voltage maps showing the oscillatory nature of the ERN and sensorimotor potentials. Time is relative to a button press, which is at 0 msec. (See color plates.)

levels at channel Fz, aligned with the button press (solid black line), and sorted according to response latency. The figure on the left shows that the vertex theta component is aligned to the target onset (first dashed line to the left of response onset) and peaks after the response deadline (first dashed line to the right of response onset). This postresponse deadline peak is larger for error than for correct responses. Additionally, after the feedback, this vertex theta component again shows a burst of activity in the theta range. The frontal theta component begins to show thetalike activity prior to the response and peaks just after the response, but it does not seem to show activity related to the target or feedback stimuli (see Fig. 3).

In another study, Luu et al. (2002) separated the feedback and response-locked components of the ERN by using a delayed-feedback paradigm. Prior to the presentation of a target stimulus, subjects received a feedback on their performance from five trials previous to the current trial. This was done to separate the response-control value of the feedback from the emotional value of the feedback as a performance indicator. The grand-averaged data were then analyzed using a theta source model derived from the work of Asada et al. (1999). Luu et al. found that the ERN was made up of two components, one component was located in the rostral ACC and the other was located in the dorsal ACC (see Fig. 4). The locations of these two sources are similar to regions reported, using fMRI methods, to be active when errors are committed (Kiehl et al., 2000; Menon et al., 2001). Luu et al. found the rostral ACC source to be locked to the response whereas the dorsal source was locked to the feedback (see Fig. 4). These results are similar to those obtained by Makeig et al. (2002a) using ICA, and they suggest there may be regional specializations within the ACC that could help explain several findings in the ERN literature.

First, these regional specializations could explain why an ERN can be observed in both stimulus-locked and response locked averages; the ventral region may be more response-locked and the dorsal

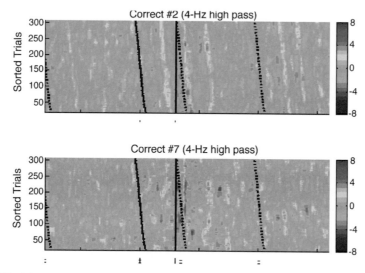

FIGURE 3 ERP of the vertex and frontal component scaled to microvolt levels at channel Fz. Left: Vertex theta component; right: frontal theta component. Plots of trials aligned to button press (solid black line). Each raster line represents a trial, and trials are sorted according to response latency. The data were filtered with a 4-Hz high pass. First dashed line to the left of the response marks target onset. First dashed line to the right of the button press marks response deadline, and second dashed line after button press marks feedback onset.

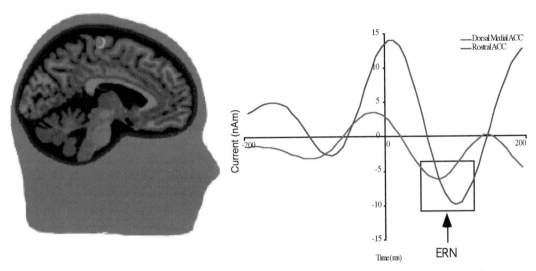

FIGURE 4   Left: Location of the generators of the ERN. Right: Source wave forms illustrating the relative contribution of each source to the scalp-recorded ERN. The box indicates the window of the ERN. (See color plates.)

region may contribute to both stimulus- and response-locked measures. Second, this evidence could explain why there are ERN and ERN-like deflections in response to a feedback stimulus when no overt motor responses are made; the more dorsal region of the ACC may provide not only response monitoring but also event monitoring generally. Third, this evidence could explain how current source density methods, which are sensitive to superficial sources, can identify a dorsal ACC (e.g., supplementary motor area or SMA) source of the ERN (Vidal *et al.*, 2000) when other ERN models have identified deep ACC sources (Dehaene *et al.*, 1994); there are indeed multiple sources, with different functional properties.

These functional properties of different ERN sources can be ascertained by considering their alignment with events in the experimental trials. In action monitoring, the execution and monitoring of the response can be separated from the monitoring of the context in which the action is executed (i.e., the context parameters that constrain the action). The source analysis study of Luu *et al.* (2002) and the ICA results reported by Makeig *et al.* (2002a)

suggest that the dorsal ACC (SMA region) monitors the context of the action (such as the target, response deadline, feedback value). In contrast, the rostroventral ACC monitors the response.

A similar differentiation may have been observed in positron emission tomography (PET) research on decision-making. Elliot and Dolan (1998) found that the dorsal ACC was active when subjects generated a hypothesis about what would constitute a correct response. In contrast, the ventral ACC was active when subjects made a choice. Elliot and Dolan proposed that the ventral ACC activation reflected emotional evaluation of the action. In action monitoring, both regions of the ACC must be functionally coupled, and it appears that this occurs through phase coupling at the theta frequency. Luu *et al.*, report that the ERN sources are at the theta frequency and are approximately 60° out of phase, which is similar to the phase relation of theta sources in the ACC reported in magnetoencephalography (MEG) research by Asada *et al.* (1999).

Thus both spatial and temporal resolution may be necessary in researching the mechanisms of self-regulation in medial frontal networks. Functional differentiation between nearby networks of the ACC is suggested by hemodynamic studies and by dense-array EEG studies. Temporal differentiation of the activity in these regions is suggested by the MEG and EEG evidence, and of course this is not apparent with hemodynamic measures. The findings of oscillatory activity contributing to the ERN and feedback-related responses may allow interpretation of the human findings in relation to the intriguing animal literature on theta dynamics that appear to coordinate learning and neural plasticity within multiple, functionally distinct corticolimbic networks. In the next section, we review models of self-regulation from neurophysiological studies that may help explain how human corticolimbic networks are integrated in motivated behavior. These neurophysiological models of learning and action regulation may provide new ways of thinking about a number of ERP measures in human research, including the no-go N2, the P3a, the P3b, and the ERN. Whereas these measures have conventionally been interpreted in a cognitive or mentalistic framework in relation to cognitive operations such as attention and memory, the neurophysiological evidence points to more elementary operations such as arousal, alerting, and orienting. By understanding how executive functions recruit subcortical as well as cortical systems, it may be possible to frame concepts of self-regulation in relation to fundamental control processes that evolved for learning and action regulation.

MECHANISMS OF ACTION REGULATION

Dopamine and Errors of Prediction

One influential model has followed from the remarkable specificity of responses in the dopamine pathway to violations of expectancy for reward cues (Schultz *et al.*, 1995, 1998). Although many researchers have assumed that dopamine projections are important to mediating responses to reward, Shultz and associates found that the dopamine response was more specific than a diffuse reward response. A property of the dopaminergic ventral tegmental area (VTA) cells is that their response can be transferred from a primary reward to a conditioned stimulus after learning. Moreover, after learning, if the expected reward is withheld, the VTA cells show a phasic depression relative to their base line activity. Such an "error signal" is particularly attractive for theoreticians interested in learning mechanisms because it is an integral component of artificial neural network models of learning, particularly those that require supervisory training to guide the learning process.

Integrating the Schultz evidence of dopamine coding of prediction errors with the human evidence of error-related negativities in the anterior cingulate cortex, Holroyd and Coles (2002) have recently proposed that the ERN reflects the transmission of an error signal from brain stem, dopaminergic cells to the ACC, and the ACC in turn uses this signal to select which motor program has access to the motor system. The Holroyd and Coles model is particularly important because it offers the opportunity to link the animal learning literature with the ACC findings in relation to human frontal lobe function, thus providing a model of the executive functions that arises not from a separate, homuncular agent, but from more intrinsic and elementary mechanisms of self-regulation.

Although the Schultz model has been highly influential in linking motivational processes to striatal and dopamine influences on action control, Redgrave *et al.* (1999) have questioned whether the response of the dopamine system may be too fast to integrate reward information with the response to prediction errors.

Rather, Redgrave *et al.* suggest that there is a more elementary role of the dopamine projections, to facilitate neostriatal behavioral switching operations in response to significant events. Others have also proposed a similar view of dopaminergic function (Spanagel and Weiss, 1999). Although the dopamine modulation is understood primarily in the neostriatum, this might be extended to dopamine targets in limbic cortex, such as the ACC. The finding that patients with Parkinson's disease exhibit smaller ERN amplitudes (Falkenstein *et al.*, 2001) is particularly relevant within this context. Gurney *et al.*, (2001) have argued that the circuits within the neostriatum may be differentiated, with certain neural populations specialized for behavioral switching functions and others for the control of those switching functions. This sort of mechanism would be well suited to motivational control of action selection.

Although the neostriatal and dopaminergic influences on the ACC are only begin-ning to be understood, they are providing important theoretical models for understanding the executive control of action. Because neostriatal loops to both limbic cortex and neocortex are closely coordinated with thalamolimbic circuits, a theoretical analysis of action regulation must extend to the limbic and thalamic mechanisms that are integral to memory formation and the control of learned behavior.

Adaptation and Context in the Papez Circuit

A novel and intriguing model of limbic and thalamic learning mechanisms has been developed by Gabriel and colleagues (Gabriel, 1990; Gabriel *et al.*, 1986, 2002). They have argued that the ACC is involved in associative attention, a conclusion based on a series of neurophysiological studies of avoidant and approach discriminant learning in rabbits. Unlike cognitive models of attention, the associative attention model of Gabriel and colleagues proposes that

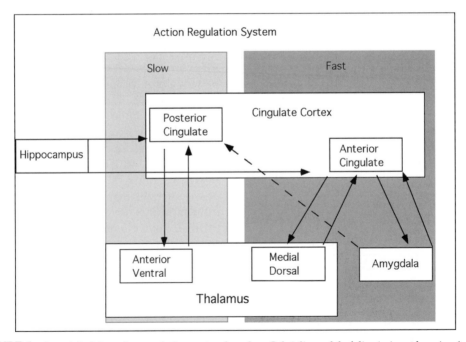

FIGURE 5   A model of the action regulation system based on Gabriel's model of discriminant learning (see text for details). The amygdala is presented in this model because it is critical to discriminant avoidance learning in the ACC and to a lesser extent in the PCC.

attention is a product of learning mechanisms. This model can thus account for at least certain attentional phenomena without recourse to an external control agent.

Gabriel *et al.* have considered the roles of both limbic and thalamic components of the Papez circuit in discrimination learning (see Fig. 5). The anterior and medial nuclei of the thalamus are central to discriminating between predictive stimuli and nonpredictive conditioned stimuli. These structures then contribute to the discriminant activity of unit responses in the cingulate cortex. The ACC is particularly important to the early stages of discrimination learning, when rapid encoding of novel reinforcement contingencies is critical to adaptive action. A key fact for understanding ventral as well as dorsal limbic inputs is that this rapid discriminative avoidant learning in the ACC is dependent on projections from the amygdala (Poremba and Gabriel, 1997). ACC cells are sufficiently responsive to the predictive value of cues such that they are able to compensate when the cues have low salience but are nonetheless predictive. Gabriel (1990) describes this as a salience compensation function.

In contrast to the ACC, the posterior cingulate cortex (PCC) is involved in later stages of discrimination learning. PCC cells are responsive to the novelty–familiarity dimension of the predictive conditioned stimulus. This suggested to Gabriel *et al.* (2002) that the PCC is involved in selecting action based on the environmental context, and that it does so with hippocampal input. The role of the hippocampal complex in action regulation is to compare inputs against an expected context for a certain action. In humans, neuroimaging studies have specifically identified hippocampal activation when expectations, particularly of an affective nature, are violated (Ploghaus *et al.*, 2000). Gabriel *et al.* reasoned that, in human cognitive studies, task-related instructions prepare the context for action, serving a purpose similar to that of reinforcement training in animal studies.

A Model of Action Regulation

In contrast to traditional Pavlovian models that attempted to explain learning in relation to associations linked to the reflex arc, modern concepts of learning emphasize the animal's prediction of behavioral outcomes (Rescorla, 1992; Schultz and Dickinson, 2000). The studies of Gabriel *et al.* suggest that the self-regulation of these predictions varies depending on the match of behavioral patterns to the current environmental context. When the environment remains stable, the hippocampus and PCC provide a regular and graded updating of the neural representation of the context, allowing actions to be determined by this representation. When more rapid changes are required, such as in emergency situations, the ACC provides a second and more rapidly adapting learning mechanism, drawing on input from the amygdala.

It may be possible to relate the Gabriel *et al.* model of limbic mechanisms with the Holroyd and Coles (2002) model of dopaminergic control by proposing that the ACC integrates striatal as well limbic circuits in its regulation of rapid adaptation. It is when the implicit prediction (i.e., the PCC context representation) is violated by unexpected events that both the ACC limbic circuit and the DA error signal are engaged. Until that point, action plans are context dependent, and very likely regulated by the ongoing hippocampal and PCC learning process. At the point that expectancies are violated, the ACC has the capacity for rapid alteration of behavior because of its unique connectivity with critical subcortical structures.

Whereas the cingulate gyrus as a whole is derived from archicortex, and thus has its predominant connectivity with the hippocampus and dorsal cortical pathways, the ACC is unique in integrating input from the amygdala, which is integral to the ventral limbic pathways (Tucker *et al.*, 2000). In addition, the ACC is closely connected with neostriatal circuits, and together with insular regions of ventral limbic cortex, receives substantial dopaminergic modulation. This pattern of connectivity may be important to both motor and motivational control. The capacity for effective switching of actions afforded by striatal circuits may be elaborated at the corticolimbic level by ACC networks, and may be extended to the role of the ACC in action selection under conditions of response conflict. The rapid emergency response to fight–flight conditions requires not only routinized action sequences but motivational control from the amygdala. In this way, the ACC integrates rapid adaptation and switching influences from striatal and ventral limbic circuits that act in opposition to the more gradual context-updating mode of self-regulation in hippocampal and posterior cingulate circuits.

Although these mechanisms of motivated action evolved as primitive mechanisms of action regulation, they seem to be important to more complex processes of human self-regulation as well. Although human executive processes may engage complex processes of reasoning, imagination, and emotional self-control that engage widespread regions of the cortex, the substantial evidence of the integral role of the ACC to these processes suggests that they may rest on a substrate of elementary mechanisms of action regulation. These mechanisms support learning which action is relevant in a given motivational context, monitoring the outcome of the action, and switching to a different set of actions when outcomes are violated.

Corticolimbic Integration and the Theta Rhythm

Through clarifying the elementary mechanisms of self-regulation in limbic,

thalamic, and striatal circuits, it may be possible to build a more accurate model of the functions of the cortex. Even the massive human cortex does not function in isolation, but requires regulatory influences from limbic cortex and diencephalic structures, such as in the process of memory consolidation (Squire, 1992). There are intriguing clues to the neurophysiological mechanisms through which limbic circuits exert regulatory control on cortical networks. A key mechanism appears to be interregional communication entrained by the theta rhythm. Given the observations above showing theta oscillations in the EEG measures of human self-monitoring and self-control, it may be useful to consider the neurophysiological mechanisms of theta modulation.

In rats, theta is observed as a rhythmic, slow activity recorded in the hippocampus under conditions in which the animal is exploring the environment (i.e., acquiring information). Cells within the hippocampal complex are easily activated at the theta frequency because they have intrinsic resonant properties tuned to this frequency (Bland and Oddie, 1998). During theta activity, most pyramidal cells are hyperpolarized (i.e., inhibited) and those that are active seem to be coding the currently relevant stimuli. This finding suggested to Buzáski (1996) that the theta rhythm may act to enhance the signal to noise ratio. Additionally, cells can be differentially active at different phases of theta, providing a mechanism for coding temporal patterns (Buzsáki, 1996; Lisman and Otmakhova, 2001). These properties suggested to Buzsáki that theta is the throughput mode of neuronal transmission, and this type of activity is centered on the input stages of the hippocampal circuit, such as the enthorinal complex and dentate gyrus. Buzsáki argues that this is the labile or temporary state of memory storage for rapidly incoming information. During the acquisition stages of discriminant learning, Gabriel and colleagues (1986) observed that cells in the hippocampus display bursting at the theta frequency. In contrast, Gabriel *et al* observed that during the inter-trial period hippocampal cells show brief bursts of activity. This appears similar to the consolidation stage of hippocampal function in which irregular sharp waves are prominent in the hippocampus (Buzsáki, 1989).

If the Papez circuit functions as an inte-grated system, in which the other struc-tures are critically dependent on information from the hippocampus, one would expect that a major mode of trans-mission of neural information to and from the hippocampus would be at the theta fre-quency. Indeed, this is the argument put forth by Miller (1991). A key finding is that bilateral lesions to the anterior nucleus of the thalamus or the cingulate gyrus reduce the duration of hippocampal theta induced by electrical stimulation. Similarly, stimu-lation to either the cingulate or the anterior thalamus induces theta activity in the ipsi-lateral hippocampus (Azzaroni and Parmeggiani, 1967). In humans, a possible parallel to the integrative role of theta in memory consolidation was suggested by the finding that coherence between differ-ent cortical regions was observed only at the theta frequency when subjects had to hold information in short-term memory (Sarnthein *et al.*, 1998).

Limbic Theta and Executive Control

In rats, hippocampal theta is seen when the animal is exploring its environment. However, in primates the most reliable method for eliciting hippocampal theta is withholding an expected reward (Crowne and Radcliffe, 1975). In humans, increased theta activity in the region of the ACC and temporal lobe is associated with increases in working memory demands (Gevins *et al.*, 1997; Raghavachari *et al.*, 2001; Slobounov *et al.*, 2000). A review by Kahana *et al.* (2001) concluded that the most parsimonious description regarding

the functional significance of theta across species is that it is related to cognitive control. More specifically, it may be that the theta rhythm reflects the control of information gathering by the hippocampal system (Buzsáki, 1996; Miller, 1991), which involves communication between multiple brain regions but particularly within the Papez circuit.

In the findings on human self-monitor-ing and attention reviewed above, we dis-cussed evidence that the ERN emerges from phase alignment of the EEG at the theta rhythm. There are also functional similarities between the ERN and theta that are important to a theory of action regulation. First, error activity in the ACC can also be induced by withholding an expected reward (Niki and Watanabe, 1979). This is similar to the condition for robustly eliciting theta in the primate hippocampus (Crowne and Radcliffe, 1975). Second, ACC error activity and hip-pocampal theta occur early in learning (Gemba *et al.*, 1986; Pickenhain and Klingberg, 1967). Once learning is well established, the error potential recorded in the primate ACC and the theta rhythm observed in the rodent hippocampus dis-appear.

MOTIVATIONAL CONTROL OF ACTION REGULATION

Phase Reset of the Theta Rhythm to Motivationally Significant Events

According to the Holroyd and Coles (2002) model of the ERN, when an error occurs dopaminergic activity is decreased, which results in a disinhibition of neurons in the ACC; the ERN is observed as a con-sequence of this disinhibition. As we have observed, however, the ERN seems to arise not as a discrete negative transient, but rather as phase shifting of mediofrontal sources that are modulated at the theta rhythm (Luu *et al.*, 2001). When an error is made, the phase of the theta rhythm is reset to the erroneous response. The question is how this phase is reset. One possibility is that the mechanism for the phase reset is the dopaminergic signal. This mechanism may occur whether the dopaminergic response carries information about reward error or whether it provides the signal to reallocate resources and switch actions, as argued by Redgrave et al. (1999). What is important is that the signal carries information about when important events occur, and this appears to be a function of dopaminergic cells that is not disputed.

Phase resetting of the theta rhythm has been observed for many years in response to a conditioned stimulus during learning trials. Adey (1967) found that, in the early stages of learning, when the animal was still trying to learn the association between the condition stimuli and reward, the theta rhythm was prominent and was phased-locked to the auditory cue. As the animal's performance indicated that it has learned the task, theta amplitude decreased, and this was due to either a loss of phase-locked activity or a modulation of the frequency. However, when the cue was reversed, theta activity reappeared and was phase-locked to the stimulus, again. Buzsáki et al. (1979) observed similar effects. When an animal has to remember whether the current stimulus is the same or different from a previous stimulus in order to determine which response to make Givens (1996) found that theta recorded in the dentate gyrus became phase-locked to the stimulus. However, when performing a much simpler, well-learned task of stimulus–response mapping, theta was not phase locked to the stimulus.

At least two studies have shown that the theta rhythm can be reset by stimulation of septohippocampal afferents. Buño et al. (1978) found that electrical stimulation of the fornix, septal nuclei, hypothalamus, and brain stem reticular formation produced an entrainment of the hippocampal theta rhythm to the stimulus. Interestingly,

the reset of the theta rhythm was not dependent on the theta phase at which the stimulus was delivered. That is, the stimulus can be delivered at any time during the theta phase and still induce a phase reset to the stimulus. These authors noted that in order for averaged, evoked responses to show rhythmic activity, the theta rhythm must be aligned at stimulus onset. Brazhnik et al. (1985) recorded the theta rhythm from the medial septum and found that stimulating the lateral septum resulted in a phase locking of the theta rhythm to the stimulus. According to Brazhnik et al., the resetting of the theta rhythm could be produced by either a temporary pause of cell activity, which lasts between 40 and 90 msec, or a cellular "burst" that is time-locked to the stimulus.

Lisman and Otmakhova (2001) proposed that there are essentially two theta states, with one engaged in learning and the other in recall. Under the recall state, the animal is constantly predicting the future based on past learning. Any violation of the prediction will be relevant to ongoing behavior and will trigger the transition to the theta-learning state. According to Lisman and Otmakhova, the transition between the recall and theta state is initiated by a dopaminergic signal. However, the evidence for dual theta states (i.e., two theta pacemakers) is inconclusive (Miller, 1991). What we have proposed above for the dopaminergic function in action regulation may be similar to the model put forth by Lisman and Otmakhova. However, instead of switching theta states, we propose that the dopaminergic response provides the marker that allows for the theta phase to be reset to the relevant event (such as an error response). Input from multiple sources may be funneled to the ventral tegmental area to elicit this reset effect, such as from the brain stem reticular formation (Brazhnik et al., 1985; Buño et al., 1978).

The observation that long-term potentiation depends on the theta phase (Buzsáki,

1996) may suggest that limbic theta facilitates the coordination of synaptic modification across multiple networks of the Papez circuit. If so, then resetting the phase of the theta rhythm, such as through error or switching signals under dopaminergic or striatal control, may coordinate the response of multiple networks to important events.

Although we have considered the possibility that dopaminergic activity may contribute to phase-resetting of the theta rhythm, the exact locus of action remains to be clarified. One candidate is the medial septum–diagonal band complex. Cells from the VTA and substantia nigra have been shown to project to cholinergic cells of the medial septum–diagonal band complex (Gaykema and Zaborszky, 1996), which is believed to be the pacemaker of the theta rhythm. Miura *et al.* (1987) injected dopamine into the medial septum and found an increase in hippocampal theta activity. Therefore, it is possible that during an error response, a decrease of dopaminergic input into the medial septum or diagonal band results in a pause (or reduction) in cholinergic activity. This pause results in a phase resetting of the theta rhythm to the error event. Interestingly, this mechanism would involve a dopamine influence at the basal forebrain rather than in the ACC. It is entirely possible, however, that phase resetting can be initiated intrinsically within the circuit, such as by the ACC. We suspect that signals from multiple brain regions may also be able to reset the phase of the theta rhythm based on error information. Shultz and Dickinson (2000) reviewed evidence that multiple regions, including the noradrenergic cells of the locus coeruleus and the cerebellum, have been shown to be responsive to errors. Moreover, human neuroimaging studies have found the insula and frontal operculum to be sensitive to errors (Menon *et al.*, 2001).

Modulating the Amplitude of the Theta Rhythm

The hippocampal theta rhythm can be altered by opiate activity. Cells in the medial septum are especially responsive to noxious stimulation, whether mechanical or thermal (Dutar *et al.*, 1985). The receptive fields of these cells are broad, a characteristic feature of cells found in the medial pain system that encode affective significance of painful stimuli (Vogt *et al.*, 1993b). The pain-responsive cells of the medial septum project to the hippocampus to produce changes in the activity of pyramidal neurons. Lesions of the medial septum, or administration of a cholinergic antagonist, abolish this pain-induced effect (Khanna, 1997).

In the hippocampus, painful stimuli produce a depression of the population spikes with a concomitant increase in theta activity (Khanna, 1997). This effect appears to result specifically from medial septal projections, which act on the γ-aminobutyric acid (GABA)ergic hippocampal interneurons. The GABAergic interneurons inhibit most of the pyramidal cells, resulting in broad suppression of population spikes accompanied by increases in theta activity. In the midst of this inhibitory influence, the activity of a small population of pyramidal neurons is enhanced, giving rise to a signal-to-noise increase that may facilitate specific processes of associative learning.

An early study by Vanderwolf *et al.* (1978) showed that, in researching the effects of multiple neuromodulators, only opiates were effective at attenuating hippocampal theta activity [but see results by Miura *et al.* (1987)]. Khanna and colleagues (Khanna, 1997; Khanna and Zheng, 1998; Zheng and Khanna, 1999) showed that intraperitoneal injections of opiates attenuate the hippocampal nociceptive response (i.e., the characteristic population suppression and increase in theta activity in response to a painful

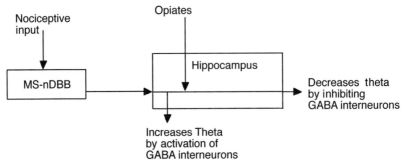

FIGURE 6 A model of nociceptive influence on the functioning of the hippocampus based on the work of Khanna (1997, 1998) (see text for details). Nociceptive input activates cells in the medial septum, which then project to the hippocampus. If the input is not moderated by the opiates, the net effect in the hippocampus is a suppression of pyramidal cells by GABAergic interneurons and an increase in theta activity. If the input is moderated by the opiates, this hippocampal nociceptive response is attenuated. MS-nDBB, Medial septum and nucleus of the diagonal band of Broca.

stimulus). Furthermore, this effect was naloxone reversible. The opiates appear to reduce the hippocampal nociceptive either by inhibiting the GABAergic hippocampal interneurons (Zieglagänsberger *et al.*, 1979) or by inhibiting the function of the medial septum (see Fig. 6).

Affective Modulation of Action Regulation

The findings on pain and opiate modulation of limbic mechanisms provide further perspective on the neural framework for learning and self-regulation. From an information-processing perspective, pain is a signal that tells the organism something is amiss in the environment, such that information must be acquired to determine what is wrong and what action is required. This signal demands that attention, and the associated limbic, striatal, and thalamic mechanisms, be engaged quickly and effectively. The evidence of opiate modulation of the theta rhythm suggests how the organism's motivational context frames the multiple processes of action regulation. We think this neurophysiological evidence is consistent with the proposal that the ongoing evaluation of action, as indexed by the ERN, reflects the individual's subjective distress, which is in turn regulated by opiate activity

(Luu *et al.*, 2000a). Furthermore, individual differences in opiate modulation and subjective distress may help explain why ERN amplitude varies as a function of anxiety (Dikman and Allen, 2000; Gehring *et al.*, 2000; Johannes *et al.*, 2001a,b). Further research on individual differences in the mechanisms of action regulation may help explain why individuals who have low levels of anxiety, such as psychopaths, are unconcerned about their errors and do not learn from their mistakes.

In summary, it appears that the ERN reflects at least two mechanisms. One is an immediate signal for action change. The other is a more general motivational state of the organism. First, the ERN arises from limbic theta that has been phase-reset by the process of response monitoring and detection of a prediction discrepancy. This discrepancy could be created by error detection, or conflict detection, but may reflect a more elementary mechanism than would be supposed by attributing the monitoring process to a higher executive function. One candidate for the phase-resetting mechanism would be mesencephalic dopaminergic projections, and their locus of action could be in the forebrain cholinergic nuclei (targeting the septohippocampal pacemaker directly) or in the ACC (targeting the cortical control of limbic output to the motor system), or both. In essence, phase resetting of the theta rhythm prepares the action regulation system for processing of significant events.

Second, the ERN and related medial frontal responses reflect the individual's current motivational state. This motivational state is a system-wide function, with multiple influences, a critical one of which is the current level of opiate modulation. The opiate activity moderates the signal-to-noise function of the theta rhythm. If the rhythm is not attenuated by the opiates, the signal-to-noise ratio is high. This may reflect the state in which the animal "cares" enough to react adaptively and learn. If the signal-to-noise ratio is reduced because of a high level of opiate modulation, it may reflect the situation in which the animal does not "care" and the signal has little effect on action and learning.

ELECTROPHYSIOLOGICAL SIGNS OF HUMAN EXECUTIVE CONTROL

Although we can assemble only a sketchy outline of self-regulatory mechanisms at this point, we propose that a more complete model of the neural mechanisms of motivated self-regulation will eventually explain a number of ERP phenomena that are known to be integral to cognitive processing, but that cannot be understood within current theory. In the following section, we will review evidence that several key ERP components can be understood to arise from the modulation of limbic theta activity, and that these components may provide key insights into the frontolimbic mechanisms of action regulation.

Electrophysiology of Action Regulation

A negative deflection over frontal sites is observed approximately 250–350 msec after a no-go stimulus in a go/no-go para-digm (Jodo and Kayama, 1992). In this paradigm, subjects either make or withhold a response according to stimulus properties. This negative deflection is referred to as the no-go N2. It has a mediofrontal distribution and has been shown by dense-array EEG recordings to be generated by a source in the anterior cingulate cortex (Bokura, et al., 2001). The N2 has been proposed to reflect response inhibitory processes (Jackson et al., 1999; Jodo and Kayama, 1992; Kopp et al., 1996b).

Kopp et al. (1996a) have proposed that in addition to appearing over frontal sites, the N2 and ERN are also similar in wave form morphology and latency. Therefore, they conclude that the N2 and ERN may reflect the same underlying process: motor inhibition. However, Falkenstein et al. (1999) found that whereas the latency and amplitude of N2 varied as a function of stimulus modality, the ERN amplitude did not. Therefore, these authors concluded that the N2 and ERN do not reflect the activity of a common inhibition mechanism. Bokura and colleagues (2001) do not believe that the N2, as reflected in the ACC activity, is involved in response inhibition. Rather, they propose that it is related more generally to the monitoring of behavior that requires control, i.e., nonroutinized behavior.

As a result of their findings, Falkenstein et al. (1999) proposed that the N2 might reflect stimulus-locked processes whereas the ERN might index response-locked processes. Luu et al. (2002) have observed N2-like (in terms of morphology, topography, and latency) ERP deflections for feedback stimuli indicating that neither a response had to be withheld nor that the response was in error. The source analysis result reported by Luu et al. is particularly interesting in light of the suggestion by Falkenstein et al. that the N2 reflects stimulus-locked activity. In the Luu et al. (2002) analysis, the N2-like deflection arose from phase locking of dorsal ACC activity to the stimulus. In contrast, the ERN was found to arise primarily from phase locking of rostral ACC activity to the response (with a lesser contribution from the source in dorsal ACC). Although no previous report has noted the frequency characteristic of the N2, the Luu *et al.* findings suggest that it may be at the theta frequency; this suggestion would be consistent with the finding that theta increases in response to a no-go stimulus in a go/no-go paradigm (Miller, 1991).

Novelty and Distraction

Another ERP component that appears to index aspects of executive control is the P3a. The P3a is a positive deflection in the EEG that has a frontocentral distribution and peaks approximately 250–350 msec after novel stimulus onset. Traditionally, the P3a is elicited using paradigms in which a distractor (or novel stimulus) is presented within a stream of target and nontarget stimuli. It has been proposed to be an index of a multimodal, corticolimbic orienting system that is responsive to novel events (Knight and Scabini, 1998). However, work by Polich and colleagues (Katayama and Polich, 1998; Polich, 2002) has shown that the critical parameter for the elicitation of the P3a may not be stimulus novelty per se. Rather, these researchers find that the experimental context appears to be the important parameter. When the discrimination between target and nontargets was difficult, a distractor stimulus that was strongly deviant from the target and nontarget stimuli elicited a large P3a. Katayama and Polich interpreted this as demonstrating that the context sets up the attentional requirements that must be redirected, by the frontal lobe (e.g., executive processes), to the distractor.

Although Katayama and Polich (Katayama and Polich, 1998) showed that novelty is not the only determinant of the P3a response, novelty is still relevant to many of the findings with this component. Demiralp *et al.* (2001) demonstrated that both typical and novel distractors presented within a target/nontarget stream of stimuli elicited P3a responses with similar topographies. However, applying wavelet analysis to the P3a, these researchers found a significant power increase at the theta frequency for the novel but not the typical distractors. Similar to the findings that the ERN is part of an ongoing theta process, the results obtained by Demiralp *et al.* may suggest that the P3a is composed of multiple frequencies (mainly delta and theta bands) of ongoing EEG rhythms. An important question for further research is whether the P3a, like the ERN, arises from phase resetting of limbic theta rhythms, similar to the finding for other averaged event-related potential components (Makeig *et al.*, 2002b).

The neural substrate of the P3a is believed to include multiple cortical and subcortical structures (Knight and Scabini, 1998; Polich, 2002). Of particular relevance are findings that implicate the frontal lobe (ACC) and hippocampus in the generation of the P3a (Ebmeier *et al.*, 1995; Knight, 1984, 1996). Based on its functional characteristics and the underlying neural generators, we propose that the P3a may be another index of the ACC response in the rapid encoding of significant and discrepant signals (Gabriel *et al.*, 2002). Thus, whereas the posterior cingulate regularly updates its representation of the context (with a P3b-like response), the more rapid alteration by the ACC appears to signal a switching mechanism, in response to predictive control violations, possibly mediated by dopamine projections.

Of course, although they share a medial frontal distribution, the P3a reflects a positive-going potential in the stimulus-locked averaged data, whereas the ERN reflects a negative-going potential in the response-locked averaged data. Could their different polarities reflect phase resetting at different phases of the theta wave? Considering the long-term potentiation findings in the hippocampus, could these opposite polarities reflect functional mechanisms such as potentiation and depotentiation of synaptic connections? Perhaps the enhancement of P3a to distractors with increased attention to the foreground task (Katayama and Polich, 1998) could reflect dopaminergic control of the ACC that inhibits the switching, i.e., that avoids the distraction. In other words, dopaminergic activity preserves the current context at the expense of ignoring potentially important stimuli. Such an action could be consistent with the "winner take all" mechanisms of switching described for dopaminergic modulation of neostriatal circuits (Redgrave *et al.*, 1999): if it is not selected, the distractor stimulus does not receive consolidation within working memory that can be provided by mechanisms of limbic theta (Buzsáki, 1996).

There is an opposite interpretation that is consistent with what is known about the theta rhythm. Gabriel *et al.* (2002) find cells in the cingulate cortex that respond with greater activity to condition stimuli (those that predict the presence or absence of a reinforcer) that are of short duration when compared to those that are of long duration. They proposed that the cingulate cortex participates in a process of *salience compensation* that allows for non-salient, yet associatively significant, stimuli to receive processing. These cells do not index stimulus duration because they increase their firing during the stimulus and not after stimulus offset. Rather, these cells may be prepared to process low-salient stimuli based on context information provided by hippocampal input (Gabriel and Taylor, 1998). Of particular importance is the observation that prior to enhanced firing these cells show a brief pause (40–80 msec) in their activity after presentation of the low-salience stimuli. Gabriel and Taylor proposed that this pause is a resetting mechanism that allows for the recruitment of neurons that would otherwise not have been available for the processing of the low-salience stimulus. The pause of

these neurons is reminiscent of the pause function identified by Brazhnik *et al.* (1985) for phase resetting of the theta rhythm. As noted previously, these researchers demonstrated that one mechanism of theta phase resetting is a 40- to 90-msec pause in neuronal activity after an electrical stimulus delivery.

The observations on rabbit learning and theta phase reset may provide insight into the human electrophysiological responses described by Katayama and Polich. Because of the effort required to distinguish between targets and standards when the differentiating feature is small, incoming distractors are not as salient. The P3a may reflect for humans a compensation process for the distractors that is similar to what is described by Gabriel *et al.* as salience compensation in their study of rabbits. In essence, the novel distractors produce a phase resetting of the ACC–hippocampal theta rhythm. Functionally, the effect is that the context is overcome by a phase reset of the theta rhythm to the distractor. Like phase resetting of the theta rhythm that gives rise to the ERN, phase resetting that gives rise to the P3a may be initiated by multiple sources, which may include dopaminergic and noradrenergic cell groups or other cortical structures.

Context Updating

Although much of the interesting evidence seems to focus on the rapid mechanisms of self-regulation in the ACC, it is also important to consider the more gradual representation of the context in the PCC and associated posterior brain networks. The P3b may provide an index to modification of this representation in human studies. The P3b component is an amodal response to voluntary detection of an infrequent target within a stream of frequent nontargets. Compared to the P3a, the P3b has a longer latency and a distribution over parietal rather than frontocentral recording sites. However, like the P3a, the P3b is not a unitary phenomenon. Rather, it reflects activity from multiple sources and contains EEG power in both delta and theta frequencies. Reviews by Polich (2002) and Knight and Scabini (1998) summarize the evidence on the neural generators of the P3b. The most consistent finding is that bilateral temporoparietal cortices are major contributors to the scalp-recorded P3b (e.g., see Ebmeier et al., 1995; Menon et al., 1997). In the frequency domain, Demiralp et al. (2001) showed with wavelet analysis that the P3b component also has contribution from the delta and theta frequencies. Similar frequency findings for the P3b have been found by others using different methods (Basar, 1998; Basar-Eroglu et al., 1992; Spencer and Polich, 1999).

The most influential theory of the P3b is that it reflects context updating processes that are engaged when an internal model of the context for action must be revised (Donchin and Coles, 1988). For Donchin and Coles, the P3b reflects strategic processes that are involved in planning action rather than immediate "tactical" processes that are concerned with immediate response control. Knight and Scabini (1998) speculated that the P3b might index the transfer of information from cortical structures, such as the temporoparietal junction, to limbic regions, such as the hippocampus, for memory updating. These proposals could align the functional significance of the P3b with the PCC–hippocampal action regulation system that is involved in context-sensitive, late-stage learning (Gabriel et al., 2002).

CONCLUSION: ELECTROPHYSIOLOGICAL CLUES TO EXECUTIVE CONTROL

Research on the error-related negativity component has provided one of the closest links between data obtained from animal experiments and electrophysiological and hemodynamic data obtained from human studies. The PET and fMRI findings of ACC activity in tasks requiring motivation, attention, and self-control have emphasized the importance of the limbic base of the frontal lobe for the human executive functions. The ERN findings not only provide temporal resolution to sharpen the psychological analysis of self-regulatory operations, but their dynamic nature also provides important clues to system-wide functions, including multiple subcortical circuits, each with unique neurophysiological properties. Because the ERN appears to arise from ongoing limbic theta activity, and because the theta rhythm reflects the functional activity of closely integrated networks of the limbic system, Luu et al. (2002) proposed that the ERN indexes not just the activity of the ACC, but the function of the rapid-learning system identified by Gabriel et al. (2002). Among the critical inputs to the ACC, the hippocampus and posterior cingulate are essential to the self-regulatory process, but the ventral limbic structures, including the amygdala, temporal pole, and caudal orbital frontal cortex, appear to be particularly important to fast adaptation. Similarly, we propose that the N2, P3a, and P3b reflect system-wide activity involving an entire network that is coordinated by theta activity.

From this perspective, functional interpretations become more complicated but perhaps more realistic. Not only is it important to consider the properties of each brain region or site, but also the functional operation of large-scale networks. To understand such an operation, one must understand how the network is coordinated and how this coordination can be measured. With these factors in mind, it becomes difficult to develop an adequate theory based on measuring activity in one subunit of the network (e.g., the ACC), even though important clues to the coordination of the wider network (e.g., corticolimbic and corticothalamic, and corticostriatal systems) are clearly gained by measuring activity in the particular subunit. It must be recognized that activity in any subunit can be modulated through influences with multiple entry points into the system-wide network.

Because no part of the network can be understood in isolation, the complexity of the neurophysiology of mammalian self-regulation thus poses a formidable theoretical challenge. Nonetheless, a theory of self-regulation built from neurophysiological mechanisms could provide unique insights not available to mentalistic theories that begin with constructs of cognitive processes and attempt to localize them in the brain. We propose that, when considered within the framework of integrated cortical and subcortical systems, executive control can be seen to arise out of primitive processes of action regulation (Gabriel *et al.*, 2002). Furthermore, these processes may provide unique insights into electrophysiological signs, including the N2, P3a, and P3b, that have proved difficult to map onto operations of a cognitive theory, such as attention and memory, because they seem to point to more elementary processes of orienting, alerting, and arousal. From the perspective of neurophysiology, it is just these elementary mechanisms that are required to explain how an organism self-regulates behavior. Considered in this way, and analyzed with modern methods providing both temporal and spatial resolution, human scalp electrophysiological measures may provide important clues to how the brain adapts behavior to a rapidly changing environment, while maintaining a context reflecting both past experience and the current motivational state.

Acknowledgments

This work was supported by National Institues of Mental Health grants MH42129 and MH42669 and an Augmented Cognition project grant funded by DARPA to Don M. Tucker.

References

Adey, W. R. (1967). Intrinsic organization of cerebral tissue in alerting, orienting, and discriminative responses. *In* (G. C. Quarton and T. Melnechuck and F. O. Schmitt, eds.), pp. 615–633. "The Neurosciences" Rockefeller University Press, New York.

Allman, J. M., Hakeem, A., Erwin, J. M., Nimchinsky, E., and Hof, P. (2001). The anterior cingulate cortex: The evolution of an interface between emotion and cognition. *Ann. N.Y. Acad. Sci.* **935**, 107–117.

Asada, H., Fukuda, Y., Tsunoda, S., Yamaguchi, M., and Tonoike, M. (1999). Frontal midline theta rhythms reflect alternative activation of prefrontal cortex and anterior cingulate cortex in humans. *Neurosci. Lett.* **274**, 29–32.

Azzaroni, A., and Parmeggiani, P. L. (1967). Feedback regulation of the hippocampal theta-rhythm. *Helv. Physiol Pharmacol. Acta* **25**, 309–321.

Badgaiyan, R. D., and Posner, M. I. (1998). Mapping the cingulate cortex in response selection and monitoring. *Neuroimage* **7**, 255–260.

Barris, R. W., and Schuman, H. R. (1953). Bilateral anterior cingulate gyrus lesions. *Neurology* **3**, 44–52.

Basar, E. (1998). "Brain Function and Oscillations." Springer, Berlin.

Basar-Eroglu, C., Basar, E., Demiralp, T., and Schürmann, M. (1992). P300-response: Possible psychophysiological correlations in delta and theta frequency channels. A review. *Int. J. Psychophysiol.* **13**, 161–179.

Bernstein, P. S., Scheffers, M. K., and Coles, G. H. (1995). "Where did I go wrong?" A psychophysiological analysis of error detection. *J. Exp. Psychol.* **21**, 1312–1322.

Bland, B. H., and Oddie, S. D. (1998). Anatomical, electrophysiological and pharmacological studies of ascending brain stem hippocampal synchronizing pathways. *Neurosci. Biobehav. Rev.* **22**, 259–273.

Bokura, H., Yamaguchi, S., and Kobayashi, S. (2001). Electrophysiological correlates for response inhibition in a Go/NoGo task. *Clin. Neurophysiol.* **112**, 2224–2232.

Brazhnik, E. S., Vinogradova, O. S., and Karanov, A. M. (1985). Frequency modulation of neuronal theta-bursts in rabbit's septum by low-frequency repetitive stimulation of the afferent pathways. *Neurosci.* **14**, 501–508.

Buño, W. J., Garcia-Sanchez, J. L., and Garcia-Austt, E. (1978). Reset of hippocampal rhythmical activities by afferent stimulation. *Brain Res. Bull.* **3**, 21–28.

Bush, G., Luu, P., and Posner, M. I. (2000). Cognitive and emotional influences in anterior cingulate cortex. *Trends Cogn. Sci.* **4**, 215–222.

Buzsáki, G. (1989). Two-stage model of memory trace formation: A role for "noisy" brain states. *Neurosci.* **31**, 551–570.

Buzsáki, G. (1996). The hippocampal–neocortical dialogue. *Cereb. Cortex* **6**, 81–92.

Buzsáki, G., Grastyán, E., Tveritskaya, I. N., and Czopf, J. (1979). Hippocampal evoked potentials and EEG changes during classical conditioning in the rat. *Electrocencephalogr. Clin. Neurophysiol.* **47**, 64–74.

Carter, C. S., Braver, T. S., Barch, D. M., Botvinick, M. M., Noll, D., and Cohen, J. D. (1998). Anterior cingulate cortex, error detection, and the online monitoring of performance. *Science* **280**, 747–749.

Carter, C. S., Botvinick, M. M., and Cohen, J. D. (1999). The contribution of the anterior cingulate cortex to executive processes in cognition. *Rev. Neurosci.* **10**, 49–57.

Coles, M. G. H., Scheffers, M. K., and Holroyd, C. B. (2001). Why is there an ERN/Ne on correct trials? Response representations, stimulus-related components, and the theory of error-processing. *Biol. Psychol.* **56**, 173–189.

Crowne, D. P., and Radcliffe, D. D. (1975). Some characteristics and functional relations of the electrical activity of the primate hippocampus and a hypothesis of hippocampal function. *In* "The Hippocampus: Neurophysiology and Behavior" (R. L. Isaacson and K. H. Pribram, eds.), Vol. 2, pp. 185–206. Plenum, New York.

Damasio, A. R., Tranel, D., and Damasio, H. (1990). Individuals with sociopathic behavior caused by frontal damage fail to respond autonomically to social stimuli. *Behav. Brain Res.* **41**, 81–94.

Dehaene, S., Posner, M. I., and Tucker, D. M. (1994). Localization of a neural system for error detection and compensation. *Psychol. Science,* **5**, 303–305.

Demiralp, T., Ademoglu, A., Comerchero, M., and Polich, J. (2001). Wavelet analysis of P3a and P3b. *Brain Topog.* **13**, 251–267.

Devinsky, O., Morrell, M. J., and Vogt, B. A. (1995). Contributions of anterior cingulate cortex to behavior. *Brain* **118**, 279–306.

Dikman, Z. V., and Allen, J. J. B. (2000). Error monitoring during reward and avoidance learning in high and low-socialized individuals. *Psychophysiology* **37**, 43–54.

Donchin, E., and Coles, M. G. H. (1988). Is the P300 component a manifestation of context updating? *Behav. Brain Sci.* **11**, 357–374.

Dutar, P., Lamour, Y., and Jobert, A. (1985). Activation of identified septo-hippocampal neurons by noxious peripheral stimulation. *Brain Res.* **328**, 15–21.

Ebmeier, K. P., Steele, J. D., MacKenzie, D. M., O'Carroll, R. E., Kydd, R. R., Glabus, M. F., Blackwood, D. H. R., Rugg, M. D., and Goodwin, G. M. (1995). Cognitive brain potentials and regional cerebral blood flow equivalents during two- and three-sound auditory "oddball tasks." *Electroencephalogr. Clin. Neurophysiol.* **95**, 434–443.

Elliot, R., and Dolan, R. J. (1998). Activation of different anterior cingulate foci in association with hypothesis testing and response selection. *Neuroimage* **8**, 17–29.

Eslinger, P. J., and Damasio, A. R. (1985). Severe disturbance of higher cognition after bilateral frontal lobe ablation. *Neurology* **35**, 1731–1741.

Falkenstein, M., Hohnsbein, J., Hoormann, J., and Blanke, L. (1991). Effects of crossmodal divided attention on late ERP components. II. Error processing in choice reaction tasks. *Electroencephalogr. Clin. Neurophysiol.* **78**, 447–455.

Falkenstein, M., Hoorman, J., and Hohnsbein, J. (1999). ERP components in Go/Nogo tasks and their relation to inhibition. *Acta Psychol.* **101**, 267–291.

Falkenstein, M., Hoorman, J., Christ, S., and Hohnbein, J. (2000). ERP components on reaction errors and their functional significance: A tutorial. *Biol. Psychol.* **51**, 87–107.

Falkenstein, M., Hielscher, H., Dziobek, I., Schwarzenau, P., Hoormann, J., Sundermann, B., and Hohnsbein, J. (2001). Action monitoring, error detection, and the basal ganglia: An ERP study. *Neuroreport* **12**, 157–161.

Ford, J. M. (1999). Schizophrenia: The broken P300 and beyond. *Psychophysiology* **36**, 667–682.

Gabriel, M. (1990). Functions of anterior and posterior cingulate cortex during avoidance learning in rabbits. *Prog. Brain Res.* **85**, 467–483.

Gabriel, M., Sparenborg, S. P., and Stolar, N. (1986). An executive function of the hippocampus: Pathway selection for thalamic neuronal significance code. *In* "The Hippocampus" (R. L. Isaacson and K. H. Pribram, eds.), pp. 1–39. Plenum, New York.

Gabriel, M., and Taylor, C. (1998). Prenatal exposure to cocaine impairs neuronal coding of attention and discriminative learning. *Ann. N.Y. Acad. Sci.* **846**, 194–212.

Gabriel, M., Burhans, L., and Scalf, P. (2002). Cingulate cortex. *In* "Encyclopedia of the Human Brain" (V. S. Ramachandran, ed.), Academic Press, New York. (In press.)

Gaykema, R. P., and Zaborszky, L. (1996). Direct catecolaminergic-cholinergic interactions in the basal forebrain. II. Substantia nigra-ventral tegmental area projections. *J. Compar. Neurol.* **374**, 555–577.

Gehring, W. J., and Fensik, D. E. (2001). Functions of the medial cortex in the processing of conflict and errors. *J. Neurosci.* **21**, 9430–9437.

Gehring, W. J., Goss, B., Coles, M. G. H., Meyer, D. E., and Donchin, E. (1993). A neural system for error detection and compensation. *Psychol. Sci.* **4**, 385–390.

Gehring, W. J., Himle, J., and Nisenson, L. G. (2000). Action monitoring dysfunction in obsessive–compulsive disorder. *Psychol. Sci.* **11**, 1–6.

Gemba, H., Sasaki, K., and Brooks, V. B. (1986). "Error" potentials in limbic cortex (anterior cingulate area 24) of monkeys during motor learning. *Neurosci. Lett.* **70**, 223–227.

George, M. S., Ketter, P. I., Rosinsky, N., Ring, H., Casey, B. J., Trimble, M. R., Horwitz, B., Herscovitch, P., and Post, R. M. (1994). Regional brain activity when selecting a response despite interference: An $H_2^{15}O$ Pet study of the stroop and emotional stroop. *Hum. Brain Mapping* **1**, 194–209.

Gevins, A., Smith, M. E., McEvoy, L., and Yu, D. (1997). High-resolution EEG mapping of cortical activation related to working memory: Effects of task difficulty, type of processing, and practice. *Cereb. Cortex* **7**, 374–385.

Givens, B. (1996). Stimulus-evoke resetting of the dentate theta rhythm: Relation to working memory. *NeuroReport* **8**, 159–163.

Gurney, K., Prescott, T. J., and Redgrave, P. (2001). A computational model of action selection in the basal ganglia. I. A new functional anatomy. *Biol. Cybern.* **84**(6), 401–410.

Holroyd, C., and Coles, M. G. H. (2002). The basis of human error processing: Reinforcement learning, dopamine, and the error-related negativity. *Psychol. Rev.*

Holroyd, C. B., Dien, J., and Coles, M. G. H. (1998). Error-related scalp potentials elicited by hand and foot movements: Evidence for an output-independent error-processing system in humans. *Neurosci. Lett.* **242**, 65–68.

Jackson, S. R., Jackson, G. M., and Roberts, M. (1999). The selection and suppression of action: ERP correlates of executive control in humans. *NeuroReport* **10**, 861–865.

Jodo, E., and Kayama, Y. (1992). Relation of a negative ERP component to response inhibition in a Go/No-go task. *Electroencephalogr. Clin. Neurophysiol.* **82**, 477–482.

Johannes, S., Wieringa, B. M., Nager, W., Dengler, R., and Münte, T. F. (2001a). Oxazepam alters action monitoring. *Psychopharmacology* **155**, 100–106.

Johannes, S., Wieringa, B. M., Nager, W., Rada, D., Dengler, R., Emrich, H. M., Münte, T. F., and Dietrich, D. E. (2001b). Discrepant target detection and action monitoring in obsessive–compulsive disorder. *Psychiatr. Res.* **108**, 101–110.

Kahana, M. J., Seelig, D., and Madsen, J. R. (2001). Theta returns. *Curr. Opin. Neurobiol.* **11**, 739–744.

Katayama, J., and Polich, J. (1998). Stimulus context determines P3a and P3b. *Psychophysiology* **35**, 23–33.

Khanna, S. (1997). Dorsal hippocampus field CA1 pyramidal cell responses to a persistent versus an acute nociceptive stimulus and their septal modulation. *Neurosci.* **77**, 713–721.

Khanna, S., and Zheng, F. (1998). Morphine reversed formalin-induced CA1 pyramidal cell suppression via an effect on septohippocampal neural processing. *Neurosci.* **89**, 61–71.

Kiehl, K. A., Liddle, P. F., and Hopfinger, J. B. (2000). Error processing and the rostral anterior cingulate: An event-related fMRI study. *Psychophysiology,* **37**, 216–223.

Knight, R. T. (1984). Decreased response to novel stimuli after prefrontal lesions in man. *Electrocencephalogr. Clin. Neurophysiol.* **59**, 9–20.

Knight, R. T. (1996). Contribution of human hippocampal region to novelty detection. *Nature* **383**, 256–259.

Knight, R. T., and Scabini, D. (1998). Anatomic bases of event-related potentials and their relationship to novelty detection in humans. *J. Clin. Neurophysiol.* **15**, 3–13.

Kopp, B., Mattler, U., Goertz, R., and Rist, F. (1996a). N2, P3 and the lateralized readiness potential in a nogo task involving selective response priming. *Electrocencephalogr. Clin. Neurophysiol.* **99**, 19–27.

Kopp, B., Rist, F., and Mattler, U. (1996b). N200 in the flanker task as a neurobehavioral tool for investigating executive control. *Psychophysiology* **33**, 282–294.

Lehrmitte, F. (1986). Human autonomy and the frontal lobes. Part II: Patient behavior in complex and social situations: The "environmental dependency syndrome." *Ann. Neurol.* **19**, 335–343.

Lehrmitte, F., Pillon, B., and Serdaru, M. (1986). Human autonomy and the frontal lobes. Part I: Imitation and utilization behavior: A neuropsychological study of 75 patients. *Ann. of Neurol.* **19**, 326–334.

Lisman, J. E., and Otmakhova, N. A. (2001). Storage, recall, and novelty detection of sequences by the hippocampus: Elaborating on the SOCRATIC model to account for normal and aberrant effects of dopamine. *Hippocampus* **11**, 551–568.

Luu, P., and Tucker, D. M. (2001). Regulating action: Alternating activation of human prefrontal and motor cortical networks. *Clin. Neurophysiol.* **112**, 1295–1306.

Luu, P., Collins, P., and Tucker, D. M. (2000a). Mood, personality, and self-monitoring: Negative affect and emotionality in relation to frontal lobe mechanisms of error monitoring. *J. Exp. Psychol. Gen.* **129**, 43–60.

Luu, P., Flaisch, T., and Tucker, D. M. (2000b). Medial frontal cortex in action monitoring. *J. Neurosci.* **20**, 464–469.

Luu, P., Tucker, D. M., Derryberry, D., Reed, M., and Poulsen, C. (2002). Activity in human medial frontal cortex in emotional evaluation and error monitoring. *Psychol. Sci.* (in press).

MacDonald, A. W., Cohen, J. D., Stenger, V. A., and Carter, C. S. (2000). Dissociating the role of the dorsolateral prefrontal and anterior cingulate cortex in cognitive control. *Science* **288**, 1835–1838.

MacLean, P. D. (1993). Introduction: Perspectives on cingulate cortex in the limbic system. *In* "Neurobiology of the Cingulate Cortex and Limbic Thalamus" (B. A. Vogt and M. Gabriel, eds. pp. 1–15). Birkhauser, Boston.

MacLean, P. D., and Pribram, K. H. (1953). Neurographic analysis of medial and basal cerebral cortex. I. Cat. *J. Neurophysiol.* **16**, 312–323.

Makeig, S., Jung, T.-P., Ghahremani, D., Bell, A. J., and Sejnowski, T. J. (1997). Blind separation of auditory event-related brain responses into independent components. *Proc. Natl. Acad. Sci.* **94**, 10979–10984.

Makeig, S., Luu, P., Briggman, K., Visser, E., Sejnowski, T. J., and Tucker, D. M. (2002a). Oscillatory sources of human error-related brain activity. In preparation.

Makeig, S., Westerfield, M., Jung, T.-P., Enghoff, S., Townsend, J., Courchesne, E., and Sejnowski, T. J. (2002b). Dynamic brain sources of visual evoked responses. *Science* **295**, 690–694.

Masaki, H., Tanaka, H., Takasawa, N., and Yamazaki, K. (2001). Error-related brain potentials elicited by vocal errors. *NeuroReport* **12**, 1851–1855.

Menon, V., Ford, J. M., Lim, K. O., Glover, G. H., and Pfefferbaum, A. (1997). Combined event-related fMRI and EEG evidence for temporalparietal cortex activation during target detection. *NeuroReport* **8**, 3029–3037.

Menon, V., Adleman, N. E., White, C. D., Glover, G. H., and Reiss, A. L. (2001). Error-related brain activation during a go/nogo response inhibition task. *Hum. Brain Mapping* **12**, 131–143.

Miller, R. (1991). "Cortico-hippocampal Interplay and the Representation of Contexts in the Brain." Springer-Verlag, New York.

Miltner, W. H. R., Braun, C. H., and Coles, M. G. H. (1997). Event-related brain potentials following incorrect feedback in a time-estimation task: Evidence for a "generic" neural system for error detection. *J. Cogn. Neurosci.* **9**, 787–797.

Miura, Y., Ito, T., and Kadokawa, T. (1987). Effects of intraseptally injected dopamine and noradrenaline on hippocampal synchronized theta wave activity in rats. *Jpn. J. Pharmacol.* **44**, 471–479.

Nauta, W. J. H. (1971). The problem of the frontal lobe: A reinterpretation. *J. Psychiatr. Res.* **8**, 167–187.

Nieuwenhuis, S., Ridderinkhof, K. R., Blom, J., Band, G. P., and Kok, A. (2001). Error-related brain potentials are differentially related to awareness of response errors: Evidence from an antisaccade task. *Psychophysiology* **38**, 752–760.

Niki, H., and Watanabe, M. (1979). Prefrontal and cingulate unit activity during timing behavior in the monkey. *Brain Res.* **171**, 213–224.

Norman, D. A., and Shallice, T. (1986). Attention to action: willed and automatic control of behavior. *In* "Consciousness and Self-regulation" (R. J. Davidson and G. E. Schwartz and D. Shapiro, eds. pp. 1–18). Plenum, New York.

Pandya, D. N., Van Hoesen, G. W., and Mesulam, M.-M. (1981). Efferent connections of the cingulate gyrus in the rhesus monkey. *Exp. Brain Res.* **42**, 319–330.

Pandya, D. N., Seltzer, B., and Barbas, H. (1988). Input-output organization of the primate cerebral cortex. *Comp. Primate Biol.* **4**, 39–80.

Pardo, J. V., Pardo, P. J., Janer, K. W., and Raichle, M. E. (1990). The anterior cingulate cortex mediates processing selection in the stroop attentional conflict paradigm. *Proc. Natl Acad. Sci.* **87**, 256–259.

Paus, T. (2001). Primate anterior cingulate cortex: Where motor control, drive and cognition interface. *Nat. Rev.* **2**, 417–424.

Pickenhain, L., and Klingberg, F. (1967). Hippocampal slow wave activity as a correlate of basic behavioral mechanisms in the rat. *Prog. Brain Res.* **27**, 218–227.

Ploghaus, A., Tracey, I., Clare, S., Gati, J. S., Rawlins, J. N. P., and Matthews, P. M. (2000). Learning about pain: The neural substrate of the prediction error for aversive events. *Proc. Natl. Acad. Sci.* **97**, 9281–9286.

Polich, J. (2002). Neuropsychology of P3a and P3b: A theoretical overview. *In* "Advances in Electrophysiology and Clinical Practice and Research" (K. Arikan and N. Moore, eds.). In press.

Poremba, A., and Gabriel, M. (1997). Amygdalar lesions block discriminative avoidance learning and cingulothalamic training-induced neuronal plasticity in rabbits. *J. Neurosci.* **17**, 5237–5244.

Posner, M. I. (1978). "Chronometric Explorations of Mind." Erlbaum, Hillsdale, N J.

Posner, M. I., and Dehaene, S. (1994). Attentional networks. *Trends Neurosci.* **17**, 75–79.

Posner, M. I., and DiGirolamo, G. (1998). Executive attention: Conflict, target detection and cognitive control. *In* "The attentive brain" (R. Parasuraman, ed., pp. 401–423). MIT Press, Cambridge, Massachusetts.

Posner, M. I., Petersen, S. E., Fox, P. T., and Raichle, M. E. (1988). Localization of cognitive operations in the human brain. *Science* **240**, 1627–1631.

Pribram, K. H., and MacLean, P. D. (1953). Neurographic analysis of medial and basal cerebral cortex. II. Monkey. *J. Neurophysiol.* **16**, 324–340.

Raghavachari, S., Kahana, M. J., Rizzuto, D. S., Caplan, J. B., Kirschen, M., Bourgeois, D., Madsen, J. R., and Lisman, J. E. (2001). Gating of human theta oscillations by a working memory task. *J. Neurosci.* **21**, 3175–3183.

Redgrave, P., Prescott, T. J., and Gurney, K. (1999). Is the short-latency dopamine response too short to signal reward error? *Trends Neurosci.* **22**, 146–151.

Rescorla, R. A. (1992). Hierarchical associative relations in pavlovian conditioning and instrumental training. *Curr. Directions Psychol. Sci.* **1**, 66–70.

Rylander, G. (1947). Personality analysis before and after frontal lobotomy. *In* "Research Publications

Association for Research in Nervous and Mental Disease: The Frontal Lobes" (J. F. Fulton and C. D. Aring and B. S. Wortis, eds). pp. 691–705. Williams and Wilkins, Baltimore.

Sanides, F. (1970). Functional architecture of motor and sensory cortices in primates in the light of a new concept of neocortex evolution. In "The Primate Brain: Advances in Primatology" (C. R. Noback and W. Montagna, eds.) Vol. 1, pp. 137–208. Appleton-Century-Crofts, New York.

Sarnthein, J., Petsche, H., Rappelsberger, P., Shaw, G. L., and von Stein, A. (1998). Synchronization between prefrontal and posterior association cortex during human working memory. Proc. Natl. Acad. Sci. U.S.A. 95, 7092–7096.

Scheffers, M. K., and Coles, M. G. H. (2000). Performance monitoring in a confusing world: error-related brain activity, judgments of response accuracy, and types of errors. J. Exp. Psychol.: Hum. Percept. Perform. 26, 141–151.

Scheffers, M. K., Coles, M. G. H., Bernstein, P., Gehring, W. R., and Donchin, E. (1996). Event-related brain potentials and error-related processing: An analysis of incorrect responses to go and no-go stimuli. Psychophysiology 33, 42–53.

Schultz, W., and Dickinson, A. (2000). Neuronal coding of prediction errors. Ann. Rev. Neurosci. 23, 473–500.

Schultz, W., Apicella, P., Romo, R., and Scarnati, E. (1995). Context-dependent activity in primate striatum reflecting past and future behavioral events. In "Models of information processing in the basal ganglia" (J. C. Houk and J. L. Davis and D. G. Beiser, eds.) pp. 11–27. MIT Press, Cambridge, Massachusetts.

Schultz, W., Tremblay, L., and Hollerman, J. F. (1998). Reward prediction in primate basal ganglia and frontal cortex. Neuropharmacology 37, 421–429.

Slobounov, S. M., Fukada, K., Simon, R., Rearick, M., and Ray, W. (2000). Neurophysiological and behavioral indices of time pressure effects on visuomotor task perfomance. Cogn. Brain Res. 9, 287–298.

Spanagel, R., and Weiss, F. (1999). The dopamine hypothesis of reward: Past and current status. Trends Neurosci. 22, 521–527.

Spencer, K. M., and Polich, J. (1999). Poststimulus EEG spectral analysis and P300: Attention, task, and probability. Psychophysiology 36, 220–232.

Squire, L. R. (1992). Memory and the hippocampus: A synthesis from findings with rats, monkeys, and humans. Psychol. Rev. 99, 195–231.

Tellegen, A., and Waller, N. G. (1996). Exploring personality through test construction: Development of the multidimensional personality questionnaire. In "Personality Measures: Development and Evaluation" (S. R. Brigg and J. M. Cheek, eds.), pp. 133–161. JAI Press, Greenwich, Connecticut.

Tucker, D. M., Hartry-Speiser, A., McDougal, L., Luu, P., and deGrandpre, D. (1999). Mood and spatial memory: Emotion and the right hemisphere contribution to spatial cognition. Biol. Psychol. 50, 103–125.

Tucker, D. M., Derryberry, D., and Luu, P. (2000). Anatomy and physiology of human emotion: Vertical integration of brain stem, limbic, and cortical systems. In "The Neuropsychology of Emotion" (J. C. Borod, ed.), pp. 56–79: Oxford University Press, Oxford.

Vanderwolf, C. H., Kramis, R., and Robinson, T. E. (1978). Hippocampal electrical activity during waking behavior and sleep: Analyses using centrally acting drugs. In "Functions of the Septohippocampal System," Vol. 58, pp. 199–221. Elsevier, Amsterdam.

Van't Ent, D., and Apkarian, P. (1999). Motoric response inhibition in finger movement and saccadic eye movement: A comparative study. Clin. Neurophysiol. 110, 1058–1072.

Vidal, F., Hasbroucq, T., Grapperon, J., and Bonnet, M. (2000). Is the "error negativity' specific to errors? Biol. Psychol. 51, 109–128.

Vogt, B. A., Pandya, D. N., and Rosene, D. L. (1987). Cingulate cortex of the rhesus monkey: I. Cytoarchitecture and thalamic afferents. J. Comp. Neurol. 262, 256–270.

Vogt, B. A., Finch, D. M., and Olson, C. R. (1993a). Functional heterogeneity in the cingulate cortex: The anterior executive and posterior evaluative regions. Cereb. Cortex 2, 435–443.

Vogt, B. A., Sikes, R. W., and Vogt, L. J. (1993b). Anterior cingulate cortex and the medial pain system. In "Neurobiology of the Cingulate Cortex and Limbic Thalamus" (B. A. Vogt and M. Gabriel, eds.), pp. 314–344. Birkhäuser, Boston.

Ward, A. A. (1948a). The anterior cingular gyrus and personality. Res. Publ. Assoc. Res. Nervous Mental Dis. 27, 438–445.

Ward, A. A. (1948b). The cingulate gyrus: Area 24. J. Neurophysiol. 11, 13–24.

Zheng, F., and Khanna, S. (1999). Hippocampal field CA1 interneuronal nociceptive responses: Modulation by medial septal region and morphine. Neuroscience 93, 45–55.

Zieglagänsberger, W., French, E. D., Siggins, G. R., and Bloom, F. E. (1979). Opioid peptides may excite hippocampal pyramidal neurons by inhibiting adjacent inhibitory neurons. Science 205, 415–417.

9

Effects of Age and Experience on the Development of Neurocognitive Systems

Teresa V. Mitchell and Helen J. Neville

INTRODUCTION

Progress in cognitive science and the development of noninvasive techniques such as electrophysiology have permitted extensive, ongoing mapping and differentiation of sensory and cognitive systems in the mature human brain. This progress presents a challenging opportunity for cognitive neuroscience: to characterize the processes that lead to the development of the differentiation of the mature brain.

The event-related potential (ERP) technique has been, and will continue to be, indispensable in informing us about development and how age and experience contribute to the adultlike mosaic of neurocognitive systems. It is a powerful technique to use with infants and children because, although it requires attention to the stimuli presented, it does not require overt responses. It is also powerful because there are times when evidence of cognitive and perceptual skills can be observed in ERP responses, but not in overt behavioral measures such as looking time. Thus, the ERP technique can reveal aspects of perception and cognition that occur independently of response preparation and execution.

There are important issues to take into consideration when using the ERP technique with infants and children. Multiple factors interact to make ERP components recorded from infants and children look very different from those recorded from adults. Developmental changes in anatomy have a significant impact on both the latency and amplitude of ERP components. For example, thickness of the skull has been shown to influence the amplitude of ERPs recorded on the scalp (Frodl *et al.*, 2001) such that a thicker skull is correlated with smaller amplitude. A substantial increase in skull thickness occurs over infancy and early childhood and this change is likely to affect amplitudes recorded from scalp electrodes. The developmental effects of increasing skull thickness may not affect all ERP components in the same way; adult ERP components are differently affected by scalp thickness (Frodl, *et al.*, 2001). Another substantial anatomical change across development is the increase in myelination of white matter. Myelin serves to increase conduction velocities along neuronal axons. For example, in early infancy there is a progressive shortening of the latencies of the auditory brain stem response that is linked to an increasing myelination of the brain stem (Starr *et al.*, 1977; Eggermont, 1988).

Myelin is present in different thicknesses in different brain regions and pathways, and the development of myelination proceeds along nonidentical timelines across regions and pathways. Because of this, the effects of myelination on the development of ERP components are likely to vary across brain regions and neurocognitive systems. Finally, regional variability in synaptogenesis and loss of synapses occur throughout the first two decades of life, the time period of greatest changes in ERP morphologies and latencies. These changes in neural development are likely to be an additional factor contributing to the differences in infant and adult ERPs (Aslin, 1987; Vaughan and Kurtzberg, 1992; Huttenlocher and Dabhoklar, 1997; Neville, 1998).

In addition to changes associated with these anatomical and physiological factors, changes are observed in ERPs across the life span that are due to the factors that interest psychologists the most: the development of cognitive and perceptual skills. Perceptual and cognitive development is heterochronous and research has shown that these skills, and the neural systems that underlie them, develop at different rates and have different sensitive periods (see Bailey *et al.*, 2001). Thus, multiple interactions between anatomical and physiological factors and cognitive and perceptual factors serve to produce significant changes in scalp ERPs from infancy to adulthood.

In this chapter we describe four domains in which electrophysiological data illustrate that development proceeds at different rates in different systems and that structural and functional plasticity as expressed by early atypical experience differs across neurocognitive systems. Within each domain we briefly describe the typical findings from adult studies, then we review evidence demonstrating the effects of age and of experience on the emergence of the adult-like state.

DEVELOPMENT OF THE DORSAL AND VENTRAL VISUAL STREAMS

Within the visual system there is a structural and functional segregation of motion and location information from color and form information along "dorsal" and "ventral" processing streams, respectively. Visual motion is processed principally by a population of cell types (magno) (M) in the lateral geniculate nucleus (LGN) that project to particular layers in the primary visual cortex (Ungerleider and Mishkin, 1982; Ungerleider and Haxby, 1994). Those layers, in turn, project to the middle temporal (MT) gyrus, a cortical region that specializes in the processing of visual motion (Maunsell and van Essen, 1983). Color and form information, on the other hand, are processed by a population of cell types (parvo) (P) in the LGN that are separate from those that process motion, and these cells project to different layers in primary visual cortex (Ungerleider and Mishkin, 1982; Ungerleider and Haxby, 1994). These layers project to cortical regions within the ventral temporal and occipital cortices that are dedicated to processing color, form, and faces (Maunsell and Newsome, 1987). Little is known about the plasticity of the dorsal and ventral visual streams in humans, but evidence from special populations suggests that dorsal stream functions, such as motion processing, are more affected by atypical experience, compared to ventral stream functions, such as color and form processing. Studies of patients with glaucoma report behavioral (Anderson and O'Brien, 1997) and anatomical (Quigley *et al.*, 1989) evidence of specific magnocellular (M)-layer deficits. Similarly, behavioral, physiological, and anatomical studies of dyslexic individuals report deficits in dorsal stream functions such as motion perception (Stein and Walsh, 1997), and functional magnetic resonance imaging (fMRI) data show reduced activation of area MT by motion in dyslexic adults (Eden *et al.*, 1996; Demb *et al.*, 1998). Psychophysical studies of adults with Williams Syndrome also report spared functioning of the ventral pathway relative to deficits observed in dorsal pathway functions (Atkinson *et al.*, 1997; Bellugi *et al.*, 1999). In sum, available evidence is consistent with the idea that the dorsal visual pathway may be more modifiable by altered early input than is the ventral visual pathway.

Effects of Atypical Early Experience

In our laboratory, we have studied the effects of congenital deafness on visual functions. Our functional MRI studies have shown that auditory deprivation affects processing of visual motion. Congenitally, genetically deaf and hearing participants were presented with a moving random-dot field and were asked to attend to changes in the brightness of the dots and changes in the velocity of the motion (Bavelier *et al.*, 2000, 2001). When attending to the center of the flow field, the two groups produced similar activation. By contrast, when attending the periphery of the flow field, deaf adults displayed more activation within dorsal stream area MT, the posterior parietal cortex (PPC), and the superior temporal sulcus (STS) than did hearing

adults. The increased recruitment of areas MT, PPC, and STS with attention to peripheral motion appears to stem from auditory deprivation rather than the use of a signed language: hearing adults who learned sign language as their first language produced similar activation in these regions when attending to motion in the visual periphery (Bavelier *et al.*, 2001).

These results raise the hypothesis that auditory deprivation specifically affects dorsal visual functions, but not ventral stream functions. To test this hypothesis, we presented normally hearing adults and congenitally, genetically deaf adults with stimuli designed to activate differentially the two visual streams (Armstrong *et al.*, 2002). The dorsal stream or "motion" stimulus was a low-spatial-frequency grayscale grating. ERPs to this stimulus were time-locked to a rightward movement of the bars that lasted 100 msec. The ventral stream or "color" stimulus was a high-spatial-frequency grating of blue and green bars. ERPs to this stimulus were recorded when the green bars of the stimulus turned red for 100 msec. Participants responded by button press to occasional presentations of a black square, thus color and motion were task-irrelevant features. Two prominent components were observed: a P1 that was largest over posterior, lateral temporal

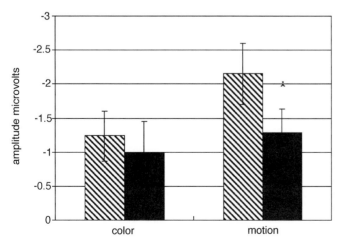

FIGURE 1 Average N1 amplitudes of deaf (hatched bars) and hearing (solid bars) adults in response to color and motion stimuli. Asterisk denotes significant population difference in response to motion only ($p > 0.05$) (from Armstrong *et al.*, 2002).

scalp sites and peaked at roughly 120 msec, and an N1 that was observed across the scalp and peaked at roughly 180 msec. Motion stimuli evoked a minimal P1 and a prominent N1 that was larger in response to central than peripheral presentations. Color stimuli evoked a prominent P1 and N1. Amplitudes and latencies of the P1 component were similar for deaf and hearing participants across both stimulus types. Amplitudes and latencies of the N1 were also similar for the two groups in response to color stimuli. By contrast, N1 amplitudes recorded in response to motion stimuli were reliably larger in the deaf than in the hearing participants (see Fig. 1). Furthermore, the distribution of N1 responses to motion stimuli was more medial and anterior in deaf than in hearing participants. The results of this ERP study show that, even when participants are not required to attend to the features of visual motion, motion stimuli evoke greater neural activity in deaf than in hearing adults.

Effects of Age

An understanding of the normal development of the dorsal and ventral visual streams could provide clues as to how and why auditory deprivation affects dorsal stream functions more than ventral stream functions. What little data exist are fairly equivocal. Behavioral studies of infant vision suggest that the development of the dorsal stream may outpace the development of the ventral stream cells in the lateral geniculate nucleus (Dobkins *et al.*, 1999). By contrast, anatomical studies suggest that dorsal stream cells have a more protracted developmental trajectory compared to the ventral stream (Hickey, 1977). Studies of macaques show that face-selective regions in temporal and occipital cortex are form and face selective by 6 months of age (Rodman *et al.*, 1991, 1993), but do not display the specificity of tuning that is observed in adults until roughly 1 year of age (Rodman, 1994). We hypothesized that although basic stimulus selectivity may be observed early in development, adultlike functioning and tuning in the ventral stream will be observed at a younger age than in the dorsal stream. To test this hypothesis, normally developing children ages 6 to 7 years of age and 8 to 10 years of age, and adults, were tested using the same color and motion stimulus paradigm described above. Children and adults produced similar componentry: a prominent P1 and N1 in response to color stimuli, and a smaller P1 and prominent N1 in response to motion stimuli. Although age-related decreases in amplitude were observed in response to both stimulus types, decreases in latency were observed only in response to motion (see Fig. 2). Thus, significant development occurs across the early school years in both

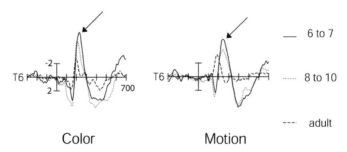

FIGURE 2 Averaged ERP traces for age groups 6 to 7 years old, 8 to 10 years old, and adults, in response to color and motion stimuli. Arrows point to the N1 component. Significant reductions in amplitude with age were observed for both stimulus types, whereas significant changes in latency with age were observed only in response to motion stimuli (from Mitchell and Neville, 2002).

visual streams, but speed of processing undergoes greater changes in response to motion as compared to response to color. The relatively longer maturation of dorsal stream pathways may render them more likely to be changed by altered early sensory experience.

When in development do the effects of auditory deprivation on motion processing emerge? The few studies that have investigated higher order attentional differences between deaf and hearing children report mixed results. A study of texture segmentation and visual search revealed evidence of enhanced featural attention in deaf as compared to hearing adults, but no such evidence emerged from studies on children (Rettenbach *et al.*, 1999). Two studies employing continuous-performance tasks reported significantly poorer performance in deaf as compared to hearing children (Quittner *et al.*, 1994; Mitchell and Quittner, 1996). An additional study investigated the effects of motion and color as distractors in a visual search task (Mitchell and Smith, 1996; Mitchell, 1996). This study was designed to test the hypothesis that if enhanced attention to motion is obligatory in the deaf, then suppression of attention to task-irrelevant motion should be difficult. On the other hand, if attention to color is not obligatory in this population, suppression of attention to task-irrelevant color should be observed. The developmental prediction was that population differences would not be observed during early school years but would emerge by adulthood. To test these hypotheses, deaf and hearing children ages 6 to 9 and adults performed two visual search tasks that required attention to shape in the presence of both color and motion distractors. In the first task, stimuli were presented in a circle in the center of the visual field. In this task, deaf and hearing children performed similarly but deaf adults were affected more by both distractor types compared to hearing adults. In the second task, stimuli were presented across the central and peripheral

visual fields. In this task, both deaf children and adults were more distracted by task-irrelevant motion and color than were hearing children and adults. Thus, deaf and hearing children in this study performed differently only when required to attend to stimuli that extended into the periphery (Mitchell, 1996).

To further investigate the development of effects of auditory deprivation on visual motion processing, we collected data from 20 congenitally, genetically deaf children and 20 hearing children ages 6 through 10 using the same color and motion ERP paradigm described above. Analyses of the N1 show that amplitudes and latencies in response to color stimuli were similar across the two groups. In response to motion, on the other hand, some group differences were observed. For central visual field presentations, deaf children produced larger N1 amplitudes than did their hearing age mates in right-hemisphere electrodes. For peripheral visual field presentations, overall amplitudes from deaf children were marginally larger compared to those from hearing children. Together, these studies suggest that some population differences emerge in early school years, but these differences vary across spatial location and stimulus features. Across behavioral and ERP studies, it appears that population differences are observed more often in response to peripheral than to central stimulation and are observed more often in response to motion than to color, but these group effects in children are not as robust as those observed in adults (Mitchell and Neville, 1999, 2002).

Results from these studies raise the hypothesis of greater modifiability within dorsal than in ventral stream areas. This difference may be due to several factors, some intrinsic to the system and some extrinsic. Results from normally developing children suggest that the development of the ventral stream may reach adultlike levels earlier than in dorsal stream areas. If this is so, then atypical experience across the lifespan may have greater opportunity to affect the structure and function of the dorsal than the ventral stream. The specific pattern of plastic changes may also be due in part to functional demands placed on the visual system when auditory information is absent. Dorsal stream visual areas may become more activated in deaf individuals, for example, because in the absence of auditory input, the system would need to attend more to dynamic visual information to navigate throughout the environment. These functional needs then interact with intrinsic developmental timetables and levels of plasticity within each neurocognitive system.

SPATIAL ATTENTION: CENTRAL VERSUS PERIPHERAL VISUAL AND AUDITORY SPACE

Selective spatial attention is the ability to focus attention on specific locations in space, which involves either increased processing of stimuli within the attended location or inhibition of processing of stimuli outside the attended location, or both. Both visual and auditory spatial attention are distributed along a gradient, with the sharpest and most efficient localization and processing in the center of attention and a gradual degradation of processing with increasing distance from the center (Downing and Pinker, 1985; Mondor and Zatorre, 1995; Teder-Salejarvi et al., 1999). In this section, we review studies that investigate the effects of unimodal sensory deprivation on the structure and function of spatial attention.

Effects of Auditory Deprivation on Spatial Attention

Functional MRI data reviewed above show that auditory deprivation leads to enhanced activation by motion and that this effect is greater for the periphery than

for the center of the visual field. Studies employing the ERP technique have also shown that, whereas centrally presented stimuli elicit similar responses in deaf and hearing adults, peripherally presented stimuli elicit larger responses from deaf than from hearing adults (Neville and Lawson, 1987). In that study, participants were presented with alternating small white squares that displayed apparent motion. ERPs were recorded as participants attended to the central or peripheral squares and responded to indicate their direction of motion. Deaf participants were faster and more accurate in detecting the direction of motion than were hearing participants, and amplitudes of the N1 in response to peripheral stimuli were reliably larger in deaf than in hearing participants. These results together suggest that effects of auditory deprivation on spatial attention are greater on the representation of the periphery than of the center of visual space.

Effects of Visual Deprivation on Spatial Attention

Attention to central and peripheral auditory space was compared in sighted and blind individuals in a similar paradigm. This study tested the hypothesis that effects of sensory deprivation on spatial attention are similar across modalities. The prediction was that the representation of auditory peripheral space would be modified more than the representation of central auditory space in blind individuals. In this ERP study, congenitally blind and sighted, blindfolded adults attended selectively to noise bursts from speakers arranged either directly in front or in an arc in the far right periphery of the participant (Röder et al., 1999). ERPs were recorded as participants localized the noise bursts. A prominent N1 was elicited that was larger in amplitude to attended as compared to unattended locations. Behavioral results showed that blind and sighted participants

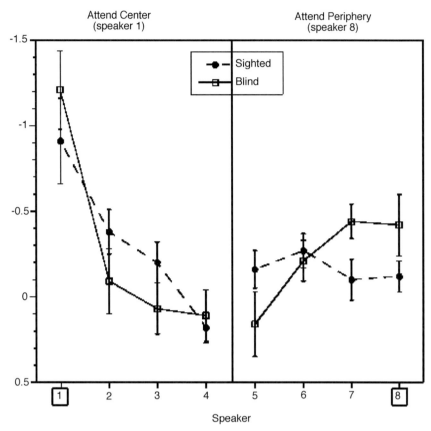

FIGURE 3 Gradients of mean N1 amplitudes (±SE; microvolts) to standard stimuli at speakers within the attended central and attended peripheral arrays. The early attention mechanism indexed by N1 was more sharply tuned in the blind than in the sighted subjects when they were attending to targets at the peripheral speaker 8. Reprinted by permission from *Nature*, Röder *et al.*, 1999; copyright 1999 Macmillan Publishers Ltd.

were equally accurate at localizing sounds presented within central space, but blind participants were more accurate than sighted participants at localizing sounds played from the peripheral speakers. ERPs recorded to the sounds further demonstrated that spatial tuning in peripheral space was sharper in blind than in sighted participants. As shown in Fig. 3, N1 amplitude was similar across the two groups with attention to the center, whereas with attention to the periphery, amplitudes from blind participants displayed a steeper gradient compared to those from sighted participants.

Together, these studies suggest that spatial attention to peripheral space is more modified by sensory deprivation than is spatial attention to central space, irrespective of the deprived sensory modality. It may be that aspects of sensory systems that are specialized for high acuity are less modifiable by atypical input, compared to those displaying less acuity and precision (see Chalupa and Dreher, 1991). In this instance, the neural representation of central space is more precisely mapped and displays higher acuity, compared to peripheral space, and it is less affected by auditory and visual deprivation than is peripheral space. The representation of peripheral space may also be more affected by sensory deprivation because it receives more converging inputs across sensory modalities than does central space. Anatomical studies provide evidence for this hypothesis (Rockland and Ojima, 2001; Falchier *et al.*, 2001). In intact organisms, the senses work in concert to develop maps of extrapersonal space; input from one modality contributes to the organization of spatial representation in the other modality. These data show that the absence of input in one modality produces sharper, rather than coarser, spatial tuning, particularly in the periphery.

THE DEVELOPMENT OF FACE PERCEPTION

Face perception calls on a set of highly complex skills that adult humans perform rapidly and with great precision and accuracy. It includes the recognition of individual faces as well as the differentiation and interpretation of facial expressions. Among the neural substrates of face processing in adults are the ventral occipital and lateral temporal lobes. Functional MRI and subdural electrophysiological measures have shown that although many categories of objects activate ventral temporal/occipital cortex, a region along the fusiform gyrus is activated primarily by face stimuli (Sergent *et al.*, 1992; Puce *et al.*, 1995; Kanwisher *et al.*, 1997). Event-related potential studies of basic face processing in adults have shown that faces, but not other objects, evoke an N170, a negative component that is prominent at temporal scalp electrode sites and is larger over the right than the left hemisphere (Bentin *et al.*, 1996). This component is also prominent in response to face components, especially isolated eyes. Intracranial electrophysiology reveals an N200 component that is recorded directly from the posterior fusiform gyrus and from the lateral middle temporal gyrus/superior temporal sulcus (Allison *et al.*, 1999; McCarthy *et al.*, 1999; Puce *et al.*, 1999). These components are recorded from subdural electrode arrays on the

ventral portion of the occipital lobes and lateral temporal lobes in patients with epilepsy (Allison *et al*, 1999). A prominent N200 can be observed only in response to face stimuli, and is observed in the fusiform gyrus, occipitotemporal sulcus, inferior temporal gyrus, and the lateral middle temporal gyrus/superior temporal sulcus. This component is relatively insensitive to habituation, and electrical stimulation of the region that generates it produces a transient inability to name familiar faces (Allison *et al.*, 1994). The scalp N170 component is believed to be generated in the lateral regions (superior temporal sulcus and/or occipitotemporal sulcus), rather than the ventral fusiform region (Bentin *et al.*, 1996), because of its distribution and because it is prominent in response to eyes, unlike the N200. Overall, both the scalp N170 and the intracranial N200 are hypothesized to be involved more in discriminating faces from other stimuli (i.e., identification of "facedness") and less in identification of individual faces (McCarthy, 2001).

The development of this neural substrate of face perception is relatively unknown. A two-phase theory has been proposed for the development of the neural substrate of face perception (Morton and Johnson, 1991). During the first phase of development, the theory proposes that subcortical mechanisms drive infants to fixate on faces. Newborn infants prefer to look at faces and facelike stimuli longer than many other visual stimuli (Fantz, 1963). This tendency to fixate on faces is hypothesized to train and tune cortical regions downstream to respond to faces and eventually to play a role in distinguishing one face from another. In the second phase of development, experience in perceiving faces, learning to recognize familiar faces, and differentiating facial expressions drives the establishment of the adultlike cortical substrate, including the fusiform gyrus and lateral temporal regions. This initial setting up of cortical regions is hypothesized to take place within the first year of life, but the long-term developmental trajectory and plasticity of these regions are only beginning to be mapped out. In this section, we review ERP studies that shed light on the development of the neural substrates of face perception.

Infant Face Recognition

A basic measure of infant face recognition is the ability to discriminate the face of one's own mother from the face of another woman. In behavioral paradigms, evidence of recognition of the mother's face can vary both with age and with dependent measure. De Haan and colleagues studied the ability of 6-month-old infants to recognize their own mother (de Haan and Nelson, 1997). In a preferential looking paradigm, 6-month-old infants spent an equivalent amount of time fixating on their own mother's face and on a stranger's face. However, ERP measures in this same age group showed that processing of the mother's face was different from that of a stranger's face. Specifically, the amplitude of the Nc component, a negative deflection occurring between 400 and 800 msec post-stimulus, was larger in response to photographs of the infant's own mother, compared to a photograph of another infant's mother (de Haan and Nelson, 1997). This effect was observed over midline and right anterior electrodes.

de Haan and colleagues further investigated effects of category and familiarity on face processing in 6-month-old infants (de Haan and Nelson, 1999). In this study, infants were presented with two categories of photographs and two levels of familiarity: photographs of familiar and unfamiliar toys and photographs of the infant's own mother or another infant's mother. Two components displayed category effects, a positivity occurring around 400 msec (the P400) and a middle latency negative ERP (the Nc) occurring around 600 msec. A cat-egory effect was observed for the P400 such that it was faster in response to faces than to objects. Both category and familiarity effects were observed for the Nc. Familiar stimuli, regardless of category, produced larger Nc amplitudes than did unfamiliar stimuli across frontal sites. Further, this familiarity effect displayed a right frontal distribution for faces, but was bilaterally distributed for objects. This replicates the right frontal distribution of the Nc, in response to faces, that was observed in the study described above (de Haan and Nelson, 1997). This more focal distribution may be early evidence of a basic right hemisphere asymmetry, or it may be due to infants' greater experience with faces than with toys. The authors conclude that basic encoding of faces in infants occurs by 400 msec and is indexed by the P400, whereas recognition processes occur by 600 msec and are indexed by the Nc. Together, these studies demonstrate that faces evoke a different pattern of neural activity compared to other visual objects by 6 months of age.

Face Processing across the Early School Years

One developmental question is whether the mechanisms involved in face processing undergo qualitative or quantitative change from early school years to adulthood. Despite the precociousness of infant face processing, the performance of young children on a variety of face recognition and discrimination tasks is far below adult levels (Carey and Diamond, 1994; Baenninger, 1994). At issue is whether children perform poorly on these tasks because the way they process faces is different from the way adults do, or whether the same processes are at work but are simply slower and less proficient.

To begin addressing this developmental issue, Taylor and colleagues have studied the developmental characteristics of the scalp N170 in children and adults. In an early study, participants, ages 4 to adult, viewed a series of individual black and white photographs of faces, cars, scrambled cars, scrambled faces, and butterflies (Taylor *et al.*, 1999). Butterflies were the target stimulus to which participants responded with a button press. An N170 was observed in response to faces in all age groups. Latencies of this component decreased linearly with age, accompanied by variable changes in amplitude. A large increase in amplitude occurred between subjects 12–14 years old and adult subjects. The typical right-greater-than-left hemispheric asymmetry of the N170 amplitude observed in adults emerged with age, from a bilateral distribution in the younger children. This was mainly due to an increase in amplitudes with age recorded from right-hemisphere sites. In sum, the N170 is prominent in response to faces even in 4-year-old children, its latency decreases with age, and the right hemispheric asymmetry of this component also emerges with age.

In a similar study, Taylor and colleagues investigated the effects of face inversion [hypothesized to elicit "featural" processing of faces in contrast to the "configural" processing typical of upright faces; (Carey and Diamond, 1994)] and the presentation of isolated eyes on the N170 in participants ages 4 to adult (Taylor *et al.*, 2001). Participants viewed upright faces, inverted faces, scrambled faces, eyes, and flowers (and checkerboards, to which they responded as the target). The N170 was observed in all age groups in response to eyes, upright faces, and inverted faces. Overall latencies of the N170 decreased linearly across age groups, with the greatest decrease observed in response to upright faces. As in the study described above, the youngest age groups displayed a bilateral distribution in response to faces, whereas older age groups displayed an adultlike right-greater-than-left hemispheric asymmetry. By contrast, the N170 in response to eyes produced a right-greater-than-left hemispheric asymmetry in all age groups. As shown in Fig. 4, amplitudes in response to eyes decreased significantly across the early school years; overall amplitudes in response to upright faces were relatively consistent across all age groups but amplitudes in response to inverted faces increased with age. Latencies were shorter in response to inverted compared to upright faces in the younger age groups, but this reversed around the onset of puberty. In sum, responses to eyes reached an adultlike profile around age 11, whereas responses to inverted faces were not adultlike until after puberty. These differences

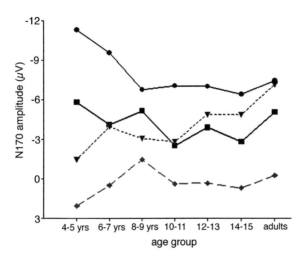

FIGURE 4   Average N170 amplitudes across age groups for eyes (●), faces (■), inverted faces (▼), and scrambled faces (♦). Amplitudes in response to eyes decreased significantly across the early school years whereas overall amplitudes in response to upright faces were relatively consistent across all age groups. Amplitudes in response to inverted faces increased with age, and amplitudes to upright faces were stable across age. Reprinted from *Clinical Neurophysiology*, Vol. 110; M. J. Taylor, G. McCarthy, E. Saliba, and E. Degiovanni; ERP evidence of developmental changes in processing of faces, pp. 910–915. Copyright 1999 with permission from Elsevier Science.

raise the hypothesis that there are differences in the development of the neural representation of eyes as compared to faces, and upright versus inverted faces.

Additional research with school-aged children similarly reports differing developmental trends for ERPs recorded in response to upright and inverted faces. Alvarez and colleagues recorded ERPs in response to upright and inverted faces in participants aged 9, 13, and 16 years, and adults, during a face recognition matching task (Alvarez and Neville, 1995). Participants were presented with one face, followed by a second, and were asked to respond to indicate whether the second face matched the first. Behavioral data indicated that all age groups were better at recognizing upright compared to inverted faces, and accuracy and reaction time (RT) improved steadily with age. Electrophysiological data revealed a negativity between 250 and 450 msec (the N320) in response to the second face that was larger for mismatched than for matched faces at all ages. Two developmental changes were observed in this component. First, although adults produced larger N320 amplitudes in the right hemisphere compared to the left hemisphere, children produced similar amplitudes across hemispheres. Second, in adults N320 amplitudes were larger for upright than for inverted faces, whereas in children similar amplitudes were observed across face orientations. Adultlike ERPs were observed only in participants ages 16 and older. Thus, the developmental changes in the N320, an index of face recognition, mirror those observed in the N170: the right-hemisphere asymmetry and face inversion effects emerge slowly with age.

Face Processing in Williams Syndrome

Williams Syndrome (WS) is a genetic disorder that produces severe deficits in many aspects of cognitive processing, but leaves face processing and verbal skills relatively spared (Bellugi *et al.*, 2000). In order to investigate whether face processing relies on the same neural substrates in adult Williams patients and controls, Mills and colleagues (2000) compared face recognition using the same paradigm as in the Alvarez study described above. All participants were faster and more accurate in response to upright compared to inverted faces. Participants with WS were slower and less accurate overall than control subjects, but most of the individual subjects performed within the range of the controls. Differences in the amplitude and distribution of the N320 were observed between the two subject groups. Normal adults displayed larger amplitudes to the mismatched targets compared to the matched targets for upright, but not inverted, faces. In contrast, the WS subjects displayed a match/mismatch effect for both face orientation conditions. Further, the overall match/mismatch effect tended to be larger from the right hemisphere in controls, but larger from the left hemisphere in WS adults. These results suggest that WS adults, like normal children and unlike normal adults, do not employ different brain systems for recognizing upright and inverted faces.

These studies show that although there is overlap in the systems involved in face processing from early school years to adulthood, age and experience affect the functioning and distribution of this network in significant ways. Effects of face orientation and a right-hemisphere asymmetry can be observed in behavioral measures (de Schonen and Mathivet, 1990) as well as ERP measures early in normal development, but an adultlike profile is not attained until puberty across many studies. This suggests that increasing skill and experience in perceiving faces may be one factor that drives the differentiation of the substrates for processing upright and inverted faces.

DEVELOPMENTAL NEUROPLASTICITY OF LANGUAGE FUNCTIONS

The neural systems important for language functions are distributed across several brain regions, and these regions are differentially involved in the processing of different aspects of language. Observations of varying rates of differentiation and degrees of specification can contribute to the identification and characterization of different functional subsystems within language. In a series of experiments, we have studied the development of the neural systems important in lexical, semantic, and grammatical processing. In normal, right-handed, monolingual adults, nouns and verbs ("open class" words) that provide lexical/semantic information elicit a different pattern of brain activity (as measured by ERPs) than do function words, including prepositions and conjunctions ("closed class" words), which provide grammatical information in English (Neville et al., 1992; Nobre and McCarthy, 1994). In addition, sentences that are semantically nonsensical but are grammatically intact elicit a different pattern of ERPs compared to sentences that contain a violation of syntactic structure but leave the meaning intact (Neville et al., 1991; Osterhout et al., 1997). These results are consistent with other types of evidence that suggest that different neural systems mediate the processing of lexical/semantic and grammatical information in adults. Specifically, they imply a greater role for more posterior temporal-parietal systems in lexical/semantic processing and for frontal-temporal systems within the left hemisphere in grammatical processing. This overall pattern appears ubiquitous in adults, and many investigators have suggested that the central role of the left hemisphere in language processing is strongly genetically determined. Certainly the fact that most individuals, regardless of the language they learn,

display left-hemisphere dominance for that language indicates that this aspect of neural development is strongly biased. Nonetheless, it is likely that language-relevant aspects of cerebral organization are dependent on and modified by language experience.

Studies of Bilingual Adults

Many investigators have studied the effects of language experience on neural development by comparing cerebral organization in individuals who learned a second language at different times in development (Dehaene et al., 1997; Kim et al., 1997; Perani et al., 1996). In general, age of exposure to language appears to affect cerebral organization for that language. Moreover, there appears to be specificity in these effects. In Chinese–English bilinguals, delays of as long as 16 years in exposure to English had very little effect on the organization of the brain systems active in lexical/semantics processing. In contrast, delays of only 4 years had significant effects on those aspects of brain organization linked to grammatical processing (Weber-Fox and Neville, 1996). These results and parallel behavioral results from the same study suggest that aspects of semantic and grammatical processing differ markedly in the degree to which they depend on language input. Specifically, grammatical processing appears more vulnerable to delays in language experience.

Studies of Deaf Adults

Further evidence of the plasticity of language systems was provided by ERP studies of English sentence processing in congenitally deaf individuals who learned English late and as a second language [American Sign Language (ASL) was the first language of these individuals (Neville et al., 1992)]. These deaf participants displayed ERP responses to nouns and to semantically anomalous sentences in written English that were indistinguishable from those of normally hearing participants who learned English as a first language. These data are consistent with the hypothesis that some aspects of lexical/semantic processing are largely unaffected by the many different aspects of language experience that differ between normally hearing and congenitally deaf individuals. By contrast, deaf participants displayed aberrant ERP responses to grammatical information such as that presented in function words in English. Specifically, they did not display the specialization of the anterior regions of the left hemisphere that is characteristic of native, hearing/speaking learners. These data suggest that the systems that mediate the processing of grammatical information are more modifiable and vulnerable in response to altered language experience than are those associated with lexical/semantic processing.

Studies of ASL

We have employed the ERP and fMRI techniques to further pursue this hypothesis and also to obtain evidence on the question of whether the strongly biased role of the left hemisphere in language occurs independently of the structure and modality of the language first acquired (Neville et al., 1997, 1998). ERPs were recorded from hearing and deaf adults who learned ASL as a first language and from hearing subjects who acquired ASL late or not at all, as they viewed ASL signs that formed sentences. The results were compared across these groups and with those from hearing subjects reading English sentences. ERPs recorded to response to open and closed class signs in ASL sentences displayed similar timing and anterior/posterior distributions to those observed in previous studies of English. However, whereas in native speakers of English responses to closed class English words were largest over anterior regions of the left hemi-

sphere, in native signers closed class ASL signs elicited activity that was bilateral and that extended posteriorly to include parietal regions of both the left and right hemispheres. These results imply that the acquisition of a language that relies on spatial contrasts and the perception of motion may result in the inclusion of right-hemisphere regions into the language system. Both hearing and deaf native signers displayed this effect. However, hearing people who acquired ASL in the late teens did not show this effect, suggesting there may be a limited time (sensitive) period during which this type of organization for grammatical processing can develop (Newman et al., 2002). By contrast the response to semantic information was not affected by age of acquisition of ASL, in keeping with the results from studies of English that suggest that these different subsystems within language display different degrees of developmental plasticity.

In fMRI studies comparing sentence processing in English and ASL, we also observed evidence for biological constraints and effects of experience on the mature organization of the language systems of the brain. As in the study described above, hearing adults with no ASL background, hearing native signers and deaf native signers, were imaged while observing written English sentences and while observing sentences signed in ASL (Neville et al., 1998). When hearing adults read English, their first language, there was robust activation within the left but not the right hemisphere and in particular within the inferior frontal (Broca's) regions. When deaf people read English, their second language, learned late and imperfectly, these regions within the left hemisphere were not activated. Is this lack of left-hemisphere activation in the deaf linked to lack of auditory experience with language or to incomplete acquisition of English grammar? ASL is not sound based but displays each of the characteristics of all formal languages, including a complex grammar that makes extensive use of spatial location and hand motion (Klima and Bellugi, 1988). When deaf subjects viewed sentences in their native ASL, we observed activation within the same inferior frontal regions of the left hemisphere that become active when native speakers of English process English. These data suggest that there is a strong biological bias for these neural systems to mediate grammatical language, regardless of the structure and modality of the language acquired. However, if the language is not acquired within the appropriate time window this strong bias is not expressed. The fMRI data also indicate a robust role for the right hemisphere in processing ASL. These results suggest that the nature of the language input, in this case the co-occurrence of location and motion information with language, shape the organization of the language systems of the brain. Further research is necessary to specify the different times in human development when particular types of input are required for optimal development of the many systems and subsystems important in language processing.

Effects of Primary Language Acquisition on Cerebral Organization

The research summarized above implies that language experience determines the development and organization of language-relevant systems of the brain. A strong test of this hypothesis would be to chart the changes in brain organization as children acquire their primary language and to separate these from more general maturational changes. We compared patterns of neural activity relevant to language processing in 13- and 20-month-old infants to determine whether changes in cerebral organization occur as a function of specific changes in language development when chronological age is held constant (Mills *et al.*, 1993, 1997; Neville and Mills, 1997). ERPs were recorded as children lis-

tened to words they knew, words they did not know, and backward words. Specific and different ERP components discriminated comprehended words from unknown and from backward words. Distinct lateral and anterior/posterior distributions were apparent in ERP responses to the different types of words. At 13 months of age, the effects of word comprehension were apparent over anterior and posterior regions of both the left and right hemispheres. However, at 20 months of age, these effects occurred only over temporal and parietal regions of the left hemisphere. This increasing specialization of language-relevant systems was not solely dependent on chronological age. Comparisons of children of the same age who differed in size of vocabulary demonstrated that language experience and knowledge were strongly predictive of the maturity of cerebral organization; 13-month-old infants with large vocabularies displayed more focal left temporal/parietal effects of word meaning than did those with small vocabularies.

A similar effect is found in the development of the differential processing of open and closed class words. We compared ERPs to open and closed class words in infants and young children from 20 to 42 months of age (Mills *et al.*, 1997; Neville and Mills, 1997). All children understood and produced both the open and closed class words presented. At 20 months, ERPs in response to open and closed class words did not differ (see Fig. 5). However, both types of words elicited ERPs that differed from those elicited by unknown and backward words. These data suggest that in the earliest stages of language development, when children are typically speaking in single-word utterances or beginning to put two words together, open and closed class words elicit similar patterns of brain activity. At 28–30 months of age, when children typically begin to speak in short phrases, ERPs to open and closed class words elicited different patterns of brain activity.

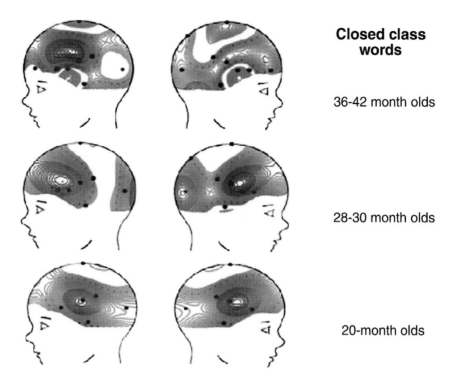

Closed class words

36-42 month olds

28-30 month olds

20-month olds

FIGURE 5 Current source density (CSD) analyses of neural activity to closed class words at 200 msec. The CSDs illustrate sinks (i.e., activity flowing into the head, shown in purple) and sources (i.e., activity flowing out of the head, shown in orange), at three age groups. At 36–42 months the CSD shows a sink over left anterior regions. At 28–30 months the CSD shows sinks that are bilateral but slightly more prominent over the right compared to the left hemisphere. At 20 months the CSD shows sinks over both the left and the right hemispheres (from Neville and Mills, 1997). (See color plates.)

However, the more mature left-hemisphere asymmetry to closed class words was not observed. By 36 months of age most children speak in sentences and use closed class words appropriately to specify grammatical relations and, like adults, ERPs from 36-month-old children displayed a left-hemisphere asymmetry to closed class words. The results across the three age groups are consistent with the hypothesis that open and closed class words are processed initially by similar brain systems and that these systems become progressively specialized with increasing language experience. Further evidence on this hypothesis comes from an examination of ERPs from children who were the same age but who differed in language abilities. The 20-month-old children who scored below

the 50th percentile for vocabulary size did not show ERP differences to open and closed class words. In contrast, those with vocabulary sizes above the 50th percentile displayed ERP differences to open and closed class words that were similar to the 28- to 30-month-old patterns. These data strongly suggest that the organization of brain activity is linked to language abilities rather than to chronological age.

Across these studies we have shown that the cerebral organization of language is the product of interactions between biological constraints and language experience across the life span, as has been described for many other systems in developmental biology. Left-hemisphere involvement in language processing appears to be highly biologically determined and is relatively unaffected by language modality. However, markedly different language experience, such as learning a manual, spatial language as one's native language, recruits the right hemisphere into language processing to an extent not observed in spoken and written languages. These results suggest that the nature of the language input, in this case the co-occurrence of location and motion information with language, shapes the organization of the language systems of the brain. Finally, the developmental data illustrate the role of language abilities in establishing the canonical organization of the language systems of the brain. Thus, similar principles govern the development and organization of neural systems important in perception and language.

SUMMARY

Factors That Influence the Development and Plasticity of Neurocognitive Systems

The studies reviewed in this chapter illustrate that the development of neurocognitive systems is influenced by factors both intrinsic and extrinsic to the child. For example, evidence of a left-hemisphere asymmetry for language processing and a right-hemisphere asymmetry for face processing is observed early in development. However, the left-hemisphere asymmetry for language appears to be driven, at least in early development, by the accumulation of words in the vocabulary. The right-hemisphere asymmetry for faces does not reach an adultlike profile until well into puberty. Although these features of language and face processing may be relatively stable in the face of atypical experience, other aspects of perception and cognition display greater plasticity. Right-hemisphere involvement is more heavily recruited with early acquisition of a signed language. Attention to peripheral space is heightened by both auditory and visual

deprivation, but attention to central space is not. Processing along the dorsal visual stream is enhanced following auditory deprivation, but processing along the ventral stream is not. These complexities reveal the need for careful characterization of developmental events within the specific neurocognitive systems and subsystems.

The variation in the effects of atypical experience may be due, in part, to differing rates of development across neural regions and neurocognitive systems. This fact has important consequences for plasticity and development because different types of atypical early experience may affect early developing, as compared to late-developing, systems differently. Systems that undergo an early and short sensitive period are strongly affected, both structurally and functionally, by atypical early experience. For example, binocular vision requires competing input from the two eyes in order for ocular dominance columns to be set up normally in primary visual cortex (Wiesel and Hubel, 1965; Tychsen, 2001). If input to one eye is disrupted within the first months of life, the pruning and branching necessary for ocular dominance columns does not occur to the extent that it does with normal, binocular input, and there are lifelong consequences for visual acuity even when input from the deprived eye is restored. In these systems with early and short sensitive periods, deprivation of the input necessary to lay down the basic wiring and function will prevent the typical developmental outcome from emerging. On the other hand, systems that undergo protracted periods of development may be less affected by acute atypical early experience if input is restored. If the developmental window is long enough, the restored input may be sufficient to establish relatively normal developmental outcomes. However, these systems with longer sensitive periods may be more affected by chronic atypical experience, even when the atypical experience is not thought of as "necessary." One example is the impact of auditory deprivation on visual functions. Although auditory input is not thought of as necessary in establishing the neural substrates of visual functions, deprivation of this input across the life span can have an impact on specific visual subsystems. In this case, when atypical input is provided throughout the developmental time course, this may be sufficient to induce plastic changes in the structure and function of these subsystems. We hypothesize that this is the case with the cross-modal developmental effects we report here.

In this chapter we have presented evidence that biological constraints and experience interact epigenetically to produce the neural substrates of perception and cognition. Further research is necessary to specify the different times in human development when particular types of input are required for optimal development of the many systems and subsystems important in cognition and perception and to understand to what degree these systems are modifiable by atypical experience and the mechanisms that underlie and permit this modifiability.

References

Allison, T., Ginter, H., McCarthy, G., Nobre, A. C., Puce, A., Luby, M., and Spencer, D. D. (1994). Face recognition in human extrastriate cortex. *J. Neurophysiol.* **71**, 821–825.

Allison, T., Puce, A., Spencer, D. D., and McCarthy, G. (1999). Electrophysiological studies of human face perception. I: Potentials generated in occipitotemporal cortex by face and non-face stimuli. *Cereb. Cortex* **9**, 415–430.

Alvarez, T. D., and Neville, H. J. (1995). The development of face discrimination continues into adulthood: An ERP study. *Soc. Neurosci. Abstr.* **21**, 2086.

Anderson, R. S., and O'Brien, C. (1997). Psychophysical evidence for a selective loss of M ganglion cells in glaucoma. *Vis. Res.* **37**(8), 1079–1083.

Armstrong, B., Neville, H., Hillyard, S., and Mitchell, T. (2002). Effects of auditory deprivation on motion and color processing. *Cogn. Brain Res.* (in review).

Aslin, R. N. (1987). Visual and auditory development in infancy. *In* "Handbook of Infant Development" (J. D. Osofsky, ed.), pp. 5–97. Wiley, New York.

Atkinson, J., King, J., Braddick, O., Nokes, L., Anker, S., and Braddick, F. (1997). A specific deficit of dorsal stream function in Williams' syndrome. *NeuroReport* **8**(8), 1919–1922.

Baenninger, M. (1994). The development of face recognition: Featural or configurational processing? *J. Exp. Child Psychol.* **57**, 377–396.

Bailey, D. B., Bruer, J. T., Symons, F. J., and Lichtman, J. W. (eds.) (2001). "Critical Thinking about Critical Periods: Perspectives from Biology, Psychology and Education." Paul H. Brookes Publ. Co., Baltimore.

Bavelier, D., Tomann, A., Hutton, C., Mitchell, T., Corina, D., Liu, G., and Neville, H. (2000). Visual attention to the periphery is enhanced in congenitally deaf individuals. *J. Neurosci.* **20**, RC93, 1–6.

Bavelier, D., Brozinsky, C., Tomann, A., Mitchell, T., Neville, H., and Liu, G. (2001). Impact of early deafness and early exposure to sign language on the cerebral organization for motion processing. *J. Neurosci.* **21**(22), 8931–8942.

Bellugi, U., Lichtenberger, L., Mills, D., Galaburda, A., and Korenberg, J. R. (1999). Bridging cognition, the brain and molecular genetics: Evidence from Williams syndrome. *Trends Neurosci.* **22**(5), 197–207.

Bellugi, U., Lichtenberger, L., Jones, W., Lai, Z., and St. George, M. (2000). The neurocognitive profile of Williams Syndrome: A complex pattern of strengths and weaknesses. *J. Cogn. Neurosci.* **12**(Suppl. 1), 7-29.

Bentin, S., Allison, T., Puce, A., Perez, E., and McCarthy, G. (1996). Electrophysiological studies of face perception in humans. *J. Cogn. Neurosci.* **8**, 551–565.

Carey, S., and Diamond, R. (1994). Are faces perceived as configurations more by adults than children? *Vis. Cogn.* **1**, 253–274.

Chalupa, L., and Dreher, B. (1991). High precision systems require high precision 'blueprints': a new view regarding the formation of connections in the mammalian visual system. *J. Cogn. Neurosci.* **3**, 209–219.

de Haan, M., and Nelson, C. A. (1997). Recognition of the mother's face by six-month-old infants: A neurobehavioral study. *Child Dev.* **68**(2), 187–210.

de Haan, M., and Nelson, C. A. (1999). Brain activity differentiates face and object processing in 6-month-old infants. *Dev. Psychol.* **35**(4), 1113–1121.

Dehaene, S., Dupoux, E., Mehler, J., Cohen, L., Paulesu, E., Perani, D., van de Moortele, P. F., Lehericy, S., and Le Bihan, D. (1997). Anatomical variability in the cortical representation of first and second language. *NeuroReport* **8**(17), 3809–3815.

Demb, J. B., Boynton, G. M., and Heeger, D. J. (1998). Functional magnetic resonance imaging of early visual pathways in dyslexia. *J. Neurosci.* **18**(17), 6939–6951.

de Schonen, S., and Mathivet, E. (1990). Hemispheric asymmetry in a face discrimination task in infants. *Child Dev.* **61**, 1192–1205.

Dobkins, K. R., Anderson, C. M., and Lia, B. (1999). Infant temporal contrast sensitivity functions (tCSFs) mature earlier for luminance than for chromatic stimuli: Evidence for precocious magnocellular development? *Vis. Res.* **39**(19), 3223–3239.

Downing, C. J., and Pinker, S. (eds.) (1985). "Attention and Performance." Erlbaum Assoc., Hillsdale, New Jersey.

Eden, G. F., VanMeter, J. W., Rumsey, J. M., Maisog, J. M., Woods, R. P., and Zeffiro, T. A. (1996). Abnormal processing of visual motion in dyslexia revealed by functional brain imaging. *Nature* **382**(6586), 66–69.

Eggermont, J. J. (1988). On the rate of maturation of sensory evoked potentials. *Electroencephalogr. Clin. Neurophysiol.* **70**, 293–305.

Falchier, A., Renaud, L., Barone, P., and Kennedy, H. (2001). Extensive projections from the primary auditory cortex and polysensory area stp to peripheral area V1 in the macaque. *Soc. Neurosci. Abstr.* **27**, S11.21.

Fantz, R. (1963). Pattern vision in newborn infants. *Science* **140**, 296–297.

Frodl, T., Meisenzahl, E. M., Muller, D., Leinsinger, G., Juckel, G., Hahn, K., Moller, H. J., and Hegerl, U. (2001). The effect of the skull on event-related P300. *Clin. Neurophysiol.* **112**, 1173–1176.

Hickey, T. L. (1977). Postnatal development of the human lateral geniculate nucleus: Relationship to a critical period for the visual system. *Science* **198**, 836–838.

Huttenlocher, P. R., and Dabhoklar, A. S. (1997). Regional differences in synaptogenesis in human Cerebral cortex. *J. Comp. Neurol.* **387**, 167–178.

Kanwisher, N., and McDermott, J., Chun, M. (1997). The fusiform face area: A module in human extrastriate cortex specialized for face perception. *J. Neurosci.* **17**, 4302-4311.

Kim, K. H. S., Relkin, N. R., Lee, K.M., and Hirsch, J. (1997). Distinct cortical areas associated with native and second languages. *Nature* **388**, 171-174.

Klima, E. S., and Bellugi, U. (1988). "The Signs of Language." Harvard University Press, Cambridge, Massachusetts.

Maunsell, J. H. R., and Newsome, W. T. (1987). Visual processing in monkey extrastriate cortex. *Annu. Rev. Neurosci.* **10**, 363-401.

Maunsell, J. H., and van Essen, D. C. (1983). The connections of the middle temporal visual area (MT) and their relationship to a cortical hierarchy in the macaque monkey. *J. Neurosci.* **3**(12), 2563-2586.

McCarthy, G. (2001). Physiological studies of face processing in humans. "The New Cognitive Neurosciences" (M. S. Gazzaniga, ed.), pp. 393-409. MIT Press, Cambridge, Massachusetts.

McCarthy, G., Puce, A., Belger, A., and Allison, T. (1999). Electrophysiological studies of human face perception. II: Response properties of face-specific potentials generated in occipitotemporal cortex. *Cereb. Cortex* **9**, 431-444.

Mills, D. L., Coffey-Corina, S. A., and Neville, H. J. (1993). Language acquisition and cerebral specialization in 20-month-old infants. *J. Cogn. Neurosci.* **5**(3), 317–334.

Mills, D. L., Coffey-Corina, S., and Neville, H. J. (1997). Language comprehension and cerebral specialization from 13 to 20 months. *Dev. Neuropsychol.* **13**(3), 397-445.

Mills, D. L., Alvarez, T. D., St. George, M., Appelbaum, L. G., Bellugi, U., and Neville, H. (2000). Electrophysiological studies of face processing in Williams Syndrome. *J. Cogn. Neurosci.* **12** (Suppl.), 47-64.

Mitchell, T. V. (1996). "How Audition Shapes Visual Attention". *Department of Psychology*, Indiana University, Bloomington.

Mitchell, T., and Neville, H. (1999). The electrophysiology of motion and color perception from early school years to adulthood. *Soc. Res. Child Dev.*

Mitchell, T., and Neville, H. J. (2002). Asynchrony in the development of electrophysiological responses to motion and color. In preparation.

Mitchell, T. V., and Quittner, A. L. (1996). A multimethod study of attention and behavior problems in hearing-impaired children. *J. Clin. Child Psychol.* **25**, 83-96.

Mitchell, T. V., and Smith, L. B. (1996). Deafness drives development of attention to change. "Proceedings of the Eighteenth Annual Conference of the Cognitive Science Society." Erlbaum Assoc., Hillsdale, New Jersey.

Mondor, T. A., and Zatorre, R. J. (1995). Shifting and focusing auditory spatial attention. *J. Exp. Psychol. Hum. Percept. Perform.* **211**, 387-409.

Morton, J., and Johnson, M. H. (1991). CONSPEC and CONLERN: A two-process theory of infant face recognition. *Psychol. Rev.* **98**(2), 164-181.

Neville, H. J. (1998). Human brain development. "Fundamental neuroscience" (M. Posner and L. Ungerleider, eds.). Academic Press, New York.

Neville, H. J., and Lawson, D. (1987). Attention to central and peripheral space in a movement detection task: An event-related potential and behavioral study. II. Congenitally deaf adults. *Brain Res.* **405**, 268-283.

Neville, H. J., and Mills, D. L. (1997). Epigenesis of language. *Mental Retard. Dev. Disabil. Res. Rev.* **3**(4), 282-292.

Neville, H. J., Nicol, J., Barss, A., Forster, K., and Garrett, M. (1991). Syntactically based sentence classes: Evidence from event-related brain potentials. *J. Cogn. Neurosci.* **3**: 155-170.

Neville, H. J., Mills, D. L., and Lawson, D. S. (1992). Fractionating language: Different neural subsystems with different sensitive periods. *Cereb. Cortex* **2**(3), 244-258.

Neville, H. J., Coffey, S. A., Lawson, D. S., Fischer, A., Emmorey, K., and Bellugi, U. (1997). Neural systems mediating American Sign Language: effects of sensory experience and age of acquisition. *Brain Lang.* **57**(3), 285-308.

Neville, H. J., Bavelier, D., Corina, D., Rauschecker, J., Karni, A., Lalwani, A., Braun, A., Clark, V., Jezzard, P., and Turner, R. (1998). Cerebral organization for language in deaf and hearing subjects: Biological constraints and effects of experience. *Proc. Natl. Acad. Sci. U.S.A* **95**(3), 922-929.

Newman, A. J., Bavelier, D., Corina, D., Jezzard, and P., Neville, H.J. (2002). A critical period for right hemisphere recruitment in American Sign Language processing. *Nat. Neurosci.* **5**(1), 76-80.

Nobre, A. C., and McCarthy, G. (1994). Language-related ERPs: Scalp distributions and modulation by word type and semantic priming. *J. Cogn. Neurosci.* **6**, 233-255.

Osterhout, L., McLaughlin, J., and Bersick, M. (1997). Event-related brain potentials and human language. *Trends Cogn. Sci.* **1**(6), 203-209.

Perani, D., Dehaene, S., Grassi, F., Cohen, L., Cappa, S. F., Dupoux, E., Fazio, F., and Mehler, J. (1996). Brain processing of native and foreign languages. *NeuroReport* **7**(15–17), 2439–2444.

Puce, A., Allison, T., Gore, J., andMcCarthy, G. (1995). Face-sensitive regions in human extrastriate cortex studied by functional MRI. *J. Neurophysiol.* **74**, 1192-1199.

Puce, A., Allison, T., and McCarthy, G. (1999). Electrophysiological studies of human face perception. III: Effects of top-down processing on face-specific potentials. *Cereb. Cortex* **9**, 445-458.

Quigley, H. A., Dunkelberger, G. R., and Green, W. R. (1989). Retinal ganglion cell atrophy correlated with automated perimetry in human eyes with glaucoma. *Am. J. Opthalmol.* **107**(5), 453-464.

Quittner, A. L., Smith, L. B., Osberger, M. J., Mitchell, T. V., and Katz, D. B. (1994). The impact of audition on the development of visual attention. *Psychol. Sci.* **5**(6), 347-353.

Rettenbach, R., Diller, G., and Sireteanu, R. (1999). Do deaf people see better? Texture segmentation and visual search compensate in adult but not in juvenile subjects. *J. Cogn. Neurosci.* **11**(5), 560-583.

Rockland, K. S., and Ojima, H. (2001). Calcarine area V1 as a multimodal convergence area. *Soc. Neurosci. Abstr.* **27**, S11.20.

Röder, B., Teder-Salejarvi, W., Sterr, A., Rosler, F., Hillyard, S. A., and Neville, H. J. (1999). Improved auditory spatial tuning in blind humans. *Nature* **400**, 162-166.

Rodman, H. R. (1994). Development of inferior temporal cortex in the monkey. *Cereb. Cortex* **5**, 484-498.

Rodman, H. R., Skelly, J. P., and Gross, C. G. (1991). Stimulus selectivity and state dependence of activity in inferior temporal cortical visual areas of infant monkeys. *Proc. Natl. Acad. Sci. U.S.A.* **88**, 7572-7575.

Rodman, H. R., and O'Scalaidhe, S. P., and Gross, C. G. (1993). Visual response properties of neurons in temporal cortical visual areas of infant monkeys. *J. Neurophysiol.* **70**, 1115-1136.

Sergent, J., Ohta, S., and MacDonald, B. (1992). Functional neuroanatomy of face and object processing: A positron emission tomography study. *Brain* **115**, 15-36.

Starr, A., Amlie, R. N., Martin, W. H., and Sanders, S. (1977). Development of auditory function in newborn infants revealed by auditory brainstem potentials. *Pediatrics* **60**, 831-838.

Stein, J., and Walsh, V. (1997). To see but not to read. The magnocellular theory of dyslexia. *Trends Neurosci.* **20**(4), 147–152.

Taylor, M. J., McCarthy, G., Saliba, E., and Degiovanni, E. (1999). ERP evidence of developmental changes in processing of faces. *Clin. Neurophysiol.* **110**, 910-915.

Taylor, M. J., Edmonds, G. E., McCarthy, G., and Allison, T. (2001). Eyes first! Eye processing develops before face processing in children. *NeuroReport* **12**(8), 1671-1676.

Teder-Salejarvi, W. A., Hillyard, S., Roder, B., Neville, H.J. (1999). Spatial attention to central and peripheral auditory stimuli as indexed by event-related potentials (ERPs). *Cogn. Brain Res.* **8**(3), 213-227.

Tychsen, L. (2001). Critical periods for development of visual acuity, depth perception and eye tracking. In "Critical Thinking about Critical Periods: Perspectives from Biology, Psychology and Education" (D. B. Bailey, J. T., Bruer, F. J., Symons, and J. W. Lichtman, eds.) pp. 67-80. Paul H. Brookes Publ. Co., Baltimore.

Ungerleider, L. G., and Haxby, J. V. (1994). "What" and "where" in the human brain. *Cur. Opin. Neurobiol.* **4**, 157-165.

Ungerleider, L. G., and Mishkin, M. (1982). Two cortical visual systems. In "Analysis of Visual Behavior" (M. A. G. D. J. Ingle, and R. J. W. Mansfield, eds.), pp. 579-586. MIT Press, Cambridge, Massachusetts.

Vaughan, H. G., and Kurtzberg, D. (1992). Electrophysiologic indices of human brain maturation and cognitive development. In "Developmental Behavioral Neuroscience: The Minnesota

Symposia on Child Psychology" (M. A. Gunnar, and C. A. Nelson, eds.), Vol. 24, pp. 1–36. Erlbaum Assoc., Hillsdale, New Jersey.

Weber-Fox, C., and Neville, H. J. (1996). Maturational constraints on functional specializations for language processing: ERP and behavioral evidence in bilingual speakers. *J. Cogn. Neurosci.* **8**(3), 231–256.

Wiesel, T. N., and Hubel, D. H. (1965). Comparison of the effects of unilateral and bilateral eye closure on cortical unit responses in kittens. *J. Neurophysiol.* **28**(6), 1029-1040.

NEURAL MECHANISMS OF SELECTIVE ATTENTION

10

Neural Mechanisms
of Attention

George R. Mangun

INTRODUCTION

Evolution has crafted powerful brain mechanisms for attending and ignoring objects and events in the visual environment. The consequences of these mechanisms include alterations in the perceptual processing of otherwise equivalent visual inputs. Whether these mechanisms involve top-down or bottom-up control over attention, they are engaged by innate mechanisms shaped by natural selection, learned strategies for survival, and the momentary pressures to interact efficiently with a complex world. An elementary form of visual selective attention is based upon location in the visual scene, and is termed *spatial attention* (e.g., Posner, 1980).

The properties of spatial attention have been contemplated for hundreds of years, and experimental observations can be traced back at least to the end of the nineteenth century. Herman Von Helmholtz, the great German scientist, dabbled in studies of visual spatial attention. In a series of studies aimed at investigating the limits of perception, Helmholz sought to determine how much information could be derived from the brief presentation of a complex display. In one study he built a crude tachistoscope by using a battery to create a brief flash of light (spark) that illu-minated an otherwise dark scene. The scene Helmholtz constructed was of a series of letters painted onto a sheet hung at one end of his lab. When he triggered the spark in the dark it provided a short lived illumination of the sheet of letters. Helmholtz quickly realized that he had difficulty accurately perceiving all the letters on the sheet during one brief illumination. But he was able to perceive the letters accurately in one portion of the screen, and moreover, he discovered that if he decided which portion of the sheet of letters to attend to in advance, then he could perceive those letters, but had trouble perceiving letters at other locations. Importantly, this could be done without moving his eyes around the screen; he maintained fixation on a central pinhole illumination on the screen. That is, Helmholtz invoked what we now call *covert visual attention* to a region of the sheet of letters. Helmholtz wrote about his observations in these experiments, and in his book "Treatise on Physiological Optics" (1924), he commented that "by a voluntary kind of intention, even without eye movements, ... one can concentrate attention on the sensation from a particular part of our peripheral nervous system and at the same time exclude attention from all other parts."

Helmholtz and others of his era, such as American psychologist William James, were apt at describing the phenomena of attention, but provided little support for their views through direct experimental tests. It was not until the middle of the next century that researchers began successfully to quantify attention effects on stimulus processing. One particularly successful approach involves the chronometric method. By measuring the time it takes to respond to a target stimulus when it occurs at attended versus unattended regions of visual space, it has been possible to quantify precisely spatial attention effects, as reflected in performance. For example, Posner and colleagues (Posner *et al.*, 1980) used target-location expectancy to manipulate spatial attention, and then acquired reaction times (RTs) to expected-location targets and compared those to the same targets when they occurred at unexpected locations. The paradigm that has been modified and used in hundreds of studies over the past 30 years is shown in Fig. 1.

In trial-by-trial spatial cuing paradigms subjects receive a cue, in this case an arrow at fixation, that indicates the most likely location (right or left field) of a subsequent target stimulus. The cue predicts the arrow with some high probability, such as 0.80 (valid trials). The remaining trials include incorrect (invalid) cues/targets (e.g., the arrow points left but the target occurs on the right), and may also include so-called neutral trials in which the cue does not predict the location of the target (under these conditions the cues might consist of double-headed arrows or other nonpredictive symbols). Posner and colleagues found that reaction times were significantly faster in response to targets appearing at precued locations in comparison to targets at uncued locations. They interpreted these effects to be evidence for early selection models of attention, models that posit that selection could occur prior to complete stimulus analysis. However, these methods do not permit the mechanisms of attention to be unambiguously related to specific stages of information processing. In order to investigate early stages of sensory analysis directly, many researchers have turned to physiological methods in humans and animals.

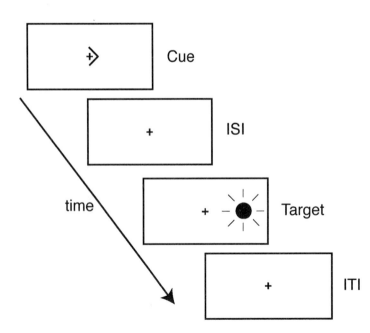

FIGURE 1 Posner cuing paradigms. An arrow presented at fixation predicts the most likely location of an impending target stimulus that follows several hundred milliseconds later. Displayed is a so-called valid trial in which the cue accurately predicts the location of the upcoming target.

ELECTROPHYSIOLOGICAL MEASURES OF SPATIAL ATTENTION

In studies in humans, event-related brain potentials have been used to investigate what stage(s) of information processing could be influenced by top-down attentional factors. We investigated the neural bases of the spatial cuing effects in healthy persons using event-related potentials (ERPs) in a series of studies (Mangun *et al.*, 1987; Mangun and Hillyard, 1991). The logic was that using ERPs we could provide indices of information processing in the human visual system at various early (sensory) and later (postperceptual and decision) stages of processing, and then could investigate whether stimuli that were precued (and elicited speeded reaction times) also showed faster or more robust sensory responses.

The design used in our studies followed that of Posner and colleagues (1980). Each trial began with an arrow, presented at fixation for 200 msec, that pointed to either the left or right visual field. Following each arrow by about 800 msec was a lateralized target (a briefly flashed vertical bar). The arrow indicated the side on which the target would occur with high probability (0.75), but on some (0.25) of the trials the target occurred in the opposite visual field location (invalid trial). This spatial priming paradigm produces an "endogenous orienting," because attention is directed by voluntary processes. Voluntary orienting is to be contrasted with "exogenous orienting" in which attention is captured reflexively to the location of a sensory signal (e.g., Klein *et al.*, 1992). We shall return to a discussion of reflexive attention below.

As noted, precuing by predictive cues has been shown to lead to faster reaction times to precued targets. If such effects are due to changes in the perceptual processing of validly and invalidly cued targets, then the early sensory-evoked ERP components should show expectancy-related (attention-related) changes in either amplitude or latency. If, on the other hand, the cuing effects on RT are the result of changes in decision and/or response bias, then one would expect stability of those early ERP components that reflect the sensory-perceptual stages of processing, and instead, changes in the longer latency ERP components related to decision or

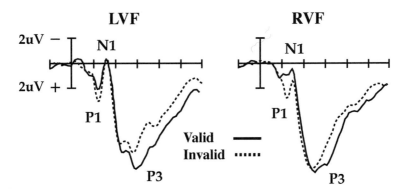

FIGURE 2 Modulations of ERPs with voluntary attention, showing group-average visual ERPs recorded to target stimuli in a trial-by-trial spatial cuing paradigm like that illustrated in Fig. 1. Modulations of the sensory evoked P1 component can be seen at right and left occipital scalp sites. When a left field stimulus (LVF) was corrected, indicated by the preceding vertical bar cue, the P1 at contralateral (right) occipital scalp sites was larger (solid more positive than dotted) from 90 to 130 msec after the onset of the target stimulus. Negative voltage is plotted upward, and stimulus onset occurs at the vertical calibration bar in each plot. After Mangun and Hillyard (1991).

action. We found that when a simple speeded response to target onset was required, an early sensory response in the ERPs (P1) was larger in peak amplitude when the evoking stimulus had been precued (Fig. 2). In other experiments, we also observed that the later N1 component (180 msec) could also be modulated when the task required discrimination of the target features (i.e., height judgment of a bar stimulus). These effects were not the result of eye movements toward the cued location because the eyes remained fixed at a central fixation point, and eye movements were rigorously monitored.

These amplitude modulations of early visual ERP components produced by trial-by-trial cuing are similar, if not identical, to those observed in tasks in which attention is sustained on a single visual field location throughout a block of trials while comparable stimuli are flashed to that location and other unattended locations in the visual field (e.g., Eason et al., 1969; Eason 1981; Van Voorhis and Hillyard, 1977). Such effects have been interpreted as evidence that early sensory processing is affected by spatially directed attention (e.g., Eason, 1981; Mangun, 1995). Thus, the evidence obtained in the trial-by-trial cuing experiment is consistent with the proposal of Posner and others that expectancy-induced facilitation of reaction time might be the result of improvements in early sensory and perceptual processing.

These data do not, however, tell us whether the effects observed in behavioral studies of spatial priming are causally dependent on early selection mechanisms. For example, it is possible that the reaction time effects of Posner and others might result from changes in decision and response criteria alone (Luck et al., 1994), or that other factors such as perceptual load might influence the relationship between physiological mechanisms and behavioral effects (e.g., Handy, 2000; Handy et al., 2001; Lavie and Tsal, 1994). Nonetheless, the finding of amplitude modulations of

ERP components with as short a latency as 80–100 msec poststimulus during expectancy-based cuing strongly suggests a link between sensory-perceptual sensitivity and RT effects. Thus, these data converge with behavioral findings of changes in perceptual sensitivity (d') for precued targets (e.g., Hawkins et al., 1990; Luck et al., 1994) and provide information about human neural mechanisms and levels of information processing involved in attentional processing that is consistent with studies in animals (e.g., McAdams and Maunsell, 1999; Moran and Desimone, 1985).

LOCUS OF SELECTION

It remains unclear precisely how early, during visual processing, top-down attention influences may be manifest; however, most selective processes appear to be operating at the cortical sensory level. Whether this can occur at the level of primary sensory cortex to act on the incoming sensory signal is still under debate. Some studies have reported that attention can influence processing in V1 (striate cortex) during spatial [e.g., McAdams and Maunsell (1999) and Motter (1993)—in monkeys] and nonspatial attention [e.g., Zani and Proverbio (1995)—in humans], but the electrophysiological findings to date remain inconsistent with other workers arguing against effects in striate cortex for visual attention (e.g., Clark and Hillyard, 1996; Heinze et al., 1994; Luck et al., 1997; Mangun et al., 1993). In part, some of the difficulty in understanding where in sensory processing attention may influence perceptual analyses comes from the fact that it is difficult to localize where in the brain a particular scalp-recorded ERP is generated; this will be discussed in detail later.

Some neuroimaging data in humans suggest that changes in neuronal processing in striate cortex may occur with selective attention (e.g., Tootell *et al.*, 1998), but these findings do not specify the time course of the activations. As a result it is not clear whether evidence of neuronal activations in striate cortex during attention reflect gating of stimulus inputs or changes in longer latency activity mediated by reafferent (top-down) modulations of striate neurons (e.g., Martinez *et al.*, 1999; see also Roelfsema *et al.*, 1998). Similarly, there is no evidence at present for subcortical modulations of ascending sensory inputs in the lateral geniculate nucleus during selective attention, although subcortical systems are clearly influenced by attention, and may participate in attentional control circuitry. For example, the pulvinar nucleus of the thalamus, though not a sensory relay nucleus per se, is known to have visually responsive neurons that are affected by attention (see Posner and Petersen, 1990; LaBerge, 1995).

REFLEXIVE ATTENTIONAL ORIENTING

Attention can be directed by voluntary, top-down processes (Kastner and Ungerleider, 2000), but may also be "captured" by sensory events. This automatic orienting of attention has been called reflexive (or exogenous) to indicate that control over attention was externally controlled (e.g., Posner *et al.*, 1980). These two types of attentional orienting have been shown to have different characteristics. Top-down voluntary attention leads to a facilitation in response times, accuracy, and sensory-evoked ERP components for attended-location stimuli, and these are not manifest until some time after the decision to orient. In the case of voluntary orienting to a symbolic cue (arrow), this may take more than 250 msec from cue onset. Some of this time involves that required to decode the cue information and then to orient attention.

Reflexive orienting also leads to faster and more accurate behavioral responses to stimuli at previously cued locations, but the effects occur more rapidly than for voluntarily oriented attention. Reflexive attention shifts may begin by 50 msec after an attention-capturing event, and compared to the effects of voluntary attention, reflexive orienting is more resistant to interference and dissipates more quickly (e.g., Cheal and Lyon, 1991; Jonides, 1981; Müller and Rabbitt, 1989). That is, the facilitation in reaction times at a reflexively cued location is replaced by inhibition at that same cued location, by a few hundred milliseconds after cue onset (e.g., Posner and Cohen, 1984). This phenomenon, known as inhibition of return (IOR), may facilitate the ability efficiently to reorient attention away from potentially distracting events (Posner and Cohen, 1984).

These differences between voluntary and reflexive attention may indicate that reflexive attention is controlled by separate neural systems from those controlling top-down voluntary attention (e.g., Kustov and Robinson, 1996; Rafal, 1996). Given that voluntary attention involves modulations of visual sensory processing (reviewed above), one might ask whether there are any changes in the perceptual processing of visual stimuli as a result of reflexive shifts of attention.

We have demonstrated that reflexive attention is indeed able to modulate early visual processing at the same neural locus as voluntary attention (Hopfinger and Mangun, 1998). Targets were preceded by an uninformative flash (the "cue") at the same location (cued-location target) or opposite field location (uncued-location target). The subjects knew that the cue was completely uninformative of the location of the upcoming target, and therefore did not invoke any voluntary orienting in response to the cue. The cue-to-target interstimulus interval (ISI) ranges were either long or short in order to measure the rapid and changing time course of reflexive attention ("short" ISI = 34–234 msec; "long" ISI = 600–800 msec).

When the cue-to-target ISI was short (34–234 msec), targets at the cued location elicited visual ERPs with significantly enhanced amplitudes compared to targets at an uncued location (Fig. 3). This enhancement was observed for a positive polarity

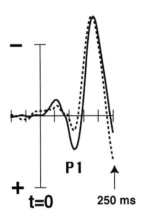

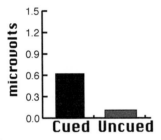

FIGURE 3 Modulations of ERPs with reflexive attention. Group-average visual ERPs to target stimuli from lateral occipital scalp sites (collapsed across left and right occipital sites when contralateral to the hemifield of the target stimulus). The P1 component was enhanced (solid line) when the eliciting target stimulus had been preceded recently at the same location by a brief sensory event (four location marking dots were turned off and on surrounding the location to which the target was subsequently presented). The amplitude changes in the P1 component are summarized in bar graphs; these amplitude differences were highly statistically significant. In order to remove the overlapping ERP potentials from cue to target at the short interstimulus interval (ISI) shown here, the ADJAR filter of Woldorff (1993) was employed to estimate and subtract away the ERPs to the cue from the ERPs to the target. After Hopfinger and Mangun (1998).

sensory ERP peak, the occipital P1 component. Topographic voltage maps during the time period of the P1 component showed that the location of the maximal response at the scalp corresponding to the P1 component was highly similar for cued- versus uncued-location targets (not shown in Fig. 3). This pattern is consistent with the view that the same neural process was invoked in both cases, with the primary difference being the strength of the response. Because the occipital P1 component represents the earliest stage of visual processing to be reliably modulated by *voluntary* spatial attention (e.g., Heinze et al., 1994; Mangun, 1995; Mangun and Hillyard, 1991), the present findings indicate that, although separate control circuitry may be involved, reflexive attention leads to modulations at this same stage of visual cortical processing.

In line with the reflexive cuing literature using reaction times, the longer cue-to-target ISI's (566–766 msec), showed the effect of the cues on the P1 component was reversed—targets at cued locations now elicited significantly smaller responses than did targets at uncued-locations (see Hopfinger and Mangun, 1998). This pattern is similar to that of reaction time IOR; however, in this study, it was actually the case that no differences were found in RTs, at the long ISIs. Moreover, in a follow-up study in which subjects speeded the reactions to the reflexively cued targets (rather than the discrimination required here), at long ISIs, the P1 showed no IOR-like pattern, but reaction times did (Hopfinger and Mangun, 2001). Thus, because of P1 and the reaction time, it is premature to suggest that IOR, as defined by reaction time inhibition, is related to the inhibition sometimes seen in the P1 at long ISIs. Nonetheless, the highly consistent findings for the short ISI facilitation effects on P1 indicate that when attention is reflexively captured by a sensory event, cortical visual processing is modulated at the same or similar stage of visual processing as the shortest latency effects of voluntary attention.

LOCALIZATION OF VOLUNTARY ATTENTION PROCESSES

The recording of ERPs from human scalps provides a powerful means for tracking the time course and, to some extent, the functional anatomy of brain attentional processes. However, limitations in the anatomical resolution of scalp-recorded ERPs make it difficult to infer functional anatomy with precision. For example, whether ERPs showing attention effects are generated in striate versus extrastriate cortex has proved to be a difficult question to answer (see section above Locus of Selection). What are the limitations in scalp recordings, and how can these limitations be overcome?

Modeling ERP Generators

Studies of the intracranial generators of scalp-recorded ERPs all suffer from the same general limitation—the recordings are being made relatively far from their site of generation. Active neurons in the brain are causing currents to flow passively through the tissues of the brain, skull, and scalp, where they can be recorded. Thus, tiny signals deep in the brain can become visible to us as they are passively conducted to the surface of the scalp. However, this fact also creates some difficulties for estimating where in the brain an ERP is generated. That is, one cannot assume that the brain tissue directly underneath a recording electrode has generated the recorded signal.

Another aspect of the problem stems from what is known as the "inverse problem." The inverse problem refers to the difficulty that exists in inferring the brain generators of scalp activity based on the pattern of voltages over the scalp (given some assumptions about generator configuration, head and brain structure, and conductivity). Although a given distribution of charges inside the head specifies a unique pattern on the scalp (the so-called forward solution), the inverse is not true. A particular pattern on the scalp might be caused by a large number of possible configurations of currents flowing inside the volume of the head. Thus, no unique solution can be obtained when going in the inverse direction from scalp recordings to neural generators. Although models can be derived from the exercise of inverse modeling, the concern remains that it is difficult to falsify such models.

If ERPs are not the method of choice of localization of brain activity, how can we achieve this localization while not losing the temporal advantage of ERPs? One approach is the integration of methods having complementary strengths for measuring the timing and localization of brain processes (e.g., Fox and Woldorff, 1994). For example, we have combined neuimaging using positron emission tomography (PET) or functional magnetic resonance imaging (fMRI) with ERP recordings in normal human subjects in several recent studies in order to investigate human brain attention mechanisms.

LOCALIZATION USING COMBINED ERP AND NEUROIMAGING

In three studies combining ERP recording and PET imaging (Heinze *et al.*, 1994; Mangun *et al.*, 1997, 2001), we investigated the neural mechanisms of visual spatial attention. Stimuli were flashed bilaterally in the visual field at a rate of about two per second, and subjects were instructed to focus attention selectively on the stimuli in one visual field in order to discriminate their features. The stimuli were nonsense symbols, two in each hemifield, and matching pairs of symbols at the attended

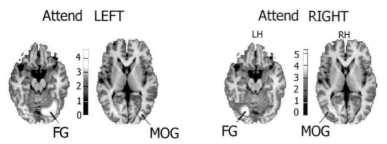

FIGURE 4   PET activations during spatial attention. Group-averaged changes in regional cerebral blood flow (activation) during attention to left versus right visual field stimuli (see text). The activations are overlaid onto horizontal sections of brain from MRI. The sections pass through ventral visual areas at lower slices on the left of the figure ($z = -16$), and at slightly higher slices on the right ($z = 4$). Activations in the hemisphere contralateral to the attended field were observed in the posterior fusiform gyrus (FG) and middle occipital gyrus (MOG). After Mangun *et al.* (1997).

location were targets that required a button press response.

In these studies we showed for the first time that spatial selective attention results in increased regional blood flow in extrastriate cortical areas in the hemisphere contralateral to the attended stimuli (Fig. 4). Modulations of occipital, sensory-evoked activity in the ERPs were also produced by spatial selective attention, in the same subjects performing the same task (Fig. 5).

The PET activations provided the possible locations and number of active cortical neurons that were related to attentional selection. This information was then incorporated as constraints for subsequent modeling of the ERP data, in order to permit us to ask whether electrical activity within the anatomical locus defined by PET imaging

could have generated the electrical patterns that were recorded from the scalp. These models are termed "seeded forward solutions," given that we placed (i.e., seeded) the model sources (equivalent current dipoles) at the PET-defined brain loci in the computer models.

Based on the evidence from Mangun *et al.* (1997), two candidate regions in each hemisphere were defined by functional imaging (see Fig. 4), it was possible to seed dipoles to either the fusiform gyrus or the middle occipital gyrus and to ask which of these produced the best forward-solution model of the recorded ERP data for any time range. For the modeling procedures we used a boundary element approach in a realistic head model (rather than a simpler spherical head model). The details of the

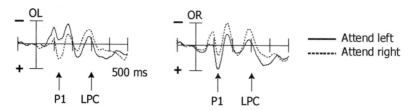

FIGURE 5   Attentional modulations of ERPs to bilateral stimuli. Grand-average visual ERPs to the bilateral stimulus arrays when the subjects attended the left half of the arrays and the right half of the arrays. The P1 and the longer latency range, the late positive component (LPC), are indicated. Attention to the left half of the array produced larger P1 components over the right hemisphere (top), whereas over the left hemispheres, larger P1 components were elicited by attention to the right. During the LPC latency range, attention to the left visual hemifield produces larger amplitude (more positive) components over both hemispheres. OL, Left occipital sites; OR, right occipital sites.

brain, skull, and scalp anatomy were derived from anatomical MR images of the subjects in the experiment, and then the ERP data were coregistered with the MR-derived realistic head model.

When dipoles were placed in the fusiform gyrus, the model provided a better explanation (lower residual variance) for the recorded data in the time range from 110 to 140 msec latency (P1 time range) than did placement of the dipoles in the more lateral brain PET activations in middle occipital gyrus. Interestingly, the reverse pattern was true for ERP activity in a later time range, that between 260 and 300 msec latency. In this time range of the ERP effects, the middle occipital gyrus dipoles produced a better model solution than did those in fusiform gyrus.

The relationship between the recorded and modeled data is illustrated in Fig. 6 as topographic maps. The topographies are displayed on the surface of the realistic head model viewed from the rear. Topographies of the model data are more similar to those of the recorded data in the time range 110–140 msec, when the dipoles were placed in the medial [fusiform gyrus (FG)] activation see Fig. 6; compare A (recorded) to B (modeled) data] than when place in the lateral [middle occipital gyrus (MOG) activation] (compare A and C, Fig. 6). Although the maps in Fig. 6C bear a superficial similarity to the recorded data, subtle differences in the magnitudes and scalp locations of maxima and minima can be discerned. The inverse pattern is the case for the longer latency effects, modeled here for the 260- to 300- msec latency range. The topography of the model data is more similar to that of the recorded data for dipoles place at the loci of the middle occipital gyrus activation (compare Daud

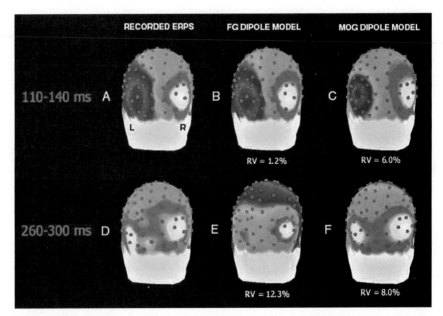

FIGURE 6 Recorded and model topographic maps of attention effects. Group-averaged topographic maps for recorded data (A and D), and model data for dipoles in fusiform gyrus (FG) only (B and E) or dipoles in middle occipital gyrus (MOG) only (C and F). The maps are for the time period of the P1 component (110–140 msec) in the D–F, and for the leading edge of the late positive component (260–300 msec) in A–C. See text for description. The difference between the recorded and model data expressed as percent residual variance (RV) is shown below each model head. The view of the heads is from the rear (left of brain, on left). Electrode locations are indicated by gray disks. (See color plates.)

F, Fig. 6) than when the dipoles are placed in the more medial, fusiform location (compare Daud E, Fig. 6). These findings support our prior conclusion that activity in the region of the fusiform location is related to attentional modulations of early sensory processing, and extend this result by showing that activations in more lateral regions of visual cortex are related to attention modulations at longer latencies, in line with the organization of the ventral visual processing stream (e.g., Tootell *et al.*, 1998).

Functional MRI

By taking advantage of the improved spatial resolution afforded by fMRI, our studies now look at covariations between ERPs and blood flow in single subjects (e.g., Mangun *et al.*, 1998). Fig. 7 shows data from six individual subjects in an attention paradigm similar to that described above. Subjects were alternately cued for 16-sec periods to attend to either the left half or the right half of bilaterally flashed stimulus arrays. The stimuli were nonsense symbols, and targets at the attended location were matching symbols. The brain sections in Fig. 7 are coronal sections of high-resolution anatomical MRIs with the statistically significant activations superimposed (correlations of voxel time series with a boxcar function that defined the attend-left and attend-right conditions). When the subjects attended the left field (keeping their eyes fixed centrally, as in all these studies) there were activated regions (yellow color) in the right hemisphere in the ventral visual cortex, and when they attended right these activations were primarily in the left hemisphere (red color). These data replicate closely the group-averaged PET effects shown in Fig. 4,

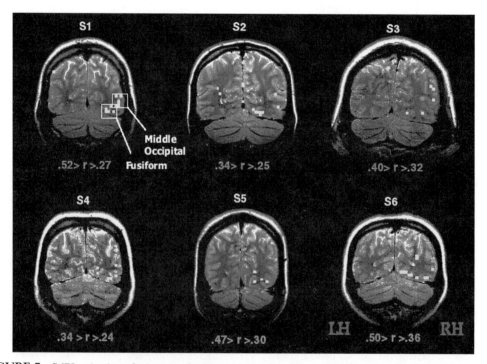

FIGURE 7   fMRI activations during visual attention in single subjects. Data from six volunteers during selective attention to bilateral stimulus arrays. See text for description. The correlation range for the correlation of voxel signal intensity and the attention conditions is shown below each coronal slice. Left of the brain is shown on the left of each image. (See color plates.)

although obtained in a very different manner. This approach could also be combined with electrical modeling, as we are doing, in order to provide fully integrated spatiotemporal models of visual analysis. The individual variations in brain anatomy and physiology that plague group approaches actually turn out to be an important source of information when working in individual subjects, because anatomy can be used to constrain dipole models for each subject as defined by their anatomical organization.

SUMMARY

Attention involves top-down processes that influence the gain of sensory transmission early in visual cortex. These effects observed in ERPs in humans are highly consistent with studies of single neuron recordings while monkeys attend and ignore visual stimuli. In a similar fashion, though presumably via different control circuitry, bottom-up reflexive control over attention can modulate visual cortical processing in humans. Neuroimaging can be brought to bear on the question of which brain structures are involved in attentional processing of visual signals, and when combined with ERP recordings, a detailed spatiotemporal model can be developed that permits a finer grained analysis of attentional selection than any single method. The view that emerges from the literature on human spatial attention indicates that within visual cortex, powerful modulations of incoming signals alter the scene one observes. Behavioral analyses tell us that these changes in visual brain processing have significant effects on how we perceive and respond to the world around us.

Acknowledgments

The author is grateful for the contributions of J. Hopfinger, M. Buonocore, M. Girelli, C. Kussmaul, M. Soltani, S. Rash, and Evan Fletcher to the work described here. Supported by grants from the NINDS, NIMH, and HFSP to G.R.M.

References

Cheal, M. L., and Lyon, D. R. (1991). Central and peripheral precuing of forced-choice discrimination. *Q. J. Exp. Psychol.* **43A**, 859–880.

Clark, V. P., and Hillyard, S. A. (1996). Spatial selective attention affects extrastriate but not striate components of the visual evoked potential. *J. Cogn. Neurosc.* **8**, 387–402.

Eason, R. G. (1981). Visual evoked potential correlates of early neural filtering during selective attention. *Bull. Psychonom. Soc.* **18**, 203–206.

Eason, R. G., Harter, M., and White, C. (1969). Effects of attention and arousal on visually evoked cortical potentials. *Physiol. Behav.* **4**, 283–289.

Fox, P., and Woldorff, M. (1994). Integrating human brain maps. *Curr. Opin. Neurobiol.* **4**, 151–156.

Handy, T. C. (2000). Capacity theory as a model of cortical behavior. *J. Cogn. Neurosc.* **12**, 1066–1069.

Handy, T. C., Soltani, M., and Mangun, G. R. (2001). Perceptual load and visuocortical processing: ERP evidence for sensory-level selection. *Psychol. Sci.* **12**, 213–218

Hawkins, H. L., Hillyard, S. A., Luck, S. J., Mouloua, M., Downing, C. J., and Woodward, D. P. (1990). Visual attention modulates signal detectability. *J. Exp. Psychol. Hum. Percept. Perform.* **16**, 802–811.

Heinze, H. J., Mangun, G. R., Burchert, W., Hinrichs, H., Scholz, M., Münte, T. F., Gös, A., Johannes, S., Scherg, M., Hundeshagen, H., Gazzaniga, M. S., and Hillyard, S. A. (1994). Combined spatial and temporal imaging of spatial selective attention in humans. *Nature* **392**, 543–546.

Hopfinger, J., and Mangun, G. R. (1998). Reflexive attention modulates processing of visual stimuli in human extrastriate cortex. *Psychol. Sci.* **9**, 441–447.

Hopfinger, J. B., and Mangun, G. R. (2001). Tracking the influence of reflexive attention on sensory and cognitive processing. *Cogn. Affect. Behav. Neurosci.* **1**, 56–65.

Jonides, J. (1981). Voluntary versus automatic control over the mind's eye movement. In "Attention and Performance IX" (J. B. Long, and A. D. Baddeley, eds.), pp. 187–203. Erlbaum Assoc., Hillsdale, New Jersey.

Kastner, S., and Ungerleider, L. (2000). Mechanisms of visual attention in the human cortex. *Annu. Rev. Neurosci.* **23**, 315–341.

Klein, R. M., Kingstone, A., and Pontefract, A. (1992). Orienting of visual attention. In "Eye Movements and Visual Cognition: Scene Perception and

Reading" (A. Raynor, ed. by), pp. 46–65. Springer-Verlag, New York.

Kustov, A. A., and Robinson, D. L. (1996). Shared neural control of attentional shifts and eye movements. *Nature* **384**, 74–77.

LaBerge, D. (1995). Computational and anatomical models of selective attention in object identification. In "The Cognitive Neurosciences" (M. Gazzaniga, ed.) , pp. 649–665. MIT Press, Cambridge, Massachusetts.

Lavie, N., and Tsal, Y. (1994). Perceptual load as a major determinant of the locus of selection in visual attention. *Percept. Psychophys.* **56**, 183–197.

Luck, S. J., Hillyard, S. A., Mouloua, M., Woldorff, M. G., Clark, V. P., and Hawkins, H. L. (1994). Effects of spatial cuing on luminance detectability: Psychophysical and electrophysiological evidence for early selection. *J. Exp. Psychol. Hum. Percept. Perform.* **20**, 887–904.

Mangun, G. R. (1995). Neural mechanisms of visual selective attention. *Psychophysiology* **32**, 4–18.

Mangun, G. R., and Hillyard, S. A. (1991). Modulations of sensory-evoked potentials indicate changes in perceptual processing during visual-spatial priming. *J. Exp. Psychol. Hum. Percept. Perform.* **17**, 1057–1074.

Mangun, G. R., Hansen, J. C., and Hillyard, S. A. (1987). The spatial orienting of attention: Sensory facilitation or response bias? In "Current Trends in Event-Related Potential Research" (R. Johnson, Jr., J. W. Rohrbaugh, and R. Parasuraman, eds.), pp. 118–124. Elsevier, Amsterdam.

Mangun, G. R., Hillyard, S. A., and Luck, S. J. (1993). Electrocortical substrates of visual selective attention. In "Attention and Performance XIV" (D. Meyer, and S. Kornblum, eds.), pp. 219–243. MIT Press, Cambridge, Massachusetts.

Mangun, G. R., Hopfinger, J., Kussmaul, C., Fletcher, E., and Heinze, H. J. (1997). Covariations in PET and ERP measures of spatial selective attention in human extrastriate visual cortex. *Hum. Brain Mapping* **5**, 273–279.

Mangun, G. R., Buonocore, M., Girelli, M. and Jha, A. (1998). ERP and fMRI measures of visual spatial selective attention. *Hum. Brain Mapping.* **6**, 383–389.

Mangun, G. R., Hinrichs, H., Scholz, M., Mueller-Gaertner, H. W., Herzog, H., Krause, B. J., Tellman, L., Kemna, L., and Heinze, H. J. (2001). Integrating electrophysiology and neuroimaging of spatial selective attention to simple isolated visual stimuli. *Vision Res.* **41**,1423–1435.

Martinez, A., Anllo-Vento, L., Sereno, M. I., Frank, L. R., Buxton, R. B., Dubowitz, D. J., Wong, E. C., Heinze, H. J., and Hillyard, S. A. (1999). Involvement of striate and extrastriate visual corti-cal areas in spatial attention. *Nat. Neurosci.* **2**, 364–369.

McAdams, C. J., and Maunsell, J. H. R. (1999). Effects of attention on orientation-tuning functions of single neurons in macaque cortical area V4. *J. Neurosci.* **19**, 431–441.

Moran, J., and Desimone, R. (1985). Selective attention gates visual processing in the extrastriate cortex. *Science* **229**, 782–784.

Motter, B. C. (1993). Focal attention produces spatially selective processing in visual cortical areas V1, V2 and V4 in the presence of competing stimuli. *J. Neurophysiol.* **70**, 909–919.

Müller, H. J., and Rabbitt, P. M. (1989). Reflexive and voluntary orienting of attention: Time course of activation and resistance to interruption. *J. Exp. Psychol. Hum. Percept. Perform.* **15**, 315–330.

Posner, M. I. (1980). Orienting of attention. *Q. J. Exp. Psychol.* **32**, 3–25.

Posner, M. I., and Petersen, S. E. (1990). The attention system of the human brain. *Annu. Rev. Neurosci.* **13**, 25–42.

Posner, M. I., Snyder, C. R. R., and Davidson, B. J. (1980). Attention and the detection of signals. *J. Exp. Psychol. Gen.* **109**, 160–174.

Posner, M. I., and Cohen, Y. (1984). Components of visual orienting. In "Attention and Performance X" (H. Bouma, and H. Bouwhuis, eds.), pp. 531–554. Erlbaum Assoc., Hillsdale, New Jersey.

Rafal, R. (1996). Visual attention: Converging operations from neurology and psychology. In "Converging Operations in the Study of Visual Selective Attention" (A. F. Kramer, M. G. H. Coles, and G. D. Logan, eds.), pp. 139–192. American Psychological Association, Washington, D.C.

Roelfsema, P. R., Lamme, V. A. F., and Spekreijse, H. (1998). Object-based attention in the primary visual cortex of the macaque monkey. *Nature* **395**, 376–381.

Tootell, R. B., Hadjikhani, N., Hall, E. K., Marrett, S., Vanduffel, W., Vaughan, J. T., and Dale, A. M. (1998). The retinotopy of visual spatial attention. *Neuron* **21**, 1409–22.

Van Voorhis, S. T., and Hillyard, S. A. (1977). Visual evoked potentials and selective attention to points in space. *Percept. Psychophys.* **22**, 54–62.

Von Helmholtz, H. (1924). "Treatise on Physiological Optics." Optical Society of America, Rochester, New York.

Woldorff, M. G. (1993). Distortion of ERP averages due to overlap from temporally adjacent ERPs: Analysis and correction. *Psychophysiology* **30**, 98–119.

Zani, A., and Proverbio, A. M. (1995). ERP signs of early selective attention effects to check size. *Electroencephalogr. Clin. Neurophysiol.* **95**, 277–292.

11

Steady-State VEP and Attentional Visual Processing

Francesco Di Russo, Wolfgang A. Teder-Sälejärvi, and Steven A. Hillyard

INTRODUCTION

The vast majority of studies that investigated attentional modulation of the visual evoked potential (VEP) have been confined to the transient responses evoked by isolated stimuli. This class of potentials is evoked by stimuli having an asynchronous and low repetition rate (not faster than 2 stimuli per second). These potentials are called "transient" because the slow rate of stimulation allows the sensory pathways to recover or "reset" before the next stimulus appears. When visual stimuli are presented at a constant rate that is rapid enough to prevent the evoked neural activity from returning to base line state, the elicited response becomes continuous and is called the steady-state visual evoked potential (SSVEP). With steady-state stimulation the typical VEP wave form is markedly changed. For instance, the transient VEP includes three major early components: the C1 at 60–80 msec, the P1 at 80–120 msec, and the N1 at 120–180 msec. (see Fig. 1). At more rapid stimulation rates, the brain response to the same stimulus becomes sinusoidal and is typically modulated at

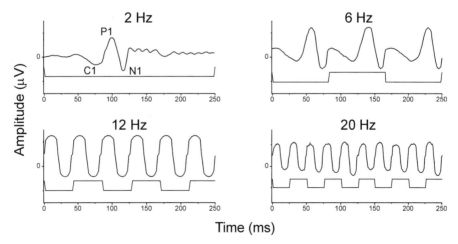

FIGURE 1 Pattern-reversal VEP wave form as a function of stimulation frequency. Note that the wave form is basically modulated at the second harmonic of the stimulus frequency. At the slowest rate (2 Hz) the components of the transient VEP can be seen.

---

the fundamental stimulus frequency in the case of an unstructured stimulus (e.g. flash) or at the second harmonic (double the stimulation frequency) if the stimulus is a pattern-reversal (Regan, 1989).

Like any sinusoidal wave form, the SSVEP can be measured in terms of its amplitude and phase. The phase is a joint function of the stimulus frequency and the time delay between stimulus and brain response. The amplitude indicates the relative magnitude of a given harmonic of the response and, as for transient evoked potentials, is measured in microvolts. The amplitude and phase of the SSVEP vary as function of the temporal frequency, spatial frequency, contrast, luminance, and hue of the driving stimulus (Regan, 1989).

SSVEP AND COGNITIVE PROCESSES

The SSVEP offers certain advantages over the transient VEP for the study of sensory and cognitive processes in that its signal is easily recorded and quantified and can be rapidly extracted from background noise (Regan, 1989). It is somewhat surprising, therefore, that only a few studies have attempted to relate SSVEP parameters to cognitive processes. One of the first such studies was by Wilson and O'Donnell (1986), who found that individual differences in reaction time in mental rotation and memory matching tasks were correlated with the conduction speed ("apparent latency") of the SSVEP recorded in a separate session. These investigators did not find any reliable relationships between SSVEP latency and mental workload, however (Wilson and O'Donnell, 1986).

In a visual vigilance task, Silberstein et al. (1990) found that the SSVEP amplitude to an irrelevant flicker was reduced during a period when the subject was actively searching for a target shape as compared to when no target was expected.

This effect was interpreted in line with the authors' hypothesis that the SSVEP to such an irrelevant probe would be reduced in brain areas as a function of how actively engaged those brain areas were in performing the ongoing task. Accordingly, they concluded that during the period of active vigilance there was increased brain activity in parietooccipital regions, leaving fewer neurons available to respond to the irrelevant background 13-Hz flicker.

The use of the SSVEP as a probe of cognitive function was extended by Silberstein et al. (1995) in a study of the Wisconsin Card Sorting Task. They found that the SSVEP amplitude to a continuous irrelevant background flicker was attenuated over prefrontal, central, and right parietotemporal regions in the interval following a cue to change the card-sort criterion. These SSVEP reductions were interpreted as reflecting an increase in task-related cortical activity in those brain regions during task performance.

SSVEP AND SPATIAL ATTENTION

The neural mechanisms of visual–spatial attention have been studied extensively by means of transient VEPs (reviewed in Hillyard and Anllo-Vento, 1998; Martinez et al., 2001). The general finding has been that paying attention to a specific region of the visual field is associated with increased amplitudes of the early components of VEPs to stimuli flashed at the attended location. This attentional modulation of the transient VEP includes amplitude enhancements of the sensory-evoked P1 (80–120 msec) and N1 (140–200 msec) components, which have been localized by dipole modeling techniques to specific zones of extrastriate visual cortex (Martinez et al., 2001). It has been proposed that these P1 and N1 modulations reflect a sensory gain control mechanism, whereby visual information falling within the spotlight of spatial attention is facilitated and passed along to

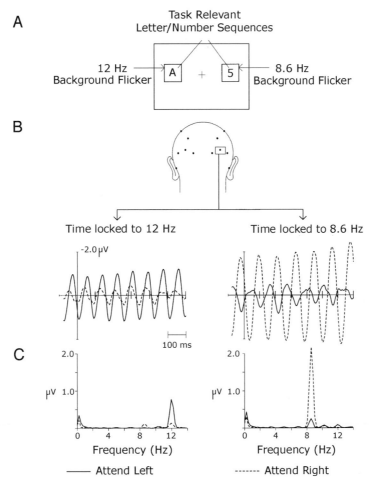

FIGURE 2 Overview of experimental design and results from the study of Morgan *et al.* (1996). (A) Subjects monitored the character sequence in one visual field while ignoring the contralateral sequence. (B) Time domain averages of SSVEP responses to flickering squares in the left (12 Hz) or right (8.6 Hz) visual field recorded from the right occipitotemporal scalp (site PO8) in a typical subject. Wave forms shown were obtained by averaging the responses to successive flashes over the first 6 sec of the flickering sequence, time locked to either the 12- or the 8.6-Hz flashes, and then averaging across all the trials of that type. Dashed wave forms correspond to the attend-left condition and solid waveforms to the attend-right condition. (C) Frequency domain analysis of the SSVEPs illustrated in B. Amplitude values were derived from fast Fourier transforms. Reprinted from Morgan, Hansen & Hillyard; *Proc. Nat. Acad. Sci. USA* **93**, 4770–4774. Copyright 1996 National Academy of Sciences, USA.

higher levels of processing (Hillyard and Anllo-Vento, 1998).

The effects of spatial attention on the SSVEP in response to flickering stimuli was studied by Morgan *et al.* (1996) in a task in which subjects were cued to attend to a letter/number sequence in one visual field and to ignore a similar, concurrent sequence in the opposite field (Fig. 2A). The letter/number sequences in the two fields were superimposed on small background squares flickering at 8.6 Hz in one field and 12 Hz in the other. Representative SSVEP waveforms (averaged in the time domain) from one subject are shown in Fig. 2B for the condition in which the 12-Hz background flicker was presented in the left visual field and the 8.6-Hz flicker was presented in the right visual field. Recordings shown are from the right occipital scalp, where consistent attention– related enhancement was observed for SSVEPs at both frequencies. The amplitude of the SSVEP elicited by the 12-Hz flicker was much larger when attention was directed to the left stimulus sequence rather than the right, whereas the SSVEP in response to the concurrently presented 8.6-Hz flicker showed the reverse. This amplitude enhancement of the SSVEP in response to the irrelevant background flashes at the attended location was also evident in the frequency domain (fast Fourier) analysis of these wave forms (Fig. 2C). These findings indicate that the relative amplitudes of the frequency-specific SSVEPs elicited by each stimulus may index the allocation of attention among the flickering stimulus locations.

To gain information about the cortical regions responsible for generating the enhanced SSVEP to attended stimuli, a further study used functional magnetic resonance imaging (fMRI) to localize active brain regions while subjects performed the same task shown in Fig. 2 (Hillyard et al., 1997). Two specific zones of extrastriate visual cortex were found to be activated during attention to the lateralized flickering stimuli, one in the fusiform gyrus/inferior occipital area and the other in more lateral occipitotemporal cortex. Dipole modeling of the grand-average SSVEP that was recorded in the same subjects revealed dipolar sources in occipitotemporal cortex just medial to the fMRI activations.

These findings of increased SSVEP amplitudes to irrelevant flicker at attended versus unattended locations might at first appear to conflict with the finding of Silberstein et al. (1990), that the SSVEP to irrelevant flicker was decreased during a period of active vigilance. This difference in outcome can be explained, however, by differences in the size and location of the irrelevant flickering stimuli between the two studies. Whereas the flickering backgrounds in the study of Morgan et al. (1996) were discrete and superimposed on the

task-relevant stimulus locations, the flickering background in the Silberstein et al. study was large and diffuse, subtending 30° by 80° of visual angle. Thus, focusing attention on the relevant stimulus sequence in the design of Morgan et al. would result in enhanced processing of the discrete flicker because it fell within the attentional spotlight, whereas in the Silberstein et al. study very little of the diffuse flicker would be included in the attentional spotlight. Indeed, if the attentional spotlight was narrowly focused on the relevant stimuli, the SSVEP response to the diffuse surrounding flicker may actually have been suppressed

The SSVEP was also found to be a sensitive index of spatial attention to stimuli flickering in the range of 20–28 Hz (Müller et al., 1998a). In this experiment, subjects were asked to attend to a flickering light-emitting diods (LED) display in one visual field while ignoring a similar display flickering at a different frequency in the other visual field. For example, when subjects attended to an array of LEDs flickering at 27.8 Hz in one visual field and ignored an array flickering at 20.8 Hz in the opposite field, the SSVEP at the attended frequency was more than doubled in amplitude (Fig. 3). Modeling of the neural generators of the higher frequency SSVEP using a current estimation technique indicated focal sources in dorsal occipital cortex in the hemisphere contralateral to the stimulus position.

In further studies, the SSVEP response to these high-frequency flickers was used to provide an electrophysiological index of the speed of attention switching (Müller et al., 1998b). In this study, each trial began with concurrent flickering of LED displays in the left (at 20.8 Hz) and right (at 27.8 Hz) visual fields. A central cue then appeared adjacent to the fixation point to indicate whether the left or right display was to be attended on that trial. It was found that the SSVEP amplitude at the attended frequency (measured by moving-window

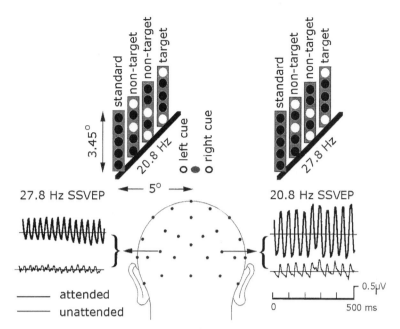

FIGURE 3 Schematic diagram of stimulus array and SSVEP wave forms from one subject shown for the attended (bold line) and unattended (thin line) conditions recorded from occipitotemporal sites (TO2 and TO1) contralateral to the flickering stimulus. The flicker rates were 20.8 Hz for the left row and 27.8 Hz for the right row of LEDs. The four possible color configurations are shown for each row, with all five LEDs being red in the standard configuration. Target and nontarget color changes (two LEDs changed to green) occurred in random order on both sides with a stimulus-onset asynchrony of 400 to 700 msec (onset to onset). Gray oval is the fixation point. The SSVEPs were obtained by a sliding-average technique in the time domain and were time-locked to either the left or the right flickering stimulus. From Müller et al. (1998b). Reprinted from Müller, Teder-Sälejärvi, & Hillyard; Nature Neuroscience **1**, 631–634, 1998.

Fourier analysis) increased abruptly after the cue (Fig. 4); it was calculated that steady-state cortical activity evoked by the attended-side stimulus was facilitated by about 500 msec after the onset of the cue to shift attention. This estimate of attention switching time corresponded with the time at which behavioral target detection within the attended display was reaching its maximum. Moreover, the SSVEP rise times were substantially faster in those subjects who switched attention more rapidly, as indicated by their earlier target detections. Also of interest was the finding that the attention effect on the SSVEP was purely facilitatory; that is, the SSVEP elicited by the attended flicker was enhanced following the attention-directing cue, but the SSVEP to the unattended-location flicker in the opposite visual field was not attenu-

ated. Müller et al. (1998b) proposed that this facilitation reflects the operation of a gain-control mechanism that boosts the discriminability of attended-location stimuli by enhancing their signal-to-noise ratio. They concluded that the SSVEP provides a continuous measure of the time course of attention switching and the facilitation of the cortical processing of the newly attended stimulus.

A further study investigated the effects of spatial attention on concurrently recorded transient and steady-state visual ERP responses to the flickering arrays (Müller and Hillyard, 2000). Consistent with previous findings, SSVEP amplitude was enlarged for attended flicker stimuli at posterior electrode sites contralateral to the attended visual hemifield. Significant correlations were found between the N1 and

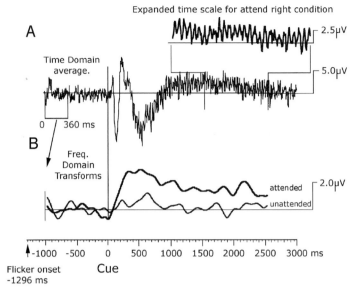

FIGURE 4 Representative time- and frequency-domain wave forms from a single subject in the study of Müller *et al.* (1998b). (A) Averaged time-domain wave form following the cue to attend right, time-locked to the right flickering stimulus. SSVEP activity to this attended flicker can be seen at the expanded time scale. (B) Time course of SSVEP amplitude in the frequency domain obtained from the wave form shown in (A) by a moving-window fast Fourier transform at the stimulus frequency; successive window steps were 4 msec. Thin horizontal line is drawn through precue base line. Bold tracing is attended wave form; thin tracing shows unattended wave form elicited by the same flickering stimulus when the cue directed the attention to the left. Note that the last 500 msec were not analyzed because the moving window reached the end of the epoch. Reprinted from Muller, Teder-Sälejärvi, & Hillyard; *Nature Neuroscience* **1**, 631–634, 1998.

N2 components of the transient ERP response to color-change target stimuli and the SSVEP attention effects, suggesting that the SSVEP and transient ERP reflect partially overlapping attentional mechanisms that facilitate the discriminative processing of stimuli at attended locations.

ATTENTION EFFECTS ON SSVEP PHASE

The aforementioned studies found that spatial attention strongly increased the amplitude of the SSVEP, but attention effects on response phase were not analyzed in detail. Morgan and colleagues (1996), using 8.6- and 12-Hz flickering stimuli, observed substantial phase shifts between attended and unattended wave forms in some subjects (e.g., Fig. 2), but

these shifts were inconsistent across subjects and electrode sites. In the studies of Müller and colleagues (1998a,b) that used stimulus frequencies of 20.8 and 27.8 Hz, phase shifts were observed at many scalp sites between the attended and unattended wave forms. Statistical analysis, however, failed to demonstrate any consistent phase shifts across subjects as a function of attention

The phase of the SSVEP depends in part on the transmission time between the stimulus and the evoked brain activity but does not give a direct measure of this transmission time. The steady-state phase can be expressed in terms of the ratio of the sine/cosine components of the Fourier analysis (see Regan, 1989; Porciatti *et al.*, 1992), but this solution is not unique and includes a group of phase values separated by multiples of 2p radians. For instance, a

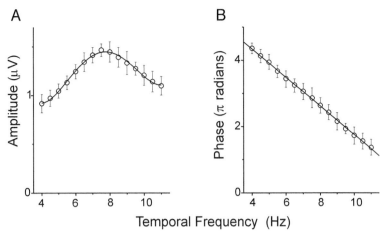

FIGURE 5 The dynamics of the SSVEP can be described by two graphs, one (A) representing the amplitude of the harmonic component analyzed as function of the stimulation frequency, and another (B) representing the phase as function of the stimulation frequency. In this example the graphs describe the second harmonic amplitude and phase as a function of the stimulation frequency (from 4 to 11 Hz) in response to a sinusoidal pattern-reversal grating having a spatial frequency of 0.6 cycle/degree (unpublished data).

45° phase shift with respect to stimulus onset for the first harmonic of a 20-Hz SSVEP corresponds to a time shift of 12.5 msec, but it is impossible to know whether the response is delayed by additional whole cycles. Thus, in this example the response latency could be 12.5, 62.5 or 102.5 msec, etc., depending on how many cycles may have occurred.

The true latency of the SSVEP cannot usually be determined unequivocally, but its "apparent latency" can be estimated as the slope of the function relating phase change to the stimulation frequency (Regan, 1989). In other words, if the SSVEP is recorded over a range of several different stimulation frequencies (for example, from 4 to 11 Hz with 0.5-Hz steps), the phase value will linearly decrease as function of the frequency (see Fig. 5b). The VEP latency for that frequency range can then be estimated in terms of the slope of the phase-frequency function. As demonstrated in numerous studies (e.g., Spekreijse et al., 1977; Riemslag et al., 1982; Spinelli et al., 1994; Spinelli and Di Russo, 1996; Di Russo and Spinelli, 1999a,b), the apparent SSVEP latency estimated in this way is around 100–150 msec, which corresponds with the latency of the P100 component of the transient VEP.

The first study to systematically analyze the SSVEP phase and apparent latency in a visuo spatial attention experiment was by Di Russo and Spinelli (1999a). In this study the SSVEP was recorded in response to a task-irrelevant grating that was phase-reversed at nine temporal frequencies ranging from 5 to 9 Hz with 0.5-Hz steps. This background grating (11° wide by 18° high) was continuously displayed in the left visual field with its medial edge 1.5° from fixation. A target (a light changing color) was presented either in the left or in the right visual field (eccentricity 7°). The task was to count the number of target color changes, without moving the eyes from the central fixation point. Thus, attention was directed either to the left or to the right visual field. The results in a single subject (Fig. 6) and averaged over all subjects (Fig. 7) confirmed that the amplitude of the early sensory activity was modulated by spatial attention. Moreover, they showed that the speed of stimulus processing in an attended region of the visual field was facilitated; i.e., the SSVEPs in the attended condition had a shorter apparent

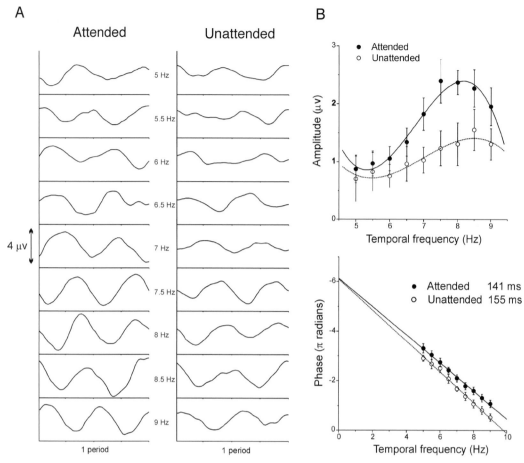

FIGURE 6 (A) SSVEP phase and amplitude variation as a function of stimulation frequency can be observed in recordings obtained from a typical subject in the attended and unattended conditions in the study of Di Russo and Spinelli (1999a). Stimuli were contrast-reversed at increasing frequencies (5–9 Hz) and SSVEPs were recorded over corresponding time epochs. (B) The resulting apparent latencies estimated from the slope of the phase-frequency function are shown below and the SSVEP amplitude-frequency function is shown above. Bars represent the standard deviations of the amplitudes and phases. Reprinted from *Vision Research* **39**; F. Di Russo and D. Spinelli; Electrophysiological evidence for an early attentional mechanism in visual processing in humans, pp. 2975–2985. Copyright 1999, with permission from Elsevier Science.

latency than SSVEPs in the unattended condition. The difference in latency produced by attention ranged from 5 to 20 msec. Similar results were obtained in this study with transient VEPs; stimuli at the attended location elicited VEPs with shorter latencies for the N60, P100, and N140 components and larger amplitudes for the P100 and N140

As mentioned before, the apparent latency of the SSVEP was calculated from the slope of the function relating phase to stimulation frequency. In control experiments, the effect of varying stimulus eccentricity on SSVEP amplitude and latency was measured (Fig. 8). It was found that the amplitude was dramatically increased when the eccentricity was reduced, but the latency was little affected. This ruled out the possibility that the attention effect on SSVEP latency was an artifact of the subjects' shifting their gaze toward the stimulus.

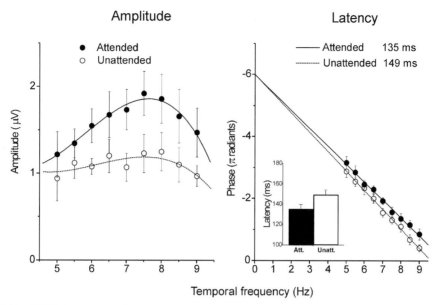

FIGURE 7 SSVEP data averaged across subjects under attended and unattended conditions in the study of Di Russo and Spinelli (1999a). Left: Mean amplitudes (and standard errors) are plotted as a function of stimulation frequency. Right: Mean phase values in radians are plotted as a function of stimulus frequency. Note the difference in phases between the two conditions. Apparent latencies are derived from the slopes of the regression lines. Mean latencies (and standard errors) across subjects are shown in the bar graph. Reprinted from *Vision Research* **39**; F. Di Russo and D. Spinelli; Electrophysiological evidence for an early attentional mechanism in visual processing in humans, pp. 2975–2985. Copyright 1999, with permission from Elsevier Science.

EFFECT OF ATTENTION ON THE MAGNOCELLULAR AND PARVOCELLULAR VISUAL PATHWAYS

A subsequent experiment (Di Russo and Spinelli, 1999b) examined the effect of spatial attention on the magno- and parvocellular components of the visual pathways. The so-called p (parvo) pathway originates predominately in the foveal region of the retina from ganglion cells that are characterized by low conduction velocity, small receptive fields, strong center surround inhibition, high-contrast sensitivity, and a tendency to adapt slowly to stationary stimuli. The optimal visual stimulus for this system is a sinusoidally modulated pattern having a low temporal frequency (1–5 Hz) and high spatial frequency. Another important feature of the p system

is its processing of color information (Eskin and Merigan, 1986). The second m (magno) pathway is so labeled because its ganglion cells are larger than the parvo cells. The magno ganglion cells are widely distributed throughout the retina and are characterized by high conduction velocity, large receptive fields, low contrast sensitivity, and rapid adaptation to stationary stimuli. This system responds over a wide range of temporal frequencies (5–40 Hz), but the optimal stimulus is a sinusoidal luminance modulation with high temporal frequency (6–10 Hz) and low spatial frequency (e.g., Bodis-Wollner, 1992; Spinelli et al., 1994).

As in the previous study, attention was directed to the left or to the right of the fixation point, but this time the stimulus gratings were modulated either in luminance or color contrast. Different temporal frequencies (from 2 to 6 Hz for color and 5

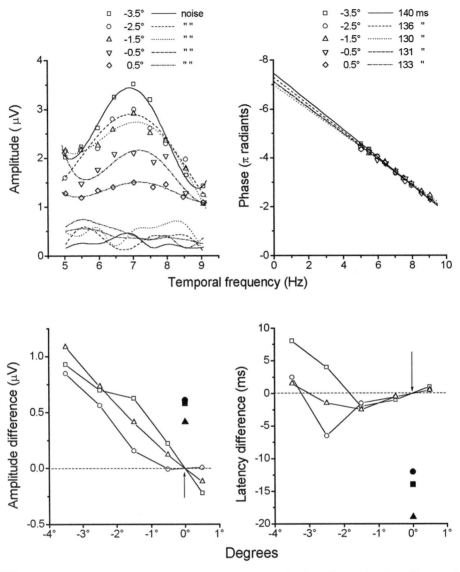

FIGURE 8 Effect of stimulus eccentricity on the SSVEP. Top graphs show the amplitude and latency data for one subject at various eccentricities. Increasing negative degree values (in the upper labels) indicate fixation points closer to the stimulus. Note the systematic increment of amplitude (top left graph) and the small variation of latency (top right graph) with decreasing eccentricity. Data from three subjects are reported with different symbols in the lower graphs. The positions of the different fixation points are shown on the abscissa. The arrow indicates the location of the fixation point used in the attention experiment. At –1.5°, the fixation point was on the edge of the grating. The SSVEP amplitudes recorded at the nine temporal frequencies were averaged to obtain a mean value for each eccentricity for each subject. The differences of the mean amplitude (bottom left graph) or the latency (bottom right graph) with respect to the reference values of each subject are showed on the ordinate. The reference values were the amplitude and the latency recorded when the fixation point was in the same position used in the attention experiment, i.e., 0° on the abscissa. For comparison, filled symbols show the increase in amplitude and the shortening of the latency observed in the same subjects when attention was manipulated. Reprinted from *Vision Research*, **39**, F. Di Russo and D. Spinelli; Electrophysiological evidence for an early attentional mechanism in visual processing in humans, pp. 2975–2985. Copyright 1999, with permission from Elsevier Science.

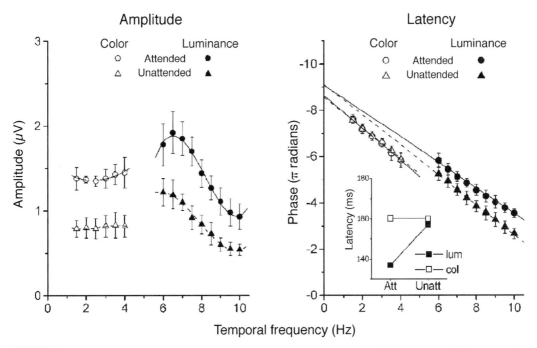

FIGURE 9 The effect of attention on SSVEPs to time-varying luminance and chromatic modulations in the study of Di Russo and Spinelli (1999b). Left: SSVEP amplitudes (and standard errors) are plotted as a function of modulation frequency. Filled symbols denote luminance gratings; open symbols denote isoluminant chromatic gratings. Attended values are shown as circles, unattended values as triangles. Right: SSVEP phases (in radians) are plotted as a function of modulation frequency. Note the differences in phase (and in apparent latency) between the attended and unattended SSVEPs for luminance gratings and the absence of such differences for chromatic gratings. From Di Russo and Spinelli (1999b).

to 10 Hz for luminance) were used in order to maximize the activation of parvocellular or magnocellular pathways, respectively. SSVEPs recorded in attended and unattended conditions were again compared. As shown in Fig. 9, both the latency and amplitude of SSVEPs to the luminance-modulated stimuli were modified by attention. For the chromatically modulated stimuli, however, attention affected only the amplitude and not the latency of the SSVEPs.

Di Russo and Spinelli (1999b) concluded that spatial attention uses different mechanisms to affect sensory transmission in the magno and parvo systems. Attention produced a decrease in latency only for evoked activity in the fast, magnocellular pathway. It was proposed that attention uses the faster signals of the magnocellular

pathways to give priority to stimuli at attended locations and to direct resource allocation and enhancement of activity of the parvosystem.

The effects of attention on SSVEP amplitude and latency suggest that attention may play a role in regulating gain control mechanisms operating in human cortex. Automatic gain control mechanisms for contrast are present at several levels in the visual system, from the retina to the visual cortex (Shapley and Victor, 1981; Bernadette et al., 1992; Reid et al., 1992). This control, specific for m but not for p pathways, is mediated by feedback loops that cause a nonlinear increment of the response amplitude and phase advance with increasing luminance contrast (Shapley and Victor, 1981; Lee et al., 1994; Bernadette and Kaplan, 1999).

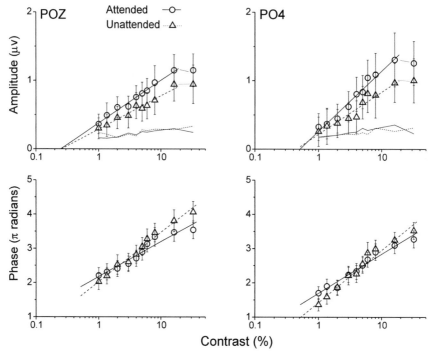

FIGURE 10 The effect of attention on SSVEP contrast-response curves for luminance gratings. Averaged data (N = 11) from the study of Di Russo *et al.* (2001). Top: SSVEP amplitudes (and standard deviations) as a function of luminance contrast recorded at two electrode sites (POz and PO4) in the attended (circles) and unattended (triangles) conditions. Noise levels recorded in the two conditions are shown as continuous (attended) and dashed (unattended) lines. Slopes of the regression lines were 0.66 (attended) vs. 0.49 (unattended) at POz, and 0.88 (attended) vs. 0.62 (unattended) at PO4. Regression lines intercepted the abscissa at 0.24% (attended) vs. 0.23% (unattended) at POz, and 0.54% (attended) vs. 0.46% (unattended) at PO4. Bottom: SSVEP phases (and standard deviations) in radians as a function of luminance contrast. The slopes of the curves were 1.09 (attended) vs. 1.42 (unattended) radians/log unit of contrast at POz, and 1.13 (attended) vs. 1.51 (unattended) radians/log unit of contrast at PO4. In other words, the phase advance with contrast was reduced in the attended condition. Reprinted from *Vision Research* **41**, F. Di Russo, D. Spinelli, and M. C. Morrone; Automatic gain control contrast mechanisms are modulated by attention in humans: Evidence from visual evoked potentials, pp. 2435–2447. Copyright 2001, with permission from Elsevier Science.

This attentional modulation of SSVEP latency is consistent with findings in patients having an attentional deficit for contralesional space (hemineglect) consequent to brain lesions. The VEPs responses to stimuli located in the contralesional, neglected hemifield have latencies longer than do those to ipsilesional, nonneglected stimuli (Spinelli *et al.*, 1994; Angelelli *et al.*, 1996; Spinelli and Di Russo, 1996); this delay was observed only for luminance-modulated stimuli, not for chromatic-modulated stimuli (Spinelli *et al.*, 1996).

ATTENTION EFFECT ON SSVEP CONTRAST RESPONSE

The effect of attention on the SSVEP response to stimuli at varying contrast levels was investigated by Di Russo *et al.*, (2001). The purpose of this study was to use SSVEPs to examine how attention may affect the cortical mechanisms that control contrast gain. Both luminance-modulated and chromatically modulated stimuli were used in order to investigate possible differ-

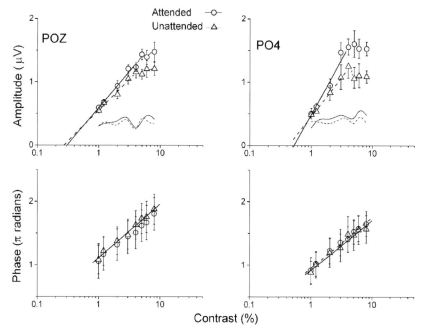

FIGURE 11 The effect of attention on SSVEP contrast-response functions for chromatic gratings. Averaged data (N = 11) from the study of Di Russo *et al.* (2001). Top: Averaged SSVEP amplitudes (and standard deviations) as a function of chromatic contrast. Slopes of the regression lines were 1.15 (attended) vs. 0.98 (unattended) at POz, and 1.77 (attended) and 1.26 (unattended) at PO4. Regression lines intercepted the abscissa at 0.29% (attended) vs. 0.25% (unattended) at POz, and 0.56% (attended) vs. 0.44% (unattended) at PO4. Bottom: Averaged VEP phases (and standard deviation) in radians as a function of chromatic contrast. The slopes of the curves were 0.79 (attended) vs. 0.86 (unattended) radians/ log unit of contrast at POz, and 0.81 (attended) vs 0.80 (unattended) radians/log unit of contrast at PO4. In other words, the phase advance with contrast was not significantly changed by attention. Reprinted from *Vision Research* **41**; F. Di Russo, D. Spinelli, and M. C. Morrone; Automatic gain control contrast mechanisms are modulated by attention in humans: Evidence from visual evoked potentials, pp. 2435–2447. Copyright 2001, with permission from Elsevier Science.

ences between the magnocellular and parvocellular pathways in their control of contrast gain (Derrington and Lennie, 1984; Merigan, 1989; Lee *et al.*, 1990).

The SSVEP was recorded in response to counterphased sinusoidal gratings modulated over a range of contrasts. The 1 cycle/degree gratings were modulated either in luminance or chromatic (red–green) contrast and were phase reversed at 9 and 2.5 Hz, respectively, to selectively activate the magno- and parvocellular systems. Attention was directed toward the gratings (displayed in the left visual field) by requiring subjects to detect and respond to randomly occurring changes in contrast. In a control condition, attention toward the

grating was minimized by requiring subjects to detect a target letter among distracters briefly flashed in the contralateral visual field. As shown in Figs. 10 and 11, attention increased SSVEP amplitudes for both luminance and chromatic stimuli, moreso at high than at low contrast levels, as reflected in steeper slopes of the contrast amplitude curves (over the nonsaturating range of contrasts).

The estimates of contrast threshold obtained by extrapolation of amplitudes to the abscissa were unaffected by attention. Attention also affected the SSVEP phases, but only for luminance gratings (Fig. 10), where it acted to reduce the magnitude of phase advance with contrast. Attention had no effect on the contrast-phase functions for chromatic gratings (Fig. 11). These results are consistent with the hypothesis that attention acts on cortical gain control mechanisms, which are known to be different for the magno- and parvocellular systems.

The contrast gain mechanism acting through a feedback loop seems to occur exclusively in the magnocellular pathway (Lee et al., 1994; Bernardete and Kaplan, 1999). Only cells of this pathway are reported to change their latency and temporal tuning with contrast, whereas parvocellular latency and temporal tuning remain constant both in response to isoluminant and luminance-modulated stimuli (Bernardete et al., 1992; Lee et al. 1994). Unfortunately, no single-cell recordings have been made to assess the cortical response to equiluminant chromatic modulations. The findings of Di Russo et al. (2001), consistent with previous results, indicate that the human SSVEP responses to chromatic modulations are subject to contrast gain control but probably only at the cortical level, although other interpretations are possible. For instance, different sources with different integration times may contribute to the overall VEP wave form, and their relative contributions may vary with contrast. However, whatever the explanation of the phase advance for isoluminant chromatically modulated gratings, attention did not affect it systematically. This result points to a possible difference between the attentional control mechanisms for the color and luminance cortical pathways.

It is interesting to compare the present luminance data with those obtained in masking experiments, where SSVEP contrast-response curves were measured in the presence of parallel or orthogonal luminance-modulated stimuli (Burr and Morrone, 1987; Morrone et al., 1987). A superimposed mask grating that was oriented orthogonally to the test grating was found to attenuate SSVEP amplitudes multiplicatively (so-called cross-orientation inhibition) and to increase the phase advance. That is, the effect of the mask mimicked the effect of engaging attention on another task, both for SSVEP amplitude and phase. It has been proposed (Burr and Morrone, 1987) that orthogonal masking effects on the SSVEP are mediated by the automatic contrast gain control mechanisms previously described. Accordingly, attention may use the same inhibitory circuitry already in place for contrast regulation to increase the processing speed and stimulus discriminability. Such a mechanism would have the advantage of improving vision without requiring any additional circuitry that was specifically dedicated to attentional processes.

CONCLUSIONS

The evidence indicates that the SSVEP provides a sensitive measure of spatial attention processes and offers certain advantages over the transient VEP. In particular, because of the high rate of stimulus presentation (4–20 times faster than for transient VEPs), it is possible to obtain reliable wave forms more rapidly. Second, with SSVEPs it is possible to study attention to stimuli that are continuously present (flickering) rather than only flashed occasionally, thereby yielding a continuous measure of attentional focusing and switching processes. Third, SSVEP measurements can reveal how attention is allocated within a complex, multielement stimulus array, because the visual response to each element can be measured individually by examining the SSVEP at its specific flicker frequency. Fourth, because the SSVEP can be elicited by an irrelevant background flicker, it can be used to study spatial attention to any type of superimposed stimulus, whether it be a rapid sequence of visual events or a stimulus that does not change over time. Finally, because of the different temporal response characteristics of the magno- and parvocel-lular visual pathways, the SSVEP provides a means of studying the mechanisms of attentional modulation of these pathways in relative isolation from one another.

References

Angelelli, P., De Luca, M., and Spinelli, D. (1996). Early visual processing in neglect patients: A study with steady state VEPs. *Neuropsychologia* **34**, 1151–1157.

Bernardete, E. A., and Kaplan, E. (1999). The dynamics of primate M-retinal ganglion cells. *Vis. Neurosci.* **16**, 355–368.

Bernardete, E. A., Kaplan, E., and Knight B. W. (1992). Contrast gain control in the primate retina: P cells are not X-like, some M cells are. *Vis. Neurosci.* **8**, 483–486.

Bodis-Wollner, I. (1992). Sensory evoked potentials: PERG, VEP, and SEP. *Curr. Opin. Neurol. Neurosurg.* **5**(5), 716–26.

Burr, D. C., and Morrone, M. C. (1987). Inhibitory interactions in the human visual system revealed in pattern visual evoked potentials. *J. Physiol.* **389**, 1–21.

Derrington, A. M, and Lennie, P. (1984). Spatial and temporal contrast sensitivities of neurones in lateral geniculate nucleus of macaque. *J. Physiol.* **357**, 219–240.

Di Russo, F., and Spinelli, D. (1999a). Electro-physiological evidence for an early attentional mechanism in visual processing in humans. *Vis. Res.* **39**, 2975–2985.

Di Russo, F., and Spinelli D. (1999b). Spatial attention has different effects on the magno- and parvo-cellular pathways. *NeuroReport.* **10**, 2755–2762.

Di Russo, F., Spinelli, D. and Morrone, M. C. (2001). Automatic gain control contrast mechanisms are modulated by attention in humans: Evidence from visual evoked potentials. *Vis. Res.* **41**, 2435–2447.

Eskin, T. A., Merigan, W. H. (1986). Selective acryl-lamide-induced degeneration of color opponent ganglion cells in macaques. *Brain Res.* **378**(2), 379–384.

Hillyard, S. A., and Anllo-Vento, L. (1998). Event-related brain potentials in the study of visual selective attention. *Proc. Natl. Acad. Sc. U.S.A.* **95**, 781–787.

Hillyard, S.A., Hinrichs, H., Tempelmann, C., Morgan, S.T., Hansen, J. C., Scheich, H., and Heinze, H. J. (1997). Combining steady-state visual evoked potentials and fMRI to localize brain activity during selective attention. *Hum. Brain Mapping* **5**, 287–292.

Lee, B. B., Pokorny, J., Smith, V. C., Martin, P. R. and Valberg, A. (1990). Luminance and chromatic modulation sensitivity of macaque ganglion cells and human observers. *J. Optic. Soc. Am. A* **7**, 2223–2236.

Lee, B. B., Pokorny, J., Smith, V. C. and Kremers, J. (1994). Responses to pulses and sinusoids in macaque ganglion cells. *Vis. Res.* **34**, 3081–3096.

Martinez, A., Di Russo, F., Anllo-Vento, L., Sereno, M. I., Buxton, R. B. and Hillyard, S. A. (2001). Putting spatial attention on the map: Timing and localization of stimulus selection processes in striate and extrastriate visual areas. *Vis. Res.* **41**(10–11), 1437–1457.

Merigan, W. H. (1989). Chromatic and achromatic vision of macaques: role of the P pathway. *J. Neurosci.* **9**, 776–783.

Morgan, S. T., Hansen, J. C. and Hillyard, S. A. (1996). Selective attention to stimulus location modulates the steady-state visual potential. *Proc. Natl. Acad. Sci. U.S.A.* **93**, 4770–4774.

Morrone, M. C., Burr, D. C. and Speed, H. (1987). Cross-orientation inhibition in cat is GABA mediated. *Exp. Brain Res.* **67**, 635–644.

Müller, M. M., and Hillyard, S. A. (2000). Concurrent recording of steady-state and transient event-related potentials as indices of visual-spatial selective attention. *Clin. Neurophysiol.* **111**, 1544–1552.

Müller, M. M., Picton, T. W., Valdes-Sosa, P., Riera, P., Teder-Sälejärvi, A. W., and Hillyard, S. A. (1998a). Effects of spatial selective attention on the steady-state visual evoked potential in the 20–28 Hz range. *Cogn. Brain Res.* **6**, 249–261.

Müller, M. M., Teder-Sälejärvi, A. W., and Hillyard, S. A. (1998b). The time course of cortical facilitation during cued shifts of spatial attention. *Nat. Neurosci.* **1**, 631–634.

Porciatti, V., Burr, D. C., Morrone, M. C. and Fiorentini, A. (1992). The effects of ageing on the pattern electroretinogram and visual evoked potential in humans. *Vis. Res.* **32**, 1199–1209.

Regan, D. (1989). "Human Brain Electrophysiology: Evoked Potentials and Evoked Magnetic Fields in Science and Medicine". Elsevier, New York.

Reid, R. C., Victor, J. D., and Shapley, R. M. (1992). Broadband temporal stimuli decrease the integration time of neurons in cat striate cortex. *Vis. Neurosci.* **9**, 39–45.

Riemslag, F. C., Spekreijse, H., and van Walbeek, H. (1982). Pattern evoked potential diagnosis of multiple sclerosis: A comparison of various contrast stimuli. *Adv. Neurol.* **32**, 417–426.

Shapley, R. M. and Victor, J. (1981). How the contrast gain control modifies the frequency responses of cat retinal ganglion cells. *J. Physiol. (Lond.)* **318**, 161–179.

Silberstein, R. B., Schier, M. A., Pipingas, A., Ciorciari, J., Wood, S. R., and Simpson, D. G. (1990). Steady-state visually evoked potential topography associated with a visual vigilance task. *Brain Topogr.* **3**, 337–347.

Silberstein, R. B., Ciorciari, J., and Pipingas, A. (1995). Steady-state visually evoked potential topography during the Wisconsin card sorting test. *Electroencephalogr. Clin. Neurophysiol.* **96**, 24–35.

Spekreijse, H., Estevez, O., and Reits, D. (1977). Visual evoked potentials and the physiological analysis of visual processes in man. *In* "Visual Evoked Potentials in Man: New Development" (J. E. Desmedt, ed.), pp. 16–89. Clarendon Press, Oxford.

Spinelli, D., and Di Russo, F. (1996). Visual evoked potentials are affected by trunk rotation in neglect patients. *NeuroReport* **7**, 553–556.

Spinelli, D., Burr, D. C., and Morrone, M. C. (1994). Spatial neglect is associated with increased latencies of visual evoked potentials. *Vis. Neurosci.* **11**, 909–918.

Spinelli, D., Angelelli, P., De Luca, M., and Burr, D. C. (1996). VEPs in neglect patients have longer latencies for luminance but not for chromatic patterns. *NeuroReport* **7**, 553–556.

Wilson, G. F., and O'Donnell, R. D. (1986). Steady-state evoked responses: Correlations with human cognition. *Psychophysiology* **23**, 57–61.

Visual Selective Attention to Object Features

Alice Mado Proverbio and Alberto Zani

INTRODUCTION

The recent developments in neuro-imaging techniques have provided new precious data on the cortical and subcortical neural circuits underlying selective attention mechanisms. So-called posterior and anterior attentional systems have been described. The *anterior attentional system*, composed of a neural network including the frontal and prefrontal areas, the anterior cingulate gyrus, and the basoganglia, is believed to regulate functionally the recruitment and control of the cerebral areas having the function of carrying out stimulus processing and complex cognitive tasks.

Unlike the anterior system, the *posterior attentional system*, including the parietal and occipital-temporal cortex, the pulvinar, and the superior colliculus, has been found to be actively involved in the selective processing of visual information. The mechanisms of selection are strongly dependent on the modulation of the functional activity of two neural substreams that project from the visual cortex to the posterior parietal area (the so-called dorsal stream) or to the inferior temporal area (the so-called ventral stream). The *dorsal stream*, which receives both contra- and ipsilateral collicular afferents, is believed to handle information on spatial location and movement of visual stimuli. Conversely, the *ventral stream* is thought to analyze stimulus features such as orientation, color, spatial frequency, and texture.

In the present chapter, findings from both our and other labs studying event-related potentials (ERPs) are reviewed and discussed in order to reveal the functional mechanisms of the anterior attentional system in regulating the selective processing of visual information. We also focus on neural mechanisms of the posterior system involved in the selection of nonspatial features as investigated by means of ERPs, with specific reference to the possible electrocortical generators of these potentials. We discuss evidence in favor of, or against, a possible segregation of the substreams of this system. Furthermore, we deal with the possibility that the primary visual areas, or striate visual cortex (whose anatomical reference in monkey is area V1), might be recruited during attentional sensory filtering of object features at the very earliest stages of information processing. In this regard, different lines of ERP research have provided robust evidence that selection of visual information based on spatial location is accomplished through the activation of extrastriate visual areas (Brodmann areas 18–19) of the contralateral hemisphere to the attended visual field starting as early as 70–80 msec poststimulus (cf. Mangun's Chapter 10 for a thorough review of this research).

Conversely, whether the selective processing of nonspatial features is fulfilled through a different neural mechanism directly modulating V1 activation, or, whether the latter view is championed, when in time—whether at the very early sensory stage of processing within the projection areas or beyond this stage—is still controversial and a matter of animated debate.

With these goals in mind, in the following discussions, a large body of recent research is reviewed and discussed, reporting ERP findings on the attentional selection of single visual features, such as orientation, and spatial frequency, as well as the conjunction of nonspatial features, such as location and frequency, and location and color. The consistency of these findings with other lines of research on attention in cognitive neuroscience, such as hemodynamic studies of the brain and intracerebral cell recordings, is also treated to some extent.

Among other main conclusions, it is proposed that neural mechanisms of attentional selection for the manifold features of visual objects, although in part functionally and anatomically distinct, strongly interact with one another, as is also suggested by comparatively recent behavioral findings obtained in brain-lesioned patients. Based on ERP findings, it is further suggested that this interaction begins at an early sensory stage of processing.

VISUAL SELECTIVE ATTENTION AND ANTERIOR AND POSTERIOR NEURAL SYSTEMS

Reviewing the body of evidence gathered so far in visual selective attention research, the main conclusion seems to be that the information selection mechanisms based on attention perform at least two distinct functions. In the first place, they permit the processing of a selected stimulus to be preferentially increased compared with others present in the surrounding environment. Without it, in fact, all stimuli would be processed at the same level (Hillyard *et al.*, 1999). In the second place, they control the recruitment of functional circuits suitable for performing a given task. This second, executive type, function is added to cognitive control functions, such as decision-making and control processes that the individual possesses vis-à-vis his own behavior and the external environment (Posner and Petersen, 1990; Aston-Jones *et al.*, 1999; Gehring and Knight, 2000).

Neurophysiological research based on recordings of single cell units (Desimone and Duncan, 1995) in animals, as well as functional anatomical studies of the brain, have provided converging evidence on the cortical and subcortical nervous circuits underlying these selection mechanisms (Hillyard *et al.*, 1998, 1999; Corbetta, 1999; Corbetta and Shulman, 1999; Haxby *et al.*, 1999). These data provide direct support for the view of the existence of two distributed functional networks: a so-called posterior attentional system and a so-called anterior attentional system (Posner and Petersen, 1990; LaBerge, 1995).

The Anterior Attentional System

The *anterior attentional system* includes the frontal and prefrontal areas, the anterior cingulate gyrus, and the basoganglia. This system is thought to be responsible for the functional recruitment and control of the cerebral areas having the function of carrying out selective information processing across all sensory modalities and complex cognitive tasks (Desimone and Duncan, 1995). Several neuroimaging and clinical studies reported in the literature confirm the crucial role played by this functional system. In particular, it has been shown that the prefrontal cortex (PFC) is involved in all kinds of top-down processing, when behavior must be guided by internal states or intentions (Gehring and Knight, 2000; Miller and Cohen, 2001).

Prior to the massive increase in these neuroimaging studies, one of the most significant research sectors supporting the view of the executive role played by the anterior intentional system is clinical neuropsychology. In general, the discoveries made in neuropsychological clinical practice have shown how the above-mentioned deficits are linked to an important disorder of the capacity to maintain a mental representation of stimulus–response mapping strategy or of the stimulus set–in other words, a combined disorder of the working memory system and the attentional system (Shimamura, 1995).

In this regard, evidence is available to show that patients with lesions of the dorsolateral prefrontal (DL/PF) cortex suffer from a set of primary (e.g., deficits of the inhibitory control of response to, or difficulties in detection of, novelty), secondary (e.g., distractibility, reduced attention, etc.), and tertiary (e.g., reduced memory and organizational planning, problems in ordering past, present, and future events) symptoms, linked to a frontal syndrome (Stuss *et al.*, 1994; Knight and Grabowecky, 1995; Swick and Knight, 1999). A body of experimental evidence to support this model has emerged from studies on patients with focal brain lesions subjected to ERP recording, a neurophysiological method to study the synchronized activity of the neuron assemblies. This technique makes it possible to evaluate the effects of specific lesions on the ERP components and provides interesting information concerning the functional role of the various brain areas in given tasks.

For this purpose, the long-latency "endogenous" components of the ERPs, which are sensitive to the cognitive and psychological variables accompanying a stimulus event (e.g., Hillyard and Kutas, 1983), were used to investigate the neural mechanisms involved in attention to, as well as memory and cognitive processing of, the stimulus material in general. A wide-ranging investigation was made, for example, of the so-called P3 of the ERPs, a positive potential associated with a number of psychological constructs, including context updating, stimulus categorization, memory, checking the correspondence of the stimulus information with an internal representation, voluntary orientation, and attention allocation (Coles, 1989). Robust evidence has accumulated to show that this component embodies different subcomponents. The best known, P3b, is greatest at central-posterior locations of the scalp, and may be observed when the observer is requested to detect relevant infrequent stimuli (Donchin, 1981) during signal detection tasks (Sutton, 1965), whenever the relevant stimulus corresponds to an internal model (Gomer *et al.*, 1976), and more generally during attentional (Proverbio *et al.*, 1994) and coding tasks as well as mnemonic tasks (Fabiani *et al.*, 1986). In addition, the P3a elicited by a new rare stimulus, irrelevant to the task, associated with automatic voluntary attentional orientation processes (Proverbio and Mangun, 1994), arousal, and response to novelty, is stronger at the frontocentral electrode sites (Squires *et al.*, 1975; Knight, 1991).

By studying DL/PF cortex patients using cognitive brain potentials it was shown that, compared with healthy control subjects, these patients displayed a dramatic reduction in P3a amplitude in the case of "novel" stimuli (that is, deviant stimuli included in a sequence of irrelevant and relevant stimuli, with the patients instructed to respond to the latter by pressing a button). This reduction was greatest at the anterior electrode sites for all the sensory modes—visual, auditory, and somatosensory—of the stimuli used in these studies (e.g., Knight, 1991; Knight and Grabowecky, 1995). It is very interesting to note that this specific reduction in frontal P3a was found to be typical only of these patients. Patients with damaged parietal and temporal lobes actually displayed P3as with amplitudes comparable to those obtained in healthy control subjects (Knight, 1991; Knight and Grabowecky, 1995).

In general, these discoveries show how crucial the prefrontal cortex is in the detection of changes in the external environment and in distinguishing derived models of the world both internally and externally (Knight, 1991; Knight and Grabowecky, 1995; Shimamura, 1995). More recent ERP data indicate that what is perhaps the most important deficit linked to a lesion of the DL/PF cortex consists of the inability to reject or suppress irrelevant information within all sensory systems, whereas the major deficit linked to a lesion of the medial prefrontal cortex is impairment of the ability to monitor behavior to guide and compensate possible behavioral errors and conflicts. These two deficits indicate that critical functions of subareas of the prefrontal cortex are the control of neural information processing through the modulation of activation of sensory systems, as shown by Barcelo *et al.* (2000) for visual extrastriate cortex, and the monitoring of behavior through direct connections to the cingulate cortex (Gehring and Knight, 2000).

We obtained P3 data supporting the neuropsychological view that prefrontal areas might also exert a function of inhibitory filter in neurologically intact volunteers (Zani and Proverbio, 1995, 1997a). In the first of the studies, we used a selective visual attention task in which the subjects were presented with random sequences of six checkerboard patterns with different check sizes. In different experimental sessions, the attentional task consisted of paying selective attention and making motor responses to one checkerboard having checks of a given size, and to ignore all the others (see also the section on space-

based and frequency-based attentional selection). ERPs were recorded from the posterior left and right mesial (O1 and O2), and lateral occipital (OL and OR), besides the anterior F7 and F8, homologous scalp sites falling over the two hemispheres of the brain. At the anterior sites, the late positive component P3b (latency between 350 and 500 msec) was found to have greater amplitude in the case of irrelevant stimuli, compared to relevant stimuli. Previous studies with a two-stimuli go/no-go task design simpler than ours also showed that suppression of the response during no-go trials elicited ERP late components, or P300 waves, of the greatest amplitude at the anterior electrode locations (e.g., Roberts *et al.*, 1994). Interestingly, similar results were also found in more structured studies requiring the information to be stored in the working memory during go/no-go tasks (e.g., Gevins and Cutillo, 1993). However, as may be inferred by observing the grand-average ERPs recorded at anterior sites in response to stimuli of different check sizes in our study (see Fig. 1), the amplitude of the late positive component displayed a clear-cut gradient as a function of attended size, in that it was larger for irrelevant stimuli more similar to the relevant target (i.e., one or more octaves within the frequency band—and thus more difficult to ignore) and decreased as the check sizes became more unlike the target (i.e., more octaves outside the frequency band—and thus easier to ignore). These findings extend those made in previous studies, in that they indicate that the larger frontal P3 effect for no-go/irrelevant stimuli does not index inhibition in simply an "all-or-none" fashion, thus enabling more than one binary separation between "irrelevant" and "relevant" stimuli. Rather, to the extent that this larger frontal positivity is indexing a suppressive process, the view is advanced that the extent of process modulation is a function of the degree of similarity of irrelevant stimuli to relevant ones. In other words, it is a function of the greater

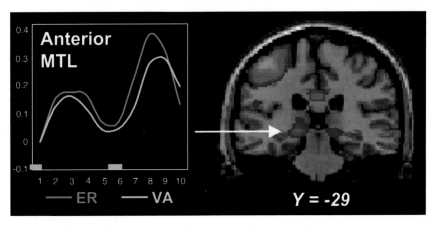

CHAPTER 3, FIGURE 10   Time courses of brain activity during episodic retrieval (ER) and visual attention (VA) in a left anterior medial temporal lobe region. Reprinted from *Neuropsychologia*; R. Cabeza, F. Dolcos, S. Prince, H. Rice, D. Weissman, and L. Nybert; Attention-related activity during episodic memory retrieval: A cross-function fMRI study. Copyright 2002, with permission from Elsevier Science.

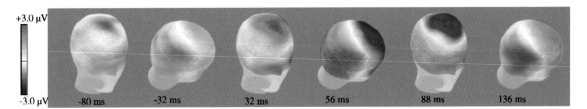

CHAPTER 8, FIGURE 2   Voltage maps showing the oscillatory nature of the ERN and sensorimotor potentials. Time is relative to a button press, which is at 0 msec.

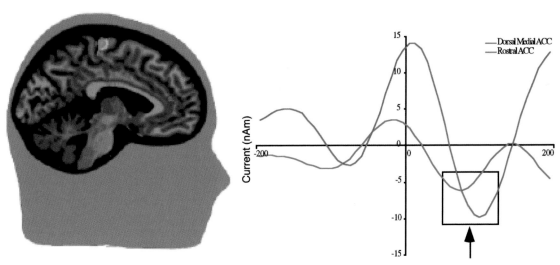

CHAPTER 8, FIGURE 4   Left: Location of the generators of the ERN. Right: Source wave forms illustrating the relative contribution of each source to the scalp-recorded ERN. The box indicates the window of the ERN.

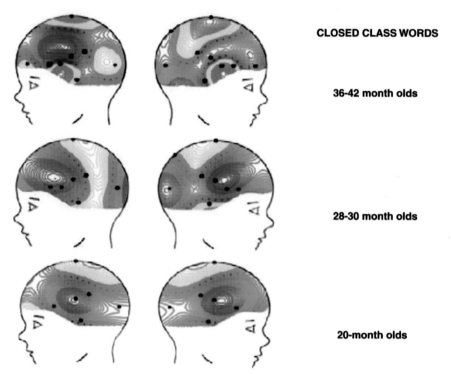

CLOSED CLASS WORDS

36-42 month olds

28-30 month olds

20-month olds

CHAPTER 9, FIGURE 5 Current source density (CSD) analyses of neural activity to closed class words at 200 msec. The CSDs illustrate sinks (i.e., activity flowing into the head, shown in purple) and sources (i.e., activity flowing out of the head, shown in orange) at three age groups. At 36–42 months the CSD shows a sink over left anterior regions. At 28–30 months the CSD shows sinks that are bilateral but slightly more prominent over the right compared to the left hemisphere. At 20 months the CSD shows sinks over both the left and the right hemispheres (from Neville and Mills, 1997).

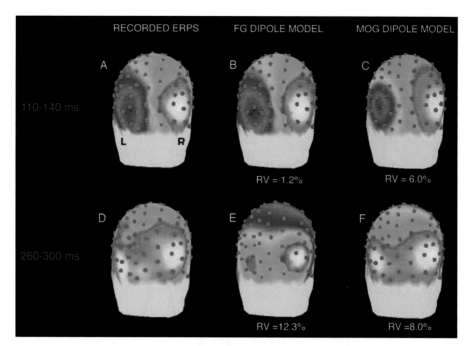

CHAPTER 10, FIGURE 6 Recorded and model topographic maps of attention effects. Group-averaged topographic maps for recorded data (A and D), and model data for dipoles in fusiform gyrus (FG) only (B and E) or dipoles in middle occipital gyrus (MOG) only (C and F). The maps are for the time period of the P1 component (110–140 msec) in the D–F, and for the leading edge of the late positive component (260–300 msec) in A–C. See text for description. The difference between the recorded and model data expressed as percent residual variance (RV) is shown below each model head. The view of the heads is from the rear (left of brain, on left). Electrode locations are indicated by gray disks.

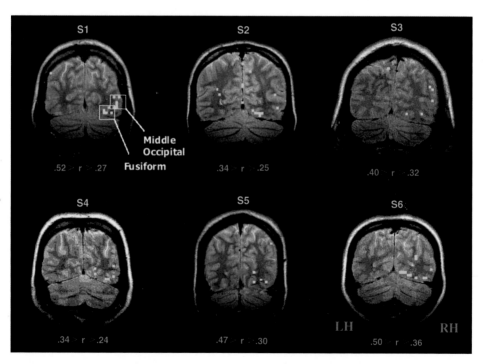

CHAPTER 10, FIGURE 7 fMRI activations during visual attention in single subjects. Data from six volunteers during selective attention to bilateral stimulus arrays. See text for description. The correlation range for the correlation of voxel signal intensity and the attention conditions is shown below each coronal slice. Left of the brain is shown on the left of each image.

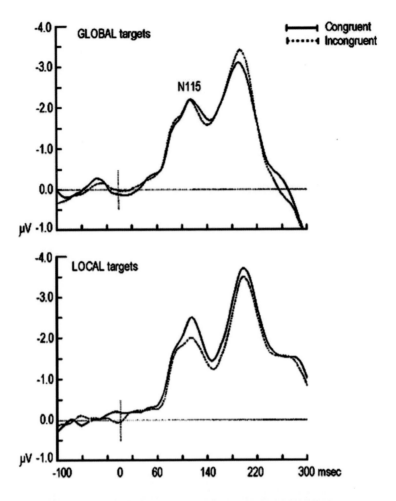

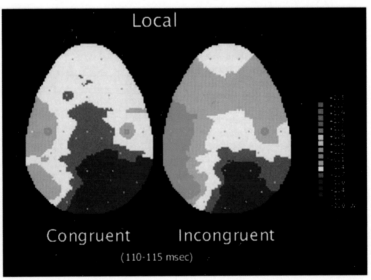

CHAPTER 12, FIGURE 5 Top: Grand-average ERPs to global and local targets as a function of congruence with the unattended level. Recordings are from Oz electrode site. Bottom: Isocolor voltage maps of early sensory response to local targets in the latency range of N115 component. Reprinted from Cognitive Brain Research, **6;** A. M. Proverbio, A. Minniti, and A. Zani; Electrophysiological evidence of a perceptual precedence of global vs. local visual information, pp. 321–334. Copyright (1998) with permission of Elsevier Science.

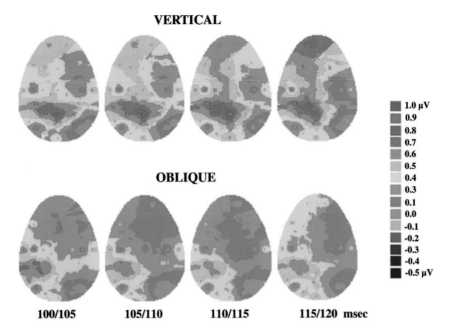

VERTICAL

OBLIQUE

100/105   105/110   110/115   115/120 msec

1.0 µV
0.9
0.8
0.7
0.6
0.5
0.4
0.3
0.1
0.0
-0.1
-0.2
-0.3
-0.4
-0.5 µV

CHAPTER 12, FIGURE 9 Top: Isocolor maps of effects of orientation selection for vertical (90°) gratings in the P1 latency range. Maps were obtained by plotting the values of the difference wave (target–nontarget) computed by subtracting the ERP to vertical gratings while oblique orientations (i.e., 50°, 70°, 110°, or 130°) were attended from the ERPs to vertical targets. Bottom: When attention was paid to oblique gratings, attention effects were still significant but somewhat smaller, and had a slightly different scalp distribution. Reprinted from *Cognitive Brain Research,* **13**; A. M. Proverbio, P. Esposito, and A. Zani; Early involvement of temporal area in attentional selection of grating orientation: An ERP study, pp. 139–151. Copyright (2002) with permission of Elsevier Science.

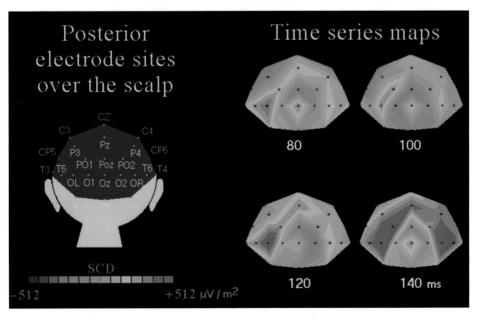

CHAPTER 12, FIGURE 10 Space selection. Scalp current density maps reflecting attention effects for spatial location selection between 80 and 140 msec poststimulus. Maps were computed on the difference wave obtained by subtracting brain response to nontargets from that to targets in the P1 latency range. Stimuli were 7-cpd black and white gratings presented in the right visual field. Note the lateral occipital-parietal flowing of currents, suggesting the activation of the *Where* system.

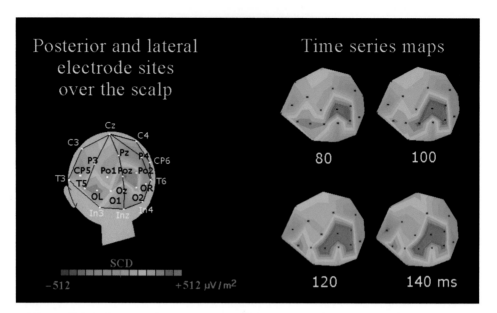

CHAPTER 12, FIGURE 14   Frequency selection. Realistic three-dimensional isocolor voltage maps for frequency (left) and location (right) selection. The maps were computed in the selection negativity latency range (i.e., 180–280 msec; peak latency, 240 msec) on difference waves obtained by subtracting brain response to nontarget gratings from that to targets in the two attend-object and attend-location tasks.

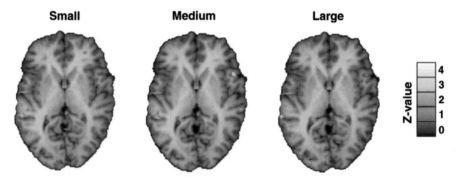

CHAPTER 14, FIGURE 2   Grand-averaged ($n = 13$) functional magnetic resonance imaging activation elicited by a small (10%), medium (30%), and large (100%) increase in frequency deviation superimposed on an individual structural MRI in Talairach space. Images were thresholded at $P < 0.01$. All deviants induced significant activation in the superior temporal gyri bilaterally, whereas the opercular part of the right frontal gyrus was significantly activated only when the large and medium deviants were presented. Adapted from Opitz *et al.* (2002).

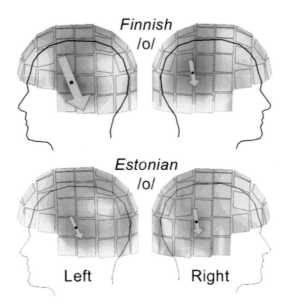

Finnish Subject

CHAPTER 14, FIGURE 3 Language-specific phoneme traces localized in the left temporal lobe reflected by the MMN. Magnetic field-gradient maps of the left- and right-hemisphere MMNs of one typical Finnish subject for Finnish and Estonian deviant vowels. The squares indicate the arrangement of the magnetic sensors. The arrows represent the equivalent current dipoles, indicating activity in the auditory cortex. The Finnish vowel prototype elicits a much larger MMN in the left (compared to the right) hemisphere, whereas the nonprototype responses to an Estonian vowel that does not exist in the Finnish language are small in amplitude in both hemispheres. Adapted from Näätänen *et al.* (1997).

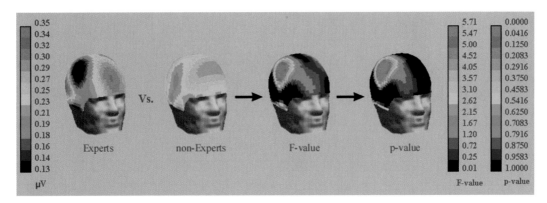

APPENDIX D, FIGURE 4 Realistic 3D color maps. Isovoltage color maps viewed from the right frontal profile for two groups of volunteers performing the same visuomotor task have been computed and projected over a 3D realistic template of the head. Before ERPs were recorded, one group received a period of training (experts) and another did not (nonexperts). Note that the rainbow color scale has been used to represent voltage changes over the scalp, and that before being plotted, the voltage levels have been normalized according to the McCarthy and Wood (1985) rescaling method. A point-by-point between-group variance comparison provided a distribution map of F-values, to which a p-values significance map corresponded, yielding a significant focus of voltage points over the right centroparietal scalp.

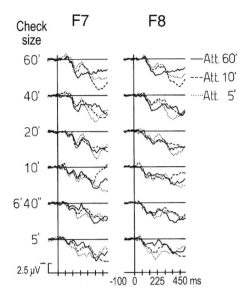

FIGURE 1   Grand-average ERPs to checkerboard patterns recorded at lateral frontal sites as a function of attended check size (in minutes of arc). The main effects of attention are an enhanced frontal positivity to relevant patterns, peaking on average at 225 msec, followed by a later P3b greater to irrelevant patterns falling outside of the band, probably reflecting an active suppression of the response to these stimuli. Reprinted from *Electroencephalography and Clinical Neurophysiology* **95**; A. Zani and A. M. Proverbio; ERP signs of early selective attention effects to check size, pp. 277–292. Copyright (1995) with permission of Elsevier Science.

or lesser interference during the task of the former with the latter, and, as a consequence, of the stronger or weaker need to suppress neural response to irrelevant stimuli within the attentional and motor channels so to avoid processing overload and incorrect responses (i.e., false alarms).

To the extent that the suppression of a response represents a gap in the primary mapping strategy between stimulus and response, the anterior distribution of this specific potential seems to be consistent with the role of the frontal lobes in the structuring of temporal events, in the mediation of preparatory processes, of programming and control on the allocation of the individual's attentional resources. It is also consistent with the hypothesis of the frontal lobes being extensively involved

in the working memory, as suggested by neurophysiological studies too (Goldman-Rakic, 1987).

In another study (Zani and Proverbio, 1997a) investigating neural mechanisms of the selective processing of multidimensional stimuli—that is, the conjoined and separate selection of spatial location and spatial frequency features—21 subjects were administered four sinusoidal gratings randomly flashed to the inferior and superior quadrants of the visual field when relevant and irrelevant. The gratings produced stimulation at 0.75, 1.5, 3, and 6 cycles per degree (cpd) of visual angle. ERPs were recorded from homologous mesial occipital O1 and O2 and lateral-occipital OL and OR, as well as mesial frontal F3 and F4 electrode sites. In different runs, volunteers either engaged in passive gazing of the gratings, or selectively attended and responded motorically to either 0.75 or 6 cpd at a relevant location (i.e., one of the visual quadrants) while ignoring all the other gratings and locations. In this way, while the physical stimuli remained unchanged, attention shifted across spatial frequency and spatial location. Thus, in separate attention conditions, one and the same stimulus could be (1) relevant both in spatial location and spatial frequency (i.e., L+F+), (2) relevant in location but irrelevant in frequency (L+F−), (3) irrelevant in location but relevant in frequency (L−F+), and (4) irrelevant in both features (L−F−). As shown in Fig. 2, regardless of the spatial frequency attended, within the 300- to 600-msec latency range, stimuli irrelevant in one (i.e., L+F− and L−F+) or in both features showed a larger P3 wave at anterior, compared to posterior, sites. The reverse was true for the targets (L+F+).

Regardless of electrode site, P3 response to targets was larger than to gratings sharing spatial location with them (L+F−). Again, the latter condition yielded larger P3s than did stimuli not sharing spatial location (L−F+) or neither feature (L−F−)

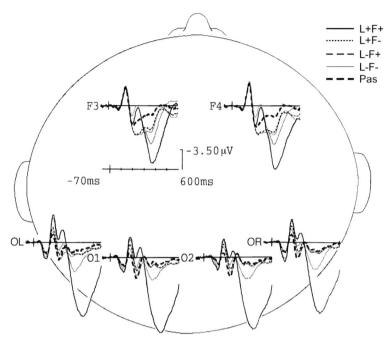

FIGURE 2 Grand-average ERPs to 7-cpd sinusoidal gratings collapsed across the four quadrants of the visual field, as recorded at homologous prefrontal and occipital scalp sites as a function of attention condition in a conjoined selection task. L, Location; F, frequency; +, relevant; –, irrelevant; Pas, passive gazing.

with targets, whereas the latter two conditions did not differ from each another. Also worth noting is that although at anterior sites the latter two conditions were significantly much larger in amplitude, compared to the passive condition, at posterior sites they were not. This finding suggests that higher level selective processing of stimuli irrelevant in location was suppressed at some previous stage of processing. ERPs displayed in Fig. 2 point to a positive activation occurring within the early latency range of 160–260 msec poststimulus as the site of the supposed suppression. Indeed, within the aforementioned latency range a large P2 component having a mean latency of 190 msec displayed a different trend across posterior and anterior electrode sites, thus indicating that this positivity might actually index different neural processes in separate districts of the brain. In actual fact, at posterior sites, P190 was largest in response to passively viewed stimuli (i.e.,

neutral), and decreased as a gradient from gratings irrelevant in both features to those irrelevant in one feature only, and, finally, to those relevant in both features. This was probably due to an overlapping effect of an increasing selection negativity as a function of feature attention conditions in the same latency range. Conversely, at anterior sites, P190 was larger in response to stimuli irrelevant in location (i.e., both L–F+ and L–F–) than to neutral stimuli. In turn, neutral stimuli yielded a larger P190 than did stimuli relevant in location (i.e., both L+F+ and L+F–).

Overall, the present findings suggest that, unlike in the passive task, during selection tasks, prefrontal areas differentially are activated to control the selective processing of stimuli falling within or outside the focus of spatial attention by the posterior areas of the brain. The view is advanced that P190 might index an early suppression operated by prefrontal cortex of stimulus perceptual processing of both relevant and irrelevant gratings falling outside the focus of spatial attention. On the other hand, the P3 might index a belated suppression mechanism of higher level stimulus processing, in particular of stimuli falling within the focus of attention.

To the extent that the same prefrontal areas exerting an executive control on selective mechanisms of attention are involved in oculomotor programming and execution, as pointed out by Corbetta and Shulman (1999), an alternative hypothesis may be advanced to explain the P190 trend at anterior sites. Indeed, it might be argued that the latter possibly index the activation of prefrontal areas suppressing eye saccades toward stimuli falling in an unattended point in space, no matter whether relevant in neither feature, or one or more features.

Sufficient evidence is still unavailable to dismiss either viewpoint, and, very likely, scalp-recorded ERPs, as well as fMRI or PET, are not enough to answer this question. Most probably, only a combining study will come up with the timing, localization, and true functional nature of the processes reflected at the scalp by P190 and P3, respectively, in this conjoined selection task. It is interesting, however, in this regard, that reviews (Knight *et al.*, 1999; Hermann and Knight, 2001) of studies on patients with prefrontal lesions engaged in goal-directed tasks show that both early (P1 and N1) and late (P3) ERP components are modulated by excitatory and inhibitory mechanisms. Based on these findings, the conclusions advanced by the authors are that, on one hand, this damage disrupts inhibitory modulation of irrelevant inputs to primary sensory cortex, and on the other, results in multimodal decreases in neural activity in the posterior association cortex in the hemisphere ipsilateral to damage.

The latter findings provide some indication in favor of the processing suppression viewpoint rather than the suppression of oculomotor saccades viewpoint in explaining P190 behavior in our study.

Briefly, the converging results of neuropsychological clinical and electrophysiological studies suggest that the maintenance of short-term behavior control strategies, together with the capacity to inhibit the processing of irrelevant stimuli or events, are among the more important functions performed by the frontal lobes of the anterior attentional system. These two functions are closely related and can account for many of the behavioral disorders deriving from lesions of the prefrontal cortex, which is part of this system.

The Posterior Attention System

Unlike the anterior system, the *posterior attentional system* includes the parietal and occipital-temporal cortex, the pulvinar and the superior colliculus. This system is actively involved in the selective processing of visual information. The selective processing strongly depends on the modulated activity of two parallel streams, or neural subsystems, which from the primary visual cortex (or V1) project to the posterior parietal area (the so-called dorsal stream) or to the inferior temporal area (the so-called *ventral stream*), first proposed by Ungerleider and Mishkin (1982) and later subjected to intense investigation (for example, see Merigan and Maunsell, 1993; Webster and Ungerleider, 1999). The dorsal stream, which receives both contra- and ipsilateral collicular afferents, manages information on stimulus spatial location and movement. Conversely, the ventral stream analyzes stimulus features such as orientation, color, spatial frequency, and texture.

Dorsal and Ventral Streams of the Posterior System

As already noted, the two streams of the posterior system involved in the selection and analysis of visual inputs project from the visual cortex onto the posterior parietal (dorsal stream) and the inferior temporal (ventral stream) areas, respectively. Evidence has accumulated to indicate that the dorsal stream handles information on spatial position and motion of stimuli, as it possesses (also ipsilateral) collicular afferents, whereas the ventral system analyzes physical features such as orientation, color, spatial frequency, and texture. (Ungerleider, and Mishkin, 1982; Webster and Ungerleider, 1999). Although the former mostly receive afferent fibers from large magnocellular gangliar cells, the latter receive afferences from small parvocellular cells. There is also further evidence that these two systems are related to scotopic and peripheral vision, as opposed to photopic and foveal vision, to the vision of low as opposed to high spatial frequencies and, more generally, to the visual attention mechanisms based on space rather than on the object (Fink *et al.*, 1997).

Hemodynamic functional anatomical studies have clearly shown that visual attention modulates the activity of both systems (Cabeza and Nyberg, 2000; Dupont *et al.*, 1998). This modulation has been observed also by measuring changes in amplitude, latency, and scalp topography of event-related potentials of the brain in response to visual stimuli as a function of task relevance and attention condition (e.g., Anllo-Vento and Hillyard, 1996; Martin-Loeches *et al.*, 1999; Näätänen, 1992; Previc, 1990; Wang *et al.*, 1999; Zani and Proverbio, 1995). [See Chapter 10, this volume, for review of attention mechanisms based on spatial location. Several additional reviews on these mechanisms have been provided by Hillyard *et al.* (1995), Martinez *et al.* (1999), and Luck *et al.* (2000).] In the remainder of this chapter, we deal primarily with neural mechanisms underlying the selection of nonspatial features as investigated with ERPs. Reference is also made to single-unit and blood-flow studies on these mechanisms concerned with their possible cortical localization to corroborate ERP findings.

DOES VISUAL SELECTIVE ATTENTION MODULATE PRIMARY VISUAL AREAS?

For a long time it was believed that the primary projection areas of brain cortex acted as simple analyzers of input features and were not directly involved in the so-called *top-down* selection mechanisms, i.e., those based on higher cognitive strategies. Only recently has this conception been opposed, thanks to the new findings provided by bioimaging and neurophysiological and electromagnetic techniques. These techniques are able, on the one hand, to determine the functional activation of the cortical and subcortical areas, and, on the other, to show up the early timing of the attentional influences on the processing stages.

Regarding auditory modality, it has been shown in selective listening tasks that attention can modulate the information flow captured by one of the ears when material is presented rapidly to both ears, right from the earliest processing stages. This was demonstrated by measuring the changes in amplitude of a small positive deflection (latency, 20–50 msec), the generator of which was identified in the primary auditory area by the combined ERP and PET study of Woldorff and colleagues (1993).

For the visual modality, there is robust evidence indicating that space-based information selection influences the extrastriate visual areas (i.e., Brodmann areas 18 and 19 of the hemisphere contralateral to the attended field) as early as 70–80 msec poststimulus (e.g., Mangun *et al.*, 1997, 2001; Martinez *et al.*, 1999).

As for nonspatial features, it has been reported that attentional selection takes place through different neural mechanisms directly affecting analysis of the specific feature (color, spatial frequency, etc.), although this view is still controversial in the literature. These findings are illus-

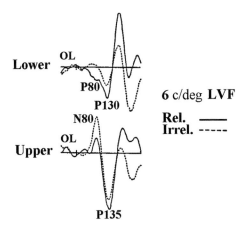

FIGURE 3 Grand-average ERPs to black and white luminance-modulated high-spatial-frequency (6 cpd) gratings as a function of task relevance. ERPs were recorded from left lateral occipital site (OL) to stimuli presented in the lower and upper quadrants of left visual field (LVF).

trated in greater detail in the following discussions.

As far as temporal onset is concerned, the attentional effect is believed to start at around 60–70 msec, corresponding in all probability to the activation of the primary visual area (V1). For example, the selection of checkerboard patterns based on their check size produces an increase in amplitude of the sensory responses P1 and N115 recorded at electrodes O1 and O2, corresponding to the primary visual areas (Zani and Proverbio, 1995). Likewise, selecting gratings on the basis of their spatial frequency (Zani and Proverbio, 1997a–e) and orientation (Karayanidis and Michie, 1997) or selecting alphanumeric characters on the basis of their shape (Skrandies, 1983) produces an increase in the evoked response at the sensory level. This means that the attentional strategy adopted by the observer to identify as rapidly and effectively as possible an interesting object in the visual environment is able to enhance the response of the visual system to that object's features by setting an early selection sensory filter.

This type of filter is seen, as well as in the attentional modulation of P1, also in

increases in amplitude of a preceding response, prominent on the hemisphere ipsilateral to stimulation, known as P/N80, so named because of its average latency of 80 msec (see Fig. 3). It has a positive or negative polarity according to the type of stimulus (for example, increasing negativity with increasing spatial frequency), type of hemifield (polarity is reversed on going from the inferior hemifield to the upper hemifield), and type of retinal eccentricity. The P/N80 is also known as C1 [Component 1, Jeffreys and Axford (1972)] and its inversion in polarity depends strongly on the crossed retinotopic organization of visual pathways and calcarine fissure in the occipital striate cortex, described as the *cruciform model*. According to this model, based on the organization of visual pathways, stimuli falling beneath the horizontal meridian of the visual field are projected to the superior lip of the calcarine fissure in the hemisphere contralateral, across the vertical meridian, to the area of the visual field affected by the stimuli. Conversely, stimuli falling above the horizontal meridian end up finding their representation in the lower lip of the same fissure with the same hemispheric logistics (see Fig. 4 A–C). The neural generator of this potential was identified in the calcarine fissure of the striate cortex using different methods, such as scalp current density (SCD) (see Appendix D for a more detailed illustration) by Proverbio *et al.* (1996), and the combining of spatiotemporal dipole modeling (this technique is described in greater detail in Chapter 2) with cortical anatomy provided by magnetic resonance (Clark and Hillyard, 1996).

Indeed, whatever the polarity of the component under passive vision conditions, we found that spatially directed selective attention was able to modulate the amplitude of this potential, generally in the direction of increased positivity (Zani and Proverbio, 1997c). The attentional modulation of P/N80 recorded in

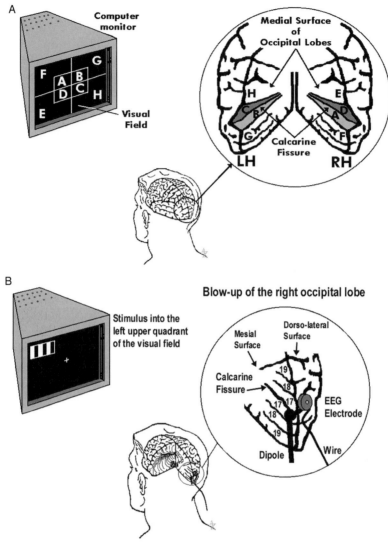

FIGURE 4 Relationships between the so-called cruciform model and the P/N80 (or C1) component. (A) Sketchy drawing of the crossed retinotopic layout of primary visual cortex versus the visual field underlying the cruciform model. On the left, the central (i.e., foveal) and peripheral (i.e., perifoveal) districts of the visual field are drawn, marked with capital letters. On the right, the occipital lobes of brain left and right hemispheres have been depicted as virtually severed and blown up, as well as pulled apart, so to expose the calcarine fissure in the mesial surface of each hemisphere. As can be seen, the various districts of the visual field find a crossed representation, across both the vertical and the horizontal meridians of the latter, in the internal and the external lips of the calcarine fissure, due to the anatomical organization of the visual pathways. (B) Downward dipole. On the right, a grating pattern is presented in the upper left visual hemifield. For the aforementioned organization of the visual pathways this stimulus is projected to the inferior lip of the contralateral calcarine fissure. This can be seen in the observer's head profile, where the posterior portions of the hemisphere ipsilateral to the stimulus have been removed to make the mesial surface of the contralateral occipital lobe visible. This lobe and its Brodmann areas may be observed more clearly, in the blow-up on the right. Observing this blow-up it can be easily evinced that the dipole localized in the inferior lip of the calcarine fissure goes downward off the scalp electrode. For this the electrode records the currents' flow inward from the head surface as a sink and early latency negativity. (C) Upward dipole. The stimulus in the lower quadrant is projected to the upper lip of the contralateral calcarine fissure. The dipole results in a *source* because the currents flow outward, approaching the electrode, which records positivity.

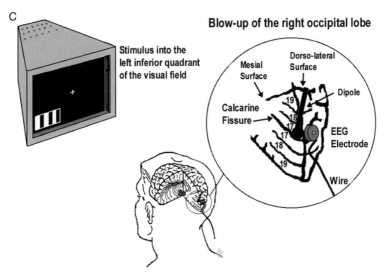

FIGURE 4 (*continued*).

human observers engaged in selective attention tasks is consistent with the neurophysiological evidence obtained using cats and monkeys (see, for instance, Motter, 1993; Lamme and Spekreijse, 2000) on the modulation of neuronal populations of V1, as well as of V2 and V4 during the selection of nonspatial features. Several different neurophysiological studies carried out on macaques also indicated a clear-cut attentional modulation of V1 for the selection of orientation (Press and Van Essen, 1997; Vanduffel *et al.*, 1997), of movement (Watanabe *et al.*, 1998), of spatial frequency and color (Metha *et al.*, 1997), and of shape (Roelfsema *et al.*, 1997, 1998). Interestingly enough, Ito and Gilbert (1999) found that the firing rate of cells in the primary visual cortex of alert monkeys was significantly modulated by attentional set during a spatial attention task. Overall, these findings provided evidence that attentional modulation of sensory responses can be observed in most areas of the visual cortex, including V1 (see Treue, 2001, for a review), and perhaps earlier in the lateral geniculate nucleus of the thalamus (Vanduffel *et al.*, 2000). Nevertheless, the literature is still controversial on this matter. Conflicting evidence concerning V1 modulation for spatial attention has been

found, for instance, by Luck *et al.*, (1997). Their macaque study, in which different spatial visual attention tasks were used, did not reveal any modulation of response of the neurons in visual area V1, as opposed to V2 and V4 modulation (Luck *et al.*, 1997). The results led the authors to conclude that the striate visual area (V1) was not modulated by spatial attention. Nevertheless, this is not a straightforward conclusion because, as the authors correctly stress, stimuli attended or ignored by the animal fell in the receptive fields of different neurons, so that it was impossible to determine whether their firing rate would also have been modulated by attention if both stimuli had fallen in their receptive field.

Somers *et al.* (1999) carried out a 3-tesla fMRI study on spatial attention modulation in humans. Very interestingly, they found a robust attentional modulation in both striate and extrastriate cortical areas during object-based spatial attention tasks. The authors concluded that neural processing in V1 can be strongly and specifically influenced by spatial attention.

Again using human subjects, a significant ERP study by McCarthy and Scabini (1991) was carried out on epileptic subjects who had microelectrodes implanted directly in the striate occipital cortex for therapeutical purposes. Because this is a direct measurement, it is interesting that an altered activation of the neurons in this area should be found during selective attention tasks. The less invasive studies of Aine *et al.* (1995), who combined MRI measures and magnetoencephalography (MEG) measures, and the metaanalysis by Shulmann *et al.* (1997), performed by making a comparative survey of a large number of studies carried out using this method, consistently indicate a modulation of visual area 17 during a large number of active tasks involving the discrimination of features. Likewise, recent electrophysiological studies (Zani and Proverbio, 1995, 1997a; Proverbio *et al.*, 1998) on healthy volunteers have shown an attentional modulation of early evoked responses selectively recorded at O1 and O2 scalp sites of mesial occipital areas, which might reflect the activity of intracranial neural generators located in the primary visual area. In particular, the study by Proverbio *et al.* (1998), using hierarchical alphanumeric stimuli that are either congruent or incongruent at local/global level, demonstrated that whenever a stimulus attended at the local level has the same shape as the global configuration (congruent condition), it elicits a greater N115 response over the mesial occipital area (as shown in the wave forms and activation map in Fig. 5), compared with the incongruent condition.

In addition to the visual cortex, attention might also modulate the functionality of subcortical structures such as the superior colliculus, and the lateral geniculate body and the pulvinar of the thalamus. They actually receive and transmit retinotopically organized projections to the striate and prestriate cortex. Indeed, data supporting this view have been reported by LaBerge and Buchsbaum (1990). An enhanced activation of these structures could also account for the increase in visual evoked potentials recorded as early as 40 msec poststimulus in an attentional task by Oakley and Eason (1990). This strongly supports the hypothesis that visual information might be subjected to a sensory filter controlled and monitored by superior centers such as the dorsolateral frontal areas, which might be capable of modulating the earliest analysis at cortical and subcortical levels.

FEATURE-DIRECTED ATTENTION

Several ERP studies have investigated the selective attending of nonspatial attributes of visual information. In these studies volunteers had to attend and select either a single attribute or a conjunction of two or more stimulus attributes. Although some studies have obtained evidence for early selection, many others have failed to find such effects (Rugg *et al.*, 1987; Hillyard *et al.*, 1998). Indeed, this has started a now long-running controversy in attention research between proponents of early versus late models of selection of an object's physical attributes. This controversy still forms the backdrop for some current electrophysiological work in attention (e.g., Martinez *et al.*, 2001; Proverbio *et al.*, 2002).

Below we illustrate the data in the literature separately for attribute and single and conjoined selection tasks. We note here that we do not review all the work carried out on visual selective attention to stimulus features; this work has been discussed exhaustively previously [see, example, the excellent review by Schroeder (1995)]. With some exceptions, our focus is mostly very recent work.

Spatial Frequency

Object recognition is known to occur in the very early stages of processing by means of *spatial frequency* analysis of the luminance configuration (see Box 1). This is made possible by the presence in visual cortex of specific frequency analyzers in

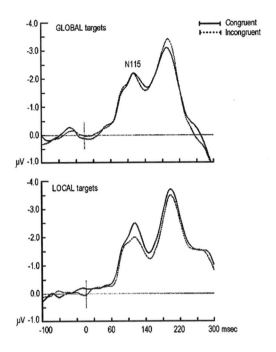

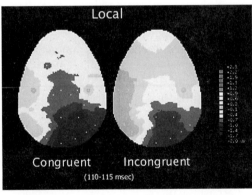

FIGURE 5 Top: Grand-average ERPs to global and local targets as a function of congruence with the unattended level. Recordings are from Oz electrode site. Bottom: Isocolor voltage maps of early sensory response to local targets in the latency range of N115 component. (See color plates.) Reprinted from *Cognitive Brain Research*, **6**; A. M. Proverbio, A. Minniti, and A. Zani; Electrophysiological evidence of a perceptual precedence of global vs. local visual information, pp. 321–334. Copyright (1998) with permission of Elsevier Science.

the form of neurons sensitive to a given range of frequencies and organized on the basis of preferences for orientation and color. The spatial frequency channels vary in sensitivity from 0.8 to 3 octaves appro-

ximately, increasing this sensitivity on average to 1.8 octaves in parafovea and 1.4–1.6 octaves in fovea. An octave is the interval between a given spatial frequency (e.g., 1° 30′) and double the frequency (in this case 3°). For example, a spatial frequency channel with a sensitivity bandwidth of 1 octave will respond significantly to the preferred frequency (e.g., 2° 15′) and to a lesser degree to limitrophe frequencies within the octave.

Harter and Previc (1978) were the first to study the spatial frequency selection mechanisms and the variation in activity of the various channels by measuring the brain's bioelectrical response to stimuli of the attended (target) or ignored (nontarget) frequency. They found that the selection negativity (onset, 150 msec) elicited by the visual cortex for target stimuli gradually decreased with the increasing gap between the frequency of the target (in the form of large checks) and those of the nontargets. These authors also showed that the amplitude of the selection bandwidth gradually shrank as the stimulus analysis proceeded down to the absolutely certain identification of the target frequency at the P300 level.

A subsequent study (Proverbio *et al.*, 1993), using 1.5, 3, 6, and 12 cpd sinusoidal foveal gratings, revealed that selective attention for spatial frequency is able to modulate the amplitude of visual evoked responses at the level of the sensory component P1, as well as N1 and N2. Fig. 6 shows the effect of attention on the first ERP components (evoked by 6 cpd gratings) manifested by a greater amplitude of the response for relevant stimuli, rather than irrelevant stimuli. The specific effect of the general state of alert, rather than that of attentional selection, is made visible by comparing the amplitude of the responses evoked by relevant and irrelevant stimuli (active condition) with those evoked by neutral stimuli (the same stimuli during passive vision), the latter being significantly lower.

Another study carried out by our research group (Zani and Proverbio, 1993, 1995) identified the first effects of spatial frequency selection in a modulation of the sensory components P90 and N115 generated on the striate and prestriate visual cortex. Fig. 7 shows the effects of attention on ERPs to target and nontarget stimuli as a function of the distance from the channel band. The effect of selection is seen to be very strong and, starting from early latencies, becomes increasingly pronounced, especially for the selection negativity (SN), which overlaps the components N1 and N2, and P300. The similarity between targets and neighboring band nontargets produced intermediate evoked responses and a certain number of false alarms (see Fig. 8).

It must be mentioned that several more recent ERP studies also dealing with selec-

---

BOX 1

SPATIAL FREQUENCY

The spatial frequency of a visual stimulus (in cycles per degrees) defines the number of variations of luminance present in a degree of visual angle. Considering that 1° of visual angle, seen from a distance of 57 cm, subtends 1 cm of visual space, it is possible to compute the stimulus spatial frequency, which will naturally vary as a function of the viewing distance, when stimulus size and viewing distance are known. The equation is as follows:

$$(1) \qquad 57 : d = 1 : s,$$

where s is stimulus size in centimeters, and d is viewing distance. For example, if the stimulus size is 2 cm (e.g., the width of a bar), and the distance from the observer is 200 cm (2 m), the stimulus spatial frequency will be:

$$(2) \qquad 57 : 200 = 1 : 2,$$
$$(3) \qquad 200 : 114 = 1.75,$$
$$(4) \qquad 1° \, 45'' \text{of spatial frequency.}$$

In psychophysics and psychophysiology of vision, simple visual configurations characterized by periodic variations of luminance such as gratings and checkerboards, defined by their spatial frequency, orientation, spatial phase, size, eccentricity, and contrast, are usually adopted as experimental stimuli. Gratings are defined as sinusoidal if their luminance varies sinusoidally (that is, smoothly from the darker to the brighter area), or square wave, if their luminance varies abruptly from the darker to the brighter area.

In principle, every complex luminance configuration is decomposable into the sum of multiple simple configurations of different phase and spatial frequency. This decomposition is based on the so-called Fourier analysis, which is a mathematical procedure used to determine the collection of sine waves, differing in phase and amplitude, that makes up a complex visual or acoustic pattern. It is named after the French mathematician Joseph Fourier (1768–1830), known chiefly for his contribution to the mathematical analysis of heat flow. This procedure is widely used in the analysis and treatment of communications signals, linear systems analysis, optics, antenna studies, acoustics, etc. In addition, this technique represents the fundamental tool underlying electroencephalogram analysis, in that it allows the raw EEG signal to be broken down into the various frequencies of oscillation of spontaneous brain bioelectrical activity (alpha, beta, theta, gamma, delta, etc).

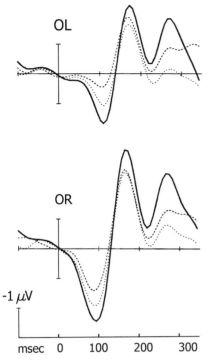

OL

OR

-1 μV

msec   0   100   200   300

FIGURE 6   Attention to spatial frequency. Grand-average ERPs to 6-cpd luminance-modulated gratings recorded at left (OL) and right (OR) lateral occipital sites as a function of attention condition: attended (—), unattended (.....), or passive (---). Stimuli were presented in the central visual field. Passive refers to a condition of passive gazing.

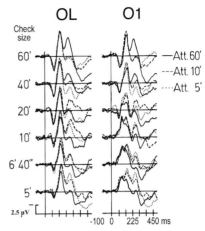

FIGURE 7   Grand-average ERPs elicited by checkerboards of different check sizes as a function of attended size (either 60, 10, or 5 minutes of arc). Recordings were taken from left (OL) and right (OR) lateral occipital sites. Reprinted from *Electroencephalography and Clinical Neurophysiology*, **95**; A. Zani and A. M. Proverbio; ERP signs of early selective attention effects to check size, pp. 277–292. Copyright (1995) with permission of Elsevier Science.

tive attention to spatial frequency did not come up with the reported early attention effects (e.g., Martinez *et al.*, 2001). Still, it is worth noting that there are many methodological differences between our studies and these others. For a review of these significant differences, possibly explaining the lack of early effects in the later studies, the reader is referred to Proverbio *et al.* (2002).

Orientation

As for spatial frequency, orientation is a visual attribute analyzed at the primary level by visual cortex neurons organized into columns. Campbell and Maffei (1970) provided electrophysiological evidence of the existence of spatial frequency channels

sensitive to stimulus orientation, and determined the amplitude of the sensitivity bandwidth in humans by measuring the amplitudes of the evoked potentials as a function of adaptation to high-contrast

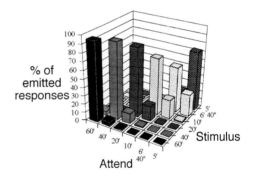

FIGURE 8   Mean percentages of emitted responses (hits plus false alarms) as a function of attention condition and check size. Note that when attention was paid to intermediate check sizes, there was a comparable high percentage of emitted responses to the patterns closer in size to the attended one. Reprinted from *Electroencephalography and Clinical Neurophysiology*, **95**; A. Zani and A. M. Proverbio; ERP signs of early selective attention effects to check size, pp. 277–292. Copyright (1995) with permission of Elsevier Science.

gratings. They showed that when the test stimulus differed in orientation at least 20° or more with respect to the adaptation gratings, the amplitude of evoked potentials dramatically increased compared to when they were elicited by stimuli closer in orientation to the adaptation gratings. These findings demonstrated that the orientation sensitivity bandwidth in humans is about 10–20° (varying as a function of stimulus spatial frequency).

So although the visual system can discriminate rather well between elementary stimuli rotated by only 20°, the vast majority of ERP studies on orientation have used only vertical and horizontal orientations for experimentation. The first electrophysiological studies on orientation selection were carried out in the early 1980s by the distinguished scholar Russell Harter (who died prematurely), together with his colleagues Guido and Previc. The results of their pioneering studies showed that the responses evoked by target grating orientations were characterized by a *selection negativity* that developed on the visual cortex beginning 150 msec poststimulus, and that indicated the existence of specific sensory filters in the visual cortex (Harter and Guido, 1980). Based on these findings, Harter advanced a *neural specificity theory* of attentional selection (Harter and Aine, 1984), according to which the SN to a given dimension of an attended stimulus (e.g., a certain orientation or spatial frequency band) reflected the increased response of neural centers normally involved in the analysis of that dimension. The latter theory, though, encountered opposition among peer electrophysiologists involved in the enterprise of investigating neural mechanisms of attention (see Hillyard and Mangun, 1986).

Although properly conducted these early studies nevertheless suffered from several methodological weaknesses, such as the use of fixed latency measurements of brain potentials (e.g., at 75 msec, at 125 msec, etc., thus not respecting the true latency of ERP peaks), and a nonoptimal signal-to-noise ratio for the evoked responses, which may have impaired the analysis of the earliest and the weakest sensory responses.

All of the relatively few studies that followed that of Harter's group continued to investigate only orthogonal orientations (e.g., Kenemans *et al.*, 1994), and oddly enough none of these studies led to knowledge of the scalp topography of the electrophysiological effects of orientation selection.

A very recent whole-head (32-channel) topographic mapping study by Proverbio *et al.* (2002a) revealed an interesting effect of early modulation of the temporal P1, with a strong lateralization over the left hemisphere (see Fig. 9), reflecting the attentional selection of grating orientation. In this study, participants were foveally stimulated using a random series of isoluminant black and white gratings (3 cpd) having an orientation of 50°, 70°, 90° (vertical), 110°, and 130° of visual angle, and a size of 2°. The task consisted of selectively attending and responding to one of the five grating orientations, while ignoring the others. Difference waves obtained by subtracting ERPs to irrelevant orientations from those to relevant orientations showed that the selection of this feature modulated neural processing at an early poststimulus latency within the P1 latency range. In addition, ERP mapping procedures yielded a focus for this effect over the posterior temporal regions.

It is worth noting that this area was indicated in both neurophysiological and hemodynamic studies as the area of final cortical projection of the ventral visual system having the function of analyzing the nonspatial features (*What* system), and thus appears to be preferentially involved in this type of task. Indeed, Vogels and Orban (1994) and Tanaka (2000) found that cells of the inferior temporal cortex in monkey are strongly activated during orientation and/or object discrimination;

the PET study by Kawashima (1998) showed a specific activation of the left inferior temporal cortex during object discrimination in humans.

In line with the aforementioned findings, our ERP results suggest that temporal area activity may be modulated by visual nonspatial attention at a very early stage of processing. Consistently, Schroeder *et al.* (1998) described an early modulatory effect in V4 and the inferior temporal region (IT), as revealed by current source density (CSD) analysis of brain single-cell potentials in awake macaques stimulated with foveally presented light flashes and black and white square-wave gratings (3 cpd). In our opinion, it is probable that the findings of our study in humans indicate that top-down attentional processes may modulate

these initial visual inputs to V4 and the IT region found in monkeys.

Besides the left-sided hemispheric asymmetry for the early attention effect, we found similar asymmetries for the attention effects concerning the later N150 and P300 components, as well as a left generator for the extrastriate posterior N150, regardless of grating relevance. All in all, these findings support the hypothesis of a predominant involvement of the left hemisphere in object features discrimination, as also supported by neuroimaging studies (Dupont *et al.*, 1998; Georgopoulos *et al.*, 2001), as well as some ERP attention studies (Eimer, 1996a; Martinez *et al.*, 2001; Zani and Proverbio, 1995).

Another very interesting result of the Proverbio *et al.* (2002a) study is the clear

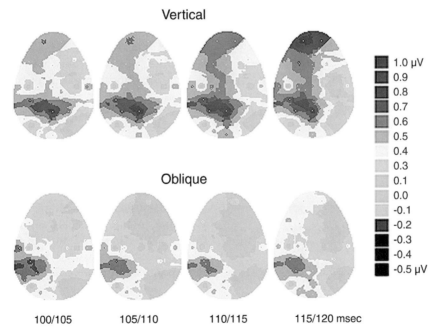

FIGURE 9 Top: Isocolor maps of effects of orientation selection for vertical (90°) gratings in the P1 latency range. Maps were obtained by plotting the values of the difference wave (target–nontarget) computed by subtracting the ERP to vertical gratings while oblique orientations (i.e., 50°, 70°, 110°, or 130°) were attended from the ERPs to vertical targets. Bottom: When attention was paid to oblique gratings, attention effects were still significant but somewhat smaller, and had a slightly different scalp distribution. (See color plates.) Reprinted from *Cognitive Brain Research*, **13**; A. M. Proverbio, P. Esposito, and A. Zani; Early involvement of temporal area in attentional selection of grating orientation: An ERP study, pp. 139–151. Copyright (2002) with permission of Elsevier Science.

difference in both performance and in the evoked responses between the attend-oblique and attend-vertical tasks (the orientations were 50°, 70°, 90°, 100°, and 130°). Indeed, the reaction times were much more rapid and the P300 and the SN much larger for the vertical targets. Taking account of the fact that all the stimuli were isoluminant, and of equal spatial frequency and dimension, this result supports the hypothesis of the so-called oblique effect phenomenon [for a description of this effect, see Regan (1989), as well as Campbell *et al.* (1996), and Arakawa *et al.* (2000)], for which the sensory response was found to be higher at configurations set in the orthogonal orientations rather than in the oblique ones. This asymmetry is believed to have a neural basis in the disproportionate representation of the two orthogonal orientations at the level of the visual cortex. In this regard the hypothesis was put forward that this asymmetry is due to the mainly perpendicular arrangement of the environmental stimuli provided by the Earth's landscape, which is subjected to the force of gravity (trees, horizon, sea, houses, human beings in erect position, etc.) The recent fMRI study by Furmanski and Engel (2000) very likely revealed the neurofunctional bases of this effect by demonstrating that the activation of neurons in V1 is greater to horizontal and vertical than to oblique orientations in humans.

SPACE-BASED AND FREQUENCY-BASED ATTENTIONAL SELECTION

Visual attention, both voluntary and automatic, can be directed either to single objects in visual space, regardless of their location, and to comparatively circumscribed regions in visual space. One example of the first mechanism is the case in which we are looking for a specific object (e.g., a pencil on our desk) on the basis of its visual features (thin, long, made of wood, brown, with a black point); an example of the second mechanism is the case in which we are monitoring (either overtly or covertly) an open door in order to see when a friend of ours comes through it. The two mechanisms of object- and space-based selective attention normally work in close interaction (in order to recognize my friend I must make a careful selection based on the features of his face and appearance). Yet, because they are partly functionally segregated, and probably based on the activation of nonoverlapping visual neural areas, to some degree it is possible to investigate the latter areas separately in order to unveil their neurofunctional activation.

We carried out a series of experiments (Zani *et al.*, 1999) in which, by adopting the same set of visual stimuli in different tasks—lateralized isoluminant gratings of two spatial frequencies, namely, 1 and 7 cpd—we were able to observe the two functionally active attentional mechanisms by inducing a different type of attentional set in the subjects. This was obtained by suitably modifying the experimental instructions—that is, the task that the observers had to perform at different times. In different sessions the same subjects were instructed to pay attention and respond to different stimulus properties while brain-evoked responses were recorded with a 32-channel montage. In this way it was possible to separate the constant effect in the ERPs due to the physical features of the stimuli from that due to the top-down attentional strategies used by our volunteers. In order to compare location selection with frequency selection mechanisms we devised two different paradigms. In the first, the subjects were requested to pay selective attention to a spatial frequency, and to respond to the target frequency whatever its spatial location, whereas in the second they had to attend and respond to all the gratings solely on the basis of their spatial location, thus ignoring the frequency. The results revealed a very early attentional selection effect in both cases, although with completely different morphology and neurofunctional activation. In particular, the selection of the location, which in agreement with the previous studies of Mangun and colleagues (Heinze et al., 1994; Mangun et al., 1997, 2001), modulated mainly the extrastriate area beginning at about 80 msec poststimulus (for the topographic distribution of our attentional effects see the color topographic maps in Fig. 10), was characterized by a prominent P1 with a peak latency of about 135–140 msec. This component was followed by a comparatively small N1 and an exceptionally early P300. Conversely, the selection of the spatial frequency determined the presence of a very early P/N80 followed by a considerable negative deflection (N1/N2 complex strongly modulated by selection negativity) and by a somewhat delayed P300 (see Fig. 11). At the same time, the response times in the spatial selection task were about 100 msec faster than those obtained in the frequency selection task. These data confirm the partial functional independence of the two visual feature selection systems, both based on a very early sensory filter (early selection) although dependent on two anatomically and functionally separate neural streams. Observation of the topographic distribution of the attentional effect of ERP differences—obtained by subtracting the response to the nontargets from that to the same stimuli when they were targets—for the selection of the spatial frequency identified a filter that is strongly linked to the visual processing first of area 17 (at the level of P80) and then of areas 18 and 19 (at the level of selection negativity; see the maps in Fig. 12), whereas the selection of the spatial position indicated it was based on the functionality of the dorsal visual pathway: "extrastriate visual area for P1 (see again Fig. 10), motor cortex for N2, and parietooccipital area for the very fast P300.

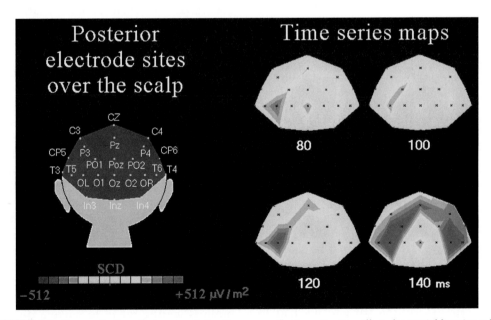

FIGURE 10 Space selection. Scalp current density maps reflecting attention effects for spatial location selection between 80 and 140 msec poststimulus. Maps were computed on the difference wave obtained by subtracting brain response to nontargets from that to targets in the P1 latency range. Stimuli were 7-cpd black and white gratings presented in the right visual field. Note the lateral occipital-parietal flowing of currents, suggesting the activation of the Where system. (See color plates.)

Location selection

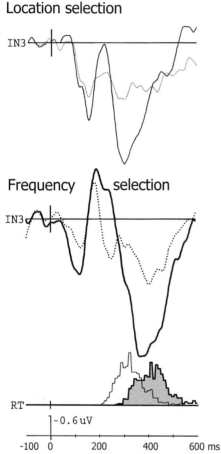

FIGURE 11 Grand-average ERPS recorded at the left inion site (IN3) in response to gratings of 7 cpd and recorded in the attend-space and attend-frequency tasks. The frequency distribution of reaction times in the two attention tasks is shown below the ERPs. RT, Response time.

FEATURES CONJUNCTION AND OBJECT PERCEPTION

Of the most interesting studies by the Harter's group, mention must be made of that of 1982 (Previc and Harter, 1982) on the mechanisms of combined selection of spatial frequency and orientation. In this pioneering study the participants had to attend and respond to target gratings having each time a given frequency and a given orientation. Spatial frequency was foveally projected and could be high or low

and the orientation vertical or horizontal. The results indicated a strong attentional effect at the level of negative deflection N2 and positive P300, the amplitudes of which are shown comparatively to the percentage of emitted responses in Fig. 13. What is interesting in this study is the attempt to gain objective measures of the allocation of attentional resources and the activation of neural mechanisms underlying sensory features selection by measuring the amplitude of the bioelectric response in the visual areas at the various stages of processing. The important findings to note in the data presented in Fig. 13 are the monotonic relations between the volunteers' conjoined and separate attentional processing of stimulus attributes and the amplitude of ERP components. At the N2 level—i.e., the timing of the first sign of sensory gating—the orientation had a lower value than spatial frequency, because the brain's response to stimuli that shared only the orientation but not the frequency with the target was significantly lower compared to when stimuli shared the spatial frequency (SF) but not the orientation (O). No attentional response is present for stimuli irrelevant in both features, whereas a large response is observable for targets. It is very important to point out that the amplitude of N2 for target stimuli (SF + O) was greater than the sum of the two responses to the single feature (SF or O), thus demonstrating a nonadditive nature and a close interaction between the mechanisms of selection of frequency and orientation. This trend was apparent for the amplitude of P300, also displayed in the central histograms in Fig. 13. At this stage of processing the response to relevant orientation in the absence of the relevant frequency is lower; in addition, the response to the individual features decreases: the brain is getting ready to make a decision concerning the presence of the target, and the conjoining of the two attributes takes on special relevance as an object. At the response time level (displayed in the lower

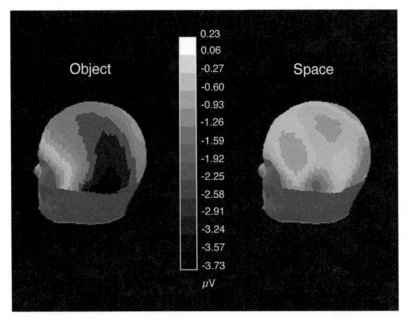

FIGURE 12 Selection negativity. Realistic three-dimensional isocolor voltage maps for frequency (left) and location (right) selection. The maps were computed in the selection negativity latency range (i.e., 180–280 msec; peak latency, 240 msec) on difference waves obtained by subtracting brain response to nontarget gratings from that to targets in the two attend-object and attend-location tasks.

block diagram, Fig. 13), this trend is even more apparent: the percentage of responses emitted to stimuli having the same frequency as the attended frequency (i.e., SF) is slightly greater than 10%. This is most relevant when thinking that the amplitude of the ERP components was as high as 50% in the case of N2 and greater than 35% in the case of P300. All in all, these findings also revealed a progressive narrowing of the attention filter band as neural processing progresses from input to motor response.

In further work on feature-conjunction selection carried out by our research group we investigated the mechanisms of the combined selection of frequency and spatial location using isoluminant gratings of variable spatial frequency (0.75, 1.5, 3 and 6 cpd) laterally presented in the inferior and superior quadrants of the left and right visual hemifields (Zani and Proverbio, 1997b). In this study we used a more advanced recording and analysis

technique than in the previous study and recorded from four occipital electrode locations, namely O1, O2, and OL, OR homologous sites. The results indicated that a much earlier selection of the frequency occurred than previously believed—that is, within 60–130 msec poststimulus. More specifically, the two features influenced the amplitude of the evoked sensory response P1, even though the effect of frequency relevance was felt only when the stimuli fell in the attended quadrant. The latter findings suggest that the selection mechanisms of the two features operate in parallel right from the earliest stages of analysis, and that object or feature selection, rather than being preceded by a space selection, is centered "on line" on precise coordinates of the attended space. This view is supported in the literature—as discussed later in this section—but can be considered straightforwardly sound *per se*, from an ecological perceptual viewpoint related to the pervasive subjective phenomena we

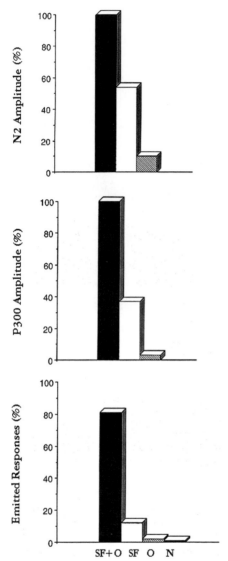

FIGURE 13 Comparative representation of the amplitudes of N2 and P300 components and percentage of emitted responses to spatial frequency gratings as a function of number of attributes shared with target (both spatial frequency and orientation, SF+O+; only spatial frequency, SF+; only orientation, O+; neither attribute, N). Reprinted from *Electroencephalography and Clinical Neurophysiology*, **45**; M. R. Harter and F. H. Previc; Size-specific information channels and selective attention: Visual evoked potentials and behavioural measures, pp. 628–640. Copyright (1978) with permission from Elsevier Science and author.

experience with objects in everyday life. Indeed, looking aimlessly and absentmindedly at the outer world, one is rather often aware of having seen something—i.e., a car, a neon sign, or whatever—automatically surfacing at the conscious level, but not being able to localize it except by means of a visual rescanning of the surrounding space, looking for its location.

In a later study (Zani and Proverbio, 1997e), carried out using exactly the same paradigm and a much higher density electrode montage (i.e., 32 electrodes). ERP data provided evidence that the effect of P1 modulation by the relevant spatial frequency presented in the attended spatial quadrant modulated the activity of the striate visual cortex, as is reported in the scalp current density maps displayed in Fig. 14. Because this does not occur when stimuli are selected solely on the basis of spatial location, this evidence indicates a strong reciprocal interaction among the various visual mechanisms of sensory analysis.

The evidence presented so far shows that object-based selective attention affects visual processing at early latency stages, as indexed by modulation of early sensory-evoked responses. To further investigate the timing of the activation of this early sensory gating and obtain further support for our findings, we have repeated the combined space–object attentional paradigm (Zani and Proverbio, 2002), using several significant methodological variants. This time, instead of measuring the amplitude of sensory-evoked responses at peak latency, we measured the mean amplitude of early potentials in four different time windows (i.e., 60–80, 80–100, 100–120, and 120–140 msec poststimulus) over both mesial and lateral occipital sites, and compared the effect of frequency relevance (F+), location relevance (L+), and the conjunction of both features (F+L+) on evoked potentials across electrodes, hemispheres, and different temporal windows. Furthermore, a larger sample of volunteers (N = 21) was tested in order to obtain the best possible signal-to-noise ratio in ERP wave forms. Results showed that stimuli relevant in frequency and/or location eli-

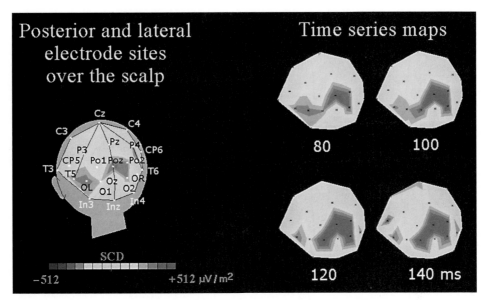

FIGURE 14 Frequency selection. Scalp current density maps reflecting attention effects for spatial frequency selection between 80 and 140 msec poststimulus. Maps were computed on the difference wave obtained by subtracting brain response to nontargets from that to targets in the P1 latency range. Stimuli were 7-cpd black and white gratings presented in the right visual field. Note the leftward occipital-temporal flowing of currents, suggesting the activation of the *What* system. (See color plates.)

cited larger evoked responses compared to irrelevant stimuli as early as 60–80 msec poststimulus (P/N80), a latency range, reflected at scalp surface by the so-called C1 component, that is acknowledged to correspond to sensory activity in the striate cortex.

Fig. 15 displays grand-average ERPs elicited by low-frequency (0.75 cpd) and high-frequency (6 cpd) luminance-modulated gratings presented for 80 msec in the left hemifield, as a function of attention condition. It is possible to see the attentional fine gradient in the form of larger responses for gratings relevant in location but not in frequency (L+F−), with respect to those relevant in frequency but not in location (L−F+). Of great interest is the finding of larger responses in the first time window (i.e., 60–80 msec) to stimuli relevant in both features compared to stimuli relevant only in location, suggesting that frequency relevance alone affects visual processing at the earliest processing stage (see Fig. 15).

So far we have seen how it is possible in the laboratory to study the way in which the visual system processes and attentionally selects one or more visual features (spatial frequency, depth, stereopsis, color, orientation, texture, luminance) of the surrounding environment, separately. Of course, in actual fact, we perceive a unitary environment and not a separate series of objects or individual attributes [see the discussion on this point in Previc (1990)]. This perception of the unitary nature derives from the interaction between the *Where* and *What* systems, which, although partially anatomically and functionally distinct, operate in parallel and in very close coordination. Clear evidence of this interdependence comes from neuroimaging and neuropsychological literature. For example, the clinical neuropsychological study by Friedman-Hill *et al.* (1995) indicated that patients with focused bilateral lesions of the parietal cortex are unable correctly to combine color and shape of stimuli presented in the two visual hemi-

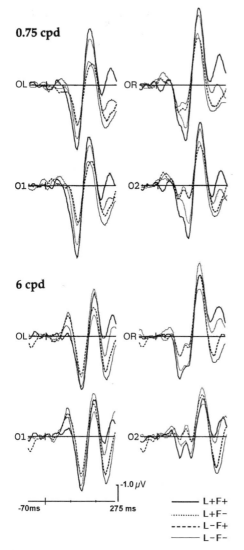

0.75 cpd

6 cpd

-1.0 μV

-70ms   275 ms

———— L+F+
············ L+F-
------ L-F+
———— L-F-

FIGURE 15 Grand-average ERPs to black and white luminance-modulated gratings of low (0.75 cpd) and high (6 cpd) spatial frequency as a function of attention condition in a conjoined selection task. ERPs were recorded from left and right lateral (i.e., OL and OR, respectively) and mesial (i.e., O1 and O2, respectively) occipital sites to stimuli presented in the lower and upper quadrants of the left visual field.

intentional mechanisms are probably not separated at all because of the existence of specific selection mechanisms centered on the object at a given spatial location (i.e., object-centered space receptive fields). In our view, our electrophysiological data on conjoined selection of frequency and space (Zani and Proverbio, 1997b,e) reported above are in line with this view derived from other research lines in cognitive neuroscience.

The extensive available neurophysiological and psychophysical literature has shown that the perceptual construction of objects takes place through the simultaneous analysis of a complex series of cues (namely luminance, color, texture, motion, and binocular disparity) at very early processing stages (Mountcastle, 1998; Regan, 2000). We shall now see how selective attention is able to modulate (that is, to optimize or ignore) the perception of objects thus constructed through the selection of illusory subjective figures. In a study carried out on healthy young controls we investigated the brain mechanisms underlying the perception of illusory contours and determined the time course of sensory and perceptual processing in the boundary completion process, analyzing the timing of ERP responses (Proverbio and Zani, 2002). The so-called illusory contours are known to be perceived edges that exist in the absence of local borders and that determine the perception of subjective figures, such as the universally known Kanizsa square or triangle (Kanizsa, 1976). They are based on the peculiar boundary alignment of inducers (simple geometric shapes in striking contrast with the homogeneous background luminance) that elicit the response of edge detectors in area 18 (Hirsch, 1995; Larsson *et al.*, 1999) and perhaps 17 (Grosof *et al.*, 1993; Lee and Nguyen, 2001; Olson, 2001), giving rise to the subjective perception of an object with partially illusory boundaries. The aim of our research was to investigate the mechanisms underlying object-based selective

fields. This suggests that the integrity of the *Where* system is absolutely essential for the correct recognition of objects. On the other hand, a large body of neuropsychological, neurophysiological, and behavioral data (see Olson and Gettner, 1996) indicates that the spatial and nonspatial

inducer

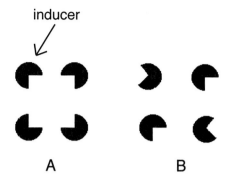

A   B

FIGURE 16 (A) Stimulus generated by thick inducers (packmen) producing the classical Kanizsa square illusion. (B) Same stimulus but with outward rotation of the packmen and no illusory perception.

attention by presenting target and non-target stimuli possessing the same amount of physical energy (luminance), differing only in the presence or absence of the subjective figure. Indeed, they consisted of the same elements presented in different orientations: the outward rotation of external inducers in nontargets cancelled the perception of illusory boundaries, and therefore of the illusory object (see Fig. 16). The object to be detected and attentionally selected thus did not actually exist for retinal photoreceptors, but was really seen by the visual cortex with the same clarity as a real object. We wondered which mechanisms underlay the attentional selection of objects mainly perceived on the basis of luminance contrast and boundary alignment, and, above all, at which stage of latency attention was able to affect visual processing. ERP results showed that the occurrence of illusory contours was associated with a strong bilateral activation of lateral occipital areas at about 145 msec poststimulus as indexed by N1 component, followed by a left-sided activation of the same region at about 250 msec of latency. Overall, our data support the view that the integration of contours arises at very early stages of visual processing, as proposed by Hess and Field (1999). Moreover, our data also indicate that object-based attention is able to affect illusory contour binding by

somewhat enhancing ERPs to the illusory percepts at lateral occipital sites.

Quite interesting, in this regard, is the Grossberg and Raizada (2000) neural model—based on neurophysiological data—indicating how visual objects are grouped, or bound together, by being connected by regions of layer 2/3 of the visual cortex. The model also proposes detailed laminar circuits to account for how top-down attentional task demands may affect the activity of V1 cells (for example, in attentional grouping) by means of a mechanism called *folded feedback*, based both on facilitatory ON-center attentional enhancements and inhibitory suppressive OFF-surround effects.

COLOR

We have seen that object features such as spatial frequency, orientation, or shape are processed in the ventral stream of the occipitotemporal visual areas (the so-called *What* system), unlike the movement and spatial position represented instead in the occipitoparietal system (the *Where* system). A separate section should be dedicated to color selection as far as aspects related to the selection of object features are concerned. This is due to the fact that several studies have dealt with the investigation of neural mechanisms underlying the selection of this feature both per se and in conjunction with other features, mostly finding a special status for this nonspatial feature with respect to others.

Neuroimaging studies have identified several human brain areas, notably the lingual and fusiform gyrus of the extrastriate cortex, which selectively respond to color (e.g., Corbetta *et al.*, 1991; Corbetta, 1999). It is interesting to note that neurological lesions in the same areas are associated with the inability to perceive the color of objects—a deficit reported as achromatopsia—which may occur also in the absence of a deficit in object recognition (i.e., visual agnosia).

Many electrophysiological studies have also been carried out in an attempt to determine how conjunctions of color and other sensory features, such as shape or orientation, are coded and selected, by recording ERPs during tasks involving attentional selection of one or more attributes of the objects. The majority of studies involved the use of simple stimuli such as geometric shapes, spatial frequency gratings, checkerboards, alphanumeric characters, colored Mondrians, or faces. In these studies, the relationship between shape and color was completely arbitrary (take, for instance, a random sequence of red or blue squares or circles), because, of course, in association with such forms, no specific representation of the color of the latter is stored in the brain.

In these ERP paradigms it has been frequently reported that the attentional selection of color takes place before that of the other nonspatial attributes such as size, shape, or orientation (e.g., Eimer, 1996b; Karayanidis and Michie, 1997). Moreover, the selection of those features often depended hierarchically on that of color (Wijers et al., 1989). In particular, the selection negativity of ERPs reflecting the attentional selection at the level of N1–N2 was absent when the color was irrelevant even when the other attribute was relevant to the task (Smid and Heinze, 1997; Rotte et al., 1996).

Yet, the data in the literature indicate that this neural logistic does not hold for the selection of color in conjunction with space location. Indeed, in an electrophysiological study by Anllo-Vento and Hillyard (1996), a comparison was made between the color- and movement-selection systems by recording ERPs to little squares displayed on a computer monitor, while individuals were involved in spatially directed attention tasks. ERP measurements and topographic mapping showed that wherever color- and movement-selection were

topographically dissociated in the two ventral and dorsal streams at selection negativity (N2) level, the selection of the spatial location in any case temporally preceded that of the two nonspatial features by modulating the early P1 and N1 components. Nonetheless, the same authors (Anllo-Vento et al., 1998), using red and blue isoluminant checkerboards, found that, as well as space selection, color selection modulated scalp-recorded potentials in the lateral occipital areas as early as 100 msec poststimulus, thus further supporting the hypothesis advanced by Zani and Proverbio (1993, 1995) of an early selection also for nonspatial attributes of sensory inputs.

To further investigate the apparent priority of color selection over that of the other sensory features, we adopted an experimental paradigm different from those used previously (Proverbio et al., 2002b). Our aim was to determine whether color processing interacted with that of shape by recording ERPs in response to familiar objects and common animals represented in their canonical color (here defined as "prototypical"), as well as in various other colors.

Because the stimuli used in our tests consisted of drawings of everyday life objects and common animals, we managed to ensure that the attribute of the objects' color was in some cases strongly associated with their shape: the combination of the two features (e.g., the color yellow and the shape of a banana) was specific to and characteristic of that particular object. The task consisted in selectively attending and responding to target images either on the basis of their color, regardless of their shape, or on the basis of their shape regardless of their color. We investigated the timing and topographic distribution of the attentional selection of both features by comparing the electrofunctional responses to target stimuli canonical in both shape and color (e.g., a yellow banana) with those to noncanonical targets (e.g., a yellow tire or swallow during color selection; a pink or blue banana during shape selection).

The results suggest that the selection of the two dimensions takes place in parallel and not separately, and that it modulates the amplitude of the occipital-temporal components N1 (N166) and N2 (N278) and of the centroparietal P300. Consistent with previous literature, both the RTs and the SN and P3 latencies were found to be more rapid in the color selection condition than in that of shape, also given that the two attentional components were much larger in the shape selection condition. This initial evidence suggests that shape selection might actually be more demanding than selection of an object's color. However, a detailed analysis of selection negativity (or N278 component) elicited by the different stimuli as a function of the attributes shared with the target indicated that color selection is affected by stimulus shape, in that greater responses were recorded to stimuli of the relevant color having a prototypical shape (e.g., a yellow banana or chick compared to a yellow tire or swallow), whereas shape selection does not depend on the color of the image presented (e.g., a piglet, whatever its color: pink, yellow, or blue—see Fig. 17).

Electrocortical topographic mapping showed that selection of the color dimension of familiar images strongly activated the posterior temporal and extrastriate cortex of the left hemisphere. These areas were found to be highly sensitive to the prototypical effect of shape with respect to color, and consequently to be able possibly to indicate the probable locus of conjoined processing of shape and color in the human visual cortex. It is interesting that in our experimental paradigm color selection is responsible for a strong activation of areas not specifically related to color but rather to information concerning shape. Indeed, this fact proves extremely important when it is taken into account that in experimental selective attentional studies

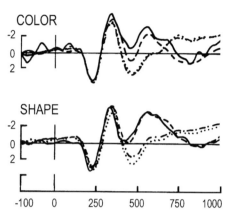

FIGURE 17 Grand-average ERPs recorded at the left inion site in response to pictures of familiar objects and animals as a function of the four target (prototypical, solid line; nonprototypical, dashed line) and nontarget (prototypical, dotted lines; non-prototypical, dot-dashed line) conditions in the two attend-color and attend-shape tasks. ERPs to shape prototypically associated to target color (such as a green artichoke in the attend-green condition) elicited a larger N2 component, as compared to nonprototypical targets (such as a *green swallow*) over the left hemisphere.

what is valid is the general assumption that the selection of one feature of the stimulus modulates the bioelectrical activity of the same brain regions that are apparently active during the perception of this feature (as suggested also by several different ERP and PET studies). In this regard it is extremely interesting that a PET study (Chao and Martin, 1999) reported, for example, that the cortical regions involved in color perception are not the same as those that convey information related to the color of objects (object color knowledge), which has many points in common with our electrophysiological results described above.

This double dissociation between color perception and object color knowledge has also been robustly supported by some very recent clinical cases reported in neuro-psychological literature. These cases show that semantic information about object colors is apparently actually grounded in neural systems distinct from those involved in form and function knowledge. Indeed, although previous neurological literature was scarce and anecdotal, Miceli *et al.* (2001) reported a straightforward case of three patients with lesions in the mesial temporal region of the left hemisphere who were unable to decide whether a color matched a given familiar object ("Can a lion be red?"), despite their essentially normal ability to name colors or to define functional properties of common objects ("Is a pencil made of glass"?). The authors concluded that mesial temporal structures of the left hemisphere are specifically involved in representing or accessing color knowledge. These findings strongly agree with our ERP topographical mapping data, notwithstanding the inherent limitations of scalp-recorded ERPs for source localization due to their scarce spatial resolution.

CONCLUSIONS

Several conclusions may be drawn on the basis of the ERP findings reviewed above on nonspatial feature selection mechanisms. One is that attentional selection of visual inputs is carried out by means of the parallel activation of a distributed neural network of the brain, made up of the anterior and posterior attentional systems, whose centers and pathways play different but synergic roles in the selection. As far as the posterior attentional system is concerned, the data indicate that, as for attention to space, attention to object features can modulate neural processing of visual areas at an early sensory level, very likely involving the primary striate cortex, with modalities that are still not clearly known and which must be further investigated. Furthermore, the data suggest that the dorsal and ventral streams of the visual system, although partially anatomically segregated, may be activated in parallel and in an independent or conjoined mode, depending on the attentional demands and task requirements. Last, but not least, there

is evidence that the perception of multidimensional objects in the visual field is accomplished through a unitary active binding process of spatial and nonspatial features. This mechanism is believed not to be based on hierarchically organized independent processes, but rather to reflect the horizontal processing of visual cells that takes place at very early stages of input analysis. This view seems to be consistent with models assuming that different stimulus attributes may be initially conjoined in a single representation, while at the same time being separately analyzed in parallel, dimension by dimension (*cf.* Treisman, 1999).

References

Aine, C. J., Supek, S., and George, J. S. (1995). Temporal dynamics of visual-evoked neuromagnetic sources: Effects of stimulus parameters and selective attention. *Int. J. Neurosci.* **80**, 79–104.

Anllo-Vento, L., and Hillyard, S. A. (1996). Selective attention to color and the direction of moving stimuli: Electrophysiological correlates of hierarchical feature selection. *Percept. Psychophys.* **58**, 191–206.

Anllo-Vento, L., Luck, S., and Hillyard, S. A. (1998). Spatio-temporal dynamics of attention to color: Evidence from human electrophysiology. *Hum. Brain Mapping* **6**, 216–238.

Arakawa, K., Tobimatsu, S., Kurita Tashima, S., Nakayama, M., Kira, J. I., and Kato, M. (2000). Effects of stimulus orientation on spatial frequency function of the visual evoked potential. *Exp. Brain Res.* **131**, 121–125.

Aston-Jones, G. S., Desimone, R., Driver, J., Luck, S. J., and Posner, M. I. (1999). Attention. In "Fundamental Neuroscience" (M. J. Zigmond, F. E. Bloom, S. C. Landis, J. L. Roberts, and L. R. Squire, eds.), pp.1385-1409. Academic Press, San Diego.

Barcelo, F., Suwazono, S., and Knight, R. T. (2000). Prefrontal modulation of visual processing in humans. Nat. Neurosci. 3, 399–403.

Cabeza, R., and Nyberg, L. (2000). Imaging cognition II: An empirical review of 275 PET and fMRI studies. *J. Cogn. NeuroSci.* **12**, 1–47.

Campbell, F. W., and Maffei, L. (1970). Electrophysiological evidence for the existence of orientation and size detectors in the human visual system. *J. Physiol.* **207**, 635–652.

Campbell, F. W., Kulikowski, J. J., and Levinson, J. (1966). The effect of orientation on the visual resolution of gratings. *J. Physiol.* **187**, 427–36

Chao, L., and Martin, A. (1999). Cortical regions associated with perceiving, naming, and knowing about colors. *J. Cogn. NeuroSci.* **11**, 25–35.

Clark, V. P., and Hillyard, S. A. (1996). Spatial selective attention affects early extrastriate but not striate components of the visual evoked potentials. *J. Cogn. Neurosci.* **8**, 387–402.

Coles, M. G. (1989). Modern mind-brain reading: Psychophysiology, physiology, and cognition. *Psychophysiology* **26**(3), 251–269.

Corbetta, M. (1999). Functional anatomy of visual attention in the human brain: Studies with positron emission tomography. *In* "The Attentive brain" (R. Parasuraman, ed.), pp. 95–122. MIT Press, Cambridge, Massachusetts.

Corbetta, M., and Shulman, G. L. (1999). Human cortical mechanisms of visual attention during orienting. *In* "Attention, Space and Action. Studies in Cognitive Neuroscience" (G. W. Humphreys, J. Duncan, and A. Treisman, eds.), pp. 183–198. Oxford University Press, Oxford.

Corbetta, M., Miezin, F. M., Dobmeyer, S., Shulman, G., and Petersen, S. E. (1991). Selective and divided attention during visual discriminations of shape color and speed: functional anatomy by positron emission tomography. *J. Neurosci.* **11**, 2383–2402.

Desimone, R., and Duncan, J. (1995). Neural mechanisms of selective visual attention. *Annu. Rev. Neurosci.* **18**, 193–222.

Donchin, E. (1981). Surprise! ... Surprise? *Psychophysiology* **9**, 493–513.

Dupont, P., Vogels, R., Vandenberghe, R., Rosier, A., Cornette, L., Bormans, G., Mortelmans, L., and Orban, G. A. (1998). Regions in the human brain activated by simultaneous orientation discrimination: A study with positron emission tomography. *Eur. J. Neurosci* **10**, 3689–3699.

Eimer, M. (1996a). The N2pc component as an indicator of attentional selectivity. *Electroencephalogr. Clin. Neurophysiol.* **99**, 225–34.

Eimer, M. (1996b). An event-related potential (ERP) study of transient and sustained visual attention to color and form. *Biol. Psychol.* **44**, 143–160.

Fabiani, M., Karis, D., and Donchin E. (1986). P300 and recall in an incidental memory paradigm. *Psychophysiology* **23**, 298–308.

Fink, G. R., Dolan, R. G., Halligan, P. W., and Marshall, J. C. (1997). Space-based and object-based visual attention: Shared and specific neural domains. *Brain* **120**, 2013–2028.

Friedman-Hill, S. R., Robertson, L., and Treisman, A. (1995). Parietal contributions to visual feature binding: Evidence from a patient with bilateral lesions. *Science* **269**, 853–855.

Furmanski, C. S., and Engel, S. A. (2000). An oblique effect in human primary visual cortex. *Nat. Neurosci.* **3**, 535–536.

Gehring, W. J., and Knight, R. T. (2000). Prefrontal-cingulate interactions in action monitoring. *Nat. Neurosci.* **3**, 421–423.

Georgopoulos, A. P., Whang, K., Georgopoulos, M. A., Tagaris, G. A., Amirikian, B., Richter, W., Kim, S. G., and Ugurbil, K. (2001). Functional magnetic resonance imaging of visual object construction and shape discrimination: Relations among task, hemispheric lateralization, and gender. *J. Cogn. Neurosci.* **13**, 72–89.

Gevins, A., and Cutillo, B. (1993). Spatiotemporal dynamics of component processes in human working memory. *Electroencephalogr. Clin. Neurophysiol.* **87**, 128–143.

Goldman-Rakic, P. (1987). Circuitry of primate prefrontal cortex and regulation of behavior by representational memory. *In* "Handbook of Physiology. The Nervous System—Higher Functions of the Brain" (F. Blum, ed.), Vol. 5, Part 1, pp. 373–417. American Physiology Association, Bethesda, Maryland.

Gomer, F. E., Spicuzza, R. J., and O'Donnell, R. D. (1976). Evoked potentials correlates of visual item recognition during memory-scanning tasks. *Physiol. Psychology* **4**, 61–65.

Grosof, D. H., Shapley, R. M., and Hawken, M. J. (1993). Macaque V1 neurones can signal "illusory" contours. *Nature* **365**, 550–552.

Grossberg, S., and Raizada, R. D. S. (2000). Contrast-sensitive perceptual grouping and object-based attention in the laminar circuits of primary visual cortex. *Vis. Res.* **40**, 10–12.

Harter, M. R., and Aine, C. J. (1984). Brain mechanisms of visual selective attention. *In* "Varieties of Attention" (R. Parasuraman, and R. Davies, eds.), pp. 293–321. Academic Press, New York.

Harter, M. R., and Guido, W. (1980). Attention to pattern orientation: Negative cortical potentials, reaction time, and the selection process. *Electroencephalogr. Clin. Neurophysiol.* **49**, 461–475.

Harter, M. R., and Previc, F. H. (1978). Size-specific information channels and selective attention: Visual evoked potentials and behavioural measures. *Electroencephalogr. Clin. Neurophysiol.* **45**, 628–640.

Haxby, J. V., Courtney, S. M., and Clark, V. P. (1999). Functional magnetic resonance imaging and the study of attention. *In* "The Attentive Brain" (R. Parasuraman, ed.), pp. 123–142. MIT Press, Cambridge, Massachusetts.

Heinze, H. J., Mangun, G. R., Burchert, W., Hinrichs, H., Scholze, M., Münte, T. F., Gös, A., Johanne, S. S., Scherg, M., Hundeshagen, H., Gazzaniga, M. S., and Hillyard, S. A. (1994). Combined spatial and temporal imaging of spatial selective attention in humans. *Nature* **372**, 543–546.

Hermann, C. S., and Knight, R. T. (2001). Mechanisms of human attention: Event-related potentials and oscillations. *Neurosci. Biobehav. Rev.* **25**, 465–476.

Hess, R., and Field, D. (1999). Integration of contours: New insights. *Trends Cogn. Sci.* **3**, 480–486.

Hillyard, S. A., and Mangun, G. R (1986). The neural basis of visual selective attention: A commentary on Harter and Aine. *Biol. Psychol.* **23**, 265–279.

Hillyard, S. A., and Anlo-Vento, L. (1998). Event-related brain potentials in the study of visual selective attention. *Proc. Natl. Acad. Sci. U.S.A.* **95**, 781–787.

Hillyard, S. A., and Kutas, M. (1983). Electrophysiology of cognitive processing. *Annu. Rev. Psychol.* **34**, 33–61.

Hillyard, S. A., Mangun, G. R, Woldorff, M. G., and Luck, S. J. (1995). Neural systems mediating selective attention. *In* "The Cognitive Neurosciences" (M. S. Gazzaniga, ed.), pp. 665–681. MIT Press, Cambridge, Massachusetts.

Hillyard, S. A., Teder-Sälejärvi, W. A., and Münte, T. F. (1998). Temporal dynamics of early perceptual processing. *Curr. Opin. Neurobiol.* **8**, 202–210.

Hillyard, S. A., Vogel, E. K., and Luck, S. J. (1999). Sensory gain control (amplification) as a mechanism of selective attention: Electrophysiological and neuroimaging evidence. *In* "Attention, Space and Action. Studies in Cognitive Neuroscience" (G. W. Humphreys, J. Duncan, and A. Treisman, eds.), pp. 31–53. Oxford University Press, Oxford.

Hirsch, J., DeLaPaz, R., Relkin, R. N., Victor, J., Kim, K., Li, T., Borden, P., Rubin, N., and Shapley, R. (1995). Illusory contours activate specific regions in human visual cortex: Evidence from functional magnetic resonance imaging. *Proc. Natl. Acad. Sci. U.S.A.* **92**, 6469–6473.

Ito, M., and Gilbert, C. D. (1999). Attention modulates contextual influences in the primary visual cortex of alert monkey. *Neuron* **22**, 593–604.

Jeffreys, D. A., and Axford, J. G. (1972). Source locations of pattern specific components of human visual evoked potentials. I. Components of striate cortical origin. *Exp. Brain Res.* **16**, 1–21.

Kanizsa, G. (1976). Subjective contours. *Sci. Am.* **234**, 48–52.

Karayanidis, F., and Michie, P. T. (1997). Evidence of visual processing negativity with attention to orientation and color in central space. *Electroencephalogr. Clin. Neurophysiol.* **103**, 282–297.

Kawashima, R., Satoh, K., Goto, R., Inoue, K., *et al.* (1998). The role of the left inferior temporal cortex for visual pattern discrimination-—a PET study. *Neuroreport* **11**, 1581–1586.

Kenemans, J. L., Kok, A., and Smulders, F. T. Y. (1994). Event-related potentials to conjunctions of spatial frequency and orientation as a function of stimulus parameters and response requirements. *Electroencephalogr. Clin. Neurophysiol.* **88**, 51–63.

Knight, R. T. (1991). Evoked potential studies of attention capacity in human frontal lobe lesions. *In* "Frontal Lobe Function and Dysfunction" (H. Levin, H. Eisenberg, and F. Benton, eds.), pp. 139–153. Oxford Univ. Press.

Knight, R. T., and Grabowecky, M. (1995). Escape from linear time: Prefrontal cortex and conscious experience. *In* "The Cognitive Neurosciences" (M. S. Gazzaniga, ed.), pp. 1357–1371. MIT Press, Cambridge, Massachussets.

Knight, R. T., Staines, W. R., Swick, D., and Chao, L. L. (1999). Prefrontal cortex regulates inhibition and excitation in distributed neural networks. *Acta Psychol.* 101, 159–178.

LaBerge, D. (1995). "Attentional Processing. The Brain's Art of Mindfulness." Harvard University Press, Cambridge, Massachusetts.

La Berge, D., and Buchsbaum, M. S. (1990). Positron emission tomographic measurements of pulvinar activity during an attention task. *J. Neurosci.* **10**, 613–619.

Lamme, V. A. F., and Spekreijse, H. (2000). Modulations of primary visual cortex activity representing attentive and conscious scene perception. *Frontiers Biosci.* **5**, 232–243.

Larsson, J., Amuntus, K., Gulys, B., Malikovic, A., Zilles, K., and Roland, P. E. (1999). Neuronal correlates of real and illusory contour perception: functional anatomy with PET. *Eur. J. Neurosci.* **11**, 4024–4036.

Lee, T. S., and Nguyen, M. (2001). Dynamics of subjective contour formation in the early visual cortex. *Proc. Natl. Acad. Sci. U.S.A.* **98**, 1907–1911.

Luck, S. J., Chelazzi, L., Hillyard, S., and Desimone, R. (1997). Neural mechanisms of spatial selective attention in areas V1, V2, and V4 of macaque visual cortex. *J. Neurophysiol.* **77**, 24–42.

Luck, S. J., Woodman, G., and Vogel, E. K. (2000). Event-related potential studies of attention. *Trends Cogn. Sci.* **4**, 432–440.

Mangun, G. R., Hopfinger, J. B., Kussmaul, C., Fletcher, E. M., and Heinze, H. J. (1997). Covariations in PET and ERP measures of spatial selective attention in human extrastriate visual cortex. *Hum. Brain Mapping* **5**, 273–279.

Mangun, G. R., Hinrichs, H., Scholz, M., Mueller-Gaertner, H. W., Herzog, H., Krause B. J., Tellman L., Kemna, L., and Heinze H. J. (2001). Integrating electrophysiology and neuroimaging of spatial selective attention to simple isolated visual stimuli. *Vis. Res.* **41**, 1423–35.

Martin-Loeches, M., Hinojosa, J. A., and Rubia, F. J. (1999). Insights from event-related potentials into the temporal and hierarchical organization of the ventral and dorsal streams of the visual system in selective attention. *Psychophysiology* **36**, 721–36.

Martínez, A., Anllo-Vento, L., Sereno, M. I., Frank, L. R., Buxton, R. B., Dubowitz, D. J., Wong, E. C., Hinrichs, H., Heinze, H. J., and Hillyard, S. A. (1999). Involvement of striate and extrastriate visual cortical areas in spatial attention. *Nat. Neurosci.* **2**, 364–369.

Martínez, A., Di Russo, F., Annlo-Vento, L., and Hillyard, S. A. (2001). Electrophysiological analysis of cortical mechanisms of selective attention to high and low spatial frequencies. *Clin. Neurophysiol.* **112**, 1980–1998.

McCarthy, G. A., and Scabini, D. (1991). Attention modifies event-related potentials recorded from human visual cortex. *IBRO World Congr. in Neurosci.* **3**,176.

Merigan, W. H., and Maunsell, J. H. R. (1993). How parallel are the primate visual pathways? *Annu. Rev. Neurosci* **16**, 396–402.

Metha, A. D., Ulbert, D., Lindsley, R. W., and Schroeder, C. E. (1997). Timing and distribution of attention effects across areas in the macaque visual system. *Soc. of Neurosci. Abstr.* **23** (121.1), 299.

Miceli, G., Fouch, E., Capasso, R., Shelton, J. R., Tomaiuolo, F., and Caramazza, A. (2001). The dissociation of color from form and function knowledge. *Nat. Neurosci.* **4**, 662–667.

Miller, E. K., and Cohen, J. D. (2001). An integrative theory of prefrontal cortex function. *Annu. Rev. Neurosci.* **24**, 167–202.

Motter, B. C. (1993). Focal attention produces spatially selective processing in visual cortical areas V1, V2, and V4 in the presence of competing stimuli. *J. Neurophysiol.* **70**, 909–919.

Mountcastle, V. B. (1998). "Perceptual Neuroscience: The Cerebral Cortex." Harvard University Press, Cambridge, Massachusetts.

Näätänen R. (1992). "Attention and Brain Function." Lawrence Erlbaum Assoc., Hillsdale, New Jersey.

Oakley, M. T., and Eason, R. G. (1990). Subcortical gating in the human visual system during spatial selective attention. *Int. J. Psychophysiol.* **9**, 105–120.

Olson, C. R. (2001). Object-based vision and attention in primates. *Curr. Opin. Neurobiol.* **11**, 171–179.

Olson, C. R, and Gettner, S. N. (1996). Brain representation of object-centered space. *Curr. Opin. Neurobiol.* **6**, 165–170.

Posner, M. I., and Petersen, S. E. (1990). The attention system of the human brain. *Annu. Rev. Neurosci.* **13**, 25–42.

Press, W. A., and Van Essen, D. C. (1997). Attentional modulation of neuronal responses in macaque area V1. *Soc. Neurosci. Abstr.* **23** (405.3), 1026.

Previc, F. H. (1990). Functional specialization in the lower and upper visual fields in humans: Its ecological origins and neurophysiological implications. *Behav. Brain Sci.* **13**, 519–575.

Previc, F. H., and Harter, M. R (1982). Electrophysiological and behavioural indicants of selective attention to multifeature gratings. *Percept. Psychophys.* **32**, 465–472.

Proverbio, A. M., and Mangun, R. G. (1994). Electrophysiological and behavioral "costs" and "benefits" during sustained visual-spatial attention. *Int. J. Neurosci.* **79**, 221–233.

Proverbio, A. M., and Zani, A. (2002). Electrophysiological indexes of illusory contour perception in humans. *Neuropsychologia* **40**, 479–491.

Proverbio, A. M., Zani A., and Mangun R. G. (1993). Electrophysiological substrates of visual selective attention to spatial frequency. *Bull. Psychonom. Soc.* **31**, 368.

Proverbio, A. M., Zani, A., Gazzaniga, M. S., and Mangun, R. G. (1994). ERP and RT signs of a rightward bias for spatial orienting in a split-brain patient. *Neuroreport* **5**, 2457–2461.

Proverbio, A. M., Zani, A., and Avella, C. (1996). Differential activation of multiple current sources of foveal VEPs as a function of spatial frequency. *Brain Topogr.* **9**, 59–68.

Proverbio, A. M., Minniti, A., and Zani, A. (1998). Electrophysiological evidence of a perceptual precedence of global vs. local visual information. *Cogn. Brain Res.* **6**, 321–334.

Proverbio, A. M., Esposito, P., and Zani, A. (2002a). Early involvement of temporal area in attentional selection of grating orientation: an ERP study. *Cogn. Brain Res.* **13** (1), 139–151.

Proverbio, A. M., Burco, F., and Zani, A. (2002b). Blue piglets? Electrofunctional evidence of how shape can affect color selection, and not vice versa. *Cogn. Brain Res.* (in revision).

Regan, D. (1989). "Human Brain Electrophysiology." Elsevier, Amsterdam.

Regan, D. (2000). "Multiple Cues for Object Perception: Early Visual Processing of Spatial Form Defined by Luminance, Color, Texture, Motion and Binocular Disparity." Sinauer Assoc. Sunderland, Massachusetts.

Roberts, L. E., Rau, H., Lutzenberger, W., and Birbaumer, N. (1994). Mapping P300 waves onto inhibition: Go/No-go discrimination. *Electroencephalogr. Clin. Neurophysiol.* **92**, 44–55.

Roelfsema, P. R., Lamme, V. A. F., and Spekreijse, H. (1997). Attentive response modulation in area V1 of the macaque during the detection of connected objects. *Soc. Neurosci. Abstr.* **23** (603.8), 1544.

Roelfsema, P. R., Lamme, V. A. F., and Spekreijse, H. (1998). Object-based attention in the primary visual cortex of the macaque monkey. *Nature* **395**, 376–381.

Rotte, M., Heinze, H. J., and Smid, H. G. O. M., (1996). Selective attention to conjunctions of color and shape of alphanumeric versus non-alphanumeric stimuli: A comparative electrophysiology study. *Biol. Psychol.* **46**, 199–221.

Rugg, M. D., Milner, A. D., Lines, C. R., and Phalp, R. (1987). Modulation of visual event-related potentials by spatial and non-spatial visual selective attention. *Neuropsychologia* **25**, 85–96.

Schroeder, C. E. (1995). Defining the neural bases of visual selective attention: Conceptual and empirical issues. *Int. J. Neurosci.* **80**, 65–78.

Schroeder, C.E., Mehta, A.D., and Givre, S. J. (1998). A spatiotemporal profile of visual system activation revealed by current source density analysis in the awake macaque *Cereb. Cortex* **8**, 575–592.

Shimamura, A. P. (1995). Memory and frontal lobe function. *In* "The Cognitive Neurosciences" (M. S. Gazzaniga, ed.), pp. 803–813. MIT Press, Cambridge, Massachusetts.

Shulman, G. L., Corbetta, M., Fiez, J. A., Buckner, R. L., Miezin, F. M., Raichle, M. E., and Petersen, S. E. (1997). Searching for activations that generalize over tasks. *Hum. Brain Mapping* **5**, 317–322.

Skrandies, W. (1983). Information processing and evoked potentials: Topography of early and late components. *Adv. Biol. Psychiatr.* **13**, 1–12.

Smid, H. G. O. M, and Heinze, H. J. (1997). An electro-physiological study of the selection of the color and shape of alphanumeric characters in response choice. *Biol. Psychol.* **44**, 161–185.

Somers, D. C., Dale, A. M., Seiffert, A. E., and Tootel, R. B. (1999). Functional MRI reveals spatially specific attentional modulation in human primary visual cortex. *Proc. Natl. Acad. Sci. U.S.A.* **96**, 1663–1668.

Squires, N. K., Squires, K. C., and Hillyard, S. A. (1975). Two varieties of long-latency positive waves evoked by unpredictable auditory stimuli in man. *Electroencephalogr. Clin. Neurophysiol.* **38**(4), 387–401.

Stuss, D. T., Eskes, G. A., and Foster, J. K. (1994). Experimental neuropsychological studies of frontal lobe functions. *In* "Handbook of Neuro-psychology" (F. Boller, and J. Grafman, eds.), Vol. 9, pp. 149–185. Elsevier, Amsterdam.

Sutton, S., Braren, M., Zubin, J., and John, E. R. (1965). Evoked-potential correlates of stimulus uncer-tainty. *Science* **26**, 1187–1188.

Swick, D., and Knight, R. T. (1999). Cortical lesions and attention. *In* "The Attentive Brain" (R. Parasuraman, ed.), pp. 143–162. The MIT Press, Cambridge, Massachusetts.

Tanaka, K. (2000). Mechanisms of visual object recog-nition studied in monkeys. *Spatial Vis.* **13**, 147–63.

Treisman, A. (1999). Feature binding, attention and object perception. *In* "Attention, Space and Action. Studies in Cognitive Neuroscience" (G. W. Humphreys, J. Duncan, and A. Treisman, eds.), pp. 91–111. Oxford University Press, Oxford.

Treue, S. (2001). Neural correlates of attention in primate visual cortex. *Trends Neurosci.* **24**, 295–300.

Ungerleider, L. G., and Mishkin, M. (1982). Two cortical visual systems. *In* "Analysis of Visual Behaviour" (D. G. Ingle, M. A. Goodale, and R. J. W. Mansfield, eds.), pp. 549–586. MIT Press, Cambridge, Massa-chusettes.

Vanduffel, W., Tootell, R. B. H., and Orban, G. A. (1997). State dependent modulation of visual pro-cessing in the macaque. *Exp. Brain Res.* **117**, S70.

Vanduffel, W., Tootell, R., and Orban, G. (2000). Attention-dependent suppression of metabolic activity in the early stages of the macaque visual system. *Cereb. Cortex* **10**, 109–126.

Vogels, R., and Orban, G. A. (1994) Activity of inferior temporal neurons during orientation discrimina-tion with successively presented gratings. *J. Neurophysiol.* **71**, 1428–1451.

Wang, J., Zhou, T. , Qiu, M., Du, A. , Cai, K., Wang, Z., Zhou, C., Meng, M., Zhuo, Y., Fan, S., and Chen, L. (1999). Relationship between ventral stream for object vision and dorsal stream for spatial vision: An fMRI + ERP study. *Hum. Brain Mapping* **8**, 170–181.

Watanabe, T., Sasaki, Y., Miyauchi, S., Putz, B., Fujimaki, N., Nielsen, M., Takino, R., and Miyakawa, S. (1998). Attention-regulated activity in human primary visual cortex. *Rapid Commun. Am. Physiol. Soc.* **22**, 2218–2221.

Webster, M. J., and Ungerleider, L. G. (1999). Neuroanatomy of visual attention. *In* "The Attentive Brain" (R. Parasuraman, ed.), pp. 19–34. MIT Press, Cambridge, Massachusetts.

Wijers, A. A., Mulder, G., Okita, T., and Mulder, L. J. M. (1989). An ERP study on memory search and selective attention to letter size and conjunctions of letter size and color. *Psychophysiology* **26**, 529–547.

Woldorff, M. G., Gallen, C. C., Hampson, S. A., Hill-yard, S. A., Pantev, C., Sobel, D., and Bloom, F. E. (1993). Modulation of early sensory processing in human auditory cortex during auditory selective attention. *Proc. Natl. Acad. Sci. U.S.A.* **90**, 8722–8726.

Zani, A., and Proverbio, A. M. (1993). ERP signs of early influences of selective attention on spatial frequency channels. Twenty-fifth Annual Meeting of the European Brain and Behaviour Society, p. 278. EBBS, Madrid.

Zani, A., and Proverbio, A. M. (1995). ERP signs of early selective attention effects to check size. *Electroencephalogr. Clin. Neurophysiol.* **95**, 277–292.

Zani, A., and Proverbio, A. M. (1997a). ERP indicants of frontal and occipital brain mechanisms mediat-ing spatially directed visual processing. *Exp. Brain Res.*, **S68**, V/18, 117.

Zani, A., and Proverbio, A. M. (1997b). Attention modulation of short latency ERPs by selective attention to conjunction of spatial frequency and location. *J. Psychophysiol.* **11**, 21–32.

Zani, A., and Proverbio, A. M. (1997c). Attention mod-ulation of C1 and P1 components of visual evoked potentials. *Electroencephalogr. Clin. Neurophysiol.* **103**, 15–3, 97.

Zani, A., and Proverbio, A. M. (1997d). ERP evidence of attentional selection in the occipital primary visual areas. *Brain Topogr.* **10**, 49–97.

Zani, A., and Proverbio, A. M. (1997e). Selective atten-tion modulates sensory activity of primary visual areas: Electrophysiological evidence in humans. *Soc. Neurosci. Abstr.* **23** (1), 121.2, p.299.

Zani, A., and Proverbio, A. M. (2002). In preparation.

Zani, A., Avella, C., Lilli, S., and Proverbio, A. M. (1999). Scalp current density (SCD) mapping of cerebral activity during object and space selection in humans. *Biomed. Tech.* **44** (Suppl. 2),162–165.

CLINICAL AND APPLIED PERSPECTIVES

13

Event-Related EEG Potential Research in Neurological Patients

Rolf Verleger

INTRODUCTION

This chapter reviews studies that have used the event-related potential (ERP) methodology to investigate patients suffering from neurological diseases. These studies have been conducted within the framework of two different points of view: one point of view assesses the utility of ERPs for the clinic, and the other perspective evaluates neurological diseases as lesion models for understanding ERPs. This review focuses on the utility of ERPs for the clinic; neurological diseases and principal neurological symptoms (*cf.* Appendix B for a synopsis of neurological diseases) will be discussed from the perspective of the degree to which ERPs have played a role in diagnosis and prognosis, in delineating and understanding impacts of diseases on cognition, and in therapy and rehabilitation

DEGENERATIVE DISEASES

For effective therapy of degenerative diseases, the mechanisms of neuronal degeneration have to be understood on a molecular level. This aim has so far not been achieved to such a degree that effec-

tive therapeutic treatment is able to ameliorate symptoms to a significant degree (except for Parkinson's disease), or even to halt the progress of the disease. The molecular level is not readily accessible to ERPs, therefore ERPs have not yet played a significant role in therapeutic research. Whether there is a role for ERPs in diagnosis and prognosis and in understanding consequences of diseases with respect to cognition is discussed in the following sections.

Alzheimer's Disease

Alzheimer's disease (AD) is the most common cause of dementia in elderly people. Pathological markers are plaques and tangles within neuronal tissue, but these markers can be identified only by postmortem neuropatholological examination. Thus, for patients, standard criteria recommend clinical diagnosis of "probable" AD by diagnosing dementia and excluding other possible causes of dementia (vascular encephalopathy, certain hormonal or vitamin deficiencies, etc.).

The Diagnostic Problem

In clinical practice, two diagnostic problems may arise in evaluating dementia: Does a patient suffer from dementing illness at all, and, if so, is it Alzheimer disease? Since the pioneering work by Goodin *et al.* (1978), the first problem has been tackled in ERP research by measuring delays of P3 latency in the "oddball" task. Such delays have been found reliably (Polich, 1991) when patients were more than mildly demented, but not in cases of mild to very mild dementia (e.g., Kraiuhin *et al.*, 1990; Verleger *et al.*, 1992; Polich *et al.*, 1986), although it is precisely in the latter cases where there is a real need for diagnostic information that would complement neuropsychological testing [cf. also the controversial exchange between Goodin (1990) and Pfefferbaum *et al.* (1990)]. In fact, the lack of P3 latency delay in mild dementia of the Alzheimer type comes as no surprise, P3 latency being a global measure of psychomotor retardation, closely covarying with response times [as long as response times are relatively fast; see review by Verleger (1997)]. Because AD patients are not mentally slow in the mild, early stage, there is no reason why their P3 latency should be delayed.

It is this author's impression that the N2 component might be a more promising candidate for distinguishing mildly demented AD patients from healthy people. This component was smaller and reliably delayed in the auditory oddball task in our study (Verleger *et al.*, 1992). Furthermore, a neurotic patient who was afraid of being demented but in fact was not had a huge N2, larger than normal and not delayed (unpublished). N2 amplitudes were also reported to be smaller even in a healthy group who had an enhanced genetic risk for AD (Green and Levey, 1999). The reason for the possible sensitivity of N2 might be its close association to response selection (Ritter *et al.*, 1979). AD patients often trouble experimenters in these tasks by continually forgetting what they have to do in response to some target event. The N2 decrease perhaps reflects such lapses of response selection even in trials in which the patients succeed in

overtly responding. Of course, these observations will have to be pursued more systematically in order to become relevant.

The second diagnostic problem, the differential diagnosis of Alzheimer disease vs. other types of dementia, has been tackled by several researchers, since Goodin *et al.* (1986) first explored the issue. Indeed, other etiologies of dementia can be delineated rather well from Alzheimer-type dementia by diagnosis-specific abnormalities, including vascular dementia (Yamaguchi *et al.*, 2000) and Huntington's disease (Goodin *et al.*, 1986) (but conflicting evidence will be discussed later). However, the relevance of these findings for diagnosing AD is limited, because in practice there is no problem in diagnosing Huntington's disease (by genetic testing), so there is no need for additional diagnostic help by ERPs; also, a positive diagnosis of reduced blood supply to the brain, leading to vascular dementia, is much easier (by computer tomography scans and transcranial Doppler measurement of cerebral blood flow) than is the positive diagnosis of AD. What is necessary is a positive marker for AD before the *postmortem* diagnosis. Positron emission tomography (PET) measurements of regional cerebral blood flow have become a promising tool, showing decreased metabolism within the temporal and parietal lobes, but PET measurements are expensive and invasive.

Measuring Hippocampal Activity

Presumably, ERPs would easily fulfill the task of providing a simple, positive marker of AD if they would allow measurement of hippocampal activity. It is well known that the hippocampus, situated in the midst of the temporal lobe, is one of the key structures for memory (see Eichenbaum, 2000), that the hippocampus is one of the structures most affected in AD, and that very large and significant P3-type potentials (peaking somewhat later than the P3 measured at the scalp) have been obtained when recordings are made intracranially from the hippocampus (from epileptic patients, to find their epileptic focus) (e.g., Grunwald *et al.*, 1995; Halgren *et al.*, 1995).

Thus, there is good reason to believe that the hippocampal potentials should be severely altered in AD. However, because the hippocampi are twisted structures, remote from the scalp surface, hippocampal potentials, whatever their strength, are unlikely to be measured by scalp electrodes (Lutzenberger *et al.*, 1987). Indeed, few changes in scalp-recorded P3 responses to target events have been found in patients whose hippocampi were severely affected (e.g., Onofrj *et al.*, 1992; Polich and Squire, 1993; Knight, 1996). However, these latter studies had focused on studying whether the scalp-recorded P3 is abolished or severely compromised by hippocampal damage (which it is not). A second look at these data might be appropriate, focusing on the questions (1) whether some reliable trace of the hippocampal activity can be found (most probably *following* the peak of the scalp-recorded P3, as it does in the intracranial recordings), (2) what recording sites would be most appropriate to measure such activity, and (3) whether this activity would be altered in AD (cf. Frodl *et al.*, 2002).

Probing the Memory Deficit

Several studies have tried to focus on cortical reflections of Alzheimer patients' memory deficit. In doing so, some of these studies pursued the discussed diagnostic problem, whereas others aimed at contributing to delineating and understanding consequences of the disease with respect to cognition. Tools used in this research were mismatch negativity, priming positivity, N400, and the P3, measured in Sternberg's task.

Mismatch negativity (MMN) can be evoked by deviant sounds even in the absence of any attention paid to the sounds and therefore serves as a measure of preconscious auditory memory (Näätänen and Winkler, 1999). Results of AD studies are somewhat ambiguous: MMN was equal in size in AD patients and in healthy controls (Gaeta *et al.*, 1999) and in the 1-sec interstimulus interval (ISI) condition of Pekkonen *et al.* (1994). On the other hand, AD patients' MMN tended to be smaller in Kazmerski *et al.* (1997) and was smaller than that of healthy controls in the 3-sec ISI condition of Pekkonen *et al.* (1994), but, as Gaeta *et al.* (1999) pointed out, this 3-sec condition always came last, so the decrease of MMN might also be due to AD patients' getting more tired or impatient with increasing time spent on the task.

Priming positivity is evoked by attended items of a large set (usually words) being repeated, either immediately or (with a usually weaker effect) with some items in between. The usual procedure is to define some targets (e.g., nonwords or animal names) and to measure priming positivity by repeating some of the nontarget words. This positivity is thought to consist of both a decrease of N400, reflecting facilitated (post)lexical processing, and an increase of P600, reflecting some conscious recollection, though this latter component might be of less relevance in elderly people (Rugg *et al.*, 1997). The amount of AD patients' priming positivity was statistically indistinguishable from age-matched healthy participants in the studies of Rugg *et al.* (1994), Kazmerski *et al.* (1995), and Kazmerski and Friedman (1997). Thus, these studies demonstrate preserved priming by earlier presentation in AD.

Ford *et al.* (1996) and Revonsuo *et al.* (1998) had AD patients listen to sentences, in order to measure whether semantic processing of naturally presented speech is still intact. This is a nearby question, in view of the patients' severe impairments of working memory, needed to integrate the meaning of heard speech. In half of the sentences, the final word did not fit the preceding words, evoking a large N400 in the healthy group. Both studies found that this difference between nonfitting and fitting final words was much reduced in AD. Less marked effects were obtained when words were primed by only one preceding word (Schwartz *et al.*, 1996), which supports the interpretation that the working-memory deficit is the important factor. Somewhat in contrast to this interpretation, Castañeda *et al.* (1997) obtained an N400 pattern similar to those of Ford *et al.* and Revonsuo *et al.* when a picture either did not fit or did fit the category of the one preceding picture.

Finally, a fourth approach to probing memory dysfunction in AD uses Sternberg's (1966) memory search task: A "memory set" of varying size (1 to 5 letters) was presented, followed by single letters that either were or were not members of the memory set, requiring an appropriate choice response. As could be expected, performance became worse in AD patients when the memory set was larger, also reflected in a disappearance of the P3 component evoked by single letters (De Toledo-Morrell *et al.*, 1991), but somewhat surprisingly, this finding was not replicated (Swanwick *et al.*, 1997). More data are needed to clarify this issue.

Conclusion

To summarize, the contribution of ERP research to problems of AD has been limited. The memory task of listening to sentences has produced the most consistent differences between AD and healthy participants (Ford *et al.*, 1996; Revonsuo *et al.*, 1998). Possible avenues for further research include the reliability of the N2 component as a diagnostic marker and the possibility of measuring traces of hippocampal activity at the scalp. The issue of diagnostic specificity, over and beyond the information obtained more easily by neuropsychological tests, and above all the issue of finding a positive marker for AD, remain a challenge.

Parkinson's Disease

The cardinal symptoms of Parkinson's disease (PD) are stiffness, lack of movement, and tremor during rest. There is often a slight diffuse impairment of cognitive functions, reminiscent of frontal lobe pathology. The main pathological mechanism is degeneration of dopamine-producing neurons in the brain stem (substantia nigra), thus the basal ganglia lack the dopamine needed for their adequate functioning. The basal ganglia project in different ways via the thalamus to cortical areas, one important target area being the supplementary motor area (SMA). There are at least two main challenges for research in PD (apart from spectacular methods such as grafting embryonic tissue). One is further precise delineation of the dopamine metabolism in order to further refine treatment beyond the global replacement of the missing dopamine. ERP research has not played a relevant role in this respect. The other challenge is precise description of the motor and nonmotor impairments of PD patients, because there is still a great gap between what is known about the neuroanatomical basis of PD and what this means in terms of behavior—in other words, the functions of the basal ganglia are still under debate. The contributions of ERP research to this endeavor will be highlighted in the following discussions. Again, as with the hippocampus in AD, a methodological obstacle for ERPs is that activity of the basal ganglia cannot be measured at the scalp. What can be measured by ERPs are cortical consequences of the basal ganglia deficit.

Movement-Related Activity

One of the cardinal symptoms in PD is the patients' problem in initiating movements. Although the problem is most obvious in global movements of the whole body, such as standing up and walking, methodological reasons (movement artifacts and immobile recording devices) have forced research to focus on finger movements, with only few exceptions (Vidailhet et al., 1993).

Self-initiated movements PD patients' Bereitschaftspotential (BP) preceding finger movements was found to differ from normal values in several studies: Dick et al. (1989) obtained weaker activation about 0.6 sec before movement onset, prior to the steep rise of activation in the remaining period until movement onset. This result was in contrast to an earlier study by Barrett et al. (1986), who measured BPs in a way similar to that of Dick et al. but did not obtain any differences between groups. On the other hand, results of Dick et al. were replicated by subsequent work published from the same lab (Touge et al., 1995; Jahanshahi et al., 1995) and by Cunnington et al. (1995) ("cues absent" condition), although other details of the results greatly differed between these studies. Touge et al. (1995) obtained no difference between groups for repetitive movements (in contrast to Dick et al. and Jahanshahi et al.), but did obtain a difference when participants had to select randomly one out of four movements. Further, in the study by Dick et al. (1989) this smaller early amplitude was compensated for by a subsequent steeper rise of activation, whereas BP amplitude remained smaller in PD patients throughout in Touge et al. (1995), Jahanshahi et al. (1995), and Cunnington et al. (1995). Studying the same PD patients by PET, Jahanshahi et al. (1995) found weaker blood flow in the PD patients' SMA (among a few other areas) during self-initiated movements, thus validating the interpretation that the smaller BP in PD patients reflects smaller involvement of the SMA. In contrast to the general trend of lower BP amplitudes, Fattaposta et al. (2000) measured larger BPs in PD patients than in healthy controls, preceding two key presses performed in quick sequence by the left and right hands. An interval of 40–60 msec was required

between the two presses to be counted as correct, which the (mildly affected) patients often failed to achieve, thus this interesting, irregular result might be due to extraordinary effort taken by the patients in order to do well.

In summary, the research on self-initiated movements showed that: (1) there is a slight but rather consistent deficit in PD patients' BP amplitude, either at an early phase of the BP or generally throughout the time course of the BP, but not focused on the immediate motor execution part; (2) in view of the severe impairment that PD may cause for movement initiation, the deficit in BP amplitude is surprisingly small; and (3) variability of results might have different reasons, including variability between patients, but probably is also due to technical limitations. For example, Barrett et al. (1986) apparently had no software available for creating grand means across groups and for overlaying those grand means of the two groups. Consequently, the measures actually taken might have been less than optimal for catching some group difference. Indeed, a difference pointed out by Cunnington et al. (1995) literally remained out of sight in other studies: at least in later stages of the disease (Cunnington et al., 1997) PD patients' BPs do not return to baseline as readily as do BPs of healthy subjects. But of course, these limitations cannot explain the findings of Fattaposta et al. (2000) of even larger BPs. Further, none of the studies used multichannel recordings in order to find subtle topographical differences. Thus, there is still need for further studies on the BP before and after self-initiated movements.

Movement preparation before imperative signals In recent years, the bulk of movement-related research in PD has turned away from the BP to the contingent negative variation (CNV), i.e., from self-initiated movements to movement preparation between some announcing

IV. CLINICAL AND APPLIED PERSPECTIVES

signal and an imperative stimulus. Empirical reasons for this turn have not been convincing so far, because two of the very few studies using both approaches [see Cunnington *et al.* (1995), though they did not use an announcing signal proper; see also Ikeda *et al.* (1997)] did not obtain a significant interaction, i.e., CNV was smaller than BP throughout and PD patients had smaller amplitudes than did healthy participants throughout, but PD patients did not have particularly reduced amplitudes in the CNV task. Another study, a short report by Oishi *et al.* (1995), even obtained no difference between groups in the movement-related (late) part of the CNV, in contrast to BP, which was smaller in the patients. But certainly the CNV situation can be better experimentally controlled, e.g., it might be argued (Rockstroh *et al.*, 1989) that the PD deficit in movement initiation actually gets out of sight in self-initiated movements because these are actually the instances in which PD patients succeeded in overcoming their deficit.

The overall finding in the studies that measured CNV before the imperative stimulus was a reduction of amplitudes in PD patients (Linden *et al.*, 1990; Wright *et al.*, 1993; Cunnington *et al.*, 1995, 1997, 1999; Pulvermüller *et al.*, 1996; Praamstra *et al.*, 1996; Wascher *et al.*, 1997; Ikeda *et al.*, 1997; Gerschlager *et al.*, 1999), with the exception of the report by Oishi *et al.* (1995) and of a study on PD patients with marked hemi-Parkinsonism (Cunnington *et al.*, 2001) (see below). The amount of CNV reduction may depend on the task: larger differences between patients and control group were found by Praamstra *et al.* (1996) after uninformative cues (four-choice response after S2) than after informative cues (limiting the response alternatives to two), but, in apparent contrast, by Linden *et al.* (1990) after fully informative cues (one response alternative) than after uninformative cues (two response alternatives). Larger differences were also found by Wascher *et al.*

(1997) in the cognitively more demanding "validity task" (brief interval between cue and imperative stimulus, possibility of wrong preparation) compared to the "clock task." Also, the topographical extent of CNV reduction on the anterior–posterior axis differed between studies and tasks: Widespread reduction was seen in Wright *et al.* (1993) and in the validity task of Wascher *et al.* (1997), only central and parietal, but not frontal reduction in Pulvermüller *et al.* (1996) and in the clock task of Wascher *et al.* (1997), only central in Praamstra *et al.* (1996), and frontally and frontocentrally focused in Gerschlager *et al.* (1999). This variability of CNV reduction by topography and task both between and within studies is hard to subsume under a general rule. It might be related to the fact that CNV is a variable mixture of activations of response preparation, stimulus expectation, and effort (van Boxtel, 1994; Verleger *et al.*, 2000a), so each of these processes might be differentially affected in Parkinson's disease, depending on the task and on the patients' status.

Effects of dopamine medication on PD patients' CNV have been published only infrequently but Gerschlager *et al.* (1999) showed that PD patients' CNV became indistinguishable from that of normal participants when their subthalamic nuclei were stimulated by implanted electrodes.

Of special interest are the topographical differences reported in studies with good topographical resolution. Praamstra *et al.* (1996) found more widespread contralateral activation; when the responding hand was already cued by the warning signal, the central site contralateral to the hand (C3 or C4) became more negative prior to the imperative stimulus than did the ipsilateral site in both healthy subjects and PD patients, but it was only in PD patients that this contralateral–ipsilateral difference extended to frontocentral and even frontal sites. Similarly, Cunnington *et al.* (2001) reported unilaterally enhanced frontocentral and frontal CNV amplitudes preceding bimanual responses in hemi-Parkinson patients contralateral to their more severely affected hand.

These results are hard to summarize, due to the large variation of the CNV difference and the topography of this difference between studies and between tasks. Again, as with the BP, these studies contribute to the overall summary that it is not movement execution that is above all impaired in PD; rather a number of processes involved in response preparation, depending on the particular task used, appear to be vulnerable to the dysfunction of the basal ganglia.

Movement preparation after ambiguous imperative signals Praamstra et al. (1998) explained their above-mentioned 1996 finding of an enlarged area of contralateral activation in PD patients by assuming that PD patients are more dependent on the lateral premotor system, making more use of visual stimulation for selecting movements, in order to compensate for the possibly deficient mesial SMA-based system or due to pathophysiological changes in the lateral premotor system. By measuring the time course of the difference between homologous sites, contralateral minus ipsilateral to the responding hand within the short time interval between stimulus and response [lateralized readiness potential (LRP); Coles, 1989], Praamstra and colleagues provided relevant data. Praamstra et al. (1998), replicated by Praamstra et al. (1999), demonstrated that PD patients were more affected, compared to healthy participants, by interfering stimuli that flanked the imperative stimulus. The LRP in PD patients went to the wrong side to a larger extent than in healthy participants when the flanking stimuli suggested a response different from the imperative stimulus. [The imperative stimulus was an arrow pointing left or right, requiring a left- or right-hand response, but was surrounded by other

arrows that also pointed left or right; cf. for LRP measurement in this task Gratton et al. (1988), Kopp et al. (1996), and Wascher et al. (1999)].

Further, Praamstra and Plat (2001) demonstrated that the fact that some relevant stimulus is presented laterally affected PD patients' motor system more than was seen in healthy participants. Lateral posterior activation contralateral to the relevant stimulus spread to a larger extent to (pre) motor sites in PD patients than in healthy participants. [Stimuli were the letters A and B, requiring a left- and right-hand response, respectively. Irrelevant to the task, but meant to induce lateral shifts of attention and response tendencies, the letters were presented left or right from fixation; cf. for measurement of posterior and central contralateral–ipsilateral differences in this task Wascher and Wauschkuhn (1996), and Wascher et al. (2001)].

Findings from both paradigms converge on the conclusion that visuomotor transmission is increased in PD. This might be interpreted as learned compensatory behavior that is applied by the patients even in inappropriate situations or, as favored by Praamstra and Plat (2001), as a pathological alteration of executive control over the motor system.

Conclusion Taken together, the ERP results on movement control in PD patients' appear to be of relevance for understanding the disease. Apart from important details, one general conclusion from these studies might be that the impairment of movement is more intimately linked to the general cognitive syndrome of PD than is commonly realized.

Other Approaches

Oddball task Beginning with Hansch et al. (1982), more than a dozen studies used the oddball task to investigate PD. Aims were (1) to establish differences among PD patients related to neuropsychological performance, to the presence of dementia, or to medication status, (2) to investigate whether PD patients differ from healthy participants, and (3) to investigate how PD patients with dementia differ from other demented patients. In retrospect, these goals do not appear to be of continuing relevance. This is not to say that they were irrelevant *a priori*. However, as with Alzheimer disease, interindividual variability proved to be too large to allow ERPs to be used for diagnosis. The main result, summarized in a review by Ebmeier (1992), was that P2, N2, and P3 peak latencies tended to be delayed in PD, more so with more cognitively impaired patients (the latter applying to N2 above all). Note that this is not so dissimilar from Alzheimer disease and, moreover, does not allow for the clinically relevant distinction between PD and multisystem atrophy.

Measures of executive control As noted in the introductory remarks on PD, some diffuse cognitive impairment is common in PD, akin to frontal lobe pathology. ERPs offer the opportunity for measuring signs of this pathology uncontaminated by impairment in overt behavior seen in PD patients. Tsuchiya *et al.* (2000) extended the auditory oddball task by interspersing occasional novel, unusual sounds among target and nontarget sounds. PD patients' orienting responses to novel sounds were impaired, reflected by reduced and delayed frontal P3 specifically to novel stimuli, not to oddball targets. Because such responses to novel sounds are drastically reduced in patients with lesions of the frontal lobe (Knight, 1984), this is evidence for impaired frontal lobe functioning. A similar argument may be made for the no-go P3, which is often larger and more anteriorly distributed than the go P3 in situations in which go and no-go stimuli are equally probable (e.g., Pfefferbaum *et al.*, 1985; Verleger and Berg, 1991), and therefore might reflect some aspect of the inhibitory function of the

frontal lobe. Indeed, the only work that compared PD patients' go and no-go P3s (Pulvermüller *et al.*, 1996) found their no-go P3s to be specifically reduced.

Stam *et al.* (1993), Vieregge *et al.* (1994), and Karayanidis *et al.* (1995) presented oddball sequences to both ears separately, instructing participants to attend to sounds in one ear only and to press a key to occasional targets presented to that ear [task introduced by Hillyard *et al.* (1973)]. Under these circumstances, the ERPs evoked by standard sounds are more negative for sounds in the attended than in the unattended ear ["Nd," Hansen and Hillyard (1980); viz. "processing negativity," Näätänen (1990)]. Nd was much smaller in PD patients than in healthy subjects in Stam *et al.* (1993). This result was replicated by Vieregge *et al.* (1994) when the interstimulus interval was 1 sec but not when the ISI was 0.5 sec and not by Karayanidis *et al.* (1995), where the ISI was 0.35 sec. Thus, it appears that PD patients have a deficit in maintaining the attentional trace of the standard sound whenever intervals between the sounds get too long [cf. Ravizza and Ivry (2001), for some converging evidence derived from performance errors]. Finally, measuring error negativity (Ne) in tasks of varying difficulty, Falkenstein *et al.* (2001) found Ne to be reduced in PD, except in very easy tasks (M. Falkenstein, personal communication), which might be interpreted either as a deficit in the very error-monitoring process or a consequence of being overloaded in moderately complex tasks. Either alternative would reflect a deficit in executive control.

Memory Mismatch negativity can be evoked by deviant sounds even in the absence of any attention paid to the sounds, and therefore serves as a measure of pre-conscious auditory memory (Näätänen and Winkler, 1999). Of particular interest to the present purpose, there is evidence for the involvement of a frontal lobe component of MMN (Deouell *et al.*, 1998). However, the report of a reduced MMN in PD (Pekkonen *et al.*, 1995) has not yet been replicated, to my knowledge (cf. Vieregge *et al.*, 1994; Pekkonen *et al.*, 1998).

Tachibana and colleagues investigated repetition priming, reflected as reduction of N400, where repetitions were either task relevant (Minamoto *et al.*, 2001) or not (Tachibana *et al.*, 1999a). A clear differential effect of priming on the N400 of PD patients and control participants could not be established. However, even at first presentation the PD patients had consistently smaller N400 amplitudes. Speculatively, this might reflect shallower processing of the presented words, reflecting the Parkinsonian frontal-patient-like attitude.

Conclusion Taken together, of the ERP approaches to investigate PD beyond movement disorders, the studies reflecting impaired frontal lobe function have provided the most consistent results. Pursuing this line of research further and making direct comparisons to patients with frontal lesions will certainly shed new light on the Parkinsonian syndrome of cognitive impairment.

Cerebellar Atrophy and Other Diseases of the Cerebellum

Cerebellar atrophy (CA) denotes a class of diseases, some idiopathic, some hereditary (some toxic, not considered here, e.g., by alcohol), which are characterized by impairments of movement precision and of balance, obviously related to shrinkage of cerebellar volume. Often, in the course of the disease, pathology progresses from the cerebellum to neighboring structures (olivo-ponto-cerebellar atrophy; OPCA).

Fortunately, CA occurs much less frequently than Parkinson's disease (PD), but similar questions can be asked about both. Like the basal ganglia, the cerebellum does not have efferent pathways of its own to the body, but rather exerts its influence by projecting via the thalamus to cortical areas, one important target area, though not the only one, being the motor cortex (Schmahmann, 1996; Middleton and Strick, 2001). Therefore, as in PD, precisely describing the motor and nonmotor impairments of CA patients is still a challenge, because the functions of the cerebellum are fervently debated. Different from the basal ganglia, the cerebellum is situated close to the scalp, so scalp-recorded ERPs might directly pick up cerebellar activity, but because the cerebellar neurons are not organized in the parallel columns formed by the cerebral neurons, they most probably do not produce fields that can be recorded from the scalp. In fact, none of the studies on CA patients cited here recorded ERP differences that can be directly ascribed to cerebellar activity. However, some data obtained more or less incidentally in basic research, e.g., by Johnson *et al.* (1998), raise some doubts as to whether recording cerebellar activity by ERPs is really impossible. In any case, this has not been done in these patient studies. What has been measured were cerebrocortical consequences of the cerebellar dysfunction.

For simplicity, studies on CA patients will here be combined with those on patients whose cerebellar damage was caused by other diseases, namely, infarctions of arteries supplying the cerebellum [the single-case studies reported by Ikeda *et al.* (1994), and Gerloff *et al.* (1996); most patients in Kitamura *et al.* (1999); some of the patients in Shibasaki *et al.* (1978) and Daum *et al.* (1993)] and tumors of the cerebellum that were resected [all patients in Akshoomoff and Courchesne (1994); one patient in Daum *et al.* (1993) and in Kitamura *et al.* (1999)].

Movement-Related Activity

The BP preceding self-initiated finger movements of CA patients drastically differs from normal by its lower amplitude (Shibasaki *et al.*, 1978; Ikeda *et al.*, 1994; Wessel *et al.*, 1994; Gerloff *et al.*, 1996), by its earlier onset (i.e., patients need more time to prepare a movement) (Shibasaki *et al.*, 1978; Wessel *et al.*, 1994), and by its diffuse topography, lacking a clear central-midline focus (Tarkka *et al.*, 1993; Wessel *et al.*, 1994; Gerloff *et al.*, 1996). Lesions of the cerebellar dentate nucleus appear to be particularly harmful (Shibasaki *et al.*, 1978, 1986; Kitamura *et al.*, 1999). Thus, differences from what is normal are more consistent and more marked than in Parkinson's disease.

These is some inconsistency about contingent negative variation developing between warning and imperative signals in CA. Ikeda *et al.* (1994) presented a single case in which the BP was entirely absent, whereas CNV was not (though amplitudes were not compared to normal values). In the same vein, CNV amplitudes of CA patients in Daum *et al.* (1993) were not significantly smaller than those of healthy participants. However, the studies by Yamaguchi *et al.* (1998) and Verleger *et al.* (1999) demonstrated drastically reduced CNV amplitudes (called late negative deflection in Yamaguchi *et al.*), and again lack of a clear central-midline focus in these patients. Thus, CNV results of CA patients do not principally differ from their BP results [cf. Verleger *et al.* (2000a), for discussing differences and similarities of these two complexes of components]. This amplitude reduction was independent of movement complexity in Verleger *et al.* (1999), i.e., although generally smaller in the patients than in normal subjects, CNV became larger by the same amount in patients and in healthy subjects preceding difficult bimanual movements, which the CA patients often failed to perform successfully, compared to simple movements. This led us to suggest that it is the motor cortex, not the cerebellum, that becomes more active in fine coordination, with the cerebellum being generally involved in any kind of preparatory and executive activity, providing the motor cortex with information needed for coordinating movements,

being used by the motor cortex for complex movements but not necessarily for simple ones.

Search for Consequences of Cerebellar Lesions for Cognition

Akshoomoff and Courchesne (1994) had participants respond to targets in either the auditory and visual modality and, having detected the target, shift their attention to the other modality. Their cerebellar patients (tumor-resected 10-year-old children) had difficulties in detecting targets when time since the preceding target in the other modality was less than 2.5 sec. This was also reflected by a lack of difference between the patients' P3 waves evoked by targets in the to-be-attended and in the to-be-ignored modalities (same modality as preceding target) when time since the preceding target was less than 2.5 sec. In a different paradigm, Yamaguchi *et al.* (1998) did not find evidence for impaired capacity for fast shifts of attention, this time of spatial attention in the visual modality. In an S1–S2 task, Yamaguchi *et al.* measured the contralateral–ipsilateral difference evoked by arrow cues or peripheral cues within the 0.8 sec S1–S2 interval. Neither the parietal difference at about 300 msec after the cue (cf. van der Lubbe *et al.*, 2000) nor the frontocentral difference at about 400 msec after the cue (cf. Verleger *et al.*, 2000b) was reduced or delayed in CA patients.

Tachibana *et al.* (1995) measured performance of CA patients in a visual oddball task (plant names written in Japanese *kana* symbols were targets; animal names were the frequent nontargets) relative to a simple-response task. Patients' Na component was delayed (measured as the difference between nontargets and simple response, peaking at about 200 msec), causing a delay of the ensuing N2 and P3 latencies in the target wave shapes. Following the Ritter *et al.* (1983) interpretation of Na, Tachibana *et al.* (1995) suggest that the cerebellar lesion causes an impairment in pattern classification, a skill that is obviously needed in reading Japanese symbols. In a subsequent study, Tachibana *et al.* (1999b) found that those patients who had delayed P3s in this task also had lower frontal blood perfusion, as measured by single-photon computed tomography (SPECT).

In summary, ERP evidence on impairment of cognitive abilities in CA is interesting but scarce.

Other Degenerative Diseases

Other degenerative diseases, fortunately occuring relatively infrequently, include Huntington's disease (HD), progressive supranuclear palsy (PSP), and amyotrophic lateral sclerosis (ALS).

Huntington's Disease

HD is a hereditary degenerative disease of the brain, focusing on parts of the basal ganglia (nucleus caudatus and putamen) and producing hyperkinesia, akinesia, and dementia. Although excess movements are a core symptom of the disease, only one study has investigated movement-related potentials in HD. In a pilot study (recordings at Cz only, without any electro-oculographic recording for artifact control), Johnson *et al.* (2001) found reduced amplitudes in movement preparation, very similar to the results obtained for Parkinson's disease in the same task studied by this group of authors (Cunnington *et al.*, 1997). The similarity to PD might seem surprising, because PD is reflected in hypokinesia, HD in hyperkinesia.

Similar to other degenerative disorders (AD and PD), P3 latency in oddball tasks is delayed in HD (Rosenberg *et al.*, 1985; Goodin and Aminoff, 1986; Filipovic *et al.*, 1990), but the finding that latencies of earlier components (N1, P2) were specifically delayed in HD (Goodin and Aminoff, 1986) was not replicated by Rosenberg *et al.* (1995) and Filipovic *et al.*, 1990). In a large study on 30 patients, on 40 of the patients' sons and daughters, and on

60 healthy controls, Hömberg *et al.* (1986) established that P3 latencies of HD patients' (as well as latencies of the earlier components N1, P2, N2) were delayed in an auditory oddball task, and that the P3 delay occurred not only in patients but also in their offspring, who are at risk of developing HD, correlating with deficits in psychometric tests. Promising as this finding was to identify those people who are at risk for developing HD, in the meantime such identification has become reliably possible by genetic testing, which is much more precise than the necessarily variable ERP measures.

Münte *et al.* (1997) used visual search tasks (modeled after Luck and Hillyard, 1990) and a continuous word recognition task (cf. Rugg *et al.*, 1997) to characterize more precisely the cognitive impairment of HD patients by means of ERPs. Several remarkable results were obtained. First, in both tasks the patients' P1 was markedly reduced and the following N1 was massively delayed. As Münte *et al.* note, this is in contrast to earlier studies. [Of the studies quoted here, Rosenberg *et al.* (1985), also used visual stimuli and did not obtain an N1 delay.] This might mean that HD patients have a deficit specifically in perceiving the complex stimuli used in these tasks [cf. below, the findings in PSP by Johnson (1992)]. Further, in both tasks the patients' ERP wave shapes were not modulated by task demands in the P3 latency range: patients displayed neither a P3 in response to targets in the visual search task nor a priming-and-recognition positivity in the word-recognition task. Although it can be argued that these missing modulations are a trivial consequence of the distorted input indicated by the P1–N1 abnormalities, at least the lack of priming positivity is remarkable, because even Alzheimer patients were shown to have priming positivity (see above). Thus, ERP studies might well contribute to understanding the specific mechanisms of impairment in HD.

Progressive Supranuclear Palsy

PSP is characterized by palsy of vertical saccades, loss of voluntary facial movements, axial dystonia, gait disturbance, and dementia, due to pathological alterations in several subcortical brain regions. As with other dementing diseases, P3 latency has been found to be delayed both in visual (Pierrot-Deseilligny *et al.*, 1989; Johnson *et al.*, 1991) and in auditory (Takeda *et al.*, 1998) oddball tasks, and P3 amplitude to be reduced (Johnson *et al.*, 1991; Wang *et al.*, 2000; Pirtošek *et al.*, 2001). In addition, anterior visual P200 components were much reduced and delayed in the patients (Johnson *et al.*, 1991) whereas occipital N1 was not altered. Johnson (1992) describes the results of a comprehensive series of tasks, including three other tasks in addition to the oddball tasks: Sternberg's (1966) memory-scanning task, a final-word verification task (sentences had to be read, with the final word being either congruent or incongruent to the preceding context) (cf. Kutas and Hillyard, 1980), and a mental-rotation task using pictures of rotated right and left hands as stimuli. Replicating the oddball results, P200 and P3 (as well as response times) were delayed. Moreover, whereas the memory-scanning task resulted in principally similar patterns of patients and controls with increasing load, the other two tasks yielded unexpected results. In the final-word verification task, no differentiation between congruent and incongruent words was visible in the patients' ERPs in the N400 time range, and in the mental-rotation task the hand stimuli elicited very large occipital N1 components in the control group but not in the patients. The deficient N400 effect is reminiscent of the finding by Minamoto *et al.* (2001) in PD, and the lack of N1 enhancement, probably related to lack of a discrimination process (Vogel and Luck, 2000), parallels the finding by Münte *et al.* (1997) in HD. More generally, Johnson's (1992) study is a nice example of applying a kind of ERP test

battery, probing several diverse but well-investigated ERP effects, from which a neurophysiological–cognitive profile can be built for the study group.

Amyotrophic Lateral Sclerosis

ALS consists of degeneration of neurons of the pyramidal tract and the consecutive spinal neurons, progressively reducing the patient's ability to move. Questions open to research include (1) how a patient's motor cortex deals with this efferent blockade, (2) whether other cognitive functions are affected by the degenerative process, and (3) whether patients' ERP responses can be used as a means for them to communicate with their environment when the disease progresses to a point at which they are no longer able to move.

Movement-related potentials Possibly the only published study on movement-related potentials in ALS patients is that of Westphal *et al.* (1998), who recorded Bereitschafts potential before self-paced movements. The total group of ALS patients did not differ from healthy controls but a subgroup of patients with increased spasticity had lower amplitudes. In our CNV study (R. Verleger, unpublished), we did not find differences between patients and healthy controls, in contrast to patients with striatocapsular infarction (see below), who also have to deal with the problem of efferent blockade. This is in contrast to the PET study by Kew *et al.* (1993), who found enlargement of the ALS patients' hand motor area, very similar to patients with striatocapsular infarction (Weiller *et al.*, 1993), interpreted in both cases as a means of compensation. Such compensatory effort might be expected to be reflected in larger movement-related potentials, which were found in neither the Westphal *et al.* study (1998) nor in our unpublished study.

Affection of cognitive functions In their study on ALS patients' performance in an auditory oddball task, Gil *et al.* (1995)

found delayed N2 and P3 latencies but no effects on earlier components. Other studies used more complex tasks. Vieregge et al. (1999) presented oddball sequences to both ears separately, instructing participants to attend to sounds in one ear only [same design as the Vieregge et al. (1994) study in PD; see above]. Nd was much reduced in ALS patients, both with slow and with fast presentation. Peculiarly, though entirely independent of any overt response, the Nd reduction correlated with the patients' motor disability but not with neuropsychological tests (in contrast to healthy subjects, in which Nd reduction did correlate with tests sensitive to frontal lobe function). In addition, the N100 amplitudes evoked by all sounds were reduced in ALS patients. [Not reported in Vieregge et al. (1999) is that N2 and P3 components to targets were unaffected by ALS, unlike Gil et al. (1995).] Similar observations of decreased amplitudes of early modality-specific components were made in the visual modality by Münte and colleagues, with ALS patients' temporo-occipital P100 components being virtually absent in response to words or to visual search displays (Münte et al., 1998a, 1999), similar to what Münte et al. (1997) had reported in these tasks for HD, but, unlike HD, visual N1 was not delayed in ALS. In addition, Münte et al. (1998b) reported recognition positivity to be absent in ALS patients, as in their HD study.

To summarize, there is surprising though still sparse evidence for abnormalities in relatively early sensory ERP components in ALS. Whether this reflects some damage of afferent pathways in ALS or the possibility that efferent pathways must be intact in order to obtain normal sensory components is an open question. In addition, a number of further findings have pointed to abnormalities of higher cognitive functions in ALS independent of motor dysfunction. How these findings relate to the fact that the world's leading astrophysicist, Stephen Hawking, has been

suffering from ALS for many years (Hawking, 1989), is certainly an open question. One might argue (S. Ravizza, personal communication) that ALS patients (as well as PD patients) are permanently distracted in such tasks by their greater difficulties with the occasional responses, which is why even their potentials to standards might be affected, but it is doubtful whether this argument indeed can account for the reported abnormalities of early components.

Communication by locked-in patients Severe ALS is a model case for the locked-in syndrome, wherein the patients' ERPs can be used as a means to communicate with their environment. Use of the P3 component evoked by target stimuli for this purpose was suggested and demonstrated in healthy subjects by Farwell and Donchin (1988). Participants might select letters to spell words and sentences by emitting enhanced P3s to arrays when these arrays contain the intended letter. Indeed, a "locked-in" patient (after ischemia of the basilar cerebral artery) studied by Onofrj et al. (1996) emitted N2–P3 complexes to target sounds, thus in principle would have been able to use this means of communication. In recent years, this line of applied research was pursued systematically by Birbaumer's group (Kübler et al., 1999; Birbaumer et al., 1999, 2000) in patients, mostly suffering from chronic ALS, whose remaining control over muscles (e.g., for moving the eyes) had become too unreliable to be used for communication. In this "thought translation device" patients select letters by enhancing the positive level measured from Cz 1.5 to 2 sec after letter presentation. In doing so, patients indeed became able to produce messages, though with a very slow speed [e.g., as reported in Kübler et al. (1999), 12 sec per letter at best, more than 3 min per letter at worst).

Alternative ways for using the EEG to help locked-in patients communicate with their environment have involved modulations of selected frequency spectra of the spontaneous EEG. These approaches (e.g., Wolpaw *et al.*, 1991; Pfurtscheller *et al.*, 1993) will not be discussed here, because they do not involve using ERPs. A comprehensive review covering all these techniques has been published (Kübler *et al.*, 2001).

LESION OF CEREBRAL TISSUE BY INFARCTION OR HEMORRHAGE

Brain tissue can be damaged by disorders of blood circulation in two ways: by infarction, i.e., some vessel is blocked such that tissue no longer has adequate blood supply, or by hemorrhage, i.e., some vessel is ruptured, causing blood to overflow into brain tissue.

Before turning to the effects of focal lesions induced by sudden ischemic events, the syndrome of "vascular dementia" (VaD) will be discussed, being more akin to the diffuse, gradually increasing effects found in degenerative diseases as discussed so far. Sudden ischemic events will be discussed according to main syndromes encountered, which will be hemiparesis, aphasia, and neglect. An alternative distinction, more down to earth at first sight, would consist in discussing the main cerebral arteries, one after the other. However, as well organized as these arteries seem at first sight (anterior, media, posterior), their winding courses and their distributed branchings blur any simple picture. Lesions of cerebellar arteries have been discussed previously.

Vascular Dementia

VaD refers to reduction of cognitive capabilities due to widespread cortical or subcortical pathological changes occurring as consequences of chronically reduced blood perfusion or microlesions brought about by hypertension. If these factors of blood circulation are treated, the progression of VaD may be stopped or delayed at least. Therefore, distinguishing VaD from Alzheimer disease has clinical relevance. A review by Looi and Sachdev (1999) concludes that VaD and AD differ in their neuropsychological profiles, with VaD patients having relatively more impairment in frontal executive functioning and AD patients in verbal memory.

Most ERP studies on VaD have been performed in Japan, VaD being more common than AD in East Asia (Looi and Sachdev, 1999). Apparently, no disease specificity for distinguishing VaD from AD can be obtained in simple oddball tasks (Neshige *et al.*, 1988), mildly affected VaD patients also having delayed N2 and normal P3 latencies (Tachibana *et al.*, 1993), similar to mildly affected AD patients (Verleger *et al.*, 1992). Also, in the more sophisticated repetition-priming paradigm (cf. above, Parkinson's disease) (Tachibana *et al.*, 1999a), very mildly affected VaD patients had normal priming positivity (Tachibana *et al.*, 1999c), similar to the findings made in AD patients (Rugg *et al.*, 1994; Kazmerski *et al.*, 1995; Kazmerski and Friedman, 1997). However, the vascular patients' N400 was generally reduced (Tachibana *et al.*, 1999c), similar to Parkinson patients (Tachibana *et al.*, 1999a), possibly likewise indicating pathology of frontal lobe function. In any case, as briefly mentioned above, in an elegant study, Yamaguchi *et al.* (2000) were able to identify VaD patients by using Knight's (1984) frontal-lobe-sensitive variant of the oddball task: in contrast to AD patients, the VaD patients lacked the anteriorly focused "novelty P3" in response to novel sounds interspersed in the oddball sequence. Thus, reliable distinction of VaD from AD by means of ERPs appears to be possible, although this is certainly of limited relevance, because reliable diagnosis of vascular encephalopathy is possible by CT scans and transcranial Doppler measurement of cerebral blood flow.

Hemiparesis

Hemiparesis, due to infarction (or hemorrhage) of the middle cerebral artery (MCA), is presumably the most well-known neurological disease, constituting the most frequent etiology of movement impairment, by disabling the contralateral arm and hand. Surprisingly, only very few papers have been published on ERPs in hemiparesis. This does not make much sense because it is easily conceivable (and in fact was expected by the patients whom we recently investigated) that studying these patients' movement-related potentials would, among other things, allow some prediction about the degree of their possible rehabilitation.

Control of hand movements may be impaired by MCA lesions in two ways—by damaging either the primary motor cortex or the subcortical course of the pyramidal tract. In the former case, movement-related potentials generated by the motor cortex can be expected to be severely altered, possibly reduced, in the latter case, the intact motor cortex has to deal with some efferent block. Three studies measured the Bereitschafts potential before self-initiated movements in MCA patients. Platz et al. (2000) investigated a relatively homogeneous group of 8 mostly subcortically affected patients, Kitamura et al. (1996) reported 2 cases of subcortical infarction, whereas the 10 patients reported in Green et al. (1999) were quite heterogeneous. When the patients of Kitamura et al. (1996) moved their affected arm, BP amplitudes were of equal size at the two hemispheres. The affected hemisphere did not reach normal, contralateral values (though being larger than when the other arm was moved) and the unaffected hemisphere was somewhat enhanced. The main finding of Platz et al. (2000) was a general reduction of BP amplitude around 600 msec before movement onset, in particular at parietal sites, causing an anterior shift of the BP topography. Unfortunately, the time course of the BP was not reported in this work. (Of

further interest, movement-related alpha and beta desynchronizations were measured, which is not within the scope of this review.) In our own study on 13 subcortically affected MCA patients (Verleger et al., 2002) in an S1–S2 task, we focused on contralateral–ipsilateral differences (LRP) (Coles, 1989) time-locked to movement onset to show the time course of interplay between the contralateral (affected) and the ipsilateral (unaffected) motor cortex. Beginning 200 msec before finger movements of the affected hand, a normal contralateral surplus of EEG activity was developing. Briefly after response onset, however, the opposite, unaffected cortex, ipsilateral to the responding hand, became additionally active, in contrast to movements of the unaffected hand and to healthy participants. This time course precludes any role of ipsilateral activity in response initiation of the affected hand but might indicate prophylactic activation of the unaffected motor system to compensate for possible failure of the affected hand.

Additionally, we found general reduction of the patients' CNV amplitudes before the imperative signal, in particular at scalp sites overlying *both* motor cortices (C3 and C4) and, similar to Platz et al. (2000), at parietal scalp sites. In summary, much more work should be done using movement-related ERPs to explore the impairments and capacities of these patients.

Aphasia

Aphasia is usually the consequence of left-side MCA infarction (in right-handers). Traditionally, Broca's area in lateral premotor cortex and Wernicke's area in superior-posterior temporal cortex have been identified as relevant to language processing. An obvious difficulty in research is the large heterogeneity between patients, both with regard to focus and extent of the lesion and with regard to language abilities.

In the first study on aphasic patients, Starr and Barrett (1987) focused on the impairment of auditory verbal short-term memory, frequently encountered as a residual symptom. Indeed, the four patients studied had a specific deficit of the P3 component in an auditory version of Sternberg's (1966) memory scanning task, using digits as stimuli, whereas their P3 amplitudes were relatively normal in an auditory oddball task with sounds as stimuli and in a visual memory-scanning task.

Perhaps coming somewhat closer to the disturbed mechanisms, Aaltonen et al. (1993) reported about a possibility to distinguish electrophysiologically between Broca and Wernicke aphasics (n = 2 patients each). Mismatch negativities were missing in the Wernicke aphasics in response to deviant synthetic vowels, whereas, as a control, all patients had MMNs in response to deviant pure tones. Ilvonen et al. (2001) presented evidence that even MMN amplitudes to pure tones deviating by their shorter duration from standard tones were smaller in Wernicke aphasics (n = 8) than in healthy controls, possibly reflecting a generalized impairment of these patients in discriminating duration of auditory stimuli. In the most systematic approach taken so far, though on only four patients with varying lesions sites, Csépe et al. (2001) compared MMNs evoked by deviating pitch, by deviating vowels, by deviating place of articulation (ga vs. ba), and by deviating voicing (pa vs. ba). MMN became more and more abnormal in this order, i.e., it was indistinguishable from normal with deviating pitch but grossly reduced with deviating voicing and place of articulation. Unfortunately, Csépe et al. had not included a pure-tone duration deviance as used by Ilvonen et al. (2001). This comparison would be of interest because the deviation of voicing was based on deviance in voice onset time, thus might be related to a general problem of duration discrimination. It should be noted here that MMN to simple pitch deviance might be a reliable marker of amusia

(deficit of music perception); according to a study by Kohlmetz et al. (2001), this might be quite common in unselected stroke patients.

Only recently has research begun to focus on the components most frequently investigated in basic research about language-related ERPs: the N400, the P600, and left-anterior negativity. A few case studies have tested the ability of patients to distinguish between semantically appropriate and inappropriate sentence endings by measuring the N400 (cf. Kutas and Hillyard, 1980). N400 effects were found (Cobianchi and Giaquinto, 2000) even in the absence of signs of explicit understanding (Revonsuo and Laine, 1996), encouraging rehabilitative treatment (Connolly et al., 1999). In contrast to these optimistic reports, on a group level, N400 amplitudes to semantically inappropriate words were found to be attenuated, both in patients with frontal lesions [Friederici et al. (1999), n = 3] and in those with parietal lesions [Reuter et al. (1994), n = 10], and in particular in patients with more severe comprehension deficits as defined by median-splitting the entire group [Hagoort et al. (1996), n = 18 aphasic patients tested; Swaab et al. (1997), n = 14; Swaab et al. (1998), n = 12], with no obvious difference between frontoparietally lesioned Broca aphasics and temporoparietally lesioned Wernicke aphasics (Hagoort et al., 1996; Swaab et al., 1997, 1998).

In addition, Friederici et al. (1999) tested sensitivity to syntactic violations (verb rather than noun presented after a preposition), measuring the left anterior negativity peaking at about 250 msec (cf. Friederici et al., 1993). Results were, however, not clear-cut, due to the small number of patients (n = 3). The P600, a second P3-type component in response to syntactic violations (e.g., Hahne and Friederici, 1999) did not differ between patients and controls.

Taking a new approach by analyzing potentials evoked by words read within stories, ter Keurs et al. (1999) focused on the difference between open- and closed-class words (i.e., articles, conjunctions, prepositions) in 14 Broca aphasics. An early frontal negativity evoked by closed-class words, peaking at 260 msec in healthy subjects, was entirely missing in the aphasic patients, and differences between the two word classes from 400 msec onward were reduced in the patients.

Thomas *et al*. (1997) recorded slow potentials during a period of several seconds during which patients had to mentally search for synonyms to a word presented at trial onset. The stable left frontal negativity evoked by this procedure in healthy subjects (cf. Altenmüller, 1989) was replaced by bilateral frontal negativity in aphasic patients tested 2–4 weeks after stroke (n = 7). When studied at a later time point, lateralization in four Broca patients had become normal, left-lateralized, whereas negativity remained bilateral in the three Wernicke patients. Cohen *et al*. (2001) measured the N400 evoked by S1 (called "slow wave" in that paper) and slow CNV negativity during the S1–S2 interval of a delayed-matching-to-sample task designed after the "token test" for aphasia, with S1 and S2 consisting of either words or symbols, from 19 aphasic patients (median time after infarction was 1 year) and 18 healthy controls. CNV preceding S2 was more clearly left-lateralized in healthy controls than in the aphasic patients. Different from Thomas *et al*. (1997), it was above all the Broca patients who lacked left lateralization in this slow CNV negativity, which might, of course, be due to differences in task or patients. The N400 evoked by S1 overlapped the posteriorly focused P3/slow wave complex and was well marked in Broca aphasics only, with an extreme left lateralization. One might ascribe this to some volume defect of these patients underlying left frontotemporal scalp sites, but both aphasics and controls had left-lateralized N400 components evoked by words as S2, rather similar to the Broca aphasics' N400 evoked by S1,

suggesting some functional meaning of this lateralization. On the other hand, this left-lateralized N400-type component was also invariably evoked in these aphasic patients by pictures that had to be classified according to either their grammatical gender or to their being natural or not [Dobel *et al*. (2001); patients largely identical to those of Cohen *et al*. (2001)]. Thus, it is still not clear whether this peculiar feature of Broca aphasics reflects some functional reorganization or some structural alteration.

In summary, research in aphasia has focused on several goals: prediction of rehabilitative success in the N400 single-case studies, finding electrophysiological markers of subtypes of aphasia in the N400 and MMN group studies, understanding mechanisms of Broca's aphasia, and mapping the course of cortical reorganization. Undoubtedly, each of these goals deserves further study.

Neglect and Extinction

Infarction (or hemorrhage) of posterior branches of the MCA, affecting parietal and superior temporal cortex, may cause "basic" disorders of somatosensory perception, which is beyond the scope of this review [for data on disordered movement-related somatosensory reafference in a few of these patients see Kopp *et al*. (1999) and Platz *et al*. (2000)]. In addition, lesions on the right (in right-handers) may result in disorders of spatial cognition and in decreased awareness for the left side of space (hemineglect). [For an introduction to and review of this fascinating syndrome, see Kerkhoff (2001) and Driver and Vuilleumier (2001).] MCA infarction is the most frequent etiology, but not the only one.

There are at least two published case studies and three group studies using endogenous ERPs. In the case study by Marzi *et al*. (2000) light flashes were presented on the left, right, or both sides, and data were averaged according to the patient's indication of what she had seen. When she reported seeing the right flash only in the case of actual bilateral stimulation, P1 and N1 components were absent at right parietal sites. When she reported seeing both flashes, or in the case of unilateral stimulation, the components were present. Thus, visual extinction appears to involve the early stages of perception. Different results were obtained by the other case study, by Vuilleumier et al. (2001), who used the same rationale as Marzi et al. (2000) but obtained N1 components of the same amplitude to extinguished and perceived left stimuli, though P1 was somewhat reduced. Moreover, using faces and shapes as stimuli rather than flashes, these authors made use of the fact that faces evoke a specific ERP signature, consisting of a temporo-occipital N170 and a central P200 [see, e.g., Eimer and McCarthy's (1999) study in a prosopagnosic patient]. Extinguished faces not only evoked the same N1 but also the same N170/P200 as perceived faces. One reason for the striking differences between these two single-case studies might be variability between patients. Furthermore, neither study used a control group [see Verleger (2001), for further discussion of Marzi et al.'s study]. Relevant to the debate of whether the early P1 and N1 components are affected in neglect patients are the studies by Spinelli and colleagues (e.g., Spinelli et al., 1994; Viggiano et al., 1995; Angelelli et al., 1996) measuring steady-state visual evoked potentials (i.e., flashes were regularly presented several times per second). Because no task was associated with these stimuli, these studies are somewhat off the focus of this review. However, their results that neglect patients' P1 latencies were delayed in response to left hemifield stimuli are certainly of interest in the present context [see the review by Deouell et al. (2000a), for more details].

The first group study using endogenous ERPs was conducted by Lhermitte et al.

(1985). Light flashes were presented left and right (not bilaterally) and P3s were found to be delayed to left stimuli. The second group study, by Verleger et al. (1996), measured potentials evoked by cues and targets in Posner et al.'s (1984) visual cueing task from 10 patients with lesions of the right parietal cortex and from age-matched healthy subjects. In essence, this task is a computerized version of the visual extinction test as used by Marzi et al. (2000), with the sequence right cue and left target leading to response delays, and therefore comparable to those bilateral stimuli in Marzi et al. that were extinguished, and the other sequences of left and right cues and targets evoking responses in time, and therefore being comparable to those bilateral stimuli in Marzi et al. that were not extinguished. The patients' N1 component evoked by left-side cues was reduced at the right parietal recording site, suggesting a general impairment in processing left-side visual input. Of more importance, the patients' EEG potentials evoked by the critical combination of right cue and left target differed in two features from the other sequences: their mean amplitude of 160–280 msec after target onset (Nd) was less negative than with other combinations of cue and target, and the following frontal P300 was enhanced. Thus, the lack of early reductions in response to extinguished stimuli confirms the results of Vuilleumier et al. (2001), but in addition we were able to describe a positive ERP sign of extinction, the missing Nd.

The third group study, by Deouell et al. (2000b), changed perspective and investigated the mismatch negativity, i.e., the (preattentive) ERP response to some changed sound in a series of unattended sounds. The neglect patients had reduced MMN amplitudes when sounds were presented on the left, in particular when stimuli deviated in location. The N100 amplitudes were not reduced to left stimuli, making a deficit in early perceptual processing improbable. Rather, as the authors suggest, a deficit appears to exist in detecting changes in the left side of the environment. Clearly, more research is promising to give further insight into this disorder.

INFLAMMATORY DISEASES

In addition to degenerative diseases or disturbances of blood supply, the brain may be damaged by inflammation. Meningoencephalitis is an acute, possibly life-threatening event caused by bacteria or viruses. ERP studies on meningo-encephalitis have been conducted primarily on patients with damage to the temporal lobe and the hippocampal system; the lesions in these patients have served as models to study ERP generators. As stated previously, this will not be discussed in detail here. The research discussed here is on the chronic, potentially deteriorating damage caused by multiple sclerosis and by the human immunodeficiency virus.

Multiple Sclerosis

Multiple sclerosis (MS), viz. encephalo-myelitis disseminata (ED), is character-ized by a diversity of symptoms due to inflammatory-type lesions of neuronal axons and the insulating myelin. Because the optical nerve is frequently affected, measurement of exogenous components of visual evoked potentials, not of interest here, is a standard diagnostic method. Similar to what occurs with degenerative diseases (as discussed previously), for effective therapy the mechanisms of destruction in MS have to be understood on a molecular level. Such information is not readily accessible via ERP studies, therefore ERPs have not played a sig-nificant role for therapeutic research. Whether there is a role for ERPs in diagno-sis and prognosis and in understanding consequences of MS on cognition will be

assessed in the following discussion. An obvious problem for research is the hetero-geneity of the disease, due to the different location of foci and due to individ-ually different courses of progression or remission.

Newton *et al.* (1989) consequently reported a large variability in the ERP responses of their 20 patients; responses were obtained for both visual and auditory (three-stimulus) oddball tasks. The sub-group of patients that had delayed or reduced N2, P3, or slow wave components also had more cerebral lesions visible in their MRI scans. Similar findings were made in auditory oddball tasks by Honig *et al.* (1992) (n = 31 patients), Triantafyllou *et al.* (1992a) (n = 47), and Gil *et al.* (1993) (n = 101). P3 latency delays tended to be related to physical disability in addition to visible brain lesions. Somewhat in contrast to these studies, van Dijk *et al.* (1992) (n = 30) and Giesser *et al.* (1992) reported normal ERP components in nondemented MS patients, but Giesser *et al.* (1992) found not only abnormal N2 and P3 but also prolonged N100 and P200 latencies in those patients diagnosed as demented. Thus, delayed ERP latencies appeared to be related to the presence of dementia only. Only six patients were included in either subgroup of this latter study; however, recordings were made in a renowned lab that has contributed much to basic research, thus it may be argued that data quality is better than in the other larger studies. But the bulk of evid-ence indicates that presence of white matter lesions and physical disability are related to ERP abnormalities in MS patients as measured in the oddball task. Initial studies on the use of oddball task-related ERPs to evaluate drug effects on cognition in MS patients are promising (Filipovic *et al.*, 1997) but not conclusive yet (Gerschlager *et al.*, 2000).

The oddball task is relatively unspecific. Using tasks that put greater demand on working memory, two studies have demonstrated ERP effects on mildly affected MS patients who would presumably have had normal results in the oddball tasks. Using Sternberg's memory-scanning task, Pelosi *et al.* (1997) found that the 8 patients (out of 24) who had somewhat lower scores in neuropsychological tests of working memory had enhanced negativity viz. reduced positivity from about 200 msec onward in their responses to memory probes. According to Pelosi *et al.*, this might reflect the extra resources required to compensate for deficits in working memory. Effects were more marked with auditory stimuli, because demands to phonological working memory were probably higher. In a task requiring visual–phonological working memory for nonsense words, Ruchkin *et al.* (1994) found that slow waves during the retention interval were larger at leftfrontal and midposterior sites in patients than in control subjects when stimuli were moderately difficult to remember (three syllables). The slow waves of healthy subjects reached these amplitudes only when stimuli were hard to remember (five syllables), whereas the increase in load from three to five syllables affected patients' slow waves much less, possibly because these amplitudes were already at their ceiling. The effect was task specific and were not present in a task requiring visual–spatial memory. These results may be interpreted as evidence for a specific deficit of MS patients in phonological memory, compensated by the patients in the case of the moderately difficult task by enhanced effort in verbal (leftfrontal) and visuospatial (midposterior) domains. Thus, using rather different paradigms and methods, these two studies lead to convergent conclusions about specific problems of working memory even in relatively healthy MS patients.

HIV Infection

The human immunodeficiency virus (HIV) may affect the central nervous system and may cause cognitive impair-ment (HIV-associated dementia), as part of the acquired immunodeficiency syndrome (AIDS). Because a principal symptom of this cognitive impairment is slowing of cognition, the measurement of ERP latency delays as an indicator of cognitive slowing makes much sense.

Goodin *et al.* (1990) reported that N1, N2, or P3 latencies were delayed in the auditory oddball task in demented AIDS patients. Delayed latencies in demented or severely symptomatic patients were generally replicated by later studies, subtle differences notwithstanding (e.g., Goodwin *et al.*, 1990; Ollo *et al.*, 1991; Messenheimer *et al.*, 1992; Arendt *et al.*, 1993; Baldeweg *et al.*, 1993; though see Connolly *et al.*, 1994), and consequently could be used as markers of medication effects in a longitudinal study (Evers *et al.*, 1998). Yet, of much interest is the question whether ERPs sensitively measure damage to the central nervous system in asymptomatic HIV-infected persons. This was indeed reported by Goodin *et al.* (1990); 12 of 41 asymptomatic men infected with HIV had prolonged latencies in the auditory oddball task, making ERPs more sensitive than the standard EEG. Evidence in support of this original finding is mixed: Schroeder *et al.* (1994) confirmed the delay of P3 latencies, and Messenheimer *et al.* (1992) similarly found increases of P3 latencies when measurements were repeated 6 or 12 months after infection. However, no abnormalities were reported by Goodwin *et al.* (1990), Ollo *et al.* (1991), and Connolly *et al.* (1994). Arendt *et al.* (1993) did not find delayed latencies but found reduced N2–P3 amplitudes (whether due to reduced N2 or reduced P3 cannot be learned from the published paper). Baldeweg *et al.* (1993) found delayed P2 but not delayed P3 latencies and a general tendency of N2 and P3 waves to be less clearly defined. Bungener *et al.* (1996) reported delayed N1 latencies but not delayed P3 latencies.

To overcome this dissatisfactory state of incongruent findings, other stimuli and tasks have been used. Ollo *et al.* (1991) reported delayed and reduced P300 components with visual stimuli, in contrast to their auditory data. However, this was not replicated by Baldeweg *et al.* (1993), who found the previously mentioned abnormalities with auditory stimuli but not with visual ones. Presenting unique novel nontargets in addition to standard nontargets and targets, Fein *et al.* (1995) measured the anteriorly distributed novelty P3 and found this to be delayed with auditory stimuli, with the delay increasing when patients were symptomatic, possibly specifically reflecting delayed function of the frontal lobe [cf. Knight (1984), for association of novelty P3 to the frontal lobe]. Finally, in a pilot study on only 13 patients, Linnville and Elliott (1997) reported smaller mismatch negativity in HIV-infected individuals; these results would also be compatible with disturbed frontal lobe functioning, in view of the evidence for the involvement of a frontal lobe component of MMN (Deouell *et al.*, 1998). Both this latter result and the findings made by Fein *et al.* (1995) need replication.

In conclusion, it appears as if, by overreliance on the unspecific oddball task, the ERP method has missed the chance of playing a more important role in HIV research. Had more specific tasks and measures been used, results would perhaps have been more consistent. A complicating factor is data quality. Many of the studies were performed by groups not renowned in ERP research and/or were published in journals whose emphasis is not on quality of ERP data, such that data quality simply cannot be judged from the published reports.

EPILEPSY

Epileptic seizures are unspecific symptoms of cerebral dysfunction. The seizure might be focal, or at least start focally, reflecting an circumscribed pathology, or alternatively might be generalized, i.e., without an identifiable focus.

ERP research has dealt with three topics in epilepsy: (1) whether a history of epileptic seizures (in combination with antiepileptic drugs) leads to cognitive slowing and to other deficits of cognitive functions, (2) whether intracranial recordings from the hippocampi can predict memory performance after surgical removal of the epileptic focus, and (3) whether seizures can be reduced by biofeedback of event-related slow waves.

Cognitive Slowing and Impairments of Memory

Not surprisingly, the issue of cognitive slowing has been investigated by measuring delays of components evoked in the auditory oddball task. In patients with focal seizures, delayed P3 latencies were found by Puce *et al.* (1989; not explicitly reported, but evident from comparing their Figs. 3a and 4b), by Triantafyllou *et al.* (1992b), and Fukai *et al.* (1990) for patients with temporal lobe seizures; by Drake *et al.* (1986) for a group of patients with different epileptic foci, and by Rodin *et al.* (1989) for patients with different types of epilepsies. Drake *et al.* (1986) and Triantafyllou *et al.* (1992b) also reported delayed N2 latencies. Moreover, Puce *et al.* (1994) reported increased variability of the time point of the P3 peak measured across single trials. In apparent contrast to these studies, Verleger *et al.* (1997) did not find significant latency delays but did find, in agreement with the general trend of these studies, that the duration of epilepsy was related to P3 latency, i.e., the longer a patient suffered from seizures the more delayed was P3.

In studying patients with idiopathic, generalized epilepsy (IGE) Triantafyllou *et al.* (1992b) found that these patients differed less than focal-seizure patients from control subjects, and Fukai *et al.* (1990) found no difference at all between IGE patients and control subjects. In contrast again, Verleger *et al.* (1997) found that these patients had already slightly delayed N1 peaks, and more and more delayed N2 and P3 peaks.

In general, the duration of epileptic symptoms was reflected in latency delays of ERP components. Puce *et al.* (1989) suggested that brains suffering from recurring seizures might be prone to advanced electrophysiological aging [be it due to epilepsy or to antiepileptic medication (Kubota *et al.*, 1998)] and, indeed, we found the patterns of delays strikingly similar between IGE patients compared to healthy age-matched controls (Verleger *et al.*, 1997) and healthy elderly compared to young adults (Verleger *et al.*, 1991).

A serendipitous finding in the visual go/no-go task used by Verleger *et al.* (1997) was a massive, isolated delay of the posterior N2, by 40 msec, in patients with temporal foci. Likewise, in patients studied by Smith and Halgren (1988), a negative complex evoked by visual stimuli, seen from 180 to 400 msec in healthy subjects at posterior sites, was either reduced or completely absent. In these patients, anterior temporal lobes were surgically removed, and were not simply functionally damaged, as was the case for patients of Verleger *et al.*, which may account for the more drastic difference from normals in this negative component. Unfortunately, other studies using visual stimuli in patients with temporal lobe epilepsy did not report data from posterior sites (Johnson, 1989; Nelson *et al.*, 1991; Rugg *et al.*, 1991; Scheffers *et al.*, 1991). Thus, there is only limited evidence that an intact temporal lobe appears to be necessary for the elicitation of the posterior N2. Because N2 is probably generated in the occipital lobe [cf. Luck *et al.* (1997) on N2pc], this is one of the few neurophysiological results in humans to support the notion of "reentrant processing" (Di Lollo *et al.*, 2000), i.e., the notion that visual information has to pass a second time through occipital areas in order to be fully processed.

Impaired memory in patients with temporal lobe epilepsy was investigated in a few studies by scalp-recorded ERPs. Smith and Halgren (1989) studied patients whose anterior right or left temporal lobe was removed, in a choice–response task in which participants had to distinguish between words presented previously and new words. "Recognition positivity" evoked by identified old words was missing in the left-resected patients but remained unchanged in the right-resected patients. This might be a specific indicator of the patients' memory impairment [as interpreted by Smith and Halgren (1989)] or might reflect the patients' ambiguity when presented with words that they could not classify with certainty [i.e., it might be an instance of the general reduction of P3 by "equivocation" (Ruchkin and Sutton, 1978)].

Rugg *et al.* (1991) used a similar though not identical task: the task was continuous, i.e., newly presented words could be presented a second time during later trials. In this task, repetition-related positivity was missing not only in left-resected patients but also in right-resected patients. Furthermore, in groups of presurgical patients with left or right foci, positivity was unilaterally reduced on the side of the focus. These reductions or complete absence of positivity must be related to conscious recollection because the same "priming positivity" as in the control group was evoked by repeated words in another task, where the fact that a word had been previously presented was not task relevant. On the other hand, the reductions were unspecific insofar as they did not correlate with response times, error rate, and a verbal memory test.

Measuring potentials evoked by probes in an auditory version of Sternberg's memory-scanning task, Grippo *et al.* (1996) found the N1 peak as well as a late positive shift to be generally reduced in patients with temporal lobe epilepsy. Specific to a subgroup of patients with worse results in neuropsychological memory tests were delays of P250 and delays and reductions of the following N290.

In conclusion, ERPs have proved to be sensitive indicators of memory deficits in epileptic patients, but the specificity of the findings has remained somewhat ambiguous. Good progress in the issue of memory specificity has been achieved in studies using intracranial recordings, as is described next.

Intracranial Recordings

In patients with intractable epilepsy, for whom surgery is chosen as treatment, electrodes are routinely inserted within the skull to gain more information about the location of the tissue to be removed and about consequences of the surgery. This has proved to be a lucky accident for basic research in ERPs and in neuroscience in general because information can be gained from within the skull, beyond the ERP components recorded from the scalp (e.g., Nobre et al., 1998; Rektor et al., 1998; Clarke et al., 1999; Yazawa et al., 2000). Of more interest in the present context, ERPs recorded by means of such intracranial electrodes have been shown to provide important information about treatment outcomes.

Grunwald et al. (1995) established sensitivity of an N400 and an N800, recorded in anterior and posterior hippocampus, respectively, to recognition of repeated words in the continuous-recognition task as used, for example, by Rugg et al. (1991) [cf. preceeding discussion; see also similar methods and results by Guillem and colleagues (e.g., Guillem et al., 1999)].

Subsequent work (Elger et al., 1997) made clear that the focus of the N400 was anterior to the hippocampus, within the anterior medial temporal lobe; another focus was situated near Wernicke's area, in the left middle temporal gyrus.

Amplitudes of this latter left-sided N400 in the continuous-recognition task correlated with the number of words immediately recalled in an auditory verbal learning test, whereas amplitudes of the former, anterior-temporal N400 correlated with number of words recalled in auditory verbal learning after a 30-min delay, also only in recordings from the left side, not from the right side. (All reported patients had left-sided language dominance). However, in those patients who underwent left-sided resection either of the anterior-temporal lobe or of the hippocampus, their right-sided anterior-temporal N400 recorded before surgery was related to the number of words recalled after 30 min in postsurgery verbal learning (Grunwald et al., 1998). That is, N400 recorded from the nondominant hemisphere allowed prediction of how much this nondominant hemisphere would compensate for the function of the resected hemisphere. Moreover, reduction of the anterior-temporal N400 on repetition of words on the side contralateral to the hemisphere to be removed predicted whether the patients would indeed become seizure free postsurgery (Grunwald et al., 1999), i.e., according to the authors, the lack of repetition effect in the hemisphere assumed to be healthy indicated that this hemisphere was likewise damaged.

Biofeedback

Event-related potentials have been used as a therapeutic means in neurological patients. Epileptic patients who are not seizure free even after careful, repeated variations of drug treatment may be able to reduce their seizure rate by learning to control their slow negative potentials. Birbaumer's group showed this in two independent studies [the first one reported in Birbaumer et al. (1991), and Rockstroh et al. (1993), and the second one reported in Kotchoubey et al. (1996, 1997, 1999, 2001)]. Specifically, patients had to control the movement of a target object on the screen during a 6-sec period. The object was in fact controlled by the amount of Cz-recorded negativity (with EOG transmission being rejected), with more or less negativity moving the object to one or the other goal. Patients had to learn this game in many training sessions and were expected to be able to use this skill to control excess amount of cortical excitation. In fact, patients needed many more sessions compared to healthy people to learn this skill, probably related to their problems in maintaining control of cortical excitation but perhaps also related to the fact that most healthy people investigated in this group's basic research (review in Rockstroh *et al.*, 1989) had higher education and were not distracted by worrying about their health problems. In favor of the disease-specific account is the finding that the absolute amount of negativity produced by patients during the first phase of biofeedback training was a negative predictor for the effectiveness of the training in reducing seizures (Kotchoubey *et al.*, 1999). On average, number of seizures could indeed be reduced by this training. A control condition in the initial report (Birbaumer *et al.*, 1991) was biofeedback of alpha wave amplitudes, and two control conditions in the most recent report (Kotchoubey *et al.*, 2001) were modifications of the drug regimen during a 6-week hospital stay and learning of a respiration technique to avoid hyperventilation in as many training sessions (n = 35) as with biofeedback. Biofeedback of slow negativity was shown to be more effective than alpha biofeedback and than the respiration technique and as effective as modification of the drug regimen. Whether this method will find wider application remains to be seen.

In summary, as evidenced by the advanced methods in intracranial recordings and in the therapeutic application just described, ERPs certainly continue being a fruitful and relevant method in epilepsy research and treatment.

CONCLUDING REMARKS

The discussions here have outlined the strengths and drawbacks of the use of event-related potentials in research on neurological patients. Not all areas could be covered, most notably migraine and headache syndromes (due to this author's lack of knowledge) and those neurological syndromes less often encountered in neurology than in neurosurgery (such as closed-head injury and coma) or in internal medicine (such as transient global ischemia and renal encephalopathy). These drawbacks notwithstanding, it is hoped that the present chapter serves as a useful guide for further research. There is still room for better application of ERPs to the three purposes emphasized at the beginning of this chapter, i.e., diagnosis and prognosis, understanding consequences of diseases on cognition, and therapy and rehabilitation.

Acknowledgments

I would like to thank my medical colleagues at our department of neurology; they taught me, a psychologist who records potentials from the scalp, to understand what the brain actually looks like. Thanks, in particular, to Detlef Kömpf, head of the department, and Wolfgang Heide, Andreas Moser, Matthias Nitschke, Peter Vieregge, Clemens Vollmer, Bernd Wauschkuhn, and Karl Wessel.

References

Aaltonen, O., Tuomainen, J., Laine, M., and Niemi, P. (1993). Cortical differences in tonal versus vowel processing as revealed by an ERP component called mismatch negativity (MMN). *Brain Lang.* **44**, 139–152.

Akshoomoff, N. A., and Courchesne, E. (1994). ERP evidence for a shifting attention deficit in patients with damage to the cerebellum. *J. Cogn. Neurosci.* **6**, 388–399.

Altenmüller, E. (1989). Cortical DC-potentials as electrophysiological correlates of hemispheric dominance of higher cognitive functions. *Int. J. Neurosci.* **47**, 1–15.

Angelelli, P., De Luca, M., and Spinelli, D. (1996). Early visual processing in neglect patients: a study with steady-state VEPs. *Neuropsychologia* **34**, 1151–1157.

Arendt, G., Hefter, H., and Jablonowski, H. (1993). Acoustically evoked event-related potentials in HIV-associated dementia. *Electroencephalogr. Clin. Neurophysiol.* **86**, 152–160.

Baldeweg, T., Gruzelier, J. H., Catalan, J., Pugh, K., Lovett, E., Riccio, M., Stygall, J., Irving, G., Catt, S., and Hawkins, D. (1993). Auditory and visual event-related potentials in a controlled investigation of HIV infection. *Electroencephalogr. Clin. Neurophysiol.* **88**, 356–368.

Barrett, G., Shibasaki, H., and Neshige, R. (1986). Cortical potential shifts preceding voluntary movement are normal in Parkinsonism. *Electroencephalogr. Clin. Neurophysiol.* **63**, 340–348.

Birbaumer, N., Elbert, T., Rockstroh, B., Daum, I., Wolf, P., and Canavan, A. (1991). Clinical-psychological treatment of epileptic seizures: a controlled study. *In* "Perspectives and Promises of Clinical Psychology" (A. Ehlers, ed.), pp. 81–96. Plenum Press, New York.

Birbaumer, N., Ghanayim, N., Hinterberger, T., Iversen, I., Kotchoubey, B., Kübler, A., Perelmouter, J., Taub, E., and Flor, H. (1999). A spelling device for the paralysed. *Nature* **398**, 297–298.

Birbaumer, N., Kübler, A., Ghanayim, N., Hinterberger, T., Perelmouter, J., Kaiser, J., Iversen, I., Kotchoubey, B., Neumann, N. and Flor, H. (2000). The Thought Translation Device (TTD) for completely paralyzed patients. *IEEE Trans. Rehab. Eng.* **8**, 190–193.

Bungener, C., Le Houezec, J. L., Pierson, A., and Jouvent, R. (1996). Cognitive and emotional deficits in early stages of HIV infection: An event-related potentials study. *Prog. Neuropsychopharmacol. Biol. Psychiatr.* **20**, 1303–1314.

Castañeda, M., Ostrosky-Solis, F., Pérez, M., Bobes, M. A., and Rangel, L. E. (1997). ERP assessment of semantic memory in Alzheimer's disease. *Int. J. Psychophysiol.* **27**, 201–214.

Clarke, J. M., Halgren, E., and Chauvel, P. (1999). Intracranial ERPs in humans during a lateralized visual oddball task: I. Occipital and peri-rolandic recordings. *Clin. Neurophysiol.* **110**, 1210–1225.

Cobianchi, A., and Giaquinto, S. (2000). Can we exploit event-related potentials for retraining language after stroke? *Disability Rehab.* **15**, 427–434.

Cohen, R., Dobel, C., Berg, P., Koebbel, P., Schönle, P.-W., and Rockstroh, B. (2001) Event-related potential correlates of verbal and pictorial feature comparison in aphasics and controls. *Neuropsychologia* **39**, 489–501.

Coles, M. G. H. (1989). Modern mind-brain reading: psychophysiology, physiology, and cognition. *Psychophysiology* **26**, 251–269.

Connolly, S., Manji, H., McAllister, R. H., Fell, M., Loveday, C., Kirkis, C., Herns, M., Sweeney, B., Sartawi, O., Durrance, P., Griffin, G. B., Boland, M., Fowler, C. J., Newman, S. P., Weller, I. V. D., and Harrison, M. J. G. (1994). Long-latency event-related potentials in asymptomatic human immunodeficiency. *Ann. Neurol.* **35**, 189–196.

Connolly, J. F., Mate-Kole, C. C., and Joyce, B. M. (1999). Global aphasia: An innovative assessment approach. *Arch. Physical Med. Rehab.* **80**, 1309–1315.

Csépe, V., Osman-Sági, J., Molnár, M., and Gósy, M. (2001). Impaired speech perception in aphasic patients: Event-related potential and neuropsychological assessment. *Neuropsychologia* **39**, 1194–1208.

Cunnington, R., Iansek, R., Bradshaw, J. L., and Phillips, J. G. (1995). Movement-related potentials in Parkinson's disease: Presence and predictability of temporal and spatial cues. *Brain* **118**, 935–950.

Cunnington, R., Iansek, R., Johnson, K. A., and Bradshaw, J. L. (1997). Movement-related potentials in Parkinson's disease: Motor imagery and movement preparation. *Brain* **120**, 1339–1353.

Cunnington, R., Iansek, R., and Bradshaw, J. L. (1999). Movement-related potentials in Parkinson's disease: External cues and attentional strategies. *Movement Disorders* **14**, 63–68.

Cunnington, R., Lalouschek, W., Dirnberger, G., Walla, P., Lindinger, G., Asenbaum, S., Brücke, T., and Lang, W. (2001). A medial to lateral shift in pre-movement cortical activity in hemi-Parkinson's disease. *Clin. Neurophysiol.* **112**, 608–618.

Daum, I., Schugens, M. M., Ackermann, H., Lutzenberger, W., Dichgans, J., and Birbaumer, N. (1993). Classical conditioning after cerebellar lesions in humans. *Behav. Neurosci.* **107**, 748–756.

Deouell, L. Y., Bentin, S., and Giard, M.-H. (1998). Mismatch negativity in dichotic listening: Evidence for interhemispheric differences and multiple generators. *Psychophysiology* **35**, 355–365.

Deouell, L. Y., Hämäläinen, H., and Bentin, S. (2000a). Unilateral neglect after right hemisphere damage: Contributions from event-related potentials. *Audiol. Neuro-Otol.* **5**, 225–234.

Deouell, L. Y., Bentin, S., and Soroker, N. (2000b). Electrophysiological evidence for an early (preattentive) information processing deficit in patients with right hemisphere damage and unilateral neglect. *Brain* **123**, 353–365.

De Toledo-Morrell, L., Evers, S., Hoeppner, T. J., Morrell, F., Garron, D. C., and Fox, J. H. (1991). A 'stress' test for memory dysfunction. Electrophysiologic manifestations of early Alzheimer's disease. *Arch. Neurol.* **48**, 605–609.

Dick, J. P. R., Rothwell, J. C., Day, B. L., Cantello, R., Buruma, O., Gioux, M., Benecke, R., Berardelli, A., Thompson, P. D., and Marsden, C. D. (1989). The Bereitschaftspotential is abnormal in Parkinson's disease. *Brain* **112**, 233–244.

Di Lollo, V., Enns, J. T., and Rensink, R. A. (2000). Competition for consciousness among visual events: The psychophysics of reentrant visual processes. *J. Exp. Psychol. Gen.* **129**, 481–507.

Dobel, C., Pulvermüller, F., Härle, M., Cohen, R., Köbbel, P., Schönle, P. W., and Rockstroh, B. (2001). Syntactic and semantic processing in the healthy and aphasic human brain. *Exp. Brain Res.* **140**, 77–85.

Drake, M. E., Jr., Burgess, R. J., Gelety, T. J., Ford, C. E. and Brown, M. E. (1986). Long-latency auditory event-related potentials in epilepsy. *Clin. Electroencephalogr.* **17**, 10–13.

Driver, J., and Vuilleumier, P. (2001). Perceptual awareness and its loss in unilateral neglect and extinction. *Cognition* **79**, 39–88.

Ebmeier, K. P. (1992). A quantitative method for the assessment of overall effects from a number of similar electrophysiological studies: Description and application to event-related potentials in Parkinson's disease. *Electroencephalogr. Clin. Neurophysiol.* **84**, 440–446.

Eichenbaum, H. (2000). A cortical-hippocampal system for declarative memory. *Nat. Rev. Neurosci.* **1**, 41–50.

Eimer, M., and McCarthy, R. A. (1999). Prosopagnosia and structural encoding of faces: Evidence from event-related potentials. *NeuroReport* **10**, 255–259.

Elger, C. E., Grunwald, T., Lehnertz, K., Kutas, M., Helmstaedter, C., Brockhaus, A., van Roost, D., and Heinze, H. J. (1997). Human temporal lobe potentials in verbal learning and memory processes. *Neuropsychologia* **35**, 657–667.

Evers, S., Grotemeyer, K. H., Reichelt, D., Luttmann, S., and Husstedt, I. W. (1998). Impact of antiretroviral treatment on AIDS dementia: A longitudinal prospective event-related potential study. *J. Acquired Immune Def. Syndr. Hum. Retrovirol.* **17**, 143–148.

Falkenstein, M., Hoormann, J., Christ, S., and Hohnsbein, J. (2000). ERP components on reaction errors and their functional significance: A tutorial. *Biol. Psychol.* **51**, 87–107.

Falkenstein, M., Hielscher, H., Dziobek, I., Schwarzenau, P., Hoormann, J., Sundermann, B., and Hohnsbein, J. (2001). Action monitoring, error detection, and the basal ganglia: An ERP study. *NeuroReport* **12**, 157–161.

Farwell, L. A., and Donchin, E. (1988). Talking off the top of your head: Toward a mental prosthesis utilizing event-related brain potentials. *Electroencephalogr. Clin. Neurophysiol.* **70**, 510–523.

Fattaposta, F., Pierelli, F., Traversa, G., My, F., Mostarda, M., D'Alessio, C., Soldati, G., Osborn, J., and Amabile, G. (2000). Preprogramming and control activity of bimanual self-paced motor task in Parkinson's disease. *Clin. Neurophysiol.* **111**, 873–883.

Fein, G., Biggins, C. A., and MacKay, S. (1995). Delayed latency of the event-related brain potential P3A component in HIV disease. *Arch. Neurol.* **52**, 1109–1118.

Filipovic, S., Kostic, V. S., Šternic, N., Marinkovic, Z., and Ocic, G. (1990). Auditory event-related potentials in different types of dementia. *Eur. Neurol.* **30**, 189–193.

Filipovic, S., Drulovic, J., Štojsavljevic, N., and Levic, Z. (1997). The effects of high-dose intravenous methylprednisolone on event-related potentials in patients with multiple sclerosis. *J. Neurol. Sci.* **152**, 147–153.

Ford, J. M., Woodward, S. H., Sullivan, E. H., Isaacks, B. G., Tinklenberg, J. R., Yesavage, J. A., and Roth, W. T. (1996). N400 evidence of abnormal responses to speech in Alzheimer's disease. *Electroencephalogr. Clin. Neurophysiol.* **99**, 235–246.

Friederici, A. D., Pfeifer, E., and Hahne, A. (1993). Event-related brain potentials during natural speech processing: Effects of semantic, morphological and syntactic violations. *Cogn. Brain Res.* **1**, 183–192.

Friederici, A. D., von Cramon, D. Y., and Kotz, S. A. (1999). Language related brain potentials in patients with cortical and subcortical left hemisphere lesions. *Brain* **122**, 1033–1047.

Frodl, T., Hampel, H., Juckel, G., Bürger, K., Padberg, F., Engel, R. R., Möller, H.-J., and Hegerl, U. (2002). Value of event-related P300 subcomponents in the clinical diagnosis of mild cognitive impairment and Alzheimer´s disease? *Psychophysiology* **39**, 175–181.

Fukai, M., Motomura, N., Kobayashi, S., Asaba, H., and Sakai, T. (1990). Event-related potential (P300) in epilepsy. *Acta Neurol. Scand.* **82**, 197–202.

Gaeta, H., Friedman, D., Ritter, W., and Cheng, J. (1999). Changes in sensitivity to stimulus deviance in Alzheimer's disease: An ERP perspective. *NeuroReport* **10**, 281–287.

Gerloff, C., Altenmüller, E., and Dichgans, J. (1996). Disintegration and reorganization of cortical motor processing in two patients with cerebellar stroke. *Electroencephalogr. Clin. Neurophysiol.* **98**, 59–68.

Gerschlager, W., Alesch, F., Cunnington, R., Deecke, L., Dirnberger, G., Endl, W., Lindinger, G., and Lang, W. (1999). Bilateral subthalamic nucleus stimulation improves frontal cortex function in Parkinson's disease. An electrophysiological study of the contingent negative variation. *Brain* **122**, 2365–2373.

Gerschlager, W., Beisteiner, R., Deecke, L., Dirnberger, G., Endl, W., Kollegger, H., Lindinger, G., Vass, K., and Lang, W. (2000). Electrophysiological, neuropsychological and clinical findings in multiple sclerosis patients receiving interferon β-1b: A 1-year follow-up. *Eur. Neurol.* **44**, 205–209.

Giesser, B. S., Schroeder, M. M., LaRocca, N. G., Kurtzberg, D., Ritter, W., Vaughan, H. G., and Scheinberg, L. C. (1992). Endogenous event-related potentials as indices of dementia in multiple sclerosis patients. *Electroencephalogr. Clin. Neurophysiol.* **82**, 320–329.

Gil, R., Zai, L., Neau, J. P., Jonveaux, T., Agbo, C., Rosolacci, T., Burbaud, P., and Ingrand, P. (1993). Event-related auditory evoked potentials and multiple sclerosis. *Electroencephalogr. Clin. Neurophysiol.* **88**, 182–187.

Gil, R., Neau, J. P., Dary-Auriol, M., Agbo, C., Tantot, A. M., and Ingrand, P. (1995). Event-related auditory evoked potentials and amyotrophic lateral sclerosis. *Arch. Neurol.* **52**, 890–896.

Goodin, D. S. (1990). Clinical utility of long latency 'cognitive' event-related potentials (P3): The pros. *Electroencephalogr. Clin. Neurophysiol.* **76**, 2–5.

Goodin, D. S., and Aminoff, M. J. (1986). Electrophysiological differences between subtypes of dementia. *Brain* **109**, 1103–1113.

Goodin, D. S., Squires, K. C., and Starr, A. (1978). Long latency event-related components of the auditory evoked potential in dementia. *Brain* **101**, 635–648.

Goodin, D. S., Aminoff, M. J., Chernoff, D. N., and Hollander, H. (1990). Long latency event-related potentials in patients infected with human immunodeficiency virus. *Ann. Neurol.* **27**, 414–419.

Goodwin, G. M., Chiswick, A., Egan, V., St.Clair, D., and Brettle, R. P. (1990). The Edinburgh cohort of HIV-positive drug users: Auditory event-related potentials show progressive slowing in patients with Centers for Disease Control stage IV disease. *AIDS* **4**, 1243–1250.

Gratton, G., Coles, M. G. H., Sirevaag, E. J., Eriksen, C. W., and Donchin, E. (1988). Pre- and post-stimulus activation of response channels: A psychophysiological analysis. *J. Exp. Psychol. Hum. Perception Performance* **14**, 331–344.

Green, J., and Levey, A. J. (1999). Event-related potential changes in groups at increased risk for Alzheimer disease. *Arch. Neurol.* **56**, 1398–1403.

Green, J. B., Bialy, Y., Sora, E., and Ricamato, A. (1999). High-resolution EEG in poststroke hemiparesis can identify ipsilateral generators during motor tasks. *Stroke* **30**, 2659–2665.

Grippo, A., Pelosi, L., Mehta, V., and Blumhardt, L. D. (1996). Working memory in temporal lobe epilepsy: An event-related potential study. *Electroencephalogr. Clin. Neurophysiol.* **99**, 200–213.

Grunwald, T., Elger, C. E., Lehnertz, K., van Roost, D., and Heinze, H.J. (1995). Alterations of intrahippocampal cognitive potentials in temporal lobe epilepsy. *Electroencephalogr. Clin. Neurophysiol.* **95**, 53–62.

Grunwald, T., Lehnertz, K., Helmstaedter, C., Kutas, M., Pezer, N., Kurthen, M., Van Roost, D., and Elger, C. E. (1998). Limbic ERPs predict verbal memory after left-sided hippocampectomy. *NeuroReport* **9**, 3375–3378.

Grunwald, T., Lehnertz, K., Pezer, N., Kurthen, M., Van Roost, D., Schramm, J., and Elger, C. E. (1999). Prediction of postoperative seizure control by hippocampal event-related potentials. *Epilepsia* **40**, 303–306.

Guillem, F., Rougier, A., and Claverie, B. (1999). Short- and long-delay intracranial ERP repetition effects dissociate memory systems in the human brain. *J. Cogn. Neurosci.* **11**, 437–458.

Hagoort, P., Brown, C. M., and Swaab, T. Y. (1996) Lexical-semantic event-related potential effects in patients with left hemisphere lesions and aphasia, and patients with right hemisphere lesions without aphasia. *Brain* **119**, 627–649.

Hahne, A., and Friederici, A. D. (1999). Electrophysiological evidence for two steps in syntactic analysis: early automatic and late controlled processes. *J. Cogn. Neurosci.* **11**, 194–205.

Halgren, E., Baudena, P., Clarke, J. M., Heit, G., Marinkovic, K., Devaux, B., Vignal, J.-P., and Biraben, A. (1995). Intracerebral potentials to rare target and distractor auditory and visual stimuli. II. Medial, lateral and posterior temporal lobe. *Electroencephalogr. Clin. Neurophysiol.* **94**, 229–250.

Hansch, E. C., Syndulko, K., Cohen, S. N., Goldberg, Z. I., Potvin, A. R., and Tourtellotte, W.W. (1982). Cognition in Parkinson disease: An event-related potential perspective. *Ann. Neurol.* **11**, 599–607.

Hansen, J. C., and Hillyard, S. A. (1980). Endogenous brain potentials associated with selective auditory attention. *Electroencephalogr. Clin. Neurophysiol.* **49**, 277–290.

Hawking, S. (1989) "Eine kurze Geschichte der Zeit." Rowohlt, Hamburg. [Originally published in English (1988). "A Brief History of Time." Bantam Books, New York.]

Hillyard, S. A., Hink, R. F., Schwent, V. L., and Picton, T. W. (1973). Electrical signs of selective attention in the human brain. *Science* **182**, 177–180.

Hömberg, V., Hefter, H., Granseyer, G., Strauss, W., Lange, H., and Hennerici, M. (1986). Event-related potentials in patients with Huntington's disease and relatives at risk in relation to detailed psychometry. *Electroencephalogr. Clin. Neurophysiol.* **63**, 552–569.

Honig, L. S., Ramsay, R. E., and Sheremata, W. A. (1992). Event-related potential P300 in multiple sclerosis. Relation to magnetic resonance imaging and cognitive impairment. *Arch. Neurol.* **49**, 44–50.

Ikeda, A., Shibasaki, H., Nagamine, T., Terada, K., Kaji, R., Fukuyama, H., and Kimura, J. (1994). Dissociation between contingent negative variation and Bereitschaftspotential in a patient with cerebellar efferent lesion. *Electroencephalogr. Clin. Neurophysiol.* **90**, 359–364.

Ikeda, A., Shibasaki, H., Kaji, R., Terada, K., Nagamine, T., Honda, M., and Kimura, J. (1997). Dissociation between contingent negative variation (CNV) and Bereitschaftspotential (BP) in patients with parkinsonism. *Electroencephalogr. Clin. Neurophysiol.* **102**, 142–151.

Ilvonen, T.-M., Kujala, T., Tervaniemi, M., Salonen, O., Näätänen, R., and Pekkonen, E. (2001). The processing of sound duration after left-hemispheric stroke: Event-related potential and behavioral evidence. *Psychophysiology* **38**, 622–628.

Jahanshahi, M., Jenkins, I. H., Brown, R. G., Marsden, C. D., Passingham, R. E., and Brooks, D. J. (1995). Self-initiated versus externally triggered movements. I. An investigation using measurement of regional cerebral blood flow with PET and movement-related potentials in normal and Parkinson's disease subjects. *Brain* **118**, 913–933.

Johnson, K. A., Cunnington, R., Iansek, R., Bradshaw, J. L., Georgiou, N., and Chiu, E. (2001). Movement-related potentials in Huntington's disease: Movement preparation and execution. *Exp. Brain Res.* **138**, 492–499.

Johnson, R., Jr. (1989). Auditory and visual P300s in temporal lobectomy patients: Evidence for modality-dependent generators. *Psychophysiology* **26**, 633–650.

Johnson, R., Jr. (1992) Event-related potential insights into progressive supranuclear palsy. In "Progressive Supranuclear Palsy: Clinical and Research Approaches" (I. Litran and Y. Agid, eds.). Oxford University Press, New York.

Johnson, R., Jr., Litvan, I., and Grafman, J. (1991) Progressive supranuclear palsy: Altered sensory processing leads to degraded cognition. *Neurology* **41**, 1257–1262.

Johnson, R., Jr., Kreiter, K., Zhu, J., and Russo, B. (1998). A spatio-temporal comparison of semantic and episodic cued recall and recognition using event-related brain potentials. *Cogn. Brain Res.* **7**, 119–136.

Karayanidis, F., Andrews, S., Ward, P. B., and Michie, P.T. (1995). ERP indices of auditory selective attention in aging and Parkinson's disease. *Psychophysiology* **32**, 335–350.

Kazmerski, V. A., and Friedman, D. (1997). Effect of multiple presentation of words on event-related potential and reaction time repetition effects in Alzheimer's patients and young and older controls. *Neuropsychiatr. Neuropsychol. Behav. Neurol.* **10**, 32–47.

Kazmerski, V. A., Friedman, D., and Hewitt, S. (1995). Event-related potential repetition effect in Alzheimer's patients: Multiple repetition priming with pictures. *Aging Cogn.* **2**, 169–191.

Kazmerski, V. A., Friedman, D., and Ritter, W. (1997). Mismatch negativity during attend and ignore

conditions in Alzheimer's disease. *Biol. Psychiatr.* **42**, 382–402.

Kerkhoff, G. (2001). Spatial neglect in humans. *Prog. Neurobiol.* **63**, 1–27.

Kew, J. J. M., Leigh, P. N., Playford, E. D., Passingham, R. E., Goldstein, L. H., Frackowiak, R. S. J., and Brooks, D. J. (1993). Cortical function in amyotrophic lateral sclerosis: A positron emission tomography study. *Brain* **116**, 655–680.

Kitamura, J. -I., Shibasaki, H., and Takeuchi, T. (1996). Cortical potentials preceding voluntary elbow movement in recovered hemiparesis. *Electroencephalogr. Clin. Neurophysiol.* **98**, 149–156.

Kitamura, J.-I., Shibasaki, H., Terashi, A., and Tashima, K. (1999). Cortical potentials preceding voluntary finger movement in patients with focal cerebellar lesion. *Clin. Neurophysiol.* **110**, 126–132.

Knight, R. T. (1984). Decreased response to novel stimuli after prefrontal lesions in man. *Electroencephalogr. Clin. Neurophysiol.* **59**, 9–20.

Knight, R. T. (1996). Contribution of human hippocampal region to novelty detection. *Nature* **383**, 256–259.

Kohlmetz, C., Altenmüller, E., Schuppert, M., Wieringa, B. M., and Münte, T. F. (2001). Deficit in automatic sound-change detection may underlie some music perception deficits after acute hemispheric stroke. *Neuropsychologia* **39**, 1121–1124.

Kopp, B., Mattler, U., Goertz, R., and Rist, F. (1996). N2, P3 and the lateralized readiness potential in a nogo task involving selective response priming. *Electroencephalogr. Clin. Neurophysiol.* **99**, 19–27.

Kopp, B., Kunkel, A., Mühlnickel, W., Villringer, K., Taub, E., and Flor, H. (1999). Plasticity in the motor system related to therapy-induced improvement of movement after stroke. *NeuroReport* **10**, 807–810.

Kotchoubey, B., Schneider, D., Schleichert, H., Strehl, U., Uhlmann, C., Blankenhorn, V., Fröscher, W., and Birbaumer, N. (1996). Self-regulation of slow cortical potentials in epilepsy: A retrial with analysis of influencing factors. *Epilepsy Res.* **25**, 269–276.

Kotchoubey, B., Blankenhorn, V., Fröscher, W., Strehl, U., and Birbaumer, N. (1997). Stability of cortical self-regulation in epilepsy patients. *NeuroReport* **8**, 1867–1870.

Kotchoubey, B., Strehl, U., Holzapfel, S., Blankenhorn, V., Fröscher, W., and Birbaumer, N. (1999). Negative potential shifts and the prediction of the outcome of neurofeedback therapy in epilepsy. *Clin. Neurophysiol.* **110**, 683–686.

Kotchoubey, B., Strehl, U., Uhlmann, C., Holzapfel, S., König, M., Fröscher, W., Blankenhorn, V., and Birbaumer, N. (2001). Modification of slow cortical potentials in patients with refractory epilepsy: A controlled outcome study. *Epilepsia* **42**, 406–416.

Kraiuhin, C., Gordon, E., Coyle, S., Sara, G., Rennie, C., Howson, A., Landau, P., and Meares, R. (1990). Normal latency of the P300 event-related potential in mild-to-moderate Alzheimer's disease and depression. *Biol. Psychiatry* **28**, 372–386.

Kübler, A., Kotchoubey, B., Hinterberger, T., Ghanayim, N., Perelmouter, J., Schauer, M., Fritsch, C., Taub, E., and Birbaumer, N. (1999). The thought translation device: A neurophysiological approach to communication in total motor paralysis. *Exp. Brain Res.* **124**, 223–232.

Kübler, A., Kotchoubey, B., Kaiser, J., Wolpaw, J., and Birbaumer, N. (2001). Brain-computer communication: Unlock the locked-in. *Psychol. Bull.* **127**, 358–375.

Kubota, F., Kifune, A., Shibata, N., Akata, T., Takeuchi, K., and Takahashi, S. (1998). Study on the P300 of adult epileptic patients (unmedicated and medicated patients). *J. Epilepsy* **11**, 325–331.

Kutas, M., and Hillyard, S. A. (1980). Reading senseless sentences: brain potentials reflect semantic incongruity. *Science* **207**, 203–205.

Lhermitte, F., Turell, E., LeBrigand, D., and Chain, F. (1985). Unilateral visual neglect and Wave P 300. *Arch. Neurol.* **42**, 567–573.

Linden, A., Bracke-Tolkmitt, R., Lutzenberger, W., Canavan, A. G. M., Scholz, E., Diener, H.-C., and Birbaumer, N. (1990). Slow cortical potentials in Parkinsonian patients during the course of an associative learning task. *J. Psychophysiol.* **4**, 145–162.

Linnville, S. E., and Elliott, F. S. (1997). Mismatch negativity: An index of subclinical neurological differences in HIV patients during rapid perceptual processing. *J. Neuropsychiatr. Clin. Neurosci.* **9**, 45–54.

Looi, J. C. L., and Sachdev, P. S. (1999). Differentiation of vascular dementia from AD on neuropsychological tests. *Neurology* **53**, 670–678.

Luck, S. J., and Hillyard, S. A. (1990). Electrophysiological evidence for parallel and serial processing during visual search. *Percept. Psychophys.* **48**, 603–617.

Luck, S. J., Girelli, M., McDermott, M. T., and Ford, M. A. (1997). Bridging the gap between monkey neurophysiology and human perception: An ambiguity resolution theory of visual selective attention. *Cogn. Psychol.* **33**, 64–87.

Lutzenberger, W., Elbert, T., and Rockstroh, B. (1987). A brief tutorial on the implications of volume conduction for the interpretation of the EEG. *J. Psychophysiol.* **1**, 81–89.

Marzi, C. A., Girelli, M., Miniussi, C., Smania, N., and Maravita, A. (2000). Electrophysiological correlates of conscious vision: Evidence from unilateral extinction. *J. Cogn. Neurosci.* **12**, 869–877.

Messenheimer, J. A., Robertson, K. R., Wilkins, J. W., Kalkowski, J. C., and Hall, C. D. (1992). Event-related potentials in human immunodeficiency virus infection. A prospective study. *Arch. Neurol.* **49**, 396–400.

Middleton, F. A., and Strick, P. (2001). Cerebellar projections to the prefrontal cortex of the primate. *J. Neurosci.* **21**, 700–712.

Minamoto, H., Tachibana, H., Sugita, M., and Okita, T. (2001). Recognition memory in normal aging and Parkinson's disease: Behavioral and electrophysiological evidence. *Cogn. Brain Res.* **11**, 23–32.

Münte, T. F., Ridao-Alonso, M. E., Preinfalk, J., Jung, A., Wieringa, B. M., Matzke, M., Dengler, R., and Johannes, S. (1997). An electrophysiological analysis of altered cognitive functions in Huntington disease. *Arch. Neurol.* **54**, 1089–1098.

Münte, T. F., Tröger, M., Nusser, I., Wieringa, B. M., Johannes, S., Matzke, M., and Dengler, R. (1998a). Alterations of early components of the visual evoked potential in amyotrophic lateral sclerosis. *J. Neurol.* **245**, 206–210.

Münte, T. F., Tröger, M., Nusser, I., Wieringa, B. M., Matzke, M., Johannes, S., and Dengler, R. (1998b). Recognition memory deficits in amyotrophic lateral sclerosis assessed with event-related brain potentials. *Acta Neurol. Scand.* **98**, 110–115.

Münte, T. F., Tröger, M. C., Nusser, I., Wieringa, B. M., Matzke, M., Johannes, S., and Dengler, R. (1999). Abnormalities of visual search behaviour in ALS patients detected with event-related brain potentials. *Amyotroph. Lateral Scler. Other Motor Neuron Disord.* **1**, 21–27.

Näätänen, R. (1990). The role of attention in auditory information processing as revealed by event-related potentials and other brain measures of cognitive function. *Behav. Brain Sci.* **13**, 201–288.

Näätänen, R., and Winkler, I. (1999). The concept of auditory stimulus representation in cognitive neuroscience. *Psychol. Bull.* **125**, 826–859.

Nelson, C. A., Collins, P. F., and Torres, F. (1991). P300 brain activity in seizure patients preceding temporal lobectomy. *Arch. Neurol.* **48**, 141–147.

Neshige, R., Barrett, G., and Shibasaki, H. (1988). Auditory long latency event-related potentials in Alzheimer's disease and multi-infarct dementia. *J. Neurol. Neurosurg. Psychiatr.* **51**, 1120–1125.

Newton, M. R., Barrett, G., Callanan, M. M., and Towell, A. D. (1989). Cognitive event-related potentials in multiple sclerosis. *Brain* **112**, 1637–1660.

Nobre, A. C., Allison, T., and McCarthy, G. (1998). Modulation of human extrastriate visual processing by selective attention to colours and words. *Brain* **121**, 1357–1368.

Oishi, M., Mochizuki, Y., Du, C., and Takasu, T. (1995). Contingent negative variation and movement-related cortical potentials in parkinsonism. *Electroencephalogr. Clin. Neurophysiol.* **95**, 346–349.

Ollo, C., Johnson, R., Jr., and Grafman, J. (1991). Signs of cognitive change in HIV disease: An event-related brain potential study. *Neurology* **41**, 209–215.

Onofrj, M., Fulgente, T., Nobilio, D., Malatesta, G., Bazzano, S., Colamartino, P., and Gambi, D. (1992). P3 recordings in patients with bilateral temporal lobe lesions. *Neurology* **42**, 1762–1767.

Onofrj, M., Melchionda, D., Thomas, A., and Fulgente, T. (1996). Reappearance of event-related P3 potential in locked-in syndrome. *Cogn. Brain Res.* **4**, 95–97.

Pekkonen, E., Jousmäki, V., Kononen, M., Reinikainen, K., and Partanen, J. (1994). Auditory sensory memory impairment in Alzheimer's disease: An event-related potential study. *NeuroReport* **5**, 2537–2540.

Pekkonen, E., Jousmäki, V., Reinikainen, K., and Partanen, J. (1995). Automatic auditory discrimination is impaired in Parkinson's disease. *Electroencephalogr. Clin. Neurophysiol.* **95**, 47–52.

Pekkonen, E., Ahveninen, J., Virtanen, J., and Teräväinen, H. (1998). Parkinson's disease selectively impairs preattentive auditory processing: An MEG study. *NeuroReport* **9**, 2949–2952.

Pelosi, L., Geesken, J. M., Holly, M., Hayward, M., and Blumhardt, L. D. (1997). Working memory impairment in multiple sclerosis. Evidence from an event-related potential study of patients with clinically isolated myelopathy. *Brain* **120**, 2039–2058.

Pfefferbaum, A., Ford, J. M., Weller, B. J., and Kopell, B. S. (1985). ERPs to response production and inhibition. *Electroencephalogr. Clin. Neurophysiol.* **60**, 423–434.

Pfefferbaum, A., Ford, J. M., and Kraemer, H. C. (1990). Clinical utility of long latency 'cognitive' event-related potentials (P3): The cons. *Electroencephalogr. Clin. Neurophysiol.* **76**, 6–12.

Pfurtscheller, G., Flotzinger, D., and Kalcher, J. (1993). Brain-computer interface—A new communication device for handicapped persons. *J. Microcomputer Appl.* **16**, 293–299.

Pierrot-Deseilligny, C., Turell, E., Penet, C., Lebrigand, D., Pillon, B., Chain, F., and Agid, Y. (1989). Increased wave P 300 latency in progressive supranuclear palsy. *J. Neurol. Neurosurg. Psychiatr.* **52**, 656–658.

Pirtošek, Z., Jahanshahi, M., Barrett, G., and Lees, A. J. (2001). Attention and cognition in bradykinetic-rigid syndromes: An event-related potential study. *Ann. Neurol.* **50**, 567–573.

Platz, T., Kim, I. H., Pintschovius, H., Winter, T., Kieselbach, A., Villringer, K., Kurth, R., and Mauritz, K.-H. (2000). Multimodal EEG analysis in man suggests impairment-specific changes in movement-related electric brain activity after stroke. *Brain* **123**, 2475–2490.

Polich, J. (1991). P300 in the evaluation of aging and dementia. *In* "Event-Related Brain Research, Electroencephalography and Clinical Neurophysiology" (C.H.M.Brunia, G.Mulder, and M. N. Verbaten, eds.), Suppl. 42, pp. 304–323. Elsevier, Amsterdam.

Polich, J., and Squire, L. R. (1993). P300 from amnesic patients with bilateral hippocampal lesions. *Electroencephalogr. Clin. Neurophysiol.* **86**, 408–417.

Polich, J., Ehlers, C. L., Otis, S., Mandell, A. J., and Bloom, F. E. (1986). P300 latency reflects the degree of cognitive decline in dementing illness. *Electroencephalogr. Clin. Neurophysiol.* **63**, 138–144.

Posner, M. I., Walker, J. A., Friedrich, F. J., and Rafal, R. D. (1984). Effects of parietal injury on covert orienting of attention. *J. Neurosci.* **4**, 1863–1874.

Praamstra, P., and Plat, F. M. (2001). Failed suppression of direct visuomotor activation in Parkinson's disease. *J. Cogn. Neurosci.* **130**, 31–43.

Praamstra, P., Meyer, A. S., Cools, A. R., Horstink, M. W. I. M., and Stegeman, D. F. (1996). Movement preparation in Parkinson's disease: Time course and distribution of movement-related potentials in a movement precueing task. *Brain* **119**, 1689–1704.

Praamstra, P., Stegeman, D.F., Cools, A. R., and Horstink, M. W. I. M. (1998) Reliance on external cues for movement initiation in Parkinson's disease: Evidence from movement-related potentials. *Brain* **121**, 167–177.

Praamstra, P., Plat, E. M., Meyer, A. S., and Horstink, M. W. I. M. (1999). Motor cortex activation in Parkinson's disease: Dissociation of electrocortical and peripheral measures of response generation. *Movement Disord.* **14**, 790–799.

Puce, A., Donnan, G. A., and Bladin, P. F. (1989). Comparative effects of age on limbic and scalp P3. *Electroencephalogr. Clin. Neurophysiol.* **74**, 385–393.

Puce, A., Berkovic, S. F., Cadusch, P. J., and Bladin, P. F. (1994). P3 latency jitter assessed using 2 techniques. II. Surface and sphenoidal recordings in subjects with focal epilepsy. *Electroencephalogr. Clin. Neurophysiol.* **92**, 555–567.

Pulvermüller, F., Lutzenberger, W., Müller, V., Mohr, B., Dichgans, J., and Birbaumer, N. (1996). P3 and contingent negative variation in Parkinson's disease. *Electroencephalogr. Clin. Neurophysiol.* **98**, 456–467.

Ravizza, S. M., and Ivry, R. B. (2001). Comparison of the basal ganglia and cerebellum in shifting attention. *J. Cogn. Neurosci.* **13**, 285–297.

Rektor, I., Louvel, J., and Lamarche, M. (1998). Intracerebral recordings of potentials accompanying simple limb movements: A SEEG study in epileptic patients. *Electroencephalogr. Clin. Neurophysiol.* **107**, 277–286.

Reuter, B. M., Schönle P. W., and Kurthen, M. (1994). Event-related potentials in aphasic patients—An N400 study. *EEG-EMG, Z. Elektroenzephalogr. Elektromyogr. Verwandte Geb.* **25**, 180–189.

Revonsuo, A., and Laine, M. (1996). Semantic processing without conscious understanding in a global aphasic: Evidence from auditory event-related brain potentials. *Cortex* **32**, 29–48.

Revonsuo, A., Portin, R., Juottonen, K., and Rinne, J.O. (1998). Semantic processing of spoken words in Alzheimer's disease: An electrophysiological study. *J. Cogn. Neurosci.* **10**, 408–420.

Ritter, W., Simson, R., Vaughan, H. G., Jr., and Friedman, D. (1979). A brain event related to the making of a sensory discrimination. *Science* **203**, 1358–1361.

Ritter, W., Simson, R., and Vaughan, H. G., Jr. (1983). Event-related potential correlates of two stages of information processing in physical and semantic discrimination tasks. *Psychophysiol.* **20**, 168–179.

Rockstroh, B., Elbert, T., Canavan, A., Lutzenberger, W., and Birbaumer, N. (1989). "Slow Cortical Potentials and Behaviour." Urban and Schwarzenberg, Baltimore, München, Wien.

Rockstroh, B., Elbert, T., Birbaumer, N., Wolf, P., Düchting-Roth, A., Reker, M., Daum, I., Lutzenberger, W., and Dichgans, J. (1993). Cortical self-regulation in patients with epilepsies. *Epilepsy Res.* **14**, 63–72 .

Rodin, E., Khabbazeh, Z., Twitty, G., and Schmaltz, S. (1989). The cognitive evoked potential in epilepsy patients. *Clin. Electroencephalogr.* **20**, 176–182.

Rosenberg, C., Nudleman, K., and Starr, A. (1985). Cognitive evoked potentials (P300) in early Huntington's disease. *Arch. Neurol.* **42**, 984–987.

Ruchkin, D. S., and Sutton, S. (1978). Equivocation and P300 amplitude. *In* "Multidisciplinary Perspectives in Event-related Brain Potential Research" (D. Otto, ed.), pp. 175–177. U.S. Government Printing Office, Washington, D.C.

Ruchkin, D. S., Grafman, J., Krauss, G. L., Johnson, R., Jr., Canoune, H., and Ritter, W. (1994). Event-related brain potential evidence for a verbal working memory deficit in multiple sclerosis. *Brain* **117**, 289–305.

Rugg, M. D., Roberts, R. C., Potter, D. D., Pickles, C. D., and Nagy, M. E. (1991). Event-related potentials related to recognition memory. Effects of unilateral temporal lobectomy and temporal lobe epilepsy. *Brain* **114**, 2313–2332.

Rugg, M. D., Pearl, S., Walker, P., Roberts, R. C., and Holdstock, J. S. (1994). Word repetition effects on event-related potentials in healthy young and old subjects, and in patients with Alzheimer-type dementia. *Neuropsychologia* **32**, 381–398.

Rugg, M. D., Mark, R. E., Gilchrist, J., and Roberts, R. C. (1997) ERP repetition effects in indirect and direct tasks: Effects of age and interitem lag. *Psychophysiology* **34**, 572–586.

Scheffers, M. K., Johnson, R., Jr., and Ruchkin, D. S. (1991). P300 in patients with unilateral temporal lobectomies: The effects of reduced stimulus quality. *Psychophysiology* **28**, 274–284.

Schmahmann, J. D. (1996). From movement to thought: Anatomic substrates of the cerebellar contribution to cognitive processing. *Hum. Brain Mapping* **4**, 174–198.

Schroeder, M. M., Handelsman, L., Torres, L., Dorfman, D., Rinaldi, P., Jacobson, J., Wiener, J., and Ritter, W. (1994). Early and late cognitive event-related potentials mark stages of HIV-1 infection in the drug-user risk group. *Biol. Psychiatr.* **53**, 54–69.

Schwartz, T. J., Kutas, M., Butters, N., Paulsen, J. S., and Salmon, D. P. (1996). Electrophysiological insights into the nature of the semantic deficit in Alzheimer's disease. *Neuropsychologia* **34**, 827–841.

Shibasaki, H., Shima, F., and Kuroiwa, Y. (1978). Clinical studies of the movement-related cortical potential (MP) and the relationship between the dentatorubrothalamic pathway and readiness potential (RP). *J. Neurol.* **219**, 15–25.

Shibasaki, H., Barrett, G., Neshige, R., Hirata, I., and Tomoda, H. (1986). Volitional movement is not preceded by cortical slow negativity in cerebellar dentate lesion in man. *Brain Res.* **368**, 361–365.

Smith, M. E., and Halgren, E. (1988). Attenuation of a sustained visual processing negativity after lesions that include the inferotemporal cortex. *Electroencephalogr. Clin. Neurophysiol.* **70**, 366–369.

Smith, M. E., and Halgren, E. (1989). Dissociation of recognition memory components following temporal lobe lesions. *J. Exp. Psychol. Learning Memory Cogn.* **15**, 50–60.

Spinelli, D., Burr, D. C., and Morrone, M.C. (1994). Spatial neglect is associated with increased latencies of visual evoked potentials. *Vis. Neurosci.* **11**, 909–918.

Stam, C. J., Visser, S. L., Op de Coul, A. A. W., De Sonneville, L. M. J., Schellens, R. L. L., Brunia, C. H. M., de Smet, D. S., and Gielen, C. (1993). Disturbed frontal regulation of attention in Parkinson's disease. *Brain* **116**, 1139–1158.

Starr, A., and Barrett, G. (1987). Disordered auditory short-term memory in man and event-related potentials. *Brain* **110**, 935–959.

Sternberg, S. (1966). High-speed scanning in human memory. *Science* **153**, 652–654.

Swaab, T., Brown, C., and Hagoort, P. (1997). Spoken sentence comprehension in aphasia: Event-related potential evidence for a lexical integration deficit. *J. Cogn. Neurosci.* **9**, 39–66.

Swaab, T. Y., Brown, C., and Hagoort, P. (1998). Understanding ambiguous words in sentence contexts: Electrophysiological evidence for delayed contextual selection in Broca's aphasia. *Neuropsychologia* **36**, 737–761.

Swanwick, G. R. J., Rowan, M. J., Coen, R. F., Lawlor, B. A., Walsh, J. B., and Coakley, D. (1997). Electrophysiologic responses to varying mnemonic demand: A "stress test" is not diagnostic in very mild Alzheimer's disease. *Biol. Psychiatr.* **42**, 1073–1075.

Tachibana, H., Toda, K., Aragane, K., and Sugita, M. (1993). Chronometrical analysis of event-related potentials and reaction time in patients with multiple lacunar infarcts. *Cogn. Brain Res.* **1**, 193–196.

Tachibana, H., Aragane, K., and Sugita, M. (1995). Event-related potentials in patients with cerebellar degeneration: Electrophysiological evidence for cognitive impairment. *Cogn. Brain Res.* **2**, 173–180.

Tachibana, H., Miyata, Y., Takeda, M., Sugita, M., and Okita, T. (1999a). Event-related potentials reveal memory deficits in Parkinson's disease. *Cogn. Brain Res.* **8**, 165–172.

Tachibana, H., Kawabata, K., Tomino, Y., and Sugita, M. (1999b). Prolonged P3 latency and decreased brain perfusion in cerebellar degeneration. *Acta Neurol. Scand.* **100**, 310–316.

Tachibana, H., Miyata, Y., Takeda, M., Minamoto, H., Sugita, M., and Okita, T. (1999c). Memory in patients with subcortical infarction—An auditory event-related potential study. *Cogn. Brain Res.* **8**, 87–94.

Takeda, M., Tachibana, H., Okuda, B., Kawabata, K., and Sugita, M. (1998). Electrophysiological comparison between corticobasal degeneration and progressive supranuclear palsy. *Clin. Neurol. Neurosurg.* **100**, 94–98.

Tarkka, I. M., Massaquoi, S., and Hallett, M. (1993). Movement-related cortical potentials in patients with cerebellar degeneration. *Acta Neurol. Scand.* **88**, 129–135.

ter Keurs, M., Brown, C. M., Hagoort, P., and Stegeman, D. F. (1999). Electrophysiological manifestations of open- and closed-class words in patients with Broca's aphasia with agrammatic comprehension: An event-related brain potential study. *Brain* **122**, 839–854.

Thomas, C., Altenmüller, E., Marckmann, G., Kahrs, J., and Dichgans, J. (1997). Language processing in aphasia: Changes in lateralization patterns during recovery reflect cerebral plasticity in adults. *Electroencephalogr. Clin. Neurophysiol.* **102**, 86–97.

Touge, T., Werhahn, K. J., Rothwell, J. C., and Marsden, C. D. (1995). Movement-related cortical potentials preceding repetitive and random-choice hand movements in Parkinson's disease. *Ann. Neurol.* **37**, 791–799.

Triantafyllou, N. I., Voumvourakis, K., Zalonis, I., Sfagos, K., Mantouvalos, V., Malliara, S., and Papageorgiou, C. (1992a). Cognition in relapsing–remitting multiple sclerosis: A multichannel event-related potential (P300) study. *Acta Neurol. Scand.* **85**, 10–13.

Triantafyllou, N. I., Zalonis, I., Kokotis, P., Anthracopoulos, M., Siafacas, A., Malliara, S., Hamburger, H. L. and Papageorgiou, C. (1992b). Cognition in epilepsy: A multichannel event-related potential (P300) study. *Acta Neurol. Scand.* **86**, 462–465.

Tsuchiya, H., Yamaguchi, S., and Kobayashi, S. (2000). Impaired novelty detection and frontal lobe dysfunction in Parkinson's disease. *Neuropsychologia* **38**, 645–654.

Van Boxtel, G. (1994). Non-motor components of slow brain potentials. Dissertation, Katholieke Universiteit Brabant, Tilburg, The Netherlands.

van der Lubbe, R. H. J., Wauschkuhn, B., Wascher, E., Niehoff, T., Kömpf, D., and Verleger, R. (2000). Event-related lateralized components with direction information for the preparation of saccades and finger movements. *Exp. Brain Res.* **132**, 163–178.

van Dijk, J. G., Jennekens-Schinkel, A., Caekebeke, J. F., and Zwinderman, A.H. (1992). Are event-related potentials in multiple sclerosis indicative of cognitive impairment? Evoked and event-related potentials, psychometric testing and response speed: A controlled study. *J. Neurol. Sci.* **109**, 18–24.

Verleger, R. (1997). On the utility of P3 latency as an index of mental chronometry. *Psychophysiology* **34**, 131–156.

Verleger, R. (2001). Comment on "Electrophysiological correlates of conscious vision: Evidence from unilateral extinction." *J. Cogn. Neurosci.* **13**, 416–417.

Verleger, R., and Berg, P. (1991). The waltzing oddball. *Psychophysiology* **28**, 468–477.

Verleger, R., Neukäter, W., Kömpf, D., and Vieregge, P. (1991). On the reasons for the delay of P3 latency in healthy elderly subjects. *Electroencephalogr. Clin. Neurophysiol.* **79**, 488–502.

Verleger, R., Kömpf, D., and Neukäter, W. (1992). Event-related EEG potentials in mild dementia of the Alzheimer type. *Electroencephalogr. Clin. Neurophysiol.* **84**, 332–343.

Verleger, R., Heide, W., Butt, C., Wascher, E., and Kömpf, D. (1996). On-line brain potential correlates of right parietal patients' attentional deficit. *Electroencephalogr. Clin. Neurophysiol.* **99**, 444–457.

Verleger, R., Lefèbre, C., Wieschemeyer, R., and Kömpf, D. (1997). Event-related potentials suggest slowing of brain processes in generalized epilepsy and alterations of visual processing in patients with partial seizures. *Cogn. Brain Res.* **5**, 205–219.

Verleger, R., Wascher, E., Wauschkuhn, B., Jaskowski, P., Allouni, B., Trillenberg, P., and Wessel, K. (1999). Consequences of altered cerebellar input for the cortical regulation of motor coordination, as reflected in EEG potentials. *Exp. Brain Res.* **127**, 409–422.

Verleger, R., Wauschkuhn, B., Van der Lubbe, R. H. J., Jaskowski, P., and Trillenberg, P. (2000a). Posterior and anterior contributions of hand-movement preparation to Late CNV. *J. Psychophysiol.* **14**, 69–86.

Verleger, R., Vollmer, C., Wauschkuhn, B., Van der Lubbe, R. H. J., and Wascher, E. (2000b). Dimensional overlap between arrows as cueing stimuli and responses? Evidence from contra-ipsilateral differences in EEG potentials. *Cogn. Brain Res.* **10**, 99–109.

Verleger, R., Adam, S., Rose, M., Vollmer, C., Wauschkuhn, B., and Kömpf, D. (2002). Synergy of hemispheres: Timing of ipsilateral activation at movement onset in patients with subcortical ischemic lesions of the pyramidal tract. Submitted for publication.

Vidailhet, M., Stocchi, F., Rothwell, J. C., Thompson, P.D., Day, B.L., Brooks, D. J., and Marsden, C. D. (1993). The Bereitschaftspotential preceding simple foot movement and initiation of gait in Parkinson's disease. *Neurology* **43**, 1784–1788.

Vieregge, P., Verleger, R., Wascher, E., Stüven, F., and Kömpf, D. (1994). Selective attention is impaired in Parkinson's disease—Event-related evidence from EEG potentials. *Cogn. Brain Res.* **2**, 117–130.

Vieregge, P., Wauschkuhn, B., Heberlein, I., Hagenah, J., and Verleger, R. (1999). Selective attention is impaired in amyotrophic lateral sclerosis — A study of event-related EEG potentials. *Cogn. Brain Res.* **8**, 27–35.

Viggiano, M. P., Spinelli, D., and Mecacci, L. (1995). Phase reversal visual evoked potentials in patients with visual neglect. *Brain Cogn.* **27**, 17–35.

Vogel, E. K., and Luck, S. J. (2000). The visual N1 component as an index of a discrimination process. *Psychophysiology* **37**, 190–203.

Vuilleumier, P., Sagiv, N., Hazeltine, E., Poldrack, R. A., Swick, D., Rafal, R. D., and Gabrieli, J. D. E. (2001). Neural fate of seen and unseen faces in visuospatial neglect: a combined event-related functional MRI and event-related potential study. *Proc. Natl. Acad. Sci. U.S.A.* **98**, 3495–3500.

Wang, L., Kuroiwa, Y., Kamitani, T., Li, M., Takahashi, T., Suzuki, Y., Shimamura, M., and Hasegawa, O. (2000). Visual event-related potentials in progressive supranuclear palsy, corticobasal degeneration, striatonigral degeneration, and Parkinson's disease. *J. Neurol.* **247**, 356–363.

Wascher, E., and Wauschkuhn, B. (1996). The interaction of stimulus- and response-related processes measured by event-related lateralisations of the EEG. *Electroencephalogr. Clin. Neurophysiol.* **99**, 149–162.

Wascher, E., Verleger, R., Vieregge, P., Jaskowski, P., Koch, S., and Kömpf, D. (1997). Responses to cued signals in Parkinson's disease: Distinguishing between disorders of cognition and of activation. *Brain* **120**, 1355–1375.

Wascher, E., Reinhard, M., Wauschkuhn, B., and Verleger, R. (1999). Spatial S-R compatibility with centrally presented stimuli: An event-related asymmetry study about dimensional overlap. *J. Cogn. Neurosci.* **11**, 214–229.

Wascher, E., Schatz, U., Kuder, T., and Verleger, R. (2001). Validity and boundary conditions of automatic response activation in the Simon task. *J. Exp. Psychol. Human Percept. Perform.* **27**, 731–751.

Weiller, C., Ramsay, S. C., Wise, R. J. S., Friston, K. J., and Frackowiak, R. S. J. (1993). Individual patterns of functional reorganization in the human cerebral cortex after capsular infarction. *Ann. Neurol.* **33**, 181–189.

Wessel, K., Verleger, R., Nazarenus, D., Vieregge, P., and Kömpf, D. (1994). Movement-related cortical potentials preceding sequential and goal-directed finger and arm movements in patients with cerebellar atrophy. *Electroencephalogr. Clin. Neurophysiol.* **92**, 331–341.

Westphal, K. P., Heinemann, H.A., Grözinger, B., Kotchoubey, B. J., Diekmann, V., Becker, W., and Kornhuber, H. H. (1998). Bereitschaftspotential in amyotrophic lateral sclerosis (ALS): Lower amplitudes in patients with hyperreflexia (spasticity). *Acta Neurol. Scand.* **98**, 15–21.

Wolpaw, J. R., McFarland, D. J., Neat, G. W., and Forneris, C. A. (1991). An EEG-based brain-computer interface for cursor control. *Electroencephalogr. Clin. Neurophysiol.* **78**, 252–259.

Wright, M. J., Geffen, G. M., and Geffen, L. B. (1993). Event-related potentials associated with covert orientation of visual attention in Parkinson's disease. *Neuropsychologia* **31**, 1283–1297.

Yamaguchi, S., Tsuchiya, H., and Kobayashi, S. (1998). Visuospatial attention shift and motor responses in cerebellar disorders. *J. Cogn. Neurosci.* **10**, 95–107.

Yamaguchi, S., Tsuchiya, H., Yamagata, S., Toyoda, G., and Kobayashi, S. (2000). Event-related brain potentials in response to novel sounds in dementia. *Clin. Neurophysiol.* **111**, 195–203.

Yazawa, S., Ikeda, A., Kunieda, T., Ohara, S., Mima, T., Nagamine, T., Taki, W., Kimura, J., Hori, T., and Shibasaki, H. (2000). Human pre-supplementary motor area is active before voluntary movement, subdural recording of Bereitschaftspotential from medial frontal cortex. *Exp. Brain Res.* **131**, 165–177.

14

Mismatch Negativity: A Probe to Auditory Perception and Cognition in Basic and Clinical Research

Risto Näätänen, Elvira Brattico, and Mari Tervaniemi

THE MMN: AN AUTOMATIC CHANGE-DETECTION RESPONSE IN AUDITION

The mismatch negativity (MMN) (Näätänen *et al.*, 1978) currently provides the only valid objective measure of the accuracy of central auditory processing in the human brain. The MMN is an electric brain response, a negative component of the event-related potential (ERP), usually peaking at 100–200 msec from change onset, to any discriminable change ("deviant") in some repetitive aspect of auditory stimulation ("standard"). Thus, an MMN is elicited when, for example, a tone changes in frequency, duration, or intensity, or a phoneme is replaced by another phoneme (Fig. 1). Importantly, the MMN can be elicited even in the absence of attention, which is of central importance in view of the possible clinical applications.

The MMN depends on the presence of a memory trace formed by the preceding stimuli; that is, the MMN cannot be attributed to "new" or "fresh" afferent elements activated by the deviant but not by the standard stimulus. Tervaniemi *et al.* (1994) found an MMN to an occasional omission

of the second tone of a tone pair (with very short intrapair intervals). MMN data consequently suggest that the first standards in the beginning of a stimulus block develop a memory trace, accurately representing each stimulus feature (including even the temporal aspects of stimulation), and, further, that if a deviant stimulus occurs while this memory trace is still active, then the automatic change-detection reaction generating an MMN occurs.

The duration of these traces (as estimated by the interstimulus interval, with which no MMN can any longer be elicited) is of the order of 10 sec (Sams *et al.*, 1993; Böttscher-Gandor and Ullsperger, 1992). This is in an agreement with the estimated duration of the long store of auditory sensory memory (Cowan, 1984). In addition, several other studies, such as those on backward masking (Winkler and Näätänen, 1992), suggest that the memory traces of the short store of auditory sensory memory (Cowan, 1984) can be probed with the MMN (see below).

The MMN has two main generator mechanisms: bilateral auditory cortex generators and a frontal cortex generator [which may also be bilateral, but such that the right hemispheric generator is consid-

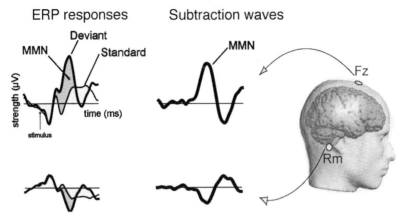

FIGURE 1 Schematic illustration of the mismatch negativity (MMN), showing the event-related potential (ERP) waveforms for the standard and deviant stimuli. On the right, difference waves are obtained by subtracting the standard stimulus response from that to the deviant stimulus response recorded at the electrode sites where the MMN is maximal.

erably stronger than the left hemispheric one (Giard *et al.*, 1990; Paavilainen *et al.*, 1991; Alho, 1995)]. The activation of the frontal generator has been associated with involuntary attention switch to sound change preperceptually detected in the auditory cortices (Giard *et al.*, 1990). Consistent with this, the frontal activation is slightly delayed in time of onset relative to the auditory cortex activation (Rinne *et al.*, 2000), supporting the assumption that the change-detection signal generated by the auditory cortex triggers the frontal mechanisms leading to attention switch to sound change (Näätänen, 1990).

Convincing behavioral evidence for the occurrence of an involuntary attention switch shortly following MMN elicitation was provided by Schröger (1996; see also Alho *et al.*, 1997). He showed that the reaction time (RT) was prolonged and the hit rate (HR) decreased in the primary task as a consequence of the occurrence of even a minor frequency change in irrelevant auditory stimulation eliciting an MMN just before the imperative stimulus (see Figs. 1 and 2).

LINGUISTIC FUNCTIONS AS REVEALED BY THE MMN

Studies have shown that in addition to short-duration traces developed in the beginning of a stimulus block, the MMN can also be used to probe long-term auditory memory traces, most typically those representing the phonemes of one's mother tongue. Näätänen *et al.* (1997) found that the Estonian vowel /õ/ elicited a much larger MMN in Estonian than in Finnish subjects when this vowel was used as a deviant stimulus (the standard stimulus being /e/, which is shared by the two languages), whereas the MMN of the two subject groups was very similar for the deviants shared by the two languages (/ö/, /o/). Subsequent magneto-encephalographic measurements in the Finnish subjects showed that the mother-tongue-related MMN (MMNm) enhancement originated from the left auditory cortex, which thus appeared to be the locus of the language-specific vowel traces of the

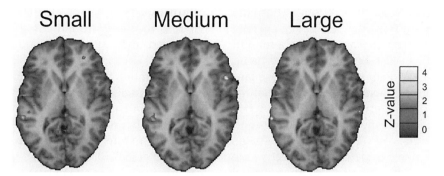

FIGURE 2 Grand-averaged ($n = 13$) functional magnetic resonance imaging activation elicited by a small (10%), medium (30%), and large (100%) increase in frequency deviation superimposed on an individual structural MRI in Talairach space. Images were thresholded at $P < 0.01$. All deviants induced significant activation in the superior temporal gyri bilaterally, whereas the opercular part of the right inferior frontal gyrus was significantly activated only when the large and medium deviants were presented. (See color plates.) Adapted from Opitz *et al.* (2002).

mother tongue (see Fig. 3). More specifically, these traces seem to be located in Wernicke's area in the posterior temporal cortex (Rinne *et al.*, 1999).

As indexed by the MMN, these language-specific memory traces for the mother tongue emerge during the first year of life (Dehaene-Lambertz and Baillet,

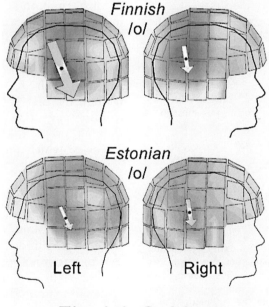

FIGURE 3 Language-specific phoneme traces localized in the left temporal lobe reflected by the MMN. Magnetic field-gradient maps of the left- and right-hemisphere MMNs of one typical Finnish subject for Finnish and Estonian deviant vowels. The squares indicate the arrangement of the magnetic sensors. The arrows represent the equivalent current dipoles, indicating activity in the auditory cortex. The Finnish vowel prototype elicits a much larger MMNm in the left (compared to the right) hemisphere, whereas the nonprototype responses to an Estonian vowel that does not exist in the Finnish language are small in amplitude in both hemispheres. (See color plates.) Adapted from Näätänen *et al.* (1997).

1998; Cheour *et al.*, 1998a). In addition, the development of the language-specific memory traces when adults learn a foreign language can also be monitored by using the MMN (Winkler *et al.*, 1999). These language-specific memory traces function as recognition patterns sequentially activated by the corresponding phonemes (and larger units) of a spoken language, enabling one to perceive correctly the speech sounds uttered (Näätänen, 2001). Consistent with this, the MMNm dipoles for phoneme changes can be modeled even when these phonemes are uttered by hundreds of speakers so that the acoustic repetition within the standard stimulus category is minimized (Shestakova *et al.*, 2002).

Findings also indicate that MMN recordings can serve as an index of the degree of auditory-processing impairment in acquired language disorders such as in Wernicke's aphasia. Ilvonen *et al.* (2001) found that in aphasic stroke patients, the MMN to duration decrement was deteriorated to right-ear stimulation as long as

approximately 2 years after the stroke, whereas the MMN to left-ear stimulation resembled that of control subjects (see Fig. 4).

Furthermore, the MMN is attenuated in developmental language disorders. In dyslexic adults, the MMN did not differ from that of control subjects when it was elicited by an interval change in a tone pair (Kujala *et al.*, 2000). In contrast, the MMN was attenuated, relative to that of controls, when this tone pair was preceded and succeeded by an extra tone. The behavioral discrimination performance was consistent with the MMN data. A subsequent study indicated that this difficulty of dyslexic subjects in discriminating temporal changes among tone patterns was caused by the masking sound following the sound change rather than by the one preceding it, suggesting their increased vulnerability to backward masking (Kujala *et al.*, 2001a).

Most importantly, the MMN also indexes the improvement of reading performance in dyslexic children receiving audiovisual training (Fig. 5). The subjects studied by Kujala *et al.* (2001b) were reading-impaired 7-year-old pupils who were in the first grade. One-half of these children played an audiovisual PC-based training program (Karma, 1999) during 7 weeks, which improved their reading skills considerably more than that of the dyslexic pupils of the control group. Furthermore, the MMN was correspondingly enhanced in the training group at the end of the training period, being clearly larger in amplitude than that of the control group. Importantly, the magnitude of the reading-skills improvement correlated with the magnitude of the MMN amplitude increase in the training group. It is noteworthy that the PC game used in training the children did not include linguistic information, which suggests that the general deterioration of central auditory processing, rather than that involving speech sounds only, is implemented in developmental dyslexia.

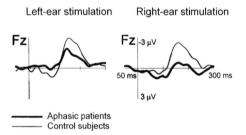

FIGURE 4 Left-hemisphere auditory dysfunction in sound-duration discrimination in Wernicke's aphasic patients. In this study, stimuli were monaurally presented in order to stimulate primarily one hemisphere (contralateral to the stimulation) at a time. Occasional duration decrements in a repetitive sound elicited a similar MMN in control subjects (thin line) when the stimuli were presented to either the left or the right ear. In contrast, in the patients (thick line), these decrements elicited a small MMN when the stimuli were presented to the right ear, and a considerably larger MMN when the stimuli were presented to the left ear. Adapted from Ilvonen *et al.* (2001).

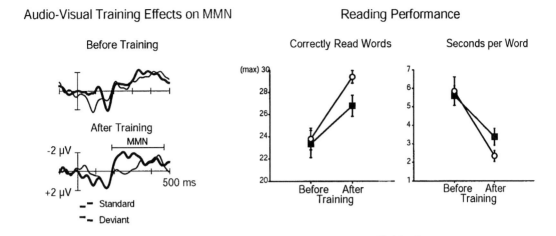

FIGURE 5   Left: MMNs recorded from dyslexic children in response to tone-order reversals. After training, the MMNs were enhanced in the trained group but not in the untrained group. Right: Reading performance [as indexed by the number of correct read words (left) and reading speed (right)]. The reading improvement was considerably greater in the trained group. Adapted from Kujala *et al.* (2001b).

MMN AS AN INDEX OF MUSIC PERCEPTION AND MUSICAL EXPERTISE

Subjects with superior performance in the pitch-discrimination task of the traditional Seashore musicality test showed an enhanced pitch MMN when compared with subjects with less accurate behavioral pitch discrimination (Lang *et al.*, 1990). Tervaniemi *et al.* (1997) studied the neural determinants underlying "cognitive musicality," defined as an ability to structure continuous sound stream into meaningful units (Karma, 1994). To this end, out of the 117 subjects tested, the MMN of 14 subjects with the best test performance ("musical" group) was compared with that recorded from 14 subjects with the poorest test performance ("nonmusical" group). It was found that, although these subjects did not differ from each other in the amount of musical training they had received, the MMN to sound-order change was considerably larger in amplitude in musical than in nonmusical subjects. This suggests that

the preattentive neural circuits as indexed by the MMN determine performance in structuring musical sounds and detecting regularities in it.

Data (Kohlmetz *et al.*, 2001) from hemispheric stroke patients showed that automatic pitch classification is selectively impaired only in those patients with music perception deficits as indexed by a new, specially created test battery. These data confirm, then, the previous results (e.g., Tervaniemi *et al.*, 1997; Koelsch *et al.*, 1999) indicating that music perception is, in part, based on the elementary discrimination processes as indexed by the MMN. The issue of whether the accuracy of automatic pitch-discrimination mechanisms differs between musicians and nonmusicians was also addressed. The subjects' pitch MMN to a tiny pitch change among chord stimuli was compared with their pitch MMN to pure tone pitch changes in both "ignore" and "attend" conditions (Koelsch *et al.*, 1999). The results demonstrated that the musically trained subjects (professional violin players) automatically detected, as indexed by the MMN elicitation, tiny pitch changes that were undetectable for non-musicians and, further, that these discriminative functions were not modified by attentional manipulations. The MMN evoked by a small or large pitch change in pure sinusoidal tones did not differentiate violinists and nonmusicians, however. Thus, the superior pitch-processing accuracy of the violinists was manifested only when the pitch change was presented among musical sounds.

In addition, musicians showed a significant MMN when infrequent omissions were interspersed among tones presented at both a faster stimulus onset asynchrony (SOA) of 100 msec or a slower SOA of 220 msec, whereas nonmusicians' brains produced an MMN only when omissions occurred within the fast-paced tone series (Rüsseler et al., 2001). Whereas the above-described pitch–MMN enhancement in musicians (Koelsch et al., 1999) could be explained merely by the more accurate tuning of frequency-specific afferent neurons in musicians, this explanation does not, of course, apply to the Rüsseler et al. data, for the activation of new afferent neurons cannot explain an MMN when no stimulus was present.

The neural mechanisms behind the musicians' superior ability to detect invariances in continuous auditory information flow was addressed by Tervaniemi et al. (2001). Musicians and nonmusicians were presented with a short melody-like sound pattern transposed to 12 frequency levels in passive (video watching) and discrimination conditions, administered in an alternating order. An MMN was elicited only in those subjects who in the discrimination condition were able to detect more than 80% of the contour-changed melodies. Even in them, the MMN was elicited only after the first discrimination condition, suggesting that conscious attention is a necessary prerequisite for complex perceptual (and preperceptual) learning to occur, as shown by Näätänen et al. (1993b).

Magnetoencephalographic (MEG) data show that the MMNs for sounds differing in their informational content are generated in slightly different parts of the auditory cortex. Alho et al. (1996) compared the frequency-MMN evoked by an identical frequency change occurring in single sinusoidal tones, parallel chords, and serial chords. It was found that the MMN elicited by chords, both parallel and serial, is generated about 1 cm medially to that elicited by single sinusoidal tones. Further, Tervaniemi et al. (1999a) compared the MMNm generator loci for phonemes and chords matched in spectral complexity and in the magnitude of frequency change embedded in them. They found that the MMNm to a frequency change of one tone within a chord (resulting in a change from A major to A minor) was generated superiorly to that generated by a frequency change of the second formant within a phoneme (resulting in a perceptual change from phoneme /e/ to /o/). In addition, in the right hemisphere, the MMNm was larger in amplitude for changes among chords than among phonemes. However, in the left hemisphere, no corresponding dominance for phoneme changes was found when compared with chord changes, which is not consistent with previous results (e.g., Näätänen et al., 1997; Rinne et al., 1999).

The issue of cerebral dominance was further investigated by Tervaniemi et al. (2000a) by using positron emission tomography (PET) and the phonetic and musical sounds developed for the MEG study described above. Subjects classified the gender of visually presented words while they were presented with sound sequences consisting of (1) both deviant and standard sounds or (2) standard sounds only (phonemes and chords in separate sequences). The data showed that the change from vowel /e/ to /o/ was processed in the middle and supratemporal gyri in the left hemisphere. In a mirrorlike manner, the change from A major to A minor chord was processed in the supra-temporal gyrus of the right auditory cortex. These data thus indicate that the hemispheric specialization for phonetic versus musical processing is present even when these stimuli are to be ignored (and a task not involving these stimuli is performed). However, this phenomenon is very vulnerable to noise (see Shtyrov et al., 1998, 1999) and is subdued to the cortico-cortical connections between the neural populations involved [see Kohlmetz et al. (2001) for hemispheric stroke patient data].

In addition, spectrally rich sounds evoked an MMN that was shorter in latency and larger in amplitude than that evoked by pure sinusoidal tones (Tervaniemi et al., 2000b). Complex sounds without the fundamental frequency do not show this advantage, however. The longer latency MMN to missing fundamental sounds rather implicates an increased difficulty in the pitch-extracting process in the presence of this spectral configuration (Winkler et al., 1997). A study by Brattico et al. (2002) addressed the effects of the sound context on pitch discrimination as indexed by the MMN. It was found that the processing of a pitch change embedded in a pattern of familiar sounds (according to the Western musical tradition) is facilitated, as indexed by the MMN amplitude, when compared with the same pitch change when embedded in an unfamiliar (arithmetically determined) sound pattern.

MMN IN CLINICAL RESEARCH

Because of its several advantages, MMN has numerous potential clinical applications. One of these advantages is its attention-independent elicitation. This is very important, in particular in studying clinical groups as well as infants and newborns. Furthermore, in interpreting the test results, it is a major advantage that the effects of attention and motivation are minimal. Data supporting MMN elicitation even in the absence of attention stem from diverse conditions, ranging from selective dichotic listening [where an MMN has been elicited even by minor changes in the unattended-ear input (Näätänen et al., 1993a; Paavilainen et al., 1993)], to certain sleep stages in adults (Campbell et al., 1991; Sallinen et al., 1994) and in newborns and infants (Cheour-Luhtanen et al., 1996, 1997), and to comatose patients [during the last days before the recovery of consciousness (Kane et al., 1993, 1996)]. Though the results of some studies (Woldorff et al., 1991, 1998; Trejo et al., 1995; Alho et al., 1992) suggest that the MMN amplitude is attenuated in the unattended channel under highly focused selective attention, no data suggest that the MMN is totally abolished by the withdrawal of attention. Moreover, the MMN amplitude is generally not affected by attention in normal (one-channel) "oddball" conditions in which the MMN is usually measured for various clinical and other applied purposes (Näätänen et al., 1982; for a review, see Näätänen, 1992).

In fact, the best way to record the MMN is to use passive conditions, with the subject or patient's attention being directed elsewhere, such as to a self-selected (silenced) video or visual computer game (Kathmann et al., 1999). If the sound sequence used for MMN elicitation is attended, then the MMN is overlapped by other ERP components such as the P165 (Goodin et al., 1978) and, most notably, the N2b [described in a visual paradigm by Renault and Lesévre (1978, 1979) and in an auditory paradigm by Näätänen et al. (1982)]. This makes the pure measurement of the MMN component very difficult or impossible. The MMNm is to a much lesser extent than the MMN overlapped by attention-related components (see Kaukoranta et al., 1989; Lounasmaa et al., 1989).

As previously mentioned, MMN can also be measured in comatose patients. An MMN elicited in an unconscious coma patient appears to provide the single most reliable predictor of the recovery of consciousness (Kane *et al.*, 1993, 1996). As for the MMN in sleep, in adults it is quite an evasive though yet well-documented effect (e.g., Campbell *et al.*, 1991; Sallinen *et al.*, 1994); it is much easier to obtain an MMN in sleeping infants and newborns, which is very helpful in evaluating their central auditory function. Consequently, one of the most promising fields of application of the MMN involves newborns and young infants. MMN is elicited even in prematurely born newborns (Cheour-Luhtanen *et al.*, 1996). In fact, the MMN is the earliest cognitive ERP component that can be recorded from the human brain. It appears that with the MMN, one could detect developmental problems in the auditory cortex early enough to treat what would otherwise prevent the normal perception of speech sounds and thus result in delayed speech development. This problem is particularly common in children with cleft palate (Cheour *et al.*, 1998b). Ceponiene *et al.* (2000) indicate that although obligatory cortical ERP components do not differentiate newborns with different types of clefts, the MMN does, even before the age of 6 months.

A multitude of studies have shown that the MMN (recorded in passive conditions) predicts the behavioral discrimination accuracy in various perceptual tasks involving the different sound types and attributes, such as the frequency of simple tones (Tiitinen *et al.*, 1994; Tremblay *et al.*, 1998; Menning *et al.*, 2000) and complex spectrotemporal patterns (Näätänen *et al.*, 1993b). Even the accuracy of speech processing can be probed with the MMN recordings; a good correspondence between MMN parameters and behavioral performance has been demonstrated for vowels of a foreign language (Winkler *et al.*, 1999), for consonant–vowel (CV) syllables of the mother tongue in school children (Kraus *et al.*, 1996), for different within-category variants of a CV syllable

(Kraus *et al.*, 1995), for toneburst and click trains (Ponton and Don, 1995), and for CV syllables after cochlear-implant installation (Kraus *et al.*, 1993a). These data open new perspectives, for example, in teaching and learning foreign languages. For instance, progress in the correct perception of foreign speech sounds can, in principle, be monitored by recording the MMN. As already mentioned, the speech-sound memory traces probed with the MMN probably serve as recognition patterns necessary for the correct perception of unfamiliar foreign speech sounds and their combinations. Furthermore, it is quite likely that the correct pronunciation of foreign speech sounds depends on the accuracy of sensory information encoded in these memory traces (Näätänen, 2001).

The MMN can also be used to measure the duration of echoic memory by varying the interstimulus interval (ISI). Here the idea is that when the decay of the memory trace of the standards has reached a certain stage, then deviants can no longer elicit an MMN. Using this logic, Pekkonen *et al.* (1994) found that Alzheimer patients had a normal MMN when stimuli were presented at a constant ISI of 1 sec but a severely attenuated one when the ISI was prolonged to 3 sec. This data pattern enabled the authors to conclude that it was sensory memory rather than discrimination in audition that was deteriorated in Alzheimer patients. Analogous results were obtained by Cheour and colleagues (1998b) in school-age children with cleft palate.

It is well-established that our sensory percepts in audition are not responses only to what is acoustically present at that moment (corrected with the perceptual latency) but to what is acoustically present during a sliding window of 150–200 msec in duration; this period is called the temporal window of integration (TWI) (see Cowan, 1984; Näätänen, 1990; Yabe *et al.*, 1998). A prime example of the TWI is the loudness summation of very brief sounds, which are heard louder as their duration is increased until about 200 msec (Scharf and Houtsma, 1986). Furthermore, backward masking is effective when the masker onset occurs within a similarly short interval from the start of the test stimulus (Hawkins and Presson, 1986; see also Winkler *et al.*, 1993). Winkler and Näätänen (1992) found that the MMN could be used to determine the duration of the TWI. Placing a masker after each (brief) stimulus of the MMN paradigm, they found that a full-size MMN could be elicited by deviants only when the silent ISI between the MMN-paradigm stimulus and the masker was 150 msec or longer. The recovery of the behavioral discrimination followed a very similar time course.

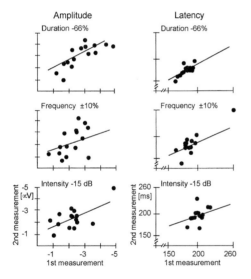

FIGURE 6 Significant test–retest reliabilities of the MMN amplitude and latency for duration, frequency, and intensity increment, or decrement deviants, measured in 15 healthy subjects. The horizontal axis indicates the amplitudes recorded in the first session and the vertical axis indicates values recorded in the second session. The 66% duration decrement elicited an MMN with the most replicable amplitude and latency. Adapted from *Clinical Neurophysiology*, **110**; M. Tervaniemi, A. Lehtokoski, J. Sinkkonen, J. Virtanen, R.J. Ilmoniemi, and R. Näätänen; Test-retest reliability of mismatch negativity for duration, frequency, and intensity changes, pp. 1388–1393. Copyright (1999), with permission of Elsevier Science.

Näätänen (1995) proposed that the TWI determines the time needed for the emergence of the central sound representation underlying sound perception.

One form of auditory pathology might be related to TWI abnormalities, such that auditory input is more vulnerable to backward-masking effects by subsequent stimuli and stimulus elements. For example, the TWI duration might be prolonged, or the backward-masking effects within the TWI might be strengthened. MMN data suggest the presence of TWI-related central auditory-processing pathology in school-aged and adult developmental dyslexics (Kujala *et al.*, 2001a,b; already reviewed above) and in chronic abstinent alcoholics (Ahveninen *et al.*, 1999).

The ERP recording and analyzing facilities are very cheap compared with those of other methodologies and are available almost in any hospital. Furthermore, for many applied purposes, only a few EEG channels are needed. Replicable MMN data can be obtained rather easily, at least when standardized methods, currently under development, become available (see Lang *et al.*, 1995; Schröger, 1998; Sinkkonen and Tervaniemi, 2000). The test–retest replicability of the MMN amplitude reaches a satisfactory level in some stimulation paradigms, especially in the duration-deviance paradigm (see Fig. 6) (Escera and Grau, 1996; Kathmann *et al.*, 1999; Tervaniemi *et al.*, 1999b, 2002). Moreover, stable MMNs have been obtained in the tone-pair paradigm (Kallio *et al.*, 2002), a result that is encouraging especially with regard to the assessment of the neurophysiological determinants of reading problems in dyslexic subjects (cf. Kujala *et al.*, 2000, 2001a,b). In addition, attempts have already been made to use the MMN as a tool for the assessment of the auditory and cognitive functions at the individual level (Kraus *et al.*, 1993b; Hämäläinen *et al.*, 2002; for methodological issues, see Ponton *et al.*, 1997; McGee *et al.*, 1997).

References

Ahveninen, J., Jääskeläinen, I. P., Pekkonen, E., Hallberg, A., Hietanen, M., Mäkelä, R., Näätänen, R., and Sillanaukee, P. (1999). Brain responses predict rapid forgetting in alcohol abusers. *Alcohol. Clin. Exp. Res.* **23**, 1507–1515.

Alho, K., Woods, D. L., Algazi, A., and Näätänen, R. (1992). Intermodal selective attention II: Effects of attentional load on processing auditory and visual stimuli in central space. *Electroencephalogr. Clin. Neurophysiol.* **82**, 356–368.

Alho, K., Tervaniemi, M., Huotilainen, M., Lavikainen, J., Tiitinen, H., Ilmoniemi, R. J., Knuutila, J., and Näätänen, R. (1996). Processing of complex sounds in the human auditory cortex as revealed by magnetic brain responses. *Psychophysiology* **33**, 369–375.

Alho, K., Escera, C., Diaz, R., Yago, E., and Serra J. M. (1997). Effects of involuntary auditory attention on visual task performance and brain activity. *NeuroReport* **8**, 3233–3237.

Alho, K. (1995). Cerebral generators of mismatch negativity (MMN) and its magnetic counterpart (MMNm) elicited by sound changes. *Ear Hear.* **16**, 38–51.

Böttscher-Gandor, C., and Ullsperger, P. (1992). Mismatch negativity in event-related potentials to auditory stimuli as a function of varying interstimulus interval. *Psychophysiology* **29**, 546–550.

Brattico, E., Tervaniemi, M., and Näätänen, R. (2002). Context effects on pitch discrimination: Evidence from ERP recordings. *Music Percept.* **19**, 1–24.

Campbell, K., Bell, I., and Bastien, C. (1991). Evoked potential measures of information processing during natural sleep. *In* "Sleep, Arousal and Performance" (R. Broughton and R. Ogilvie, eds.), pp. 88–116. Birkhauser, Boston and Cambridge, Massachusetts.

Ceponiene, R., Hukki, J., Cheour, M., Haapanen, M.-L., Koskinen, M., Alho, K., and Näätänen, R. (2000). Development of the auditory cortex persists in infants with certain cleft types. *Dev. Med. Child Neurol.* **42**, 258–265.

Cheour, M., Ceponiene, R., Lehtokoski, A., Luuk, A., Allik, J., Alho, K., and Näätänen, R. (1998a). Development of language-specific phoneme representations in the infant brain. *Nat. Neurosci.* **1**, 351–353.

Cheour, M., Haapanen, M.-L., Ceponiene, R., Hukki, J., Ranta, R., and Näätänen, R. (1998b). Mismatch negativity (MMN) as an index of auditory sensory memory deficit in cleft-palate and catch-syndrome children. *NeuroReport* **9**, 2709–2712.

Cheour-Luhtanen, M., Alho, K., Sainio, K., Rinne, T., Reinikainen, K., Pohjavuori, M., Aaltonen, O., Eerola, O., and Näätänen, R. (1996). The ontogenetically earliest discriminative response of the human brain. *Psychophysiology* **33**, 478–481.

Cheour-Luhtanen, M., Alho, K., Sainio, K., Reinikainen, K., Renlund, M., Aaltonen, O., Eerola, O., and Näätänen, R. (1997). The mismatch negativity to changes in speech sounds at the age of three months. *Dev. Neuropsychol.* **13**, 167–174.

Cowan, N. (1984). On short and long auditory stores. *Psychol. Bull.* **96**, 341–370.

Dehaene-Lambertz, G., and Baillet, S. (1998). A phonological representation in the infant brain. *NeuroReport* **9**, 1885–1888.

Escera, C., and Grau, C. (1996). Short-term replicability of the mismatch negativity. *Electroencephalogr. Clin. Neurophysiol.* **100**, 1–6.

Giard, M.-H., Perrin, F., Pernier, J., and Bouchet, P. (1990). Brain generators implicated in processing of auditory stimulus deviance: A topographic event-related potential study. *Psychophysiology* **27**, 627–640.

Goodin, D. S., Squires, K. C., Henderson, B. H., and Starr, A. (1978). An early event-related cortical potential. *Psychophysiology* **15**, 360–365.

Hämäläinen, H., Kujala, T., Kekoni, J., Hurskainen, H., Pirilä, J., Wikström, H., and Huotilainen, M. (2002). Effects of unilateral hippocampus-amygdala resection on arousal, orienting and sensory memory: A case study with EEG and MEG. Submitted.

Hawkins, H. L., and Presson, J. C. (1986). Auditory information processing. *In* "Handbook of Perception and Human Performance" (K. R. Boff, L. Kaufman, and J. P. Thomas, eds.), pp. 26.1–26.64. Wiley, New York.

Ilvonen, T. M., Kujala, T., Tervaniemi, M., Salonen, O., Näätänen, R., and Pekkonen, E. (2001). The processing of sound duration after left hemisphere stroke: Event-related potential and behavioral evidence. *Psychophysiology* **38**, 622–628.

Kallio, J., Kujala, T., Tervaniemi, M., and Näätänen, R. (2002). The test–retest replicability of the MMN in paired-tone paradigm. In preparation.

Kane, N. M., Curry, S. H., Butler, S. R., and Gummins, B. H. (1993). Electrophysiological indicator of awakening from coma. *Lancet* **341**, 688.

Kane, N. M., Curry, S. H., Rowlands, C. A., Manara, A. R., Lewis, T., Moss, T., Cummings, B. H., and Butler, S. R. (1996). Event-related potentials-neurophysiological tools for predicting emergence and early outcome from traumatic coma. *Intensive Care Med.* **22**, 39–46.

Karma, K. (1994), Auditory and visual temporal structuring: How important is sound to musical thinking? *Psychol. Music* **22**, 20–30.

Karma, K. (1999). Auditory structuring in explaining dyslexia. *In* "Proceedings of the Eight International

Workshop on the Cognitive Science of Natural Language Processing (CSNLP-8), August 9–11, 1999" (P. Mc Kevitt, C. Mulvihill, S. Ó. Nualláin, and C. O'Riordan, eds). Information Technology Centre, National University of Ireland, Galway, Ireland.

Kathmann, N., Frodl-Bauch, T., and Hegerl, U. (1999). Stability of the mismatch negativity under different stimulus and attention condition. *Clin. Neurophysiol.* **110**, 317–323.

Kaukoranta, E., Sams, M., Hari, R., Hämäläinen, M., and Näätänen, R. (1989). Reactions of human auditory cortex to changes in tone duration. *Hear. Res.* **41**, 15–22.

Koelsch, S., Schröger, E., and Tervaniemi, M. (1999). Superior attentive and preattentive auditory processing in musicians. *NeuroReport* **10**, 1309–1313.

Kohlmetz, C., Altenmueller, E., Schuppert, M., Wieringa, B. M., Muente, T. F. (2001). Deficit in automatic sound-change detection may underlie some music perception deficits after acute hemispheric stroke. *Neuropsychologia* **39**, 1121–1124.

Kraus, N., Micco, A. G., Koch, D. B., Mcgee, T., Carrell, T., Sharma, A., Wiet, R. J., and Weingarten, C. Z. (1993a), The mismatch negativity cortical evoked potential elicited by speech in cochlear-implant users. *Hear. Res.* **65**, 118–124.

Kraus, N., McGee, T., Ferre, J., Hoeppner, J.-A., Carrel, T., Sharma, A., Nicol, T. (1993b). Mismatch negativity in the neurophysiologic/behavioral evaluation of auditory processing deficits: A case study. *Ear Hear.* **14**, 223–234.

Kraus, N., McGee, T., Carrell, T., King, C., Tremblay, K., and Nicol, T. (1995). Central auditory system plasticity associated with speech discrimination training. *J. Cogn. Sci.* **7**, 27–34.

Kraus, N., Mcgee, T., Carrell, T. D., Zecker, S. G., Nicol, T. G., and Koch, D. B. (1996). Auditory neurophysiologic responses and discrimination deficits in children with learning problems. *Science* **273**, 971–973.

Kujala, T., Myllyviita, K., Tervaniemi, M., Alho, K., Kallio, J., and Näätänen, R. (2000). Basic auditory dysfunction in dyslexia as pinpointed by brain-activity measurements. *Psychophysiology* **37**, 262–266.

Kujala, T., Kallio, J., Tervaniemi, M., and Naatanen, R. (2001a). The mismatch negativity as an index of temporal processing in audition. *Clin. Neurophysiol.* **112**, 1712–1719.

Kujala, T., Karma, K., Ceponiene, R., Belitz, S., Turkkila, P., Tervaniemi, M., and Näätänen, R. (2001b). Plastic neural changes and reading improvement caused by audiovisual training in reading-impaired children. *Proc. Natl. Acad. Sci. U.S.A.* **98**, 10509–10514.

Lang, H., Nyrke, T., Ek, M., Aaltonen, O., Raimo, I., and Näätänen, R. (1990). Pitch discrimination performance and auditory event-related potentials. *In* "Psychophysiological Brain Research" (C. H. M.

Brunia, A. W. K. Gaillard, A. Kok, G. Mulder, and M. N. Verbaten, eds.), Vol. 1, pp. 294–298. Tilburg University Press, Tilburg, The Netherlands.

Lang, H., Eerola, O., Korpilahti, P., Holopainen, I., Salo, S., and Aaltonen, O. (1995). Practical issues in the clinical application of mismatch negativity. *Ear Hear.* **16**, 118–130.

Lounasmaa, O. V., Hari, R., Joutsiniemi, S.-L., and Hämäläinen, M. (1989). Multi-SQUID recordings of human cerebral magnetic fields may give information about memory processes. *Europhys. Lett.* **9**, 603–608.

McGee, T., Kraus, N., and Nicol, T. (1997). Is it really a mismatch negativity? An assessment of methods for determining response validity in individual subjects. *Electroencephalogr. Clin. Neurophysiol.* **104**, 359–368.

Menning, H., Roberts, L. E., and Pantev, C. (2000). Plastic changes in the auditory cortex induced by intensive frequency discrimination training. *NeuroReport* **11**, 817–822.

Näätänen, R. (1990). The role of attention in auditory information processing as revealed by event-related potentials and other brain measures of cognitive function. *Behav. Brain Sci.* **13**, 201–288.

Näätänen, R. (1992). "Attention and Brain Function". Lawrence Erlbaum Assoc., Hillsdale, New Jersey.

Näätänen, R. (1995). The mismatch negativity—A powerful tool for cognitive neuroscience. *Ear Hear.* **16**, 6–18.

Näätänen, R. (2001). The perception of speech sounds by the human brain as reflected by the mismatch negativity (MMN) and its magnetic equivalent (MMNm). *Psychophysiology* **38**, 1–21.

Näätänen, R., Gaillard, A. W. K., and Mäntysalo, S. (1978). Early selective-attention effect reinterpreted. *Acta Psychol.* **42**, 313–329.

Näätänen, R., Simpson, M., and Loveless, N. E. (1982). Stimulus deviance and evoked potentials. *Biol. Psychol.* **14**, 53–98.

Näätänen, R., Paavilainen, P., Tiitinen, H., Jiang, D., and Alho, K. (1993a). Attention and mismatch negativity. *Psychophysiology* **30**, 436–450.

Näätänen, R., Schröger, E., Karakas, S., Tervaniemi, M., and Paavilainen, P. (1993b). Development of a memory trace for a complex sound in the human brain. *NeuroReport* **4**, 503–506.

Näätänen, R., Lehtokoski, A., Lennes, M., Cheour, M., Huotilainen, M., Iivonen, A., Vainio, M., Alku, P., Ilmoniemi, R. J., Luuk, A., Allik, J., Sinkkonen, J., and Alho, K. (1997). Language-specific phoneme representations revealed by electric and magnetic brain responses. *Nature* **385**, 432–434.

Opitz, B., Rinne, T., Mecklinger, A., von Cramon, D. Y., and Schröger, E. (2002). Differential contribution of frontal and temporal cortices to auditory change detection: fMRI and ERP results. *NeuroImage* **15**, 167–174.

Paavilainen, P., Alho, K., Reinikainen, K., Sams, M., and Näätänen, R. (1991). Right-hemisphere dominance of different mismatch negativities. *Electroencephalogr. Clin. Neurophysiol.* **78**, 466–479.

Paavilainen, P., Tiitinen, H., Alho, K., and Näätänen, R. (1993). Mismatch negativity to slight pitch changes outside strong attentional focus. *Biol. Psychol.* **37**, 23–41.

Pekkonen, E., Jousimäki, V., Könönen, M., Reinikainen, K., and Partanen, J. (1994). Auditory sensory memory impairment in Alzheimer's disease: An event-related potential study. *NeuroReport* **5**, 2537–2540.

Ponton, C. W., and Don, M. (1995). The mismatch negativity in cochlear implant users. *Ear Hear.* **16**, 131–146.

Ponton, C. W., Don, M., Eggermont, J. J., and Kwong, B. (1997). Integrated mismatch negativity (MMN_I): A noise-free representation of evoked responses allowing single-point distribution-free statistical tests. *Electroencephalogr. Clin. Neurophysiol.* **104**, 143–150.

Renault, B., and Lesévre, N. (1978). Topographical study of the emitted potential obtained after the omission of an expected visual stimulus. *In* "Multidisciplinary Perspectives in Event-Related Brain Potential Research" (D. Otto, ed.), EPA 600/9-77–043I, pp. 202–208. U.S. Government Printing Office, Washington, D.C.

Renault, B., and Lesévre, N. (1979). A trial-by-trial study of the visual omission response in reaction time situations. *In* "Human Evoked Potentials" (D. Lehmann and E. Callaway, eds.), pp. 317–329. Plenum Press, New York.

Rinne, T., Alho, K., Alku, P., Holi, M., Sinkkonen, J., Virtanen, J., Bertrand, O., and Näätänen, R. (1999). Analysis of speech sounds is left-hemisphere predominant at 100–150 ms after sound onset. *NeuroReport* **10**, 1113–1117.

Rinne, T., Ilmoniemi, R. J., Sinkkonen, J., Virtanen, J., and Näätänen, R. (2000). Separate time behaviors of the temporal and frontal MMN sources. *NeuroImage* **12**, 14–19.

Rüsseler, J., Altenmueller, E., Nager, W., Kohlmetz, C., and Muente, T. F. (2001). Event-related potentials to sound omission differ in musicians and non-musicians. *Neurosci. Lett.* **308**, 33–36.

Sallinen, M., Kaartinen, J., and Lyytinen, H. (1994). Is the appearance of mismatch negativity during stage 2 sleep related to the elicitation of K-complex?. *Electroencephalogr. Clin. Neurophysiol.* **91**, 140–148.

Sams, M., Hari, R., Rif, J., and Knuutila, J. (1993). The human auditory sensory memory trace persists about 10 msec: Neuromagnetic evidence. *J. Cogn. Neurosci.* **5**, 363–370.

Scharf, B. D., and Houtsma, A. J. (1986). Audition II: Loudness, pitch, localization, aural distortion, pathology. *In* Handbook of Perception and Human

Performance (K. R. Boff, L. Kaufman, and J. P. Thomas, eds.), pp. 15.1–15.60. Wiley, New York.

Schröger, E. (1996). A neural mechanism for involuntary attention shifts to changes in auditory stimulation. *J. Cogn. Neurosci.* **8**, 527–539.

Schröger, E. (1998). Measurement and interpretation of the mismatch negativity. *Behav. Res. Methods Instrum. Comput.* **30**, 131–145.

Shestakova, A., Brattico, E., Huotilainen, M., Galunov, V., Soloviev, A., Sams, M., Ilmonienni, R. I., and Näätänen, R. (2002). Abstract phoneme representations in the left auditory cortex: Magnetic mismatch negativity study. *NeuroReport* (In press.)

Shtyrov, Y., Kujala, T., Ahveninen, J., Tervaniemi, M., Alku, P., Ilmoniemi, R. J., and Näätänen, R. (1998). Background acoustic noise and the hemispheric lateralization of speech processing in the human brain: Magnetic mismatch negativity study. *Neurosci. Lett.* **251**, 141–144.

Shtyrov, Y., Kujala, T., Ilmoniemi, R. J., and Näätänen, R. (1999). Noise affects speech-signal processing differently in the cerebral hemispheres. *NeuroReport* **10**, 2189–2192.

Sinkkonen, J., and Tervaniemi, M. (2000). Towards optimal recording and analysis of the mismatch negativity. *Audiol. Neuro-Otol.* **5**, 235–246.

Tervaniemi, M., Saarinen, J., Paavilainen, P., Danilova, N., and Näätänen R. (1994). Temporal integration of auditory information in sensory memory as reflected by the mismatch negativity. *Biol. Psychol.* **38**, 157–167.

Tervaniemi, M., Ilvonen, T., Karma, K., Alho, K., and Näätänen, R. (1997). The musical brain: Brain waves reveal the neurophysiological basis of musicality in human subjects. *Neurosci. Lett.* **226**, 1–4.

Tervaniemi, M., Kujala, A., Alho, K., Virtanen, J., Ilmoniemi, R. J., and Näätänen, R. (1999a). Functional specialization of the human auditory cortex in processing phonetic and musical sounds: A magnetoencephalographic (MEG) study. *NeuroImage* **9**, 330–336.

Tervaniemi, M., Lehtokoski, A., Sinkkonen, J., Virtanen, J., Ilmoniemi, R. J., and Näätänen, R. (1999b). Test-retest reliability of mismatch negativity for duration, frequency, and intensity changes. *Clin. Neurophysiol.* **110**, 1388–1393.

Tervaniemi, M., Medvedev, S. V., Alho, K., Pakhomov, S. V., Roudas, M. S., van Zuijen, T. L., and Näätänen, R. (2000a). Lateralized automatic auditory processing of phonetic versus musical information: A PET study. *Hum. Brain Mapping* **10**, 74–79.

Tervaniemi, M., Schröger, E., Saher, M., and Näätänen, R. (2000b). Effects of spectral complexity and sound duration in complex-sound pitch processing in humans—A mismatch negativity study. *Neurosci. Lett.* **290**, 66–70.

Tervaniemi, M., Rytkönen, M., Schröger, E., Ilmoniemi, R. J., and Näätänen, R. (2001). Superior formation of cortical memory traces for melodic patterns in musicians. *Learn. Mem.* **8**, 295–300.

Tervaniemi, M., Kallio, J., Sinkkonen, J., Virtanen, J., Ilmoniemi, R. J., Salonen, O., and Näätänen, R. (2002). Test-retest stability of the magnetic mismatch response (MMNm). Submitted.

Tiitinen, H., May, P., Reinikainen, K., and Näätänen, R. (1994). Attentive novelty detection in humans is governed by pre-attentive sensory memory. *Nature* **372**, 90–92.

Trejo, L. J., Ryan Jones, D. L., and Kramer, A. F. (1995). Attentional modulation of the mismatch negativity elicited by frequency differences between binaurally presented tone bursts. *Psychophysiology* **32**, 319–328.

Tremblay, K., Kraus, N., and McGee, T. (1998). The time course of auditory perceptual learning: Neurophysiological changes during speech-sound training. *NeuroReport* **9**, 3557–3560.

Winkler, I., and Näätänen, R. (1992). Event-related potentials in auditory backward recognition masking: A new way to study the neurophysiological basis of sensory memory in humans. *Neurosci. Lett.* **140**, 239–242.

Winkler, I., Reinikainen, K., and Näätänen, R. (1993). Event-related brain potentials reflect echoic memory in humans. *Percept. Psychophys.* **53**, 443–449.

Winkler, I., Tervaniemi, M., and Näätänen, R. (1997). Two separate codes for missing-fundamental pitch in the human auditory cortex. *J. Acoustic. Soc. Am.* **102**, 1072–1082.

Winkler, I., Kujala, T., Tiitinen, H., Sivonen, P., Alku, P., Lehtokoski, A., Czigler, I., Csépe, V., Ilmoniemi, R. J., and Näätänen, R. (1999). Brain responses reveal the learning of foreign language phonemes. *Psychophysiology* **36**, 638–642.

Woldorff, M. G., Hackley, S. A., and Hillyard, S. A. (1991). The effects of channel-selective attention on the mismatch negativity wave elicited by deviant tones. *Psychophysiology* **28**, 30–42.

Woldorff, M. G., Hillyard, S. A., Gallen, C. C., Hampson, S. T., and Bloom, F. E. (1998). Magnetoencephalographic recordings demonstrate attentional modulation of mismatch-related neural activity in human auditory cortex. *Psychophysiology* **35**, 283–292.

Yabe, H., Tervaniemi, M., Sinkkonen, J., Huotilainen, M., Ilmoniemi, R. J., and Näätänen, R. (1998). The temporal window of integration of auditory information in the human brain. *Psychophysiology* **35**, 615–619.

A PRIMER OF BRAIN RESEARCH TECHNIQUES AND CLINICAL SYNDROMES

Recording and Neurochemical Methods: From Molecules to Systems

Gabriele Biella, Alice Mado Proverbio, and Alberto Zani

INTRODUCTION

Most of the present volume is devoted to the analysis of relationships between mind and brain as investigated by means of scalp electrophysiological recordings, in the context of a cognitive approach. The methods and theories of cognitive electrophysiology are dealt with as large systems from the viewpoint of the brain.

To enhance comprehension of the background of neurophysiological findings, we present here basic descriptions of neuroanatomical, electrophysiological, and neurochemical techniques for investigating brain functions.

STEREOTAXIC NEUROSURGERY

Stereotaxic neurosurgery (SN) is an invasive surgical procedure that is performed on patients after a specific central nervous system region of concern has been identified. Identification of the exact area is accomplished using brain imaging methods such as magnetic resonance (MR) or computerized axial tomography (CAT), applying geometric (or stereotactic) coordinates referring to points conventionally denoted as zero points. In its classic version, SN is performed following straight-line surgical invasion trajectories that proceed from the point of access on the brain surface toward the target area. Images of the path or segment joining the point of entry to target point display a number of inclinations based on spatial ordering (or taxis) in the three spatial directions (stereology) of the final point, with reference to the surgical penetration points. Positional identification of the region is accomplished by spatial superimposition of the region using standard regions (SRs). SR position and size are based on weighted averages and supplementary measurements made using different subjects to make virtual maps, which have been published in stereotaxic atlases. The various atlases available (e.g., Schaltenbrand and Wahren, 1977; Talairach and Tournoux, 1988; Ono *et al.*, 1990) satisfy different surgical or analytical needs. Talairach and Tournoux's atlas is the reference system used in experimental research. It makes a distinction between direct and indirect localization. Direct localization refers to radiographically detectable tissue or cavity structures. Indirect localization is carried out using the method introduced by Talairach in the "reference system" based on a geometric grid made up of virtual lines projected on the anterior and posterior commissures (AC and PC) and the corresponding vertical lines (VAC and VPC) to be adjusted to suit the specific case. Stereotaxy is thus the result of a positional computation carried out in the space of the target zone relative to the reference points. In neurosurgery, the stereotactic procedure is used in a large number of cases: brain biopsies, destruction of microlesions, insertion of electrical stimulators, and interoperative guidance in the case of radiotherapy resection and targeting. In the more modern versions, which are still comparatively rare, magnetic stereotaxic systems (MSSs) are used. Using this technique it is possible to position catheters, electrodes, or small microresection instruments made of flexible materials that can follow curved trajectories. This affords fundamental advantages such as greater precision in tissue targeting and the possibility of avoiding passing through areas of particular functional interest. For this type of SN interoperative data from real-time fluoroscopic imaging are used in combination with preoperative MR images. The operation takes place under magnetic guidance, with a continuous computerized comparison made between the actual trajectory and the programmed one, and the consequent possibility of correcting the trajectory in the case of any undesirable deviation. The force pushing the magnet through the brain is provided by rapidly changing magnetic fields induced in the brain by superconductors connected to the machine.

Stereotaxic neurosurgery cannot be distinguished from the set of procedures known as functional neurosurgery (FN), which, to be performed properly, require the application of stereotaxic neurosurgery. The term *functional neurosurgery* embraces all procedures that tend to modify pathological conditions of functioning by means of electrical or neurochemical stimulation or the destruction of brain regions of varying size. Examples of FN with SN are pallidotomy, thalamotomy, deep brain stimulation, or cell transplants in brain structures. (Pallidotomy

consists of the surgical removal of the innermost part of the globus pallidus in order to reduce diskinetic disorders related to Parkinson's disease, whereas thalamotomy implies the general destruction of the intermediate ventral nucleus by thermocoagulation in order to reduce tremors.) The functional technique involves the application of cortical electrode matrixes left *in situ* for 1–2 days on average in order to determine the extent of epileptic firing, and that of the less active areas, thus reducing the likelihood of functional damage due to surgical aggression.

NEUROSURGICAL METHODS

In addition to the classical procedures of removal by cutting or aspiration of brain matter, it is also possible to use invasive procedures such as thermocoagulation and cryocoagulation, and, above all, noninvasive procedures such as gamma-knife and X-knife.

Invasive Procedures

Thermocoagulation

Used primarily all to block expansive processes by means of high-frequency electric currents, the thermocoagulation electrode is inserted until it reaches the zone to be coagulated, guided by stereotactic techniques. The size of the expansive process determines the intensity of the thermocoagulation current used. The thalamus and the Gasser (trigeminal) ganglion are elective sites for inducing thermocoagulation. Typical thermocoagulation operations are percutaneous rhizolysis or microvascular decompression.

Cryocoagulation

Cryocoagulation, using stereotactic techniques similar to those used in thermocoagulation, causes degeneration of the brain tissue by freezing.

Noninvasive Neurosurgical Techniques

Stereotaxic Neuroradiosurgery

In stereotaxic neuroradiosurgery, stereotaxic neurosurgical techniques are combined with multiple collimated (convergent) rays in the treatment of numerous kinds of brain pathologies. Collimating (arranging in parallel beams) or focusing many single radiation beams on the target point allows high doses of radiation to be brought to bear without particularly large loads along the trajectories of single rays.

The different methods available for potential use are linear accelerator irradiation or X-knife, gamma-knife, and charged-particle irradiation. Linear accelerator (LINAC) irradiation entails using of a large number of rays produced by a particle accelerator and emitted along stereotactic arcs. The gamma-knife uses 201 fixed cobalt-60 gamma ray sources distributed over a hemispherical helmet collimator. The sources emit gamma rays that are then focused on the target.

Charged-particle irradiation uses three to five rays in a configuration similar to that employed in classic radiotherapy, but also exploiting the deep-penetration characteristics of charged particles in order to obtain a highly localized dose distribution. A further innovation is represented by using frameless stereotactic methods for positioning instead of metal frame stereotaxy and involves the use of optical positioning methods based on emission diodes or lasers.

NEURONAL RECORDINGS

Multiunit Activities and Local Field Potentials

Extracellular recordings may be performed using electrodes made of different materials (e.g., tungsten, or platinum–iridium alloys) and a recording tip of variable diameter. When the tip of the probe exceeds a given diameter (e.g., >50 µm) numerous multiunit activities (MUAs) or local field potentials (LFPs) begin to be observed. MUAs and LFPs represent complex forms of integration of summation of the different cellular and synaptic components of the circuits, or in any case of the recorded neuron populations. Their form is represented graphically as slow deflections that diverge from the recording line. The deflections are formed by the various signals of simultaneously recorded individual units that are added together to form a common signal. The MUAs are used preferably to record the spontaneous activity of a neuron population (extending for about 200 µm from the electrode tip), whereas the LFPs are due to inputs activating the dendrites and the soma of the neurons within a diameter of several millimeters. It should be noted that some success has been achieved in the attempt to correlate activation recorded using functional magnetic resonance imaging (fMRI) with the various LFPs in different experimental situations. In this way it was found that fMRI activation is not linked so much to the neuron activity as to the processes of signal input and intracortical processing, and thus not to spontaneous cortical activity but to that influenced by input.

Extracellular Neuronal Recordings

The extracellular recording of individual units can be used to detect the activity of individual neurons and to provide information concerning the state of activation of the individual cell inside the circuit containing it. The activity of the recorded neurons consists of the sum total of electrochemical events taking place outside the neuronal membrane and that characterize neuron depolarization. On average, depolarizations (and repolarizations) of the neuronal membranes take place in less than 1 msec, although some neurons display faster or slower times. The graphic form used to record depolarization is known as a *spike*, that is, a rapid bipolar drop and almost equally rapid return to the isopotential base line accompanied by a short transient period of hyperpolarization (a type of mechanism that completely recharges the neuronal membrane, which may be likened to a condenser being charged and then discharged).

When the electrode tip (which of course must be particularly thin in this case) penetrates the neuronal membrane, intracellular recordings can be made. Experimental trials have been conducted involving simultaneous recording using a large number of microelectrodes (even more than 100) to allow the recording of a large number of neurons and thus obtain a complex dynamic image made up of the collective activity of individual units during normal behavior or in response to experimental tasks in experimental animals. From the conceptual point of view, this allows the gap between behavioral structures and possibly associated areas of the nervous system to be reduced. The application of sophisticated analysis techniques (correlograms, information estimates, graphs, and other geometric–algebraic methods) makes it possible to study also the characteristics of coding, stabilizing, or weakening of the synaptic forces inside a nervous circuit under different behavioral conditions.

Intracellular Neuronal Recordings

Intracellular neuronal recordings are technically more complex, compared to extracellular ones, owing to the need to maintain the electrode inside the neuron and thus guarantee the absolute stability of the recording system. To reduce the technical difficulty involved, intracellular recordings are generally performed on brain tissue regions placed *in vitro*, which can thus be manipulated under conditions of absolute mechanical stability and can guarantee long periods of recordability. The big advantage of intracellular recordings stems from the fact that it is possible to read con-

tinuously all the electrochemical events occurring inside a neuron. It should be noted that the membrane potential of a neuron at rest does not remain fixed and stable but continues to fluctuate more or less perceptibly. Each variation in potential may be the result of different events, due both to the input from other neurons and to spontaneous variations. When the potential reaches a given threshold the neuron produces a spike. The large quantities of data obtainable using intracellular recordings (concerning the electrochemical and electrodynamic aspects of the depolarization processes) *in vitro* are, however, handicapped by the unavoidable problem that the brain region (whether in the form of tissue "slices" or as neurons dissociated in a medium) is dissected and separated from the natural connections regulating many of its activities. Recent technical enhancements have made it possible to make recordings also in experimental animals during cognitive-motor tasks.

Patch-Clamp Neuronal Recordings

Patch-clamp recordings are characterized by different techniques that share the common features of using glass electrodes (very fine, hollow tubular devices) with 2– to 4-μm tips filled with solutions mimicking cytoplasm conditions. The electrode is placed in the vicinity of a cultivated cell or of *in vitro* structures and is brought up against the membrane surface. Slight suction is used to create complete contact between the membrane and the tip. In this way continuity is ensured between the interior of the cell and the liquids inside the electrode. The various techniques used in any case afford a reasonable means of studying the activity of the individual ion channels and their modulation under different experimental conditions. It becomes possible to evaluate the activity of thousands of channels when, by studying neurons or small cells, the entire cell is attracted inside the electrode, or else it is possible to study the dynamics of individual channels when only small areas of membrane are observed. It is possible to study the effect of variations in electrolyte type and concentration on the conductance behavior of the ion channels by placing a second electrode in the vicinity of the first, in order to allow rapid electrolyte renewal around the ion channel being observed.

NEURONAL RECORDINGS IN CLINICAL PRACTICE

Stereotaxic neurosurgery often involves the positioning of (stimulus and recording) electrodes in both surface and deep areas. Electrodes positioned in epidural or subdural locations, for example, may be necessary in the case of failure to obtain an accurate topographic identification of the trigger areas of a primary epileptic focus that cannot be detected even using high-resolution electroencephalographic observation. Recordings using surgically positioned electrodes may be epidural, subdural, or intracerebral. Each strategy has its own specific risks and characteristic benefits, which also depend on the therapeutic strategies following identification of the electrochemical characteristics of the regions involved. All the invasive recording techniques applied to the central nervous system have the common disadvantage of providing a representation of comparatively small volumes, but on the other hand allow much more specific and analytical data to be extracted compared to those obtained using scalp recordings (without any further artifacts produced by myograms or movement).

Epidural Electrodes

Use of epidural electrodes is very restricted. They are generally used for a more accurate localization of an epileptic focus. They are positioned on the dura mater after drilling small holes in the skull.

Through their contact with the dura, the electrodes produce a large electroencephalogram with no interference or muscular or movement artifacts. They are marked by low spatial resolution and are feasible only in the zones of cerebral convexity.

Subdural Electrodes

Subdural electrodes are made up of matrixes (networks) or multielectrode linear bands. These electrode arrays are placed in a subdural position on the cortical surface. They consist of flat contact points mounted on flexible plastic supports. Of course, because of the size of these electrodes a craniotomy is required to place them, and so their use is plausible only in the case that monolateral recordings prove sufficient. They do not penetrate the brain tissue and, in view of the size of the recording network, collect data from over a rather wide area. They are effective in the identification of focal areas and even of cortical regions of high and low functional significance. This enables mapping of the patients' most widely used cerebral areas, thus reducing the risk of significant functional lesions during resection surgery, especially in the left temporal regions (for instance, by avoiding damage to the speech areas of the brain during removal of the damaged portion).

Deep Intracerebral Electrodes

Deep intracerebral electrodes may be positioned stereotactically in the deep brain regions in general, with the help of MR, CAT, and/or angiographic imaging. Their use has gradually declined since the advent of modern noninvasive recording techniques. Recordings are generally associated with operating techniques involving the positioning of stimulus electrodes for therapeutic purposes.

The electrodes can be inserted into the brain through small trephinations in the skull. They may be positioned in the globus pallidus, subthalamic nucleus, lateral intermediate thalamic nucleus, orbitofrontal regions, cingulate gyrus, amygdala, or hippocampus. These recordings may be used in association with those of the scalp or even subdural recordings, which provide a more general picture of the activities recorded analytically by the deep electrodes.

NEUROCHEMICAL LESIONS

Experimental neurochemical lesions (to be distinguished from experimental or clinical neuroablation lesions or from thermo- or cryolesions) are used according to different experimental strategies. For example, it is possible to produce lesions selectively in one of the five nuclear groups that are interconnected to form the basal ganglia in the basal forebrain and involved in the modulation of voluntary movement. For instance, selective lesion of the substantia nigra (one of the nuclear groups of the basal ganglia) in primates has allowed partial models of Parkinson's disease to be advanced.

Drug Protection on Brain Lesioned Areas

Another strategy involving the use of experimental targeted lesions of the nervous system evaluates the protective effectiveness of certain drugs or natural factors (e.g., nerve growth factor) or of ganglioside molecules on the lesion. Molecular biology techniques have also been introduced to establish the relationship between the development of the lesion and the associated gene activation or deactivation, as well as the modulation of cell receptor synthesis. For example, injecting anti-D2 antisense oligonucleotides (anti-RNA of type 2 dopamine receptors) into the cerebral ventricles in order to study the role of type 2 dopaminergic receptors through their selective elimination in the pathological corollaries of animal models of Parkinson's disease allows a specific receptor study to be made,

because gene expression of the D-1 (type 1 dopaminergic) receptors remains intact.

Neurotoxins

Typical neurotoxic substances include 6-hydroxydopamine (6-OH-DA); ibotenic acid; 1-methyl-4-phenyl-1, 2, 3, 6-tetrahydropyridine (MPTP), a neurotoxin that is very harmful to substantia nigra neurons; and quisqualic acid, which in suitable concentration induces apoptosis (programmed cell death) of neurons through the phenomenon of excitotoxicity (that is, due to an excess of metabolic–ionic phenomena associated with supramaximal neuronal excitation). Quisqualic acid causes neuronal cell death but leaves the fibers passing inside the cerebral nuclei intact.

Strategies of causing lesions to nervous tissue during development have been used experimentally. For example, cyitosine arabinoside (Ara-C) has been used in experiments involving lesions of cortical and hippocampal stages of development. Administration of Ara-C to pregnant female mice produced disgenic microcephaly and disorder in the cell arrays in the CA1 layer of the hippocampus. Ara-C is an antimitotic drug; when used experimentally in the conditions described, it inhibits replication of neurons and progenitor glial cells during development. Lesions are created that are selective on the cell lines, leading to disorder in the constitution of correct nervous circuits.

AUTORADIOGRAPHY WITH RADIOACTIVE 2-DEOXYGLUCOSE LABELED WITH ^{14}C

Autoradiographic analysis can be based on functional data that emerge after injection of radioactive 2-deoxyglucose labeled with ^{14}C (2-[^{14}C]DG) and on the fact that 2-[^{14}C]DG is internalized by active neurons or (more probably) by the glial cells surrounding the neurons, which participate together in the glial lactic acid cycle that serves as the energy substrate for neurons. 2-[^{14}C]DG is taken up intracellularly but is not metabolized, and tends to accumulate intracellularly; 2-[^{14}C]DG is thus taken up in a quantity proportional to the state of activation of the neurons. The more active a region, the more glucose it absorbs and the more 2-[^{14}C]DG it accumulates, which marks the level of neuronal activation of the region.

The brain is extracted and cut into slices after the injection of the labeled product. The material is placed in contact with X-ray-sensitive film, which develops in proportion to the intensity of the radioactive product, thus allowing the activation of the brain areas to be mapped.

CEREBRAL MICRODIALYSIS

One of the available cerebral perfusion techniques, cerebral microdialysis (CM), can be used to perform an *in vivo* study of the brain neurochemical processes. In this system a very thin dialysis tube (less than 0.3 mm external diameter) is inserted under stereotactic guidance into the region of interest; this allows the passive transfer of substances flowing inside the capillary under the concentration gradient between the perfusion liquid and the extracellular liquid. The liquid collected by the probe electrode is subjected to standard chemical analysis, such as high-pressure liquid chromatography (HPLC), in order to assay the transmitter substances of specific interest.

Because it obviously allows specific transmitters to be investigated, CM can prove useful in the pharmacological study of conditions requiring a pharmacokinetic investigation of transmitters and drug metabolites. Microdialysis has been used in human neurosurgery to study intraoperative and posttraumatic ischemic damage online.

VOLTAMMETRY

In voltammetry a voltage wave is released through a carbon fiber electrode previously inserted in the brain under stereotactic guidance. At a specified voltage each monoamine releases electrons in the direction of the electrode due to an electrochemical oxidation mechanism. The released electrons induce a current, the intensity of which is proportional to the quantity of electrons released and thus to the quantity of transmitter present in the region of concern. Because each transmitter has its own elective oxidation current, by calibrating the currents it is possible to obtain accurate information about, as well as to quantify, the types of transmitter present in a given area, even without any *a priori* knowledge of its presence.

Voltammetry is used primarily for monoaminergic transmitters (dopamine, noradrenaline, and 5-hydroxytryptamine or serotonin) and their metabolites. Each voltammetry cycle (that is, release of current wave and measure of quantity of electronic current released, with the identification and quantification of transmitter) takes several seconds to be completed. The result is therefore not an immediate and temporally selective measure of the actual concentration at any given instant.

The same techniques, of course without any need for stereotaxy, can also be used for assaying transmitter concentration in solutions, and for *in vitro* observations of organs, especially brain slices.

Fast Cyclic Voltammetry

Fast cyclic voltammetry (FCV) allows the quantity of neurotransmitters present to be measured online. The technique allows for repeated measurement every 20 msec. For example, it is possible to record the uptake of monoamine, or rather the presynaptic internalization of the monoamines, a mechanism of presynaptic transmitter recovery.

Suggested Reading

Stereotactic Neurosurgery

Benabid, A. L. (1999). Histoire de la stereotaxie [History of stereotaxis]. *Rev. Neurol. (Paris)* **155**(10), 869–877.

Ono, M., Kubic, S., and Abernathey, C. D. (1990). "Atlas of the Cerebral Sulci." georg Thieme Verlag, Stuttgart.

Schaltenbrand, G., and Wahren, H. (1977). "Atlas of Stereotaxy of the Human Brain." Georg Thieme Verlag, Stuttgart.

Talairach, J., and Tournoux, P. (1988). "Coplanar Stereotaxic Atlas of the Human Brain." Georg Thieme Verlag, Stuttgart.

Neurosurgical Methods

Hussman, K. L., Chaloupka, J. C., Berger, S. B., Chon, K. S. , and Broderick, M. (1998). Frameless laser-guided stereotaxis: A system for CT-monitored neurosurgical interventions. *Stereotact. Funct. Neurosurg.* **71**(2), 62–75.

Nutting, C., Dearnaley, D. P., and Webb, S. (2000). Intensity modulated radiation therapy: A clinical review. *Br. J. Radiol.* **73**(869), 459–469.

Neuronal Recordings

Fox, K., Glazewski, S., and Schulze, S. (2000). Plasticity and stability of somatosensory maps in thalamus and cortex. *Curr. Opin. Neurobiol.* **10**(4), 494–497.

Logothetis, N. K., Pauls, J., Augath, M., Trinath, T., and Oeltermann, A. (2001). Neurophysiological investigation of the basis of the fMRI signal. *Nature* **412**(6843),150–157.

O'Donovan, M. J. (1999). The origin of spontaneous activity in developing networks of the vertebrate nervous system. *Curr. Opin. Neurobiol.* **9**(1), 94–104.

Schanze, T., and Eckhorn, R. (1997). Phase correlation among rhythms present at different frequencies: Spectral methods, application to microelectrode recordings from visual cortex and funtional implications. *Int. J. Psychophysiol.* **26**(1–3), 171–89.

Steriade, M., and Amzica, F. (1998). Coalescence of sleep rhythms and their chronology in corticothalamic networks. *Sleep Res. Online* **1**(1),1–10.

Neuronal Recordings in Clinical Practice

Lozano, A. M., Hutchison, W. D., Tasker, R. R., Lang, A. E., Junn, F., and Dostrovsky, J. O. (1998). Microelectrode recordings define the ventral posteromedial pallidotomy target. *Stereotact. Funct. Neurosurg.* **71**(4), 153–63.

Tasker, R. R., and Kiss, Z. H. (1995). The role of the thalamus in functional neurosurgery. *Neurosurg. Clin. N. Am.* **6**(1), 73–104.

Neurochemical Lesions

Ono-Yagi, K., Ohno, M., Iwami, M., Takano, T., Yamano, T., and Shimada, M. (2000). Heterotopia in microcephaly induced by cytosine arabinoside: Hippocampus in the neocortex. *Acta Neuropathol.* **100**(4), 403–408.

Pollack, A. E. (2001). Anatomy, physiology, and pharmacology of the basal ganglia. *Neurol. Clin.* **19**(3), 523–534.

Fast Cyclic Voltammetry

Mendelowitsch, A. (2001). Microdialysis: Intraoperative and posttraumatic applications in neurosurgery. *Methods* **23**(1), 73–81.

Stamford, J. A. (1989). *In vivo* voltammetry: Prospects for the next decade. *Trends Neurosci.* **12**, 407–412.

Stamford, J. A. (1990). Fast cyclic voltammetry: Monitoring transmitter release in real time. *J. Neurosci. Methods* **34**, 67–72.

B

A Synopsis of Neurological Diseases

Rolf Verleger

This synopsis is restricted to neurological diseases affecting the brain. This excludes disturbances affecting peripheral nerves and neural transmission within the spinal cord. Neurological diseases affecting the brain may be distinguished by their class of etiology. The disease may be (1) degenerative, (2) due to failures of blood supply, (3) due to inflammation and problems within the immune system, (4) due to tissue growth (tumors), and (5) directly due to external agents.

DEGENERATIVE DISEASES

In degenerative diseases, brain cells are damaged due to some endogenous reason affecting their metabolism or interfering with signal transmission. Some progress has been achieved in understanding the involved mechanisms, perhaps most of all in Parkinson's disease, but nevertheless the causal agents have still remained obscure. A strong hereditary component is involved in Huntington's disease and in some types of cerebellar degeneration. Some hereditary factors have also been demonstrated in Alzheimer's disease and Parkinson's disease, but only in infrequent subtypes of these diseases. The major obvious risk factor in the latter two diseases is age.

Alzheimer's Disease

Alzheimer's disease is the most common cause of dementia in elderly people. Pathological markers are plaques and tangles within neuronal tissue, above all within the temporal and parietal lobes, but these markers can so far be identified only by neuropatholological examination, i.e., not while the patients are alive. Thus, standard criteria recommend diagnosis of "probable" Alzheimer's disease by diagnosing dementia and excluding other possible causes of dementia (vascular encephalopathy, lack of certain vitamins or hormones, and other reasons). The main symptom is a deficit of working memory but, in order that Alzheimer's disease (and dementia in general) be diagnosed, some second capacity in addition to memory must be affected.

Parkinson's Disease

The cardinal symptoms of Parkinson's disease are stiffness, lack of movement, and tremor during rest. There is often a slight, diffuse impairment of cognitive functions, reminiscent of frontal lobe pathology. The main pathological mechanism is degeneration of dopamine-producing neurons in the brain stem (i.e., substantia nigra). Because of this, the basal ganglia lack the dopamine needed for their adequate functioning. The basal ganglia project in different ways via the thalamus to cortical areas. Dopamine replacement therapy may alleviate the symptoms for a number of years.

Other Degenerative Diseases

Cerebellar atrophy denotes a class of diseases, some idiopathic, some hereditary, that are characterized by impairments of movement precision and of balance, obviously related to shrinkage of cerebellar volume. Often, in the course of the disease, pathology progresses from the cerebellum to neighboring structures (olivo-ponto-cerebellar atrophy, OPCA).

Huntington's disease is a hereditary degenerative disease of the brain, focusing on parts of the basal ganglia (nucleus caudatus and putamen), producing hyperkinesia, akinesia, and dementia. A core symptom of the disease is excess movements (St. Vitus' dance).

Progressive supranuclear palsy is characterized by palsy of vertical saccades, loss of voluntary facial movements, axial dystonia, gait disturbance, and dementia. Pathological alterations in several subcortical regions form the basis for these impairments.

In amyotrophic lateral sclerosis (ALS) there is degeneration of neurons of the pyramidal tract and of the consecutive spinal neurons, progressively reducing a patient's ability to move. Different from other degenerative diseases, ALS is neither hereditary nor a disease of old age, but has its peak of incidence during the fifth decade of age.

LESION OF CEREBRAL TISSUE DUE TO FAILURE OF BLOOD SUPPLY

Brain tissue can be damaged by disorders of blood circulation in two ways: by infarction, i.e., some vessel is blocked such that tissue no longer has blood supply, or by hemorrhage, i.e., some vessel is ruptured, causing blood to overflow into brain tissue.

Infarction or hemorrhage affecting the cortex will cause well-delimited symptoms and syndromes. For example, lesions of anterior branches of the middle cerebral artery (MCA) may cause palsy of the contralateral arm, of the contralateral side of the mouth and (if in the left hemisphere in right-handers) Broca-type aphasia. Lesions of posterior branches of the MCA may cause Wernicke-type aphasia, if on the left, and disorders of spatial abilities, including neglect, if on the right.

INFLAMMATORY DISEASES

Inflammation of the brain may be acute, possibly life-threatening, in meningoencephalitis, and may be caused by bacteria and viruses (or, hard to distinguish clinically, by fungi). There are also chronic inflammatory-type processes caused by multiple sclerosis, by the human immunodeficiency virus (HIV), or by prions.

Multiple sclerosis (encephalomyelitis disseminata) is characterized by a diversity of symptoms, due to inflammatory-type lesions of neuronal axons and the insulating myelin, appearing and disappearing at a variety of cerebral, cerebellar, and spinal locations. The optical nerve is frequently affected as a first symptom.

The human immunodeficiency virus frequently affects the central nervous system and may cause cognitive impairment up to HIV-associated dementia, as part of the acquired immunodeficiency syndrome.

TUMORS

Tissue may grow within the head, thereby causing either unspecific symptoms (nausea, epileptic seizures, etc.) or symptoms specific to their location, in this case similar to consequences of infarction. Depending on the particular tissue, growth may be benign, i.e., slow and not penetrating other tissue, or malign, i.e., fast and infiltrating.

EXTERNAL AGENTS

The brain may be damaged by accidents and poisonous substances. The most important poisonous substance is alcohol, causing cerebellar dysfunction and, mediated by lack of vitamin B1, several symptoms summarized as Wernicke–Korsakow syndrome. In chronic alcoholics, acute alcohol withdrawal may lead to epileptic seizures.

C

State-of-the-Art Equipment for Electroencephalographic and Magnetoencephalographic Investigation of the Brain and Cognition

Alberto Zani and Alice Mado Proverbio

INTRODUCTION

This appendix provides basic information on the equipment necessary in a modern laboratory for recording and analyzing electromagnetic brain signals.

First is a description of a laboratory for recording electroencephalogram (EEG) and event-related potentials (ERPs) with high-density electrode placement. Very large laboratories with powerful systems of calculation can acquire and analyze signals recorded from more than 100 (e.g., 128) scalp sites. In this case, the large number of pieces of equipment are very powerful in order to manage the large number of input channels, but, in principle, a smaller laboratory would have similar equipment with similar features. There is a headbox with input wires arriving from the electrodes on the scalp, the bundles of wires to the analog digital (A/D) converter, and, above all, the amplifiers. The storage capacity and the velocity of modern computers allow sophisticated analysis algorithms to be applied and

complex calculations to be made on recorded data, even when the spatial resolution is high (large number of input channels) and when the temporal resolution is high (high sampling rate, e.g., 512 or even 1024 Hz). Whatever the size of an electrophysiology laboratory, they all have in common certain principles and standards of construction and function that ensure that recording procedures are carried out correctly with a high level of safety. For example, sound-proofing of the recording cabin, electromagnetic shielding, temperature regulation, and earthing of all equipment, as well as the recording environment, are all essential and obligatory procedures for any EEG laboratory of any level to carry out. It is not our intention to discuss these aspects [for excellent discussions of electrophysiology laboratories, see the book by Regan (1989) and the review by Greene *et al.* (2000)].

Also included here is a consideration of the characteristics of a modern magnetoencephalography laboratory.

THE ELECTROPHYSIOLOGY LABORATORY FOR RECORDING EEG AND ERPs

(Fig. 1A–C) show the typical arrangement of a modern, medium-sized, computer-based electrophysiology laboratory mainly devoted to ERP recording in healthy volunteers in order to investigate the relationships between the mind and the brain. As shown in Fig. 1A, the volunteer is made to sit in a comfortable chair, preferably one with a high back that supports the torso and head, in front of a videoscreen (A) connected by a cable to the computer responsible for managing the stimuli and experimental tasks. Both the volunteer and the screen are inside an electrically shielded cubicle (B), which functions as a Faraday cage (C in Fig. 1B). In order to allow the height of the screen to be adjusted according to the individual's height, the screen (A) shown in Fig. 1B is situated on a height-adjustable support (D) fixed to a table (E), the height of this latter also being adjustable. The table has two blockable wheels to allow the distance from the observer to be altered easily, depending on the requirements of the experiment. An infrared digital videocamera with adjustable focus (F) is fixed to the monitor of the stimulator. This videocamera photographs the volunteer and

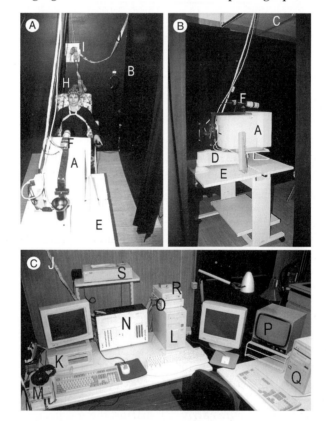

FIGURE 1   Illustration of typical equipment for EEG recording used in a modern ERP laboratory. The actual laboratory represented (with kind permission from the Director) is in the Institute of Neuroscience and Bioimaging of the National Research Council, Milan, Italy. (A) A volunteer sits inside the electrically and magnetically shielded cubicle facing a computer monitor and an infrared videocamera. (B) Entrance to the recording cabin. Part of the Faraday cage is visible on the ceiling; laterally, it is hidden behind the walls. (C) Overall view of most of the electrical devices necessary for carrying out ERP recordings and analysis. See text for explanation of letters.

sends the images to the control screen (P, in Fig. 1C) in order to allow the researcher to monitor any head, eye, or body movements throughout the recording session.

The volunteer shown in Fig. 1A wears an elastic cap (H) on her head. The electrodes are fixed to the cap, which is maintained under tension by a pair of elastic braces attached to a harness fixed around the volunteer's chest. The flat wires from the cap, with their relative connectors, allow the analog signals recorded by the single electrodes to be transmitted to the individual input channels of the EEG headbox (I), keeping the transmission channel for each electrode completely separate from those of the others. This headbox has the important function, besides merely transmitting the signals to the amplifiers through a shielded flat wire (J in Fig. 1C), of pre-amplifying the signals. During recording the curtain is kept closed and the area dimly lit. Figure 1A shows how the volunteer rests her arms on the arms of the armchair and places her index fingers on the response pads, which, if required, will record any response times during the experiment. These data can be recorded permanently on the hard disk of the stimulator (K in Fig. 1C), or can be kept in working memory (or random access memory) and subsequently sent through the COM1 or USB serial port into the local network to the so-called master (L) computer, which links the behavioral responses emitted by volunteers to single stimuli to single EEG sweeps synchronized with these latter, before permanently storing both on the hard disk.

The computer that is dedicated to presenting the acoustic, visual, or linguistic stimuli (K) is called the slave computer, because it carries out commands from another computer in the local network, the *master* computer, shown in the center of the figure (L). It is the *master* computer that stores all of the volunteer's experimental acquisition and stimulation data. The stimulator creates the sensory stimuli. In

order to do this it has a graphic program designed to produce visual stimuli, and a sound and voice synthesis board, and for online presentation of these stimuli for the experiments a device called a video splitter (M) (Fig. 1C, on the left of the *slave* computer), placed below the earphones and above the auditory interface. The video splitter allows the stimuli stored on the hard disk of the *slave* computer to be displayed on its screen as well as on a remote screen (A) connected via cable and located within the electrically shielded cubicle. This technical solution allows the researcher to monitor the correct functioning of the stimulation procedures during the recordings. Using a similar logical solution, the researcher can monitor the stream of auditory stimuli through the earphones available on the left of the stimulator (Fig. 1C). On the right of the *slave* computer the 32-channel amplifiers (N) are receiving EEG signals through the shielded flat cable (J) arriving from the headbox near the volunteer in the shielded cubicle. The amplifier shown in the photograph is powered by a ± 6-V lead battery rather than by the main electricity source (which is 220 V in most overseas countries). On the left of the amplifiers there are the *luminance-emitting devices* (LEDs) that signal any excess impedance of the EEG signal in one or more channels. On the right of the amplifier, there are controls to regulate high-pass and low-pass filters (see Appendix D for details on the regulation of these filters). The EEG signals thus amplified and filtered are transmitted to the interface (O), the "interpreter," which allows the amplifiers and A/D conversion board within the *master* computer (L) to "talk to each other" efficiently. The A/D board converts the bioelectrical analog signal into numerical values as a function of time and preselected sampling rate, set via the *master* computer's software. The values thus obtained, and expressed in microvolts, are then stored in the bulk memory of the master computer. At the end of the recording the raw EEG data, usually a very considerable quantity, can be transferred directly to another computer (Q), also part of the network, for data analysis, or can be downloaded onto a data storage system, which in the system illustrated is a CD burner (R).

The EEG signal thus recorded then undergoes a series of standard analyses by specifically designed software that allows the EEG to be divided and the procedures of artifact rejection, base line correction, averaging, digital filtering, amplitude and latency computing of the components of the signal, topographic mapping, etc. to be carried out.

Hard copies of the wave forms and the color topographic maps calculated on the basis of the wave forms can be printed by the printer (S), visible on the table behind the amplifiers.

THE MEG LABORATORY

A magnetoencephalography (MEG) laboratory is very similar to an electrophysiology laboratory but does have some

particular characteristics that distinguish it. Figure 2 offers an example of a possible setup of such a laboratory with its different components. A detail of the magnetically shielded room (A) can be seen in the upper right. The volunteer and the Dewar probe (C) are inside this room during the experiments and recordings. The walls of the room are made of sheets of aluminium, which predominantly block high-frequency fields by the currents induced in the sheets.

In order to shield out very low-frequency fields as well, several layers of "mu metal" (metal alloys of steel and nickel with an optimal permeability of $\mu > 10^4$) are overlapped on the inside walls of the room in which the recordings from the volunteer are made. This metal shields the walls extremely well and can absorb magnetic field lines. These special alloys are, however, very expensive and as a result this feature of the MEG laboratory is extremely costly.

Within the shielded room, the volunteer is made comfortable on a transformable hydraulic system (B), which allows positions intermediate between supine and

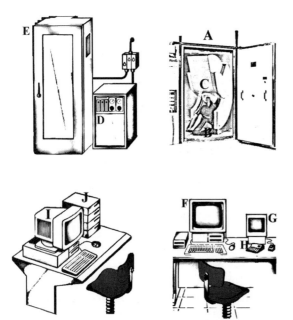

FIGURE 2 An example of a magnetoencephalography laboratory with its various pieces of equipment.

sitting straight upright. Figure 2 shows the volunteer in a seated position with his head in the helmet, which is the basis of the Dewar probe (C), in a vertical position. The sensors in the helmet send the magnetic fields picked up to the superconducting quantum interference device (SQUID) within the probe.

Before the recording, a digitalization device (not shown here) can record the cartesian coordinates in three dimensions (x, y, z) of the positions of markers (vitamin E oil capsules or digital sensors) placed on the volunteer's nasion and the two auricular depressions. Using these coordinates it is possible to superimpose the magnetic fields offline with the findings of the MRI scanning in order to locate the MEG dipoles of the anatomical brain structures.

Inside the shielded room there is a closed-circuit videocamera trained on the volunteer so that his behavior can be monitored directly. Furthermore, there are devices producing various stimuli: plastic tubes with low distortion of the auditory signal are usually used for acoustic stimuli, a liquid crystal screen may be used for visual stimuli and commercially marketed vibrotactile stimulators produce somatesthetic stimuli.

The device (D) amplifying the magnetic fields measured by the MEG probe is located outside the shielded room, together with the unit of bulk storage (E) of these fields. The experimental protocols administered to the volunteers are managed by the computer (F) at its workstation (in the lower right of Fig. 2). A videocamera films the volunteer, who can be observed on the screen (G), shown next to the computer. A two-way phone (H) allows communication with the volunteer.

Once the recording has been made, the fields can be analyzed, the dipoles computed, and these latter be recombined with the MRI tomographic images. This is carried out by a different computer (I), shown in Fig. 2 at another workstation, on the bottom left. It is essential that this computer has a large working memory and bulk memory (J). It must, in fact, perform fast mathematical recombination algorithms, as well as store and manage the files of "voxel" (Vx), which make up the MRI images. The voxel is the smallest three-dimensional graphic unit of the digital image of the MRI scanning. It is derived from progressive layers of the tomographic scanning of the MRI. This progression leads to the addition of the third dimension to the "pixel," that is, the individual square-shaped point that, together with innumerable others, will make up the digital image on a two-dimensional plane. The smaller the dimension of the voxel, the greater the resolution (or sharpness) of the MRI images because brain scanning is proceeding in thinner sections. In order to achieve a faithful reproduction of images made up of an incommensurable number of voxels, it is thus essential that the computer screen also has a high graphic resolution, or sharpness, and a high cathode scanning velocity.

Suggested Reading

Safety Standards

Greene, W. A., Turetsky, B., and Kohler, C. (2000). General laboratory safety. *In* "Handbook of Physiology" (J. T. Cacioppo, L. G. Tassinary, and G. G. Bernston, eds.), 2nd Ed., pp. 951–977. Cambridge University Press, Cambridge.

ERP Laboratory

Cacioppo, J. T., and Tassinary, L. G. (eds.) (1990). "Principles of Psychophysiology. Physical, Social, and Inferential Elements." Cambridge University Press, Cambridge.

Coles, M. G. H., Donchin, E., and Porges, S. W. (1986)." Psychophysiology: Systems, Processes and Applications." Guilford Press, New York.

Gale, A., and Smith, D. (1980). On setting up a psychophysiological laboratory. *In* "Techniques in Psychophysiology" (I. Martin, and P. H. Venables, eds.), pp. 565–582. John Wiley & Sons, Chichester.

Hugdahl, K. (1995). "Psychophysiology. The Mind-Body Perspective." Harvard University Press, Cambridge, Massachusetts.

Martin, I., and Venables, P. H. (1980). "Techniques in Psychophysiology." John Wiley & Sons, Chichester.

Regan, D. (1989). "Human Brain Electrophysiology. Evoked Potentials and Evoked Magnetic Fields in Science and Medicine." Elsevier, New York.

Stern, R. M., Ray W. J., and Davis C. M. (1980). "Psychophysiological Recording." Oxford University Press, New York and Oxford.

MEG Laboratory

Del Gratta, C., and Romani, G. L. (1999). MEG: Principles, methods, and applications. *Biomed. Technik* **44** (Suppl. 2), 11–23.

Hämäläinen, M., Hari, R., Ilmoniemi, R., Knuutila, J., and Lounasmaa, O. (1993). Magnetoencephalography—Theory, instrumentation, and applications to noninvasive studies of the working human brain. *Rev. Mod. Phys.* **65**, 413–497.

Hari, R., and Lounasmaa, O. V. (1989). Recording and interpretation of cerebral magnetic fields. *Science* **244**, 432–436.

Näätänen, R., Ilmoniemi, R. J., and Alho, K. (1994). Magnetoencephalography in studies of human cognitive brain function. *Trends Neurosci.* **17**, 389–395.

Regan, D. (1989). "Human Brain Electrophysiology. Evoked Potentials and Evoked Magnetic Fields in Science and Medicine." Elsevier, New York.

Romani, G. L., Williamson, S. J., and Kaufman, L. (1982). Biomagnetic instrumentation. *Rev. Sci. Instruments* **53**, 1815–1845.

Terbrake, H. J. M., Wieringa, H. J., and Rogalia, H. (1991). Improvement of the performance of a u-metal magnetically shielded room by means of active compensation. *Measures Sci. Technol.* **2**, 596–601.

Wieringa, H. J. (1993). "MEG, EEG and the Integration with Magnetic Resonance Images." Doctoral Thesis, CIP-Gegevens Koninklijke Bibliotheek, Den Haag.

D

Recording and Analysis of High-Density Electromagnetic Signals of the Brain

Alberto Zani and Alice Mado Proverbio

INTRODUCTION

An electroencephalogram (EEG) consists of a surface recording of the difference in electrical potential between two active sites of the scalp, or between an active scalp site and a neutral one. The difference is generated by changes in membrane potentials of large cell assemblies in the underlying brain. Excitatory and inhibitory post-synaptic potentials (EPSPs and IPSPs) of these assemblies "inwardly" (sink) and "outwardly" (source) flow through the brain, passing through the skull and the scalp. These potentials may be recorded through electrolytic contacts using external sensors, called electrodes, placed at various locations on the surface of the scalp. Due to their low magnitude, these potentials must be run through preamplifiers and amplifiers in order to increase their output magnitude. These signals are actually represented by variations of varying rapidity in the potential fields, characterized by an amplitude expressed in microvolts ($1 \ \mu V = 1/1,000,000 \ V = 1/1000 \ mV$) and by a frequency expressed in cycles/second or hertz (Hz). After passing through the amplifiers and being converted into an infinite series of digits, the EEG appears as a continuous, rhythmically "waxing and waning" wave form. By averaging a number of EEG sweeps related to an event repeatedly occurring over time (both exogenous—i.e., a stimulus from the outside world—and endogenous—i.e., an estimation of the time elapsing between one stimulus and another), an average event-related potential (ERP) is obtained. This is because the theoretical principle holds for the latter technique that, by averaging, consistent signals are enhanced and inconsistent signals are cancelled out. The following discussions provide a primer of methods and materials for ERP recording and analysis.

ELECTRODES

Electrodes normally consist of sensors made of metal, owing to the high conduction properties possessed by metals in general. However, because ferrous metals tend to develop spontaneous polarizations, the most suitable metals are platinum, gold, silver, or silver chloride (Ag/AgCl). It is essential that the construction metal be the same for all electrodes used for EEG recording and that different metals are not mixed (Davidson *et al.*, 2000). The best electrodes for ERP recording are the nonpolarizable Ag/AgCl type, which can accurately record very slow changes in potential.

Electrode Types

Electrodes may be found in different forms. They may consist of hypodermic needles, hollow or flat disks and cups, or flat disks of fine silver chloride fixed in a rigid plastic cup. For the reference electrode attached to the ear lobe, so-called clip-leads are a very practical solution because they can be clipped on like earrings. Autoadhesive electrodes prove more practical for use as ocular electrodes. With the exception of hypodermic electrodes, all electrodes have a hole in the top through which they may be filled with an electrolytic jelly, usually composed of water, talc, and salt. The electrode is filled with the jelly after being attached to the scalp. The jelly provides a "flexible" electrolytic bridge contact with the scalp tissue so that movements of scalp or jelly do not disturb the contact with the electrode metal.

Electrode Placement

Up to only a few years ago, electrodes for research purposes were affixed to the scalp by means of an adhesive. The most commonly used adhesive was collodion, which is celluloid dissolved in ether (removable only with acetone or ethyl alcohol). Collodion was available in various commercial formats, typically in small tubes or as large jars of liquid. It was enough to place a little of the tube collodion around the contour of the electrodes and to dry it using cold or warm air jets (for instance, using blasts of compressed air, or a hair dryer). With liquid collodion, a small quantity was poured into a small beaker or dish, and small gauze patches were soaked in it before being placed over the electrode. After drying by one of the methods mentioned above, the gauze patches firmly secured the electrodes in place.

Regardless of the electrode placement method used, in order to enhance electrolytic contact and conductance level, before positioning the electrode on the chosen point on the scalp it was necessary to abrade the scalp slightly. This was accomplished by rolling a blunted obsidian tip over the scalp site (so-called *skin drilling*), or by rubbing the scalp with a special abrasive paper or cotton flock soaked in abrasive paste. In general, the abrasive paste was made of water, pumice, and salt. Because of the greater sensitivity of skin, especially that of the face, compared with the scalp, electrolytic contact between electrode and skin required light abrasion of the skin using a cotton flock or, better, special commercially available preprepared abrasive wipes, soaked in an alcohol solution.

These procedures were long and tedious. Luckily, only a few electrodes, mostly affixed to few sites of the anterior–posterior midline, were used by most research groups engaged in the investigation of brain and cognition.

Electrode Caps

The modern application of recording electrodes has been greatly facilitated by the recent introduction of special elastic caps; these are kept in place by straps attached to a chest harness, on which are fixed a number of Ag/AgCl electrodes, covered by perforated plastic cups, which can accommodate a minimum of 16 or 32, and a maximum of 128, electrodes. High-density electrode arrays obviously guarantee a better spatial resolution of the EEG sampling, which can be very useful, especially when the objects are source analysis (the localization of the underlying brain generators) or the combining of ERP signals with hemodynamic or functional neuroimaging data. There is evidence that using a large number of electrodes improves spatial resolution in identifying highly localized patterns of EEG activity (Davidson *et al.*, 2000). For example, Srinivasan *et al.* (1998) showed how focal hot spots could be washed out by 19- and 32-channel recording montages as a result of spatial aliasing.

Regardless of the number of electrodes fixed to the cap, it is important for the cap to adhere tightly to the head of the individual subjected to recording, so as to ensure better contact between the electrodes and the scalp. Furthermore, it is important to ensure that the cap fits the head properly. In other words, it must not be too tight or too large as a result of excessive stretching of the elastic tissue of the cap or loose sagging over the head, because this could produce a progressive drift of the electrodes away from the initially electrolytically active scalp locations, or inadequate contact of the electrodes. In both cases, this leads to recording difficulties involving relatively noisy EEG signals, not to mention misleading localizing data when source analysis is concerned. All this may be avoided by using electrode caps of different sizes for individuals of different ages, height, or gender. Head size may actually vary considerably even among adults. For example, average head sizes are usually larger for men than for women.

After fitting the cap to the head, the electrodes are filled with electrolytic jelly using a blunted hypodermic syringe needle, which is used also for gently abrading the skin beneath the electrode by means of small rotational movements during the insertion of the jelly.

Electrode Impedance

After completing the procedure of affixing the electrodes, the effectiveness of electrode contact is assessed by measuring the resistance, defined as R, and measured in *ohms* (Ω), of the skin (or scalp) to the passage of the current; the impedance of the electrodes is measured in thousands of ohms, using special external or software-controlled impedance meters. It is common practice to keep electrode impedance well below 5000 Ω (e.g., Eimer, 1998). Indeed, the guidelines for the use of ERPs in research on cognition, prepared by the committee appointed by the Society for Psychophysiological Research (see Picton *et al.*, 2000), recommend that impedance should be reduced to less than 2000–10,000 Ω. The inverse of the resistance is conductance (defined as G). Conductance denotes the facility with which current flows, and is measured in siemens (S) (or *mho*—i.e., the inverse of ohm). As already mentioned briefly, unlike plastics, gums, and clothing, metals and salt solutions display a high conductance.

Electrode Sites

Whatever technique is used for affixing electrodes to the scalp, they are positioned following the standard coordinates introduced in the "ten–twenty" international system (IS) by the *International Federation of Electroencephalography* (*cf.* Jasper, 1958). These coordinates more or less guarantee electrode positioning in certain cortical areas regardless of the shape and size of the head of the patient for which the EEG is to be recorded. The coordinates are computed taking into account the distance between the *nasion*, which is the nasal depression at the superior end of the nose beneath the forehead, and the *inion*, the posterior apophysis at the bottom of the skull. This distance, which in an adult is usually about 34–36 cm, represents 100% of the total distance between the INz site located on the inion, and the Nz site located on the nasion (see Fig. 1).

By computing percentages varying between 10 and 20% of this distance, it is possible to position all the electrodes on the medial line of the scalp passing through these sites or lateral to it. The intersection between the nasion–inion line and the one joining the two auricular depressions, which are also positioned transversely at a distance of 100% (see Fig. 1 again), is indicated as the vertex (or Cz).

To give a concrete example, in a head with a nasion–inion distance of 35 cm, 10% will amount to about 3.5 cm and the occipital sites O1 and O2 will lie at this distance

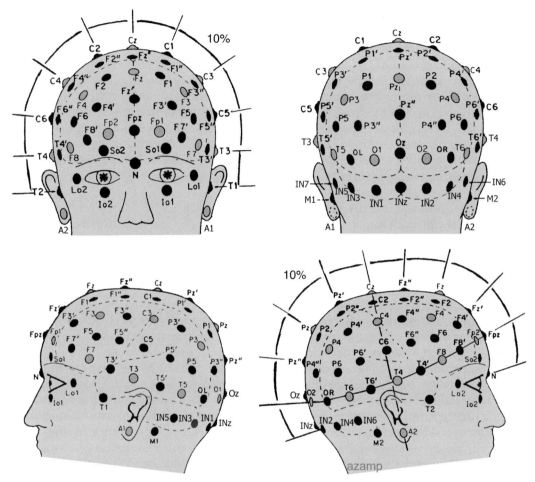

FIGURE 1 The "ten–twenty" electrode system, updated. Electrode nomenclature and positions on the scalp as viewed from the right and left sides and from the front and back. Note how the number of electrodes for topographic studies is very much increased with respect to the traditional 10–20 system originally proposed by Jasper (1958). The electrode sites reported in the traditional system are gray; all of the other electrodes are black. Because of the large increment in the electrode number, in the up-to-date system electrodes are affixed equally spaced from each other at 10% of the inion–nasion distance.

to the left and right of Oz, which is itself positioned 3.5 cm above the inion. Traditionally, a full 10–20 montage involved 19 active scalp sites, which were usually supplemented with two recording leads for the recording of the electrooculogram (EOG). However, in modern ERP laboratories recordings with as many as 32, 64, or 128 channels have become common. To deal with higher density electrode montages, an extended system, defined as the 10% system, in which electrode sites are placed halfway between each of the main 10–20 placements, was advanced by Chatrian et al. (1985), and its use was later championed (see Nuwer, 1987).

In order to allow systematic treatment of the introduction of standard arrays comprising a much larger number of electrodes than those of the traditional 10–20 IS, in 1990 the American Electroencephalographic Society commissioned an overhaul of the system described above (see Myslobodsky et al., 1990). This overhaul entailed partly reinstating the 10% method. The electrodes are indicated by an initial letter denoting the topographical area in which they are placed (for example, C, central; F, frontal; P, parietal; T, temporal; O, occipital) or by means of two or more letters denoting intermediate areas (e.g., FC, frontocentral; PO, parietooccipital). These letters are followed by a progressive number that depends on the distance of the electrode site from the medial sagittal line, indicated with the ending z, which denotes the value 0 (the *zenith*). Odd numbers refer to locations on the left side of the scalp; even numbers refer to locations on the right side of the scalp. For example, PO3 is located half way between POz and PO7 on the left of the medial line.

In this revision a number of modifications were made to the original nomenclature used for several electrodes. For example, electrodes originally indicated with T3 and T5 on the left hemisphere, and T4 and T6 on the right, in this new system are denoted as T7 and P7, and T8 and P8, respectively. More interestingly, a number of anatomotomographical research lines based on both postmortem and computer axial tomography analytic studies support the cortical localization of electrodes indicated by the aforementioned nomenclature. For an exhaustive review of these research lines, see Homan *et al.* (1987). Whenever nonstandard sites are used it is important to specify as fully as possible the position of the electrode sites used for recording so as to allow interlaboratory comparison. It is recommended (Picton *et al.*, 2000) that standard electrode positions and nomenclature be used whenever possible, and that ERPs be recorded simultaneously from regularly spaced multiple scalp electrodes. Also, the way in which the electrodes are affixed to the scalp and the type of reference should always be specified in scientific reports.

BIPOLAR AND MONOPOLAR RECORDINGS

The electrodes may be connected together into several different kinds of bipolar and monopolar montages. In *bipolar* montages all electrodes are connected together in chains, with the second input to one channel becoming the first input to the next channel. The most common use of a bipolar montage is to record the electrooculogram. In this case horizontal eye movements are recorded by means of two electrodes placed at the external canthus of the left and right eyes, and blinks and vertical eye movements are recorded by means of two electrodes placed below and above the right eye, with a bipolar montage. In a *monopolar* montage, also called a *common reference method*, one electrode is active and the other one (or two electrodes linked together) acts as a reference electrode. Typical arrangements for the reference electrode(s) are the linked ears and the linked mastoids configurations. The reference lead must be as electrically neutral as possible with regard to brain activity, while it nevertheless records the basic activity underlying the various physiological functions of the body in spite of any possible external noise (electromagnetic waves). What is actually recorded is the difference that exists between the potential of the active site and that of the reference site. The most commonly used reference leads are the left or right ear (or ear lobe), or the linked or balanced ears (or ear lobes), the left or right mastoid, or the linked or balanced mastoids, the tip of the nose, the chest, and the balanced noncephalic sternovertebral lead [see Tyner *et al.* (1983), p. 166, for a buildup scheme of this reference lead]. None of these is totally free of problems or is the best in an absolute sense. What is, however, important is the distance of these sites from the active electrode. Neighboring sites will cancel out electrical activation sites similar to the two electrodes. Conversely, distant sites will tend to capture more artifacts from many different sources. When using linked references, such as the two ear lobes (i.e., the so-called A1 and A2) or mastoids

(i. e., the so-called M1 and M2), it is advisable to use a balanced strategy to remove possible variations in impedance between the two linked reference sites. This allows a so-called balanced linked reference to be obtained. The balancing may be achieved in several different ways. For example, the same weighting (intensity) may be assigned to the two combined signals by connecting together two low-value (e.g., 5000 Ω) resistances (R1 and R2), which are

coupled in series to the electrode connectors. Alternatively, it is possible to use two variable resistances in series and to change their value as a function of possible variations in impedance during recording. Both procedures offer advantages and disadvantages.

The most important reason for making a careful choice of reference is the strong influence it has on the surface topographic distribution of the bioelectric signal (that

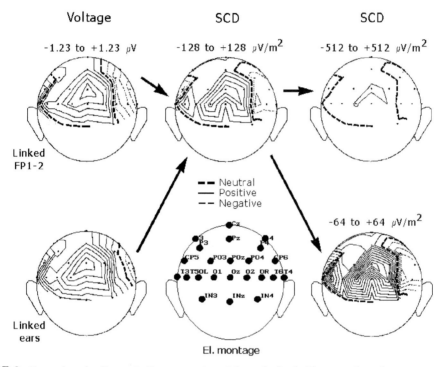

FIGURE 2 Examples of spline or isoline maps viewed from the back. The maps have been computed at P1 peak latency (120 msec) on a difference wave form obtained by subtracting ERPs to gratings relevant in location but irrelevant in spatial frequency, from ERPs to gratings relevant in both features and presented in the right visual field. Left: Changes in voltage (microvolts) isolines and, as a consequence, in scalp topography with "offline" rereferencing (linked Fp1–2) with respect to referencing during "online" ERP recording (linked ears). Note that unlike the latter, the linked Fp1–2 reference determines a decrease in positivity at occipitotemporal sites, and an increase in negativity at right temporoparietal sites. Middle: Regardless of the reference, the computation of the Laplacian operator provides the same scalp current density (SCD) (in $\mu V/m^2$) spline map. Here a larger neat positive focus, centered on O1, O2, and POz mesial-occipital scalp sites, and a smaller one, focused at the posterior-temporal (T5) site, can be observed. (For electrode locations over the posterior scalp maps, see the electrode montage insert at the bottom.) Right: Examples of misleading representations of SCD maps. Top: A too large scale has been chosen, and too few isolines have been drawn in the map to represent the currents' topography over the scalp. In this way, not much topographic information is provided. Bottom: Unlike above, here a too small scale has been chosen, and too many isolines have been drawn in the map to represent the current source topography over the scalp, providing an overload of information to the observer. It follows that an extra effort is needed to figure out the topographic information.

is, on its geographic distribution over the scalp). As we have seen, the reference must be electrically "silent" (or neutral), but unfortunately there are no absolutely silent points in a living biological system. Consequently, because the recorded signal is the result of computing the difference between the signal recorded at the active electrode and that recorded at the earthed reference, the topographic distribution of the EEG signal on the scalp will vary as the reference value varies. This is of more than trivial importance. The topography of the biolectric signal from the same individual taken as the active agent in the same psychomotor task will be found to vary as the reference varies (see Fig. 2). This raises considerable problems as regards the identification of the cerebral areas activated during the performance of the task. To get around them several reference-free signal transformation solutions have been developed. The first of these consists of using the so-called average reference, which, as its name suggests, is based on taking the average value of all the active electrodes as reference (for a detailed treatment of the advantages and disadvantages of this method see Appendix E in the present volume). An alternative to this consists of using a method that enhances the local sources (i.e., radial currents, that is, currents perpendicular to the head), which minimizes the voltage gradients (or currents tangential to the head) due to spurious correlations among the various electrodes. This is done by transforming the scalp voltage values into scalp current density (SCD) by means of a Laplacian analysis. It involves solving the Laplace equation or second derivative of the interpolated voltage area. By acting as a spatial filter, this method eliminates the distant sources contribution (or remote potential fields). In this way it is possible to obtain a reference-free topographic representation of brain activation. So no matter what reference is used during the recording, SCD mapping provides a unique topographical

solution (see Fig. 2). This procedure entails using a large number of electrodes because it is based on computing the difference between one specific electrode and many others that surround it. For a recording that takes in the entire head surface, a minimum of 32 electrodes is thus required (for further details on this method, see later, the section on "ERP Topographic Mapping").

To prevent charge accumulation during EEG recordings, participants have to be connected to charge dispersion devices by means of a ground lead linked to the security plant of the building where the lab is located, or, much better, to a small pit dug in the earth and constructed in accordance with the relevant norms. Grounded active leads, (e.g., Fz) located on the scalp are commonly used.

Amplifiers

The bioelectric signals detected by the electrodes are conveyed separately to electronic amplifying devices—one channel for each electrode site. The amplifiers are made up of a series of resistors and capacitors that have the function of filtering and amplifying the signal. Biological potentials actually have only tiny voltages—millionths of a volt—which must be stepped up to the level of several tens of volts in order to be recorded. The purpose of the amplifiers is to supply energy to tiny potential differences so that they are multiplied tens of thousands of times. For instance, with a gain of 40 the signal is magnified 40,000 times. Unlike the EEG, the EOG is given a lower amplification. Because the EOG signals are actually generated by the electrophysiological signals of the eye muscles developed during eye movement, they have a relatively high amplitude and do not require much amplification.

To distinguish physiological potentials from potential differences with reference to the ground, amplifiers amplify the potential difference between their input terminals (i.e., electrodes) and are relatively insensitive to a potential between these terminals and the ground. For this reason they are known as differential or balanced amplifiers. The voltage with respect to ground common to two electrodes is called an *in-phase* or *common mode* signal. The potential difference between the electrodes is called the *antiphase* or *differential* signal. The specific property of a balanced amplifier is to record and amplify the antiphase signals while eliminating the in-phase signals. This property is referred to as the *high common mode rejection ratio*.

"Online" Analog Filters

The electric circuits in the amplifier are equipped with filters. The main components of a filter usually consist of a resistor and a capacitor (R–C circuit). This circuit allows selective elimination of electric frequencies causing disturbance, or in any case that are extraneous to the brain's bioelectric activity, such as those due to muscle movement or to the alternating current circulating in the electrical equipment. Or else, depending on the aim of the research, filters allow the elimination of recorded physiological signals above or below a specified frequency, called the turnover or cutoff frequency (f_c). High-pass, low-pass, or band-pass filters can commonly be found on commercially available amplifiers. For any of these filters, several frequency settings can be made. With high-pass filters, the setting regulator shows the cutoff frequency above which higher frequencies are passed, and lower frequencies are attenuated. For this reason they are also called low-frequency, or "L.F. cut," filters. Conversely, for low-pass filters the cutoff frequency setting indicates the frequency above which higher frequencies are attenuated, while lower frequencies are allowed to pass. For this reason they are called high-frequency, or "H.F. cut," filters. The band-pass filters

delimit a "window" of frequencies accepted by the amplifier within two upper and lower extremes. For example, a band-pass filter suitable for recording evoked potentials could be 0.01–100 Hz for EOG and 0.1–100 Hz for EEG. However, with studies aimed at investigating cognitive processes, which develop more slowly than sensory processes (for instance, longer latency linguistic processes), a band of 0.01–100 Hz for EEG filtering is certainly more suitable. Notch filters to exclude the line frequency range (60 Hz for the United States and 50 Hz for most overseas countries) are not recommended in that they may significantly distort the recorded signal (Picton *et al.*, 2000).

Common settings for high-pass filters indicate, rather than a cutoff frequency, how long it takes for a signal to return to the base line following an exponential curve. This is a curve that approaches its final value at a decreasing rate, with a slope of attenuation that is also called the *rolloff*. This is characterized by the time— usually measured in seconds—within which the signal amplitude falls to 37% of its initial value before the filter action takes place. This value, which is independent of the magnitude of the initial step, is called the *time constant* (T_C). For these filters, then, the cutoff frequency has to be estimated through the following expression:

$$f_c = 1/2\pi T_C,$$

where T_C is the time constant and $1/2\pi$ is a constant equal to ~0.159, obtained by dividing 1 by the double of $\pi = 3.14$. Thus, $f_c = 0.159/T_C$ may also be found. For example, with $T_C = 3$ sec, $f_c = 0.053$ Hz; with $T_C = 10$ sec, $f_c = 0.0159$ Hz. Clearly, in those rare cases in which f_c, rather than T_C, is known, the latter may be obtained by simple transposition of the above-mentioned expression: namely, $T_C = 1/2\pi/f_c$. For instance with $f_c = 0.053$, $T_C = 0.159/0.053 = 3$ sec. Much care has to be taken over these inversions in order to communicate accurately the characteristics of filters used during experimental recordings. Indeed, some risks are run, not only of communicating incorrect values of T_C because of inconsistency in filter nomenclatures among amplifier manufacturers, but also of obtaining misleading data regarding signals of interest. For instance, when studies are carried out aimed at investigating late latency slow processes of the brain, these processes could be cut off by a misleading setting of the turnover frequency.

Different definitions are, in fact, reported for f_c by different manufacturers, and confusion may arise. Mostly, f_c is defined as the half-*power* frequency, that is, the frequency at which the "output power-to-input power ratio" (i.e., also called gain or sensitivity) is 0.5. The f_c setting, by allowing a gain in power of 0.5, actually determines a gain in amplitude of 0.707, the latter simply being the square root of 0.5 (i.e., power = amplitude^2). In other words, this means that the sensitivity amounts to 70.7% of its maximum value. Indeed, this is the definition of f_c that is implicitly contained in the expression used above to compute T_C. Because amplifier gain was often traditionally expressed in decibels (dB)—the logarithmic expression of frequency—this reduction in gain is the same as a "3-dB down" of the maximum value.

For some manufacturers, however, f_c indicates the half-*amplitude* frequency, which is different from the half-power, because it actually marks the frequency at which a 50% decrease in sensitivity occurs. In decibels, this entails a further halving of the power with respect to 3 dB, that is, a "6-dB down." Obviously, at this point, when, unknown to the experimenter, in setting up a filter, the half-power is confused with the half-amplitude, for example, at $f_c = 0.053$, the late-latency components—such as P300—might be partly washed out because of too fast a T_C. With half-amplitude-regulated amplifiers, in order to record ERPs with, for instance, a $T_C = 3$ sec, the f_c value should be lower, namely, 0.031.

EEG Signal Digitation Rate

Using an interface set up between the amplifiers and the computer, the EEG signals are fed into the analog/digital (A/D) converter in the computer. The computer converts the analogic variations in potential into a series of discrete digits with a given *digitation rate* as a function of time. What characterizes the strength of ERPs is their high temporal resolution, which allows the faster sensory processing of the brain to be investigated without any time lag. For example, a digitation rate of 512 Hz indicates that over a time span of 1 sec the potential value is sampled about once every 2 msec. In some cases, such as in recording auditory brain stem potentials, which reach the primary projection cortex in 10 msec, even a sampling rate of 1 or 0.5 msec may be utilized. The set of sampled points may thus be stored in the mass memory or on the hard disk (HD) of the computer and subsequently displayed and analyzed in the form of continuous oscillating signals (EEG) using dedicated graphics display software. A/D conversion should be carried out at a rate that is sufficiently rapid to allow those frequencies that reflect the EEG and ERP signals of interest to be properly recorded. The A/D conversion rate, as well as the amplifier filter set up in terms of low and high cutoff frequencies, should always be specified in scientific reports (Picton *et al.*, 2000).

ARTIFACTS IN EEG RECORDING

Electrophysiological artifacts, electric signals extraneous to the actual brain activity, overlap the brain activity signals, making them impossible to detect and rendering their recorded values unreliable [see Barlow (1986), and Pivik *et al.* (1993) for a discussion of artifact processing and minimization in EEG recordings]. For this reason artifact signals are very undesirable and should be identified at the outset in order to be remedied immediately. In order to eliminate them effectively and efficiently, it must be borne in mind that they originate from different sources inside and outside the EEG volunteer's body and that the methodological solutions adopted to avoid them differ according to their origin. The following artifacts of external origin are among the most important:

1. *Alternating current:* activity having the same frequency as the main voltage supply (50 or 60 Hz); to avoid induced alternating current it is mandatory for all metal structures and equipment in the lab be appropriately grounded.

2. *Switching artifacts:* rapid discharge spikes caused by sudden voltage oscillations associated with switching electrical equipment on and off.

3. *Radio frequencies:* preamplifiers and amplifiers can synchronize with oscillating frequencies of radio signals in the ether.

In order to avoid these artifacts the recording area must be shielded. The shielding may be provided by a Faraday cage, but can also be ensured by a simple grid made of metal or other conducting material if shielding is not already provided within the silent cabin or cubicle (see Appendix C, this volume), where data collection generally takes place. In this regard it is absolutely essential for the EEG volunteer to be properly grounded.

Internal or physiological artifacts are dealt with in a different way. The most important and easiest to detect are those originating from the following sources:

1. *Body movements:* irregular high-voltage activity due to variations in the distribution of static electrical charges can occur when the EEG volunteers rock in their chair, cough, chew, yawn, or swing their legs, or when they wear tennis shoes or when plastic surfaces are not grounded.

2. *Electrocardiograms:* slow spiked waves synchronized with the electrocardiogram are detected when a balanced sternoverte-

bral lead is used [for further details see Tyner et al. (1983)].

3. *Eye blinks:* V-shaped waves, strongly visible in the prefrontal area yield a deflection that is positive or positive/negative; during the experiment they should be reduced to less than 10/minute.

4. *Horizontal eye movements:* slow waves of variable polarity; in bipolar montages the electrode that becomes positive indicates the direction of the movement.

5. *Muscle activity:* isolated spikes caused by contraction of the neck muscles or scalp; it is a good idea to place a cylindrical cushion behind the volunteer's neck; in patients suffering from headache due to tension a continuous electromyographic activity is observed in the frontal or occipital regions.

6. *Sweating:* very slow waves due to the bioelectric activity of the sweat glands are observed when room temperature is high or when the volunteer is anxious.

In order to avoid artifactual signals special care should also be taken to avoid errors or methodological oversights during electrode assembly and during recording. Artifacts may in fact be the result of common errors such as (1) *placement asymmetries* (nonsymmetrical amplitude in derivations from homologous regions due to incorrect electrode positioning or unilateral references) and (2) *electrode movements* (irregular spike-shaped or square discharges due to momentary interruption of the electrolytic contact between the electrode and the skin).

ERP AVERAGING

The electroencephalogram recorded using the described technique is subjected to automated standard procedures, including breaking down the EEG signals into discrete epochs time-locked to stimulus or mental events, of variable duration (for example, 1 sec), depending on research goals, base line correction, and artifact rejection. When artifacts are intermittent and infrequent (for example, blinks or saccades), artifacts rejection is accomplished by removing contaminated trials from the averaging process. The rejection may be performed automatically and/or by visual inspection. Any trial showing electrical activity greater than a criterion level (e.g., ± 50 µV) in any recording channel should be rejected from averaging. All procedures used to eliminate artifacts (such as compensation or correction procedures) should be adequately documented.

The averaging technique represents the very essence of evoked or event-related potentials techniques. By means of averaging it is possible to obtain the brain's amplified response to a stimulus or event summing numerous EEG sweeps synchronized with the stimulus. In general, averaging should be sufficient to make the signal distinguishable from any noise. The more sums used the better the signal-to-noise ratio. Indeed, this ratio increases as a function of the square root of the number of EEG sweeps summed and averaged. Averaging may be computed only if the EEG is time-locked to a series of external impulses, called *triggers*, which temporally code the simultaneous onset of the stimulus and the brain response. In this case, stimulus-locked average wave forms are obtained. Conversely, in the case of response-locked ERPs, the wave forms are time-locked to mechanical signals, such as, the pressing of a button or an electromyogram (EMG) measurement. [For further details concerning averaging methods see the authoritative treatise by Regan (1989).]

"Offline" Digital Filtering

Even under ideal conditions and with a sufficient number of trials in each ERP average, EEG averaging may often leave residual noise, including high-frequency noise contaminating the unfiltered ERP record, or any EEG rhythmical activity not time-locked to any stimulus events. Appropriate digital filtering can effectively abolish these residual frequencies, which complicate component identification and measurement. This kind of filtering involves a wide range of techniques that share the fact of being grounded on mathematical algorithms applied to discrete numeric representations of continuous wave forms to selectively smooth out certain frequencies. These algorithms are of two principal types: those operating "in the time domain," and those representing signals "in the frequency domain." With the former, a time series of digital values for voltage or some other parameter as a function of time is represented. In filtering out noise, these algorithms base their computation on a template-matching procedure, where the template is determined from "past" data. Decisions concerning noisy "present" data are then made with respect to this template, which is customized for each individual. Serious caveats regarding these filters are the loss of data at the beginning and at the end of the ERP trace, as well as the introduction of phase errors distorting the final wave form.

Unlike time-based filters, frequency-based digital filters produce filtered wave forms with zero phase shift. This is accomplished by representing the data using a Fourier transform. The principle underlying this method is that any stationary wave form may be represented as the sum of a set of sinusoidal wave forms, each of a different frequency, amplitude, and phase angle. As a consequence, three successive steps must be performed in order to filter undesired frequencies.

As a first step, a direct Fourier transformation of the original time series to the frequencies that are present in the ERP trace has to be performed. Second, the frequencies of the transform to be abolished are set to zero. As a last step, an inverse Fourier transform reconverts the frequency domain to the time domain, leaving out the band of frequencies that are set to zero. In this way a filtered version of the ERP wave form is obtained.

SCALP TOPOGRAPHIC MAPPING

The average wave forms obtained separately for the different stimulus categories by means of averaging display a series of deflections (or peaks). It may seem obvious that, regardless of the possible differences among stimulus categories, the instant (i.e., latency) at which the deflection reaches its peak, and the height reached (i.e., amplitude) by the latter, will vary from electrode to electrode. In other words, in each stimulus category the parameters of amplitude and latency of these peaks (or components) will vary according to both the scalp area (i.e., space) and the poststimulus instant (i.e., time) considered. This is all the more true, the greater the number of electrodes used for the electrophysiological recording. It will thus not be easy to perceive the topographies of the underlying components with the naked eye.

In order to get some idea of the data it is thus very useful to make a visual display of the distribution of scalp potential amplitude—in other words, to map it. This mapping may be focused on a single potential value, for example, the instant in which the component reaches its maximum peak at a given cluster of electrodes, thus providing a map of the signal amplitude distribution (in microvolts) over the scalp (or spatial distribution) in that given moment (*stationary mapping*). Due to the aforementioned variations in time and space of the component latency and amplitude, however, this kind of map is often not a satisfactory substitute for the displaying of wave forms recorded at multiple electrodes.

Conversely, the mapping may involve a successive voltage time series (*dynamic mapping*) within a latency range of concern (e.g., 80–140 msec for P1 in spatial atten-

tion studies), thus allowing the computation of multiple maps indicating how the topography of brain electrofunctional activation varies as a function of time and space (space–time distribution).

There are different ways of graphically displaying or mapping voltage or current density distributions over the scalp. These may consist of *spline* or *isoline maps* representing the aforementioned measures. These types of maps are made using the same kind of technique used to mark contour lines on geographic maps. The signal amplitude value decreases from a central area of maximum amplitude (the *focus*) toward the periphery in a gradually decreasing number of concentric linear levels (see Fig. 2 for an example of these maps). The number of levels (and, therefore, of lines) depends partly on signal amplitude and partly on the scale selected for representing the amplitude. In addition, frequent use is also made of displays in which the scalp potential values are represented by different colors or by changes in color saturation of one or two hues, each corresponding to a specific range of values (see Fig. 3).

Whatever type of mapping is used, it is mandatory that, before it is carried out, a careful examination is made and a clear idea gained of the wave forms obtained. Mapping cannot be used as a tool for measuring the waves. Therefore, if we wish to make a topographic map of a maximum peak, we must know precisely at what latency the peak reaches its maximum and have some idea of which electrode or group of electrodes displays its maximum amplitude.

With all types of maps, topographic analysis is based on the mathematical interpolation of the potential or of the current density among numerous electrodes. The starting point for the mapping is the voltage measured at one instant in time at a certain number of electrodes. However numerous, the electrodes are always some distance apart and certainly

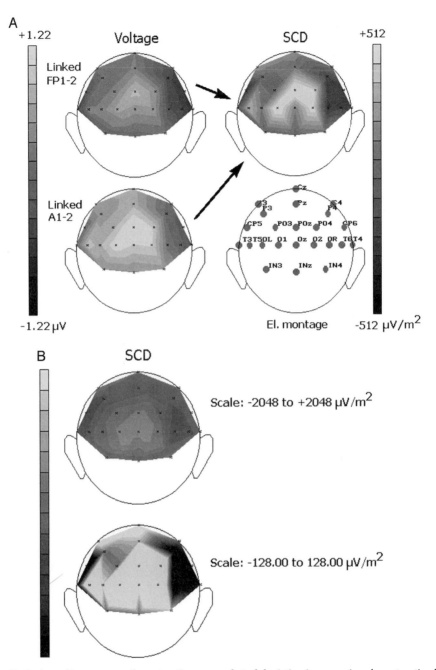

FIGURE 3 Back view of isocontour color saturation maps plotted depicting increases in color saturation levels of black and white hues. Stimulus and task conditions as well as latency of computation are the same as in Fig. 2. (A) As for spline maps, voltage-related saturation levels of the two hues change as a function of reference lead. The scalp current density (SCD) map has the advantage of providing a reference-free representation of current source density over the scalp. (B) Examples of misleading two-hue saturation maps. Top: Too few saturation levels of the black and white hues provide insufficient information on SCD topography. Bottom: The map shows too many hue saturation levels and a too small scale was used. This makes the reading of topographic information far from being straightforward. Note, for example, how the highest saturation level for the white hue covers a large cluster of electrodes without any change in saturation.

do not cover the whole scalp area. To plot a distributed color map, the gap among the electrodes must be "filled in." This means that probabilistic estimates of values "falling" between the various electrodes have to be computed, interpolating the true values measured at these sites. The interpolation may be carried out both two-dimensionally (2D) and three-dimensionally (3D). Regardless of its mathematical basis, it may be explained, with a degree of simplification, as a series of successive steps of reelaboration of the ERP data providing the above-mentioned approximate estimated values. First, the space coordinates of the electrodes attached to the scalp are reported in (or rather projected into) the circle—in the case of 2D maps—or the sphere—in the case of 3D maps—that best fits the head surface and scalp. Subsequently, over the surface of the circle or the sphere, interpolations are performed among the values obtained at the various electrodes. In interpolating a specified point (in other words, the voltage or current density to estimate), all the electrodes are taken into account. However, electrodes closer to the interpolated point

have a higher "weight" (i.e., influence) than do those more distant [a principle first advanced and applied to ERP mapping by Buchsbaum *et al.* (1982)].

Of interest, in this context, is a special interpolation method known as *triangulation*. This is performed by taking points on vertically adjacent top and bottom contours, and connecting them anticlockwise by the shortest lines between the points to form triangles. In this way, signal mapping is possible although the circumference of the head is, from top to bottom (or vice versa), smaller in some parts than in others, thus producing a different number of points per contour.

Spherical spline interpolation is very gradual and there are no abrupt variations in the interpolated values. As far as the color coding is concerned, the algorithm used is fairly simple. The minimum (V_{min}) and maximum (V_{max}) voltage values are singled out and made to correspond to the minimum and maximum indexes on a color scale. Then, for each interpolated point (V_i), a color index in the scale is computed. In practical terms, having a numerically coded scale of N colors (0, 1, 2, 3, ...,

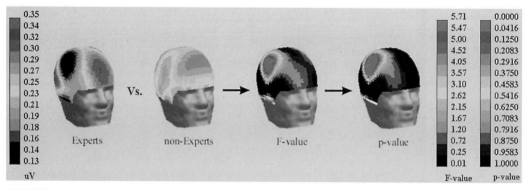

FIGURE 4 Realistic 3D color maps. Isovoltage color maps viewed from the right frontal profile for two groups of volunteers performing the same visuomotor task have been computed and projected over a 3D realistic template of the head. Before ERPs were recorded, one group received a period of training (experts) and another did not (nonexperts). Note that the rainbow color scale has been used to represent voltage changes over the scalp, and that before being plotted the voltage levels have been normalized according to the McCarthy and Wood (1985) rescaling method. A point-by-point between-group variance comparison provided a distribution map of *F*-values, to which a *p*-values significance map corresponded, yielding a significant focus of voltage points over the right centroparietal scalp. (See color plates.)

N, where 0 corresponds to the minimum and N to the maximum value), such an index may be obtained by solving the following formula:

$$\text{Index} = N (V_i - V_{min}) / (V_{max} - V_{min}).$$

Whenever V_i is equal to V_{min}, the index will be 0, and so the first color in the scale will be plotted on the map. Conversely, whenever V_i is equal to V_{max}, corresponding to N, the final color on the scale is plotted on the map. Obviously, with intermediate values of V_i, intermediate colors of the scale relatively close to the first or last color are used, depending on the index value obtained. An example of color-coded three-dimensional mapping can be seen in Fig. 4.

As we have already seen, color indexes used for plotting signal topographies are computed on the basis of interpolated measures, i.e., V_i, thus among many electrodes, the reliability of these plots depends on the degree of rigor with which other electrodes have been "weighted" in determining the index value at electrode E_n, and the immediate surroundings. This criterion must be decided before implementing the mapping procedure by choosing a value for the variable λ. The more stringent the criterion set, the lower the weights of the other electrodes and the more realistic the estimated index, because, in this way, only currents radial to the interpolated point over the sphere will be taken into account. This will increase the spatial resolution with which the map reflects on the skull the electrofunctional activation of the brain as the flow of mental processes progresses.

The use of stringent λ values to use radial currents only for signal mapping is specific to SCD mapping. The method representing SCDs derived from the spatial derivatives (cf. Perrin et al., 1987, 1989) of interpolated values is based on computing the Laplacian operator. Through this mathematical procedure the potential at each electrode is converted into an estimate of the current density entering or exiting the head at that site. In this way, data distortion due to the spatial smearing of the surface potential dependent on the volume conductive properties of the brain and surrounding tissues in general is reduced. This has the further advantage that, unlike isocontour voltage maps, SCD maps are independent of the location of the reference—that is, they are reference free. One of the interesting properties of this method is that it does not create those possibly misleading polarity reversals sometimes reported when using the "average" reference method.

It must be remembered, however, that prefixed proper values of λ do not exist. They must change dynamically as a function of electrode montage density. In practical terms, if $\lambda = 0.0008$ represents a proper criterion for mapping ERPs recorded with a 32-electrode montage, this same value is not proper when 64 or more electrodes are used. In the latter case, in fact, the surface potential would be somewhat spatially smeared because of the use of an insufficiently stringent criterion.

Obtaining a focus giving information on the maximal location of potentials recorded or SCD does not, however, mean localizing the intracranial source of electrical activity. To gain knowledge of the source, or dipole, far more complex mathematical algorithms are required. The basic principles of these algorithms may be found in Chapter 2 and Appendix E of this volume.

PROBLEMS AND LIMITS OF TOPOGRAPHIC MAPPING

We have seen that topographic mapping has the advantage of combining into a single image an overall view of the spatial relationships existing between the electrodes. This information is essential when ERP recordings have been made with such a large number of electrodes that it is somewhat difficult to grasp how the spatial data evolve. Thanks to technological advances in the field of electronics and above all the reduction in the cost of electrophysiological equipment, this is now consolidated practice. The use of topographical maps to sum the results reported in the literature has thus become increasingly widespread.

However, the types of maps used have varied widely, not only in terms of spherical splines or color isocontour voltage maps, but also in terms of which and how many colors are used to represent variations in scalp voltage. This is why Picton et al. (2000) deemed it important to tackle this matter, providing advice and suggestions to be followed in topographic mapping.

In general, problems of interpreting both spline and isocontour color maps have proved similar and arise from a lack of standards. For instance, one important question regarding spline maps is the number of isolines necessary to display potential levels or, in other words, the appropriate distance between the various isocontours. This problem arises out of the fact that, in order to highlight a voltage focus, it is possible, for graphic purposes, to modify the above-mentioned number of lines at will during mapping. Clearly, the number of lines should be sufficient to display the potential difference among the various scalp regions. However, using too many lines could be confusing (see Fig. 2 for an example). Guidelines by Picton et al. (2000) indicate that a resolution of 10 levels should generally be used.

As far as color maps are concerned, one additional problem is that of the choice of color spectrum. It would be possible, for example, to use simple gray-scale maps in which, instead of colors, there are gradual changes in the shades of gray from black to white, passing through all the intermediate levels (see Fig. 3). Again, several authors prefer to use only two colors to denote zones of positive or negative polarity. For example, the colors may vary from a bright red (representing maximum positive voltage) that gradually changes until it becomes dark blue at the other end (representing minimum negative voltage), passing through intermediate gradations. However, any other color pair can be used, for instance, blackblue or blackgreen. With this two-color representation, however, there is a risk that in the areas where the voltage turns from positive to negative, the very light gradations of the two colors may appear as white, making it difficult to distinguish between the two polarities (see, for example, Fig. 3A).

In most cases, multiple color scales have been reported. Rather than a single hue gradually changing in saturation, different hues have been used to represent consecutive levels of the scale. With this solution, grasping the various levels of the measure scale proves to be straightforward. However, it also entails the substantial risk of giving the observer the impression that significant voltage variations have occurred when this is sometimes not true at all (see Fig. 4).

Because several research journals do not accept color maps, or simply wish to avoid the heavy printing costs involved, many electrophysiologists prefer to use a gray scale. As we saw, however, this has the disadvantage of not allowing any easy immediate identification of positive and negative zones, because it practically corresponds to a coding scheme based on a single color. The maps should thus be used for noninferential but exclusively descriptive purposes, and only after having carried out statistical analyses of the data measured in electrode subarrays. Or else considerable help may be obtained from any available algorithms for statistically analyzing the significance of possible topographic differences between two maps, thus allowing the t-Student or Fisher's F-value to be mapped, together with the relative statistical probability (or p-value), as shown by way of example in Fig. 4.

The greatest drawback of maps, however, is that they may give erroneous information concerning anatomical localization. This is for two main reasons. First, because of *volume conduction*, source currents flowing in a cluster of cells give rise to extracellular currents that spread throughout the conducting volume of the head and reach the scalp surface through the skull. Because the skull varies in thickness, depending on skull region, and has several apertures, it is not a homogeneous conductor. This may cause distortion in the translation of current onto the scalp, with consequent possible distortions in scalp topography. Second, with respect to tomographic techniques, for which anatomical resolution is solidly grounded on each pixel of the tomographic image, the spatial resolution of ERP maps depends on the number of electrodes used, which, however large, is always limited with respect to the total surface of the scalp. As a result, the resolution is also limited, especially when it is considered that a very high percentage (nearly 99%) of the pixels used in the reconstruction of an ERP map derives from an interpolation of the data from a small number of closely spaced electrodes. In this regard, the larger the number of electrodes used, the greater the resolution obtained. In any case, a large number of electrodes means high costs in terms, for example, of time of application, of the management of the quantity of data recorded, and of the interpretation of the data. In spite of this, a number of laboratories today use more than 128 electrodes.

Several algorithms have been developed for the recombination of ERP voltage values with 3D anatomical MRI in order to solve the problem of the localization of this voltage in the cortical brain areas. These algorithms require the 3D digitization of the spatial coordinates of the electrode positioning on the scalp of each individual subjected to recording, which will subsequently be used for the recombination of voltage pixels interpolated with pixels of the brain computed tomographic image.

RECORDING OF MAGNETIC FIELDS (MAGNETOENCEPHALOGRAPHY)

Flowing from their source along the neural pathways of the brain, potential fields give rise "online" to magnetic fields, orthogonal to the potential fields. The electrofunctional activation of the brain is then actually reflected by its electromagnetic counterparts. The magnetic fields are extremely weak—in the order of 0.4 gauss, amounting to 10^{-15} T—very much smaller than the potential fields, the latter being in the order of microvolts to 10^{-6} V. For this reason, only highly sensitive electronic devices are able to detect and record these magnetic signals in the form of a magnetoencephalogram (MEG).

This type of device is based on the use of highly sensitive magnetic sensors called *superconducting quantum interference devices* (SQUIDs), characterized by so-called Josephson's contacts and operating at very low temperatures, in the order of –273 C° (–460 F°). These temperatures are reached by maintaining the SQUID continuously dipped in liquid helium or nitrogen. Indeed, in order to achieve superconduction, the whole device is housed inside a superinsulated cryogenic columnar structure (see Fig. 5A) mounted on a nonmetallic supporting structure. The base of the cryogenic structure is shaped like a helmet that, in more sophisticated systems, may host up to 155 ultrasensitive sensors suitable for whole-head recordings. As shown in Fig. 5, the columnar structure housing the MEG probe consists of a superinsulated double-walled dewar. The space between the walls is maintained under vacuum to prevent heat diffusion and the surfaces facing toward the interior are made of heat-insulating material to maintain the liquid gases at low temperatures.

Unlike what has been described for ERPs, for the detection of *event-related fields* (ERFs) of the brain the sensors mounted on

A

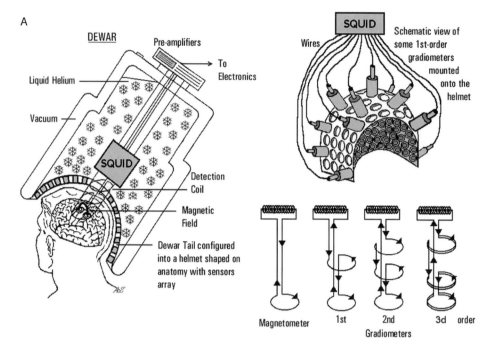

B

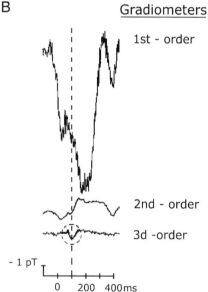

Gradiometers

1st - order

2nd - order

3d -order

- 1 pT

0   200   400 ms

FIGURE 5   (A) MEG cryostat and gradiometers. On the left, the superconducting quantum interfering device (SQUID) is shown dipped in liquid helium to guarantee the very low temperatures that allow superconductivity of the Josephson's contacts. The SQUID device is hosted within a superinsulated cryogenic columnar structure consisting of a superinsulated double-walled dewar, the base of which is configured into a helmet for whole-head recordings. On the right, a schematic view shows the features of the helmet, which has a shape based on head anatomy. Examples of some first-order gradiometers mounted on the helmet and connected to the SQUID are also portrayed. Below the helmet, flux transformers, or detection coils, are configured as a simple magnetometer or as progressively increasing nth-order gradiometers. Note how the gradiometers are constructed as increasingly complex coils and how the flux of the bias current fed through them reverts as it passes through the separate loops of the coils. (B) Output of MEG sensors. Progressive steps of the process of filtering and extraction for auditory ERFs. Conveying the signal through the progressive orders of software or hardware gradiometers allows the brain's event-related magnetic response to be enhanced.

the helmet at the bottom of the dewar do not have to be affixed directly to the scalp. In addition, the scalp does not have to be abraded to reduce skin resistance below optimal values. Instead, the magnetic sensors are simply maintained contiguous with the head, and located about 20 mm away from the head, thus making preparation and recording procedures very fast.

The SQUID detects the weak magnetic fields irradiating from the brain and converts them into electrical signals, which are much easier to measure. The electronic principle on which this conversion is based is that the current that mechanically transports the "quantum" through a weak bond (i.e., Josephson's contacts) in a small superconductor circuit is a function of the magnetic flux circulating through the circuit. The flow sensitivity of a modern SQUID can be as high as 20–30 Tm^2. To further increase its sensitivity, the SQUID is coupled to specially designed external circuits operating as flux transformers, known as detection coils. The simplest configuration for such transformers is a *magnetometer* (see Fig. 5A). This consists of a single loop of wire inductively connected to the SQUID, which detects the projections of the magnetic field along the loop.

Bearing in mind that brain magnetic fields are weak, and that many nonbiological sources of disturbance exist in the environment spatially uniform with respect to the magnetometer, it is possible to cancel out this environmental noise by building input coils with more complex configurations that respond only to the field spatial gradients. This configuration is called a *gradiometer*. Essentially, it consists of a flux transformer comprising a system of two or more subtractive loops. For hardware gradiometers, the coils may be connected to a single SQUID sensor, whereas software gradiometers are combined with signal digital filtering software routines. The linking of two magnetometers having opposite flow directions, and thus opposite polarities, goes to make up a "first-order gradiometer." Likewise, the linking of two first-order gradiometers of opposite polarity makes up a second-order gradiometer, and again, the linking of two second-order gradiometers of opposite polarity makes a third-order gradiometer. The latter is obtained by altering the distance between the coils in individual gradiometers (see Fig. 5A).

The passage of the field flux through the coils in the opposite direction cancels out more uniform fields generated by distant sources. The result is an absence of current in the gradiometer and of flow inside the SQUID. Instead, a magnetic field gradient varying in space will produce a current in the gradiometer that is equal to the difference across the opposite polarity fluxes in the various loops of the latter.

Conveying the signal through the various different progressive orders of software or hardware gradiometers allows the brain's spontaneous or event-related response to be extracted. This not only cancels out the environmental noise, but also rejects spurious signals in the order of picoteslas (1 pT = 10^{-12} T), stemming from the internal "milieu" (e.g., magnetic fields deriving from the myocardiac activity) and overlapping the aforementioned response. The steps of this progressive process of filtering and extraction for auditory *event-related fields* are shown in the example in Fig. 5B.

The pioneering investigations of MEG were carried out using a single gradiometer. It was thus extremely laborious to obtain a spatial map of the magnetic field. This was because the experimental paradigm had to be repeated many times while the gradiometer was moved over the different areas of the volunteer's head. Current commercial multichannel equipment has arrays consisting of tens of input coils, allowing whole-head recordings to be made during a single session (see Fig. 5A), even though an optimal signal-to-noise ratio is always obtained by averaging a large number of responses (for further information on modern MEG laboratory equipment, see Appendix C).

Once average ERFs have been obtained their sources may be estimated by then superimposing them on a topographical map of the field, as is done for ERPs. However, it is more satisfactory to use sophisticated computer algorithms to "merge" the estimated generators of the MEG signal with the 3D MRI images obtained from the same volunteer subjected to tomographic scanning. In order to achieve this merging, three or more landmark points (commonly, nasion and preauricular depressions) marked on the volunteer's head are used. Vitamin E capsules are placed on these landmark sites during MRI scans. Later on, during MEG recording, small coils are placed on the landmark sites as where the capsules were. The points thus marked provide a coordinate system centered on the volunteer's head in order to localize the position of the dewar probe and the gradiometers. Using computational transformations of coordinates provided by vitamin E capsules, MRI scans of the brain are first situated inside this system. Thanks to the coil-based coordinates, the MEG sources, or dipoles, can then be laid over the MRI scans, as can be observed in the image shown in Fig. 6. Further examples of this superimposition can be found in this volume in the outstanding reviews of MEG findings on visual (Chapter 5) and auditory (Chapter 14) cognition.

Before concluding this overview of MEG recording methods it is important to again

stress that, as partly anticipated in Chapter 2 and at the beginning of this section, ERP and MEG techniques are complementary and both present advantages and disadvantages. The maximum progress in our knowledge of the brain's functional activity can thus certainly be obtained only by using a combination of both recording techniques. Although still very expensive, this combination is currently made easier by the fact than many commercial MEG systems now allow the simultaneous recording of both MEG fields and ERPs, thus providing integrated amplification systems for the recording of both potentials together with only MEG equipment.

RECRUITMENT OF VOLUNTEERS

The recruitment of volunteers to participate in brain wave recording studies must be monitored very carefully in order to avoid the likelihood of interindividual

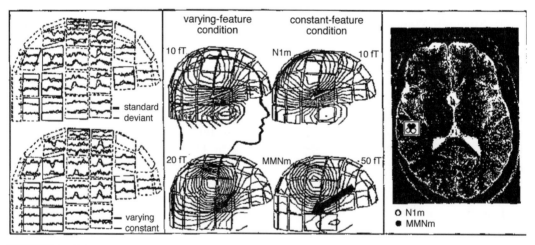

FIGURE 6 Successive steps of the superimposition of MEG dipoles over an axial MRI image of the brain for a single volunteer. Left: Examples of averaged event-related fields to standard and deviant tones in the varying-feature condition (top) and subtraction wave forms in the varying- and constant-feature conditions (bottom). Middle: isocontour field maps for N1m and MMMm, recorded in both conditions and viewed from the right-hemisphere, with superimposed equivalent current dipoles (represented by the arrows). Right: The equivalent dipoles are localized on the right hemisphere of the MRI image. Note that they are reported on the left of the brain image because by convention this is viewed from below. Reprinted from *NeuroReport* 4; M. Huotilainen, R. J. Ilmoniemi, J.Lavikainen, H. Tititen, K. Alho, J. Sinkkonen, J. Knuutila, and R. Näätänen; Interaction between representations of different features of auditory sensory memory, pp. 1279–1281. Copyright (1993) with kind permission from Oxford Ltd. and Dr. Huotilainen.

variability due to differences in anatomical and functional brain organization of various individuals; these differences may have a greater effect on ERPs than do the experimental factors of interest.

Before dealing with factors related to the recruitment of participants, a few words must be said about how to refer to volunteers. The term "experimental subject" is considered disrespectful of the human personality (see the guidelines of the *Society for Neuroscience* on the bioethics of human experimentation). The term "participants" or "volunteers" is preferred as being more respectful and more correct. [Oddly, in the guidelines of Picton *et al.* (2000) for using human event-related potentials to study cognition, the term "subjects" was extensively used.] Similarly, the use of pronouns (*he, him*) or masculine nouns (e.g., "in man") to indicate individuals of both genders should be avoided. The awkward effect due to the repeated use of the she/he formula can be avoided, for example, by using pronouns in their plural form (*they*).

It is fundamental to gather a homogeneous sample of participants when hemispheric asymmetries and handedness are concerned, in order to avoid statistical false negatives due to a misleading mixing of individuals with left- and right-sided brain asymmetries, causing a "washing out" effect. To keep this independent variable under control, prior to recording, the lateral dominance of the eye, the foot, and the hand must be measured by means of suitable motor tasks or written self-questionnaires [for example, the well-known laterality questionnaire by Oldfield (1971)]. Additionally, control should be exerted over volunteers' morningness–eveningness preference by means of self-questionnaires, such as the one by Horne and Ostberg (1976). These traits are pervasively influential, with different diurnal phases over the day, both on overt performance and psychophysiological functions (e.g., Mecacci *et al.*, 1984; Zani, 1986). Furthermore, somehow control

should be exerted over volunteers' longer span biological rhythms (e.g., Zani, 1989) as well as cognitive skills (Zani and Rossi, 1990, 1991).

In general, it is advisable to draw samples from a population as homogenous as possible in terms of age, handedness, educational level, and gender. Because gender affects many electrophysiological measurements, experimenters should generally use an equal number of female and male subjects, or subjects of one gender only.

Unless investigating brain aging or ontogenetic development, when the aim of the investigation is the study of normal cognitive brain functions in average young adults, it is advisable to test individuals in the age range of 18–40 years. In fact, before the age of 18 the frontal executive control function is still somewhat immature, whereas after the age of 40 the beginning of a faint slowing down of brain responses may be observed.

Naturally, it is crucial for participants to be able to perceive the stimuli properly. The experimenter should make sure that they have normal hearing (at 20 dB HL), normal or glasses-corrected vision, normal acuity, and color vision. Again, they should not have suffered from cranial traumas followed by coma, and should not be affected by any psychiatric syndrome (unless the study is aimed directly at individuals suffering from such syndromes, or specified groups of people with psychomotor handicaps). The investigator should also make sure that the participants are not taking prescription medications that may affect cognitive processes, and are not under the influence of alcohol or recreational drugs.

In general, it is recommended that the total number of participants recruited, which should be large enough to represent a given population, along with the mean and range of the ages of the participants, be provided in scientific reports. It is also essential to obtain the informed consent of human participants involved in any kind of experimentation (Picton *et al.*, 2000).

References and Suggested Reading

General Normative Guidelines for Using Human EEG–ERP Recordings in Research

Picton, T. W., Bentin, S., Berg, P., Donchin, E., Hillyard, S. A., Johnson, R., Miller, G. A., Ritter, W., Ruchkin, D. S., Rugg, M. D., and Taylor, M. J. (2000). Guidelines for using human event-related potentials to study cognition: Recording standards and publication criteria. *Psychophysiology* 37, 127–52.

Pivick, R. T., Broughton, R. J., Coppola, R., Davidson, R. J., Fox, N., and Nuwer, M. R. (1993). Guidelines for recording and quantitative analysis of electroencephalographic activity in research contexts. *Psychophysiology* 30, 547–558.

Basic General Techniques in Psychophysiology

Cacioppo, J. T., and Tassinary, L. G., and Bernston, G. G. (eds.) (2000). "Handbook of Psychophysiology," 2nd Ed. Cambridge University Press, Cambridge.

Coles, M. G. H., Donchin, E., and Porges, S. W. (1986). "Psychophysiology: Systems, Processes and Applications." Guilford Press, New York.

Hugdahl, K. (1995). "Psychophysiology. The Mind–Body Perspective." Harvard University Press, Cambridge, Massachusetts.

Martin, I., and Venables, P. H. (1980). "Techniques in Psychophysiology." John Wiley & Sons, Chichester.

Stern, R. M., Ray, W. J., and Davis, C. M. (1980). "Psychophysiological Recording." Oxford University Press, New York and Oxford.

Fundamentals of EEG and ERP Technology

Barrett, G. (1986). Analytic techniques in the estimation of evoked potentials. *In* "Handbook of EEG and Clinical Neurophysiology", Vol.2, Clinical Applications of Computer Analysis of EEG and Other Neurophysiological Signals" (F. H. Lopes da Silva, W. Storm Van Leeuwen, and A. Rémond, eds.), pp. 311–333. Elsevier, Amsterdam.

Davidson, R. J., Jackson, D., and Larson, C. L. (2000). Human electroencephalography. *In* "Handbook of Psychophysiology" (J. T. Cacioppo, L. G. Tassinary, and G. Berntson, eds.), pp. 27–52. Cambridge University Press, Cambridge.

Eimer, M. (1998). Methodological issues in event-related brain potential research. *Behav. Res. Methods Instrum. Comput.* 30, 3–7.

International Federation of Societies for Electroencephalography and Clinical Neuropsychology (1974). A glossary of terms commonly used by clinical electroencephalographers. *Electroencephalog. Clin. Neurophysiol.* 37, 538–548.

Nuwer, M. R. (1988). Quantitative EEG: I. Techniques and problems of frequency analysis and topographic mapping. *J. Clin. Neurophysiol.* 4, 321–326.

Srinivasan, R., Tucker, D. M., and Murias, M. (1998). Estimating the spatial Nyquist of the human EEG. *Beh. Res. Methods Instrum. Comput.* 30, 8–19.

Tyner, F. S., Knott, J. R., Mayer, W. B. (1983). "Fundamentals of EEG Technology. Vol. 1, Basic Concepts and Methods." Raven Press, New York.

Zappulla, R. A. (1991). Fundamentals and applications of quantified electrophysiology. *Ann. N.Y. Acad. Sci.* 620, 1–21.

Electrode Placement Systems for Topographic Investigation

American Electroencephalographic Society (1991). Guidelines for standard electrode position nomenclature. *J. Clin. Neurophysiol.* 8, 200–201.

Chatrian, G. E., Lettich, E., and Nelson, P. L. (1985). Ten percent electrode system for topographic studies of spontaneous and evoked EEG activities. *Am. J. Electroencephalogr. Technol.* 25, 83–92.

Jasper, H. H. (1958). The ten–twenty electrode system of the International Federation. *EEG Clin. Neurophysiol.* 10, 371–375.

Myslobodsky, M. S., Coppola, R., Bar-Ziv, J., and Weinberger, D. R. (1990). Adeguacy of the international 10–20 electrode system for computed neurophysiologic topography. *J. Clin. Neurophysiol.* 7, 507–518.

Nuwer, M. R. (1987). Recording electrode nomenclature. *J. Clin. Neurophysiol.* 4, 121–133.

Anatomical Location of EEG Electrodes

Homan, R. W., Herman, J., and Purdy, P. (1987). Cerebral location of international 10–20 system electrode placement. *EEG Clin. Neurophysiol.* 66, 376–382.

Artifact Rejection and Minimization Methods

Barlow, J. S. (1986). Artifact processing (rejection and minimization) in EEG data processing. *In* "Handbook of EEG and Clinical Neurophysiology, Vol. 2, Clinical Applications of Computer Analysis of EEG and Other Neurophysiological Signals" (F. H. Lopes da Silva, W. Storm Van Leeuwen, and A. Rémond, eds.), pp. 15–62. Elsevier, Amsterdam.

EEG Averaging

Dawson, G. D. (1951). A summation technique for detecting small signals in a large irregular background. *J. Physiol.* (Lond.) 115, 2–3.

Regan, D. (1989). "Human Brain Electrophysiology. Evoked Potentials and Evoked Magnetic Fields in Science and Medicine." Elsevier, Amsterdam.

Basic Principles of Digital Filtering

Cook III, E. W., and Miller, G. A. (1992). Digital filtering: Background and tutorial for psychophysiologists. *Psychophysiology* **29**, 350–367.

Farwell, L. A., Martinerie, J. M., Bashore, T. R., Rapp, P. E., and Goddard, P. H. (1993). Optimal digital filters for long-latency components of the event-related potentials. *Psychophysiology* **30**, 306–315.

Ruchkin, D. S. (1988). Measurement of event-related potentials: Signal extraction. *In* "Handbook of Electroencephalography and Clinical Neurophysiology" (D. Otto, ed.), Vol. 3, pp. 7–43. Elsevier, Amsterdam.

Mapping

Coppola, R. (1990). Topographic mapping of multi-lead data. *In* "Event-Related Brain Potentials" (J. W. Rohrbaugh, R. Johnson, and R. Parasuraman, eds.), pp. 37–43. Oxford University Press, Oxford.

Duffy, F. H. (1989). Topographic mapping of brain electrical activity: Clinical applications and issues. *In* "Topographic Brain Mapping of EEG and Evoked Potentials" (K. Maurer, ed.), pp. 19–52. Springer-Verlag, New York.

Hassainia, F., Medina, V., Donadey, A., and Langevin, F. (1994). Scalp potential and current density mapping with an enhanced spherical spline interpolation. *Med. Prog. Technol.* **20**, 23–30.

Kahn, E. M., Weiner, R. D., Brenner, R. P., and Coppola, R. (1988). Topographic maps of brain electrical activity—Pitfalls and precautions. *Biol. Psychiatr.* **23**, 628–636.

Perrin, F., Bertrand, O., and Pernier, J. (1987). Scalp current density mapping: Value and estimation from potential data. *Biomed. Eng.* **34**, 283–288.

Perrin F., Pernier J., Bertrand O., and Echallier J. F. (1989). Spherical splines for scalp potential and current density mapping. *Electroncephalogr. Clin. Neurophysiol.* **72**, 184–187.

Best EEG Reference for Mapping

MacGillivray, B. B., and Sawyers, F. J. P. (1988). A comparison of common reference, average and source derivations in mapping. *In* "Statistics and Topography in Quantitative EEG" (D. Samson-Dollfus, J. D. Guieu, J. Gotman, and P. Etevenon, eds.), pp. 72–87. Elsevier, Amsterdam.

Pioneering Interpolation Method for Signal Mapping

Buchsbaum, M. S., Rigal, F., Coppola, R., Cappelletti, J., King, C., and Johnson, J. (1982). A new system for gray-level surface distribution maps of electrical activity. *Electroencephalogr. Clin. Neurophysiol.* **53**, 237–242.

Pitfalls and Problems with Mapping

Lopes Da Silva, F. H. (1990). A critical review of clinical applications of topographic mapping of brain potentials. *J. Clin. Neurophysiol.* **7 (4)**, 535–551.

Perrin, F., Bertrand, O., Giard, M. H., and Pernier, J. (1990). Precautions in topographic mapping and in evoked potential map reading. *J. Clin. Neurophysiol.* **7 (4)**, 498–506.

Dipoles and Brain Sources

De Munck, J. C., Van Dijk, B. W., and Speckreijse, H. (1988). Mathematical dipoles are adequate to describe realistic generators of human brain activity. *IEEE Trans. Biomed. Eng.* BME **35**, 950–966.

Scherg, M., and Ebersole, J. S. (1993). Models of brain sources. *Brain Topogr.* **5**, 419–423.

Scherg, M., Vajsar, J., and Picton, T. W. (1989). A source analysis of the late human auditory evoked potentials. *J. Cogn. Neurosci.* **4**, 336–355.

Combining Electrophysiological and Hemodynamic Signals

Gevins, A., Brickett, P., Costales, B., Le, J., and Reutter, B. (1990). Beyond topographic mapping: Towards functional-anatomical imaging with 124-channel EEG and 3-D MRIs. *Brain Topogr.* **3**, pp. 53–64.

Gevins, A., Le, J., Brickett, P., Reutter, B., and Desmond, J. (1991). Seeing through the skull: Advanced EEGs use MRIs to accurately measure cortical activity from the scalp. *Brain Topogr.* **4**, 125–131.

McCarthy, G. (1999). Event-related potentials and functional MRI: A comparison of localization in sensory, perceptual and cognitive tasks. *In* "Functional Neuroscience: Evoked Potentials and Magnetic Fields. The 6th International Evoked Potential Symposium" (C. Barber, G. G. Celesia, I. Hashimoto, and R. Kakigi, eds.), pp. 3–12. Elsevier, Amsterdam.

Scherg, M. (1992). Functional imaging and localization of electromagnetic brain activity. *Brain Topogr.* **5**, 103–111.

Use of Statistics in Electrophysiology and Map Comparisons

Hassainia, F., Petit, D., and Montplaisir, J. (1994). Significance probability mapping: The final touch in t-statistics mapping. *Brain Mapping* **7**, 3–8.

John, E. R., Harmony, T., and Valdes-Sosa, P. (1987). The use of statistics in electrophysiology. *In* "Handbook of EEG and Clinical Neurophysiology, Vol. 1, Methods of Analysis of Brain Electrical and

Magnetic Signals" (A. S. Gevins and A. Rémond, eds.), pp. 497–540. Elsevier, Amsterdam.

McCarthy, G., and Wood, C. (1985). Scalp distribution of event-related potentials: An ambiguity associated with analysis of variance models. *Electroencephalogr. Clin. Neurophysiol.* **62**, 203–208.

MEG Recording: Principles and Methods

Del Gratta, C., and Romani, G. L. (1999). MEG: Principles, methods, and applications. *Biomed. Technik* **44** (Suppl. 2), 11–23.

Hari, R., and Lounasmaa, O. V. (1989). Recording and interpretation of cerebral magnetic fields. *Science* **244**, 432–436.

Huotilainen, M., Ilmoniemi, R. J., Lavikainen, J., Tititen, H., Alho, K., Sinkkonen, J., Knuutila, J., and Näätänen, R. (1993). Interaction between representations of different features of auditory sensory memory. *NeuroReport* **4**, 1279–1281.

Josephson, B. D. (1962). Possible new effects in superconductive tunneling. *Phys. Rev. Lett.* **1**, 251.

Näätänen, R., Ilmoniemi, R. J., and Alho K. (1994). Magnetoencephalography in studies of human cognitive brain function. *Trends Neurosci.* **17**, 389–395.

Romani, G. L., and Rossini, P. (1988). Neuromagnetic functional localization: Principles, state of the art, and perspectives. *Brain topogr.* **1**, 5–21.

Vrba, J. (1996). SQUID gradiometers in real environments. *In* "SQUID Sensors: Fundamentals, Fabrication and Application" (H. Weinstock, ed.), pp. 117–178. Kluwer Academic Publisher, New York.

Wieringa, H. J. (1993). "MEG, EEG and the Integration with Magnetic Resonance Images." Doctoral Thesis, CIP-Gegevens Koninklijke Bibliotheek, Den Haag.

Volunteer Recruitment

Horne, J. A., and Ostberg, O. (1976). A self-assessment questionnaire to determine morningness–eveningness in human circadian rhythms. *Int. J. Chronobiol.* **4**, 97–110.

Mecacci, L., Misiti, R., and Zani, A. (1984). The relevance of morningness–eveningness typology in human factor research: A review. *In* "Human Factors in Organizational Designs and Management" (H. W. Hendrick, and O. Brown, Jr., eds.), pp. 503–509. Elsevier, Amsterdam.

Oldfield, R. C. (1971). Assessment and analysis of handedness: The Edinburgh inventory. *Neuropsychologia* **9**, 97–113.

Zani, A. (1986). Time of day preference, pattern evoked potentials and hemispheric asymmetries: A preliminary statement. *Percept. Motor Skills* **63**, 413–414.

Zani, A. (1989). Brain evoked responses reflect information processing changes with the menstrual cycle in young female athletes. *J. Sport Med. Physical Fitness* **29**, 113–121.

Zani, A., and Rossi, B. (1990). Differences in attentional style in skeet and trap shooters: An Event-related brain potential study. *In* "AIESEP'88 World Congress on Humanism and New Technology in Physical Education in Sport" (J. Duran, J. L. Hernandez, and L. M. Ruiz, eds.), pp. 325–329. INEF, Madrid.

Zani, A., and Rossi, B. (1991). Cognitive psychophysiology as an interface between cognitive and sport psychology. *Int. J. Sport Psychol.* **22**, 376–398.

Topographical Analysis of Electrical Brain Activity: Methodological Aspects

Wolfgang Skrandies

INTRODUCTION

In general, human electrophysiological studies have to rely on noninvasive measurements of mass activity originating from many neurons simultaneously (the only exception being intracranial recordings in patients before surgery for epilepsy or during tumor removal). The basis for scalp recordings is the propagation of field potentials, originating in large neuronal populations, through volume conduction. For brain activity to be detected at some distance by large electrodes, many neurons must be activated synchronously, and only activity originating from "open" intracranial electrical fields can be assessed by scalp recordings. In contrast to this, "closed" electrical fields are formed by populations of neurons arranged so that electrical activity cancels. This constellation is found in many subcortical structures that consequently are inaccessible to distant mass recordings. The major neuronal sources for electrical activity on the scalp are the pyramidal cells located in the cortical layers, arranged in parallel perpendicular to the cortical surface, which, however, is folded in intricate ways so that the generators cannot be assumed to be perpendicular to the outer surface of the brain. The study of evoked (or so-called event-related) activity aims at elucidating different brain mechanisms, and it allows assessment of sensory or cognitive processing while the participant or patient is involved in perceptual or cognitive tasks.

As in most neurophysiological experiments, topographical analysis of electrical brain activity is used in order to detect covariations between experimental conditions manipulated by the investigator and features of the recorded brain activity. Evoked scalp potential fields yield information on a number of partly independent neurophysiological parameters such as component latency, which indicates neural processing time, or field strength, which indexes the amount of synchronous activation of a neuronal population engaged in stimulus processing or during the execution of cognitive tasks.

Measures derived from such data are used as unambiguous descriptors of the electrical brain activity, and they have been employed successfully to study visual information processing in humans (Skrandies, 1987, 1995, 2002). The aim of evoked potential (or event-related potential) studies is to identify subsets or so-called components of electrical brain activity that are defined in terms of latency with respect to some external or internal event and in terms of topographical scalp distribution patterns. Irrespective of whether the exact intracranial generator populations can be determined, the interpretation of scalp potential data combined with knowledge of the anatomy and physiology of the human central nervous system may allow drawing useful physiological interpretations (Skrandies, 2002; see also Chapter 3, this volume). Scalp topography is taken as a means to characterize electrical brain activity objectively in terms of latency, neural response strength, and scalp location. Comparison of scalp potential fields obtained in different experimental conditions (e.g., different physical stimulus parameters, different subjective or psychological states, or normal vs. pathological neurophysiological traits) may be used to test hypotheses on the identity or nonidentity of the neuronal populations activated in these conditions. Identical scalp potential fields may or may not be generated by identical neuronal populations, whereas nonidentical potential fields must be caused by different intracranial generator mechanisms. Thus, we can study noninvasively systematic variations of the electrical brain activity, and we are interested in variations of scalp potential fields caused by the manipulation of independent experimental parameters.

The basic ideas on topographical mapping are similar irrespective of whether spontaneous electroencephalogram (EEG) or event-related brain activity is considered. Here we are concerned only with the analysis of the scalp distribution of evoked electrical brain activity, with only little consideration of the underlying neural structures. [For a review on the localization of intracranial processes and human electrophysiological signals (EEG and event-related brain activity), the reader is referred to Skrandies (2001).]

With modern imaging techniques [computed tomography (CT), structural or functional magnetic resonance imaging (fMRI), or positron emission tomography (PET)],

the determination of anatomical brain structures or of hemodynamical responses to different processing demands is available at high spatial resolution, but typically has to rely on longer integration times in order to derive significant signals that reflect changes in metabolic responses. Different from brain imaging methods such as fMRI or PET, noninvasive electrophysiological measurements of spontaneous EEG and evoked potential fields [or measurements of the accompanying magnetic fields by magnetoencephalography (MEG)] possess high temporal resolution, in the order of milliseconds, and techniques to quantify electric brain topography are unsurpassed when functional validity is required in order to characterize central nervous processing in humans. In addition, electrical measurements are relatively easy and inexpensive to perform, and offer the possibility to assess brain function directly in real-life situations, without referring to indirect comparisons between experimental states and neutral base line conditions or between different task demands.

REASONS FOR TOPOGRAPHIC BRAIN MAPPING AND BASIC IDEAS

Electrophysiological data are recorded from discrete points on the scalp against some reference point, and conventionally have been analyzed as time series of potential differences between pairs of recording points. Multichannel recordings allow assessment of the topographical distribution of brain electrical activity. For imaging, wave form patterns are transformed to displays reflecting the electrical landscape of brain activity at discrete time points or for different frequency content of the recorded EEG signals. The results of a topographical transformation are maps that show the scalp distribution of brain activity at discrete time points or for selected frequencies of the spontaneous EEG. Such functional imaging (1) possesses the high degree of time resolution needed to study brain processes, (2) allows charac-terization of sequences of activation patterns, and (3) is very sensitive to state changes and processing demands of the organism.

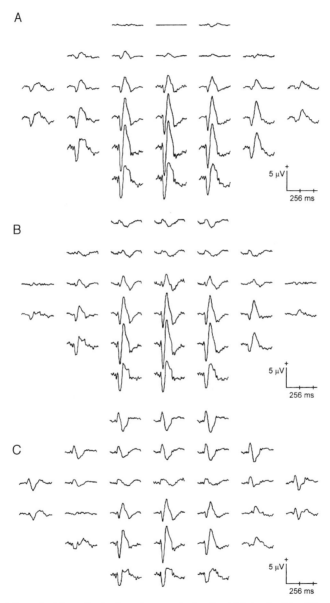

FIGURE 1 Potentials evoked by a checkerboard reversal stimulus (60' checks, 14 × 18° test field, 95% contrast) recorded from 30 electrodes over the occipital and parietal areas (see electrode scheme in Fig. 2). The same data set was computed offline for different reference electrodes. A frontal electrode in the midline (A), linked mastoids (B), or the average reference (C) yields small but significant changes in the pattern of wave forms at all recording electrodes. Note how amplitudes and latencies of all peaks differ with different reference electrodes. The calibration bars correspond to 256 msec (horizontally) and 5 μV (vertically); positive is up. Data from a healthy volunteer with normal vision.

Conventionally, electrophysiological data were displayed and analyzed as many univariate time series. Only the technical possibility of simultaneous acquisition of data in multichannel recordings allowed for the treatment of EEG data as potential distributions (Lehmanan and Skrandies, 1984; Skrandies, 1983, 1986, 1987). The strength of mapping of brain activity lies not only in the display of brain activation in a topographical form, but mapping is a prerequisite of an adequate analysis of brain activity patterns. Because EEG and evoked potentials are recorded as potential differences between recording sites, the location of a reference point will drastically influence the shape of activity recorded over time. The basic properties of scalp potential maps and adequate topographical analysis avoid the fruitless discussion about an electrically neutral reference point.

When data are recorded in many channels, at each electrode an evoked potential wave form is obtained. Figure 1 illustrates conventional checkerboard reversal visual evoked potentials (VEPs) recorded from 30 electrodes overlying the occipital and parietal brain regions. Over the occipital areas, the wave forms clearly display a negative component at about 70 msec followed by the classical P100 component occurring at a latency of about 100 msec. It is important to note that the form of the recorded activity is directly determined by the choice of the recording reference: in Fig. 1A

a frontal reference was used—a choice that is common in many laboratories when visual evoked brain activity is recorded. Of course, linked mastoids may also be employed, yielding a pattern of activity shown in Fig. 1B. Note that these are the same data, because only the reference point has been changed. Again the VEPs are dominated by two components; however, comparison to Fig. 1A reveals subtle but significant differences. Another widely used recording method is the average reference, whereby the mean of all electrodes is computed as a reference value at each time point. The resulting 30 wave forms are illustrated in Fig. 1C. As mentioned above, in this figure we are dealing with identical data seen from different view points—the evoked brain response, of course, is independent of the choice of the recording reference. The search for a so-called inactive reference point has no practical solution because evoked potential wave forms always constitute measurements of the continuously fluctuating potential gradients between two points, whether both on the scalp or not (see also Nunez, 1981).

It is evident that from identical data, different conclusions can be derived. In evoked potential research, conventional amplitude and latency measures are treated as independent variables, but from comparison of the wave forms in Fig. 1A–C, it is obvious that all amplitudes change, depending on the recording refer-

TABLE 1   P100 Latencies Measured at Five Different Electrodes[a]

Reference electrode	Recording channel				
	12	17	21	27	29
Midfrontal (Fig. 1A)	104	112	110	112	112
Linked mastoids (Fig. 1B)	102	100	108	112	102
Average reference (Fig. 1C)	80	96	110	120	102

[a]Identical data are analyzed with different reference electrodes (evoked potential data illustrated in Fig. 1). The values are peak latencies (in milliseconds); the electrode recording channel numbers refer to the electrode scheme shown in Fig. 2.

ence. In addition, the latency of a given component appears to be different. As a practical example, analysis of the amplitude peaks of channels 12, 17, 21, 27, and 29 results in significantly different P100 peak latencies, as illustrated in Table 1.

In this restricted set of electrodes, component latencies range between 80 and 120 msec. Of course, reality is even more complex because the data have been recorded in many channels. When 30 scalp electrodes are used for recording, 870 different wave forms may be obtained (435 of these are sign inverted), and many more apparently different components emerge. We also note that none of the electrode locations can be privileged as reference electrode, because there is no inactive point available (Nunez, 1981), and each of the 30 electrodes may be determined to serve as recording reference. It is impossible to evaluate such extensive data sets that contain redundant information by simple visual inspection or by wave shape comparisons, and thus the analysis of electrical activity must not deal with reference-dependent potential wave forms. The example in Fig. 1 demonstrates that conventional analysis of evoked brain activity recorded simultaneously in many channels will always result in a confusing number of individual component latencies that cannot be interpreted in a physiologically meaningful way [see also Figs. 3, 4, and 5 in Skrandies (1987), for further illustration]. Of course, all data sets illustrated in Fig. 1 carry identical information; changes of the reference does not change the underlying neural process but only the appearance of the curves. This is not obvious from Fig. 1 because the polarity and the latencies of all individual peaks may change drastically. It is also virtually impossible to see that the data of Fig. 1 represent an identical data set: with linked mastoids as reference an occipital positivity is seen around 100 msec (P100 component), which however, shows a latency range between 98 and 122 msec among the 15 most posterior channels.

With a frontal reference, all peak latencies are different, ranging from 106 to 130 msec. In a similar line, the N70 component has peak latencies between 70 and 90 msec for the linked mastoid reference, whereas the frontal reference yields latency values between 66 and 72 msec. Some of the changes may appear small. In clinical applications, however, latency differences of only a few milliseconds may determine a given patient's data as pathological. Thus small alterations may attain great importance; also, for physiological questions, time differences in the order of milliseconds are important (Skrandies, 1987).

For the analysis of the topographical aspects of electroencephalographic activity it is important to keep in mind that we are dealing with electrical fields originating in brain structures whose characteristics vary with recording time and space: the position of the electrodes on the scalp determines the pattern of activity recorded, and multichannel EEG and evoked potential data enable us to analyze topographically the electrical fields that are reconstructed from many spatial sampling points. From a neurophysiological point of view, evoked components are generated by the activation of neural assemblies located in certain brain regions with certain geometric configurations. Landscapes of electrical brain activity may give much more information than conventional wave form analysis that stresses only restricted aspects of the available electrical data (Lehmann, 1987; Skrandies, 1986, 1987).

As a response to visual stimulation the brain generates an electrical field that originates from neuronal assemblies in the visual cortex. This electrical field changes in strength and topography over time, and the data of Fig. 1 are displayed as series of potential distributions in Fig. 2. These maps simply show the potential distribution within the recording array at various time points after stimulation (between 40 and 190 msec after the presentation of a visual stimulus). At each latency time a

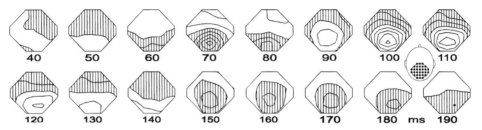

FIGURE 2   The data of Fig. 1 illustrated as maps series between 40 and 190 msec after stimulus reversal. Recordings were obtained from 30 electrodes over the occipital areas (see head inset). Lines are in steps of 1.0 μV; hatched areas are negative with respect to the average reference.

characteristic topography is elicited. Note that the structure of each map does not change when a different recording reference is employed: all topographical features remain identical when the electrical landscape is viewed from different points, similar to the constant relief of a geographical map, where the sea level is arbitrarily defined as zero level. The locations of maxima and minima, as well as the locations and strengths of potential gradients in a given map, are independent of the reference point that defines zero. It is obvious that the topography as well as the strength of the electrical field change as a function of time. Around 70 msec, or between 100 and 120 msec, the field relief is pronounced: there are high voltage peaks and troughs, associated with steep potential gradients. Obviously these time instances indicate strong synchronous activation of neurons in the visual cortex.

The maps in Fig. 2 are potential maps that were reconstructed from data recorded from the electrode array shown in the inset. The 30 electrodes are distributed as a regular grid over the brain regions under study. Because only potential differences within the scalp field are of interest, all data are referred to the computed average reference. This procedure results in a spatial high-pass filter, eliminating the direct current offset potential introduced by the necessary choice of some point as recording reference. In order to interpret the topographic patterns, more detailed analysis is needed. It is important to keep

in mind that the absolute locations of the potential maxima or potential minima in the field do not necessarily reflect the locations of the underlying generators. This fact has led to confusion in the interpretation of EEG data. A striking example for visual evoked activity is the phenomenon known as paradoxical lateralization (see below). Rather than potential maxima, the location of steep potential gradients appears to be a more adequate parameter, reflecting intracranial source locations (Skrandies, 2002).

MAPPING OF BRAIN ACTIVITY AND DEFINITION OF COMPONENTS

Topographical analyses should not be restricted to the qualitative graphical display of maps at many time points, instead of conventional time series at many recording points. It is mandatory that quantitative methods are applied to multichannel EEG and evoked potential data in order to extract relevant information from such maps series. In the following discussion, methods for quantitative topographical data analysis are illustrated, and it is shown how field strength, component latency, and topography can be used to quantify electrical brain activity.

Mapping of electrical brain activity in itself does not constitute an analysis of the recorded data, but it is a prerequisite to extract unambiguously quantitative features of the scalp recorded electrical activity. In a second step of data analysis the derived topographical measures must be employed to test statistically differences between experimental conditions or between groups of subjects.

For the analysis of evoked brain activity one of the main goals is the identification of so-called components that are commonly interpreted as steps of information processing. Multichannel recordings of electrical activity result in a large amount of data: mapping of potentials evoked by a simple checkerboard reversal stimulus sampled at 500 Hz in 30 channels over an epoch of 256 msec results in 3840 individual amplitude values. Of course, not each of these amplitude measures attains physiological meaningfulness. As is evident from the maps shown in Fig. 2, there occur potential field distributions with only very little activity (few field lines, shallow gradients between 40 and 60 msec, or at 140 msec), whereas at other latency times maps display high peaks and deep troughs with large potential gradients in the potential field distributions (at 70 or at 100 msec in Fig. 2).

It appears reasonable to define component latency as the occurrence time of maximal activity in the electrical field reflecting synchronous activation of a maximal number of intracranial neuronal elements. In order to quantify the amount of activity in a given scalp potential field we have proposed a measure of "global field power" (GFP), which is computed as the mean of all possible potential differences in the field corresponding to the standard deviation of all recording electrodes with respect to the average reference (Lehmann and Skrandies, 1984). Scalp potential fields with steep gradients and pronounced peaks and troughs will result in high global field power, whereas global field power is low in electrical fields with only shallow gradients that have a flat appearance. Thus, the maximum in a plot of global field power over time determines component latency. In a second step the features of the scalp potential field are analyzed at these component latencies. Derived measures, such as location of potential maxima and minima, and steepness and orientation of gradients in the field are by definition independent of the reference electrode, and they will give an adequate description of the electrical brain activity.

Global field power is computed as the mean potential deviation of all electrodes in the recording array (see Fig. 3). With an array of equidistant electrodes on the scalp surface, the potentials e_i, $i = 1, ..., n$, yield the measured voltages $U_i = e_i - e_{\text{common reference}}$. From this potential distribution at one time instant, a reference-independent measure of GFP is computed as the mean of all potential differences within the field

$$GFP = \sqrt{\frac{1}{2n} \sum_{i=1}^{n} \sum_{j=1}^{n} (U_i - U_j)^2}$$

(1)

GFP corresponds to the root-mean-square amplitude deviations between all electrodes of a given array recording the electrical field. Note that this measure is not influenced by the choice of the reference electrode, and allows for a reference-

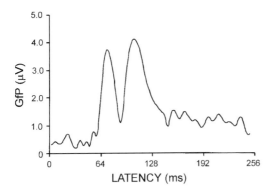

FIGURE 3 Global field power (GFP) as a function of poststimulus time computed on the data shown in Fig. 2. Field strength displays maxima at 76 and 108 msec, defining component latencies.

independent treatment of electrophysiological data.

In a similar way, GFP may be computed for EEG data referred to the average reference:

$$GFP = \sqrt{\sum_{i=1}^{n}\left(U_i - \frac{1}{n}\sum_{j=1}^{n}U_j\right)^2}$$

(2)

This is mathematically equivalent to the formula shown in Eq. (1).

Equations (1) and (2) illustrate that GFP reflects the spatial standard deviation within each map (i.e., at a given instant): pronounced potential fields with high peaks and troughs and steep gradients are associated with high GFP values whereas with flat fields GFP is small. Field strength as determined by GFP results in a single number at each latency point, and it may be plotted as a function of time. This illustrates how field strength varies over time, and the occurrence of its maximum value in a predetermined time window can be used in order to determine component latency. It is important to note that all recording electrodes contribute equally to the computation of GFP, and that at each time point it results in one value that is independent of the reference electrode that was used for recording. In this way the problems of conventional wave shape analysis are avoided.

High global field power also coincides with periods of stable potential field configurations when the spatial characteristics of the fields remain unchanged. Figure 3 illustrates GFP as a function of time, and it is evident that two components occur at 76 and at 108 msec. The brain's response to the visual stimulus resulted in electrical field distributions with maximal activity at these time points. In this way, component latency is defined topographically and independent of the reference electrode. For further topographical analysis, latency, field strength, or the complete potential fields at component latency may be compared directly between experimental conditions or between groups of subjects.

All of these derived measures can be submitted to statistical analysis and can be interpreted in a physiological context: component latency may be equated with neural processing time, whereas field strength is an index of the amount of synchronous activation or the spatial extent of a neuronal population engaged in stimulus processing. In addition, derived measures can be used to quantify the topography of potential fields. One useful parameter for the definition of topographical characteristics is the location of the centers of gravity (centroids) for the positive and negative areas within each potential field. These locations consider the information of all recording points in a given map, and they constitute a meaningful data reduction that can then be treated with statistical methods. An example is given in Fig. 4. Visual brain activity elicited by checkerboard reversal stimulation with stimuli presented to the fovea or in the left or right visual field was recorded in 30 channels from 22 healthy volunteers. Three different components were identified by the occurrence of maximal field strength (GFP) at 78.2, 118.2, and 186.7 msec latency, and the mean locations of the positive and negative centers of gravity are displayed. Because lateral visual stimuli were also employed, this figure concentrates on the effects seen in the left–right direction, giving component locations over the left or right hemisphere. With all three components (Fig. 4A–C), central stimulation results in maximal activity in the midline whereas lateral visual input yields a complex pattern of lateralization of activity over the left and right hemispheres. As is evident from Fig. 4, there is no lateralization with central stimuli, and centroids are shifted toward the left or right hemisphere when stimuli occur in the visual half-fields. Such location data can also be treated statistically, and significant effects of stimulus location on the topographic distribution

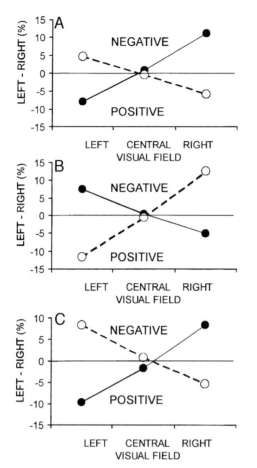

FIGURE 4   Mean centroid locations in the left–right direction on the scalp at different component latencies. (A) 78.2 msec; (B) 118.2 msec; (C) 186.7 msec. A checkerboard reversal stimulus was presented in the center or in the left or right visual half-field. Note that there is no lateralization with central stimuli, and centroids are shifted toward the left or right hemisphere when stimuli occur in the visual half-fields. Numbers give the distance from the midline in percentages of the nasion–inion distance. Positive centers of gravity are indicated by closed symbols; negative centroids are indicated by open symbols. Mean data of 22 healthy adults.

are derived from further analysis, enabling the comparison of experimental conditions.

Such differences in the topographical localization characterize the spatiotemporal distribution over longer time epochs. Skrandies (1988) illustrates how differences in visual information processing is reflected by sustained differences in topographical

features. Visual stimuli of different spatial frequency yield significant differences in the geometry of underlying neural assemblies selectively sensitive to different stimulus characteristics. This is seen not only at the occurrence time of evoked components but may persist up to 27 msec (Skrandies, 1988).

Statistical analysis may also be performed on complete scalp distribution maps when data obtained in different experimental conditions or in different groups of subjects are obtained. The procedure is straightforward: a statistical measure (such as a *t*-value) is computed at each electrode site, and its significance is then plotted as topographical distribution. Such a comparison of complete maps results in so-called significance probability maps (see Chapter 3, this volume).

STATISTICALLY DEFINED COMPONENTS: PRINCIPAL COMPONENT ANALYSIS

The Extraction of Components

Electroencephalographic data recorded from many electrodes constitute multi-dimensional observations, and wave shapes of evoked potentials have been analyzed by multivariate statistical methods (Chapman and McCrary, 1995; Donchin, 1966; Skrandies, 1981). Evoked brain potentials may be considered as the sum of independent components, and principal component analysis (PCA) has been used to extract such underlying components. The amplitudes of evoked potentials show some correlation between successive time points as well as between neighboring electrode sites. In addition to the autocorrelation inherent in evoked potential data, variation of the independent experimental variables introduces systematic variation in the data set yielding patterns of correlation caused by stimulus or subject conditions.

The use of PCA is first to find a reduced set of nonredundant wave form descriptors that explain most of the variance in the original data, and PCA has been applied to evoked potential wave forms by a number of researchers. Principal components are by definition orthogonal, and their correlation is zero. After component extraction the loading pattern may be rotated to a simple structure, maintaining orthogonal relationships between components (varimax rotation) (Harman, 1967; Glaser and Ruchkin, 1976). This procedure is used to maximize high component loading values and minimize low loading values.

In a second step the contribution of each of the derived components to the original data is determined by examining the component scores associated with each stimulus or subject condition. These scores are dependent measures like the conventional amplitude values, and experimental effects may be revealed by treating component scores with conventional statistical methods (Dillon and Goldstein, 1984).

Different from factor analysis (Harman, 1967), PCA does not consider unique factors that show high loadings only on individual variables. This appears appropriate, because, due to the autocorrelation in evoked potential data mentioned above, cortical activity modulated by experimental conditions never influences only isolated time points or electrode positions. In addition, it has been shown that a high percentage of the variance in a given data set is accounted for by only a few principal components, indicating that most of the variance of the data is related to few common factors and that unique factors can be neglected.

With evoked potential wave forms, amplitudes measured at successive time points are entered as variables, whereas different electrode positions, subjects, and experimental conditions are the observations in the input data matrix. Topographical effects may then be analyzed by testing the statistical significance of the scalp distribution of component scores obtained in different experimental or subject conditions. The topographical analysis of principal component scores has been successfully performed on both one-dimensional potential profiles and two-dimensional potential fields (Skrandies, 1981, 1983; Skrandies *et al.*, 1998).

For direct topographical analysis a spatial PCA may be used in order to reduce the dimensionality of the original data matrices, where the amplitudes at each electrode location are the variables, and time points, different subjects, or different experimental conditions serve as the observations. Then the matrix of correlations (or covariances) between electrodes is decomposed by PCA. When wave forms are used, component loadings form basic wave forms whereas with topographical maps the spatial PCA results in basic maps (i.e., scalp distributions of component loadings). The statistical method of PCA computation extracts components that are orthogonal, with the first principal component representing the maximum variation in the data; the second principal component is orthogonal to the first and represents the maximum variation of the residual data. This process is repeated several times, and because the original variables are correlated only a small number of principal components accounts for a large proportion of the variance in the original data. When PCA is performed on multichannel evoked potential wave shapes, between 6 and 10 principal components are found (Skrandies, 1981, 1983), whereas a spatial PCA results in about three to four basic field distributions that account for more than 90% of the variance (Skrandies, 1989; Skrandies and Lehmann, 1982; Skrandies *et al.*, 1998). An example is given in Fig. 5.

The general linear model of evoked potential or EEG maps reads as

$$M(i) = S_1 C_1(i) + S_2 C_2(i) + \ldots + S_n C_n(i) + X, \qquad (3)$$

or in matrix notation

$$M = SC' + X, \qquad (4)$$

where $M(i)$ is the potential map defined by i electrodes, C_n are fundamental components (maps of component loadings), S_n are component scores (gain factors) associated with subject or stimulus conditions, and X is the grand mean of the original data entered in the PCA. In this model the grand mean is added for visualization because it is removed from the original data when the covariance or correlation matrix is computed. In a similar way the matrix M of Eq. (4) contains the original amplitude values, C' represents the component loadings, S the component scores, and X contains the grand mean values. Components are extracted from the covariance or correlation matrix, thus the contribution of each component is relative to the grand mean of the original data. When the basic components derived from the correlation matrix are illustrated in the form of scalp distribution maps, the metric of each component can be restored to microvolts by multiplying component loadings by their respective standard deviations.

As a result of the spatial PCA, large numbers of electrodes are reduced to a few underlying components, each of which is weighted by a component score that indicates the contribution of each component to a given experimental condition [see Eq. (3)]. For a detailed description of the mathematical and statistical backgrounds of factor analysis, see the statistical literature by Harman (1967) or Dillon and Goldstein (1984), for example. The application of PCA to biomedical signals has been reviewed by Glaser and Ruchkin (1976), John *et al.* (1978), and Chapman and McCrary (1995).

Examples of Spatial Principal Components Analysis

After extracting principal components, their relation to stimulus conditions is of major interest, and conventional statistics such as analysis of variance (ANOVA) on the component scores may reveal significant experimental effects. An example is given in Fig. 7, where the results of an experiment on the scalp distribution of electrical brain activity elicited by visual motion stimuli in 14 healthy adults are displayed. Stimuli were square wave gratings of high or low contrast moving with a velocity of 4.9° per second on a computer monitor. Adaptation to motion was varied by changing the so-called duty cycle of stimulus presentation (i.e., the relation of motion to nonmotion time) in order to enhance motion-related activity. Data obtained with motion stimuli were compared to checkerboard pattern reversal evoked activity. Spatial principal components analysis on the data of all subjects and experimental conditions reveals four latent topographical components that accounted for 92.05% of the variance (Fig. 6).

Two components showed occipital extreme values surrounded by steep potential gradients (components 1 and 2 in Fig. 6), whereas there occurred another two statistically independent components displaying lateralized activity (components 3 and 4 in Fig. 6). From the plot of cumulative variance, it is obvious that more than 50% of the variance can be explained by the first component. It is important to note, however, that components associated with less variance also carry useful information. Analysis of the contribution of these spatial components to the observed potential fields revealed significant differences between pattern reversal- and motion-evoked activity seen with components 3 and 4 (for details see Skrandies *et al.*, 1998). Significant differences in scalp topography evoked by checkerboard reversal and by motion stimuli are revealed by the analysis of component 1 occurring at 158 msec latency. It is important to note that identical basic field configurations contribute to different experimental conditions, where, however, the relative weighting is significantly different. This further stresses that with PCA not only the extraction of components is critical but the main aim is the analysis of component

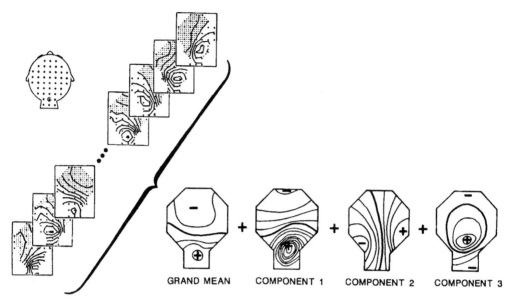

FIGURE 5   Results of a spatial PCA. Sixty visually evoked scalp distribution maps at GFP component latency (schema on the left) obtained from six participants in 45 channels were entered in a PCA. This procedure extracted three varimax-rotated components with eigenvalues greater than 1.0, which accounted for 93.4% of the variance. Thus, for each experimental condition 45 amplitude values are reduced to three components plus the grand mean field, which is computed as the mean over all subjects and stimulus conditions. Components are shown with a score (scaling factor) of 1.0, and the metric was restored to microvolts by multiplying component loadings by their respective standard deviations. Field lines are in steps of 0.3 μV. From Skrandies (1989), with permission.

scores that allows for comparisons of experimental conditions.

Results of a spatial PCA on evoked potential recordings in 45 channels obtained from six participants are shown in Fig. 5. Visual potentials were evoked by a contrast reversing checkerboard pattern in five stimulus conditions (two stimulus sizes in two lateral retinal locations and one upper hemiretinal stimulus). Further details on the experimental conditions and the VEP recordings is given by Skrandies and Lehmann (1982). The computation of GFP identified two components with mean latencies of 105.8 and 145.1 msec in all subjects and conditions. The original data consisted of 45 variables (amplitude values) by 60 cases (experimental stimulus conditions) that were entered in a spatial PCA using the correlation matrix. The amplitudes at the 45 electrodes were reduced to only three components with eigenvalues greater than 1.0, which accounted for 93.4% of the variance. As is evident from Fig. 5, component 1 shows anterior–posterior distribution differences with an extreme value in the midline over occipital areas; component 2 mainly displays lateral differences, and component 3 has a concentric distribution with a maximum at parietal sites. This appears as a meaningful numerical decomposition of the scalp field distributions. As a result of the spatial PCA the number of variables is reduced from 45 amplitude values at all electrodes to three component scores for each experimental condition. The topographic pattern of principal components illustrated in Fig. 5 is very similar to the distribution of factor scores derived from frequency analyses of spontaneous EEGs, and John *et al.* (1993) have illustrated that the topographical distribution of scores on a limited number of factors may be used successfully to quantify the abnormalities of

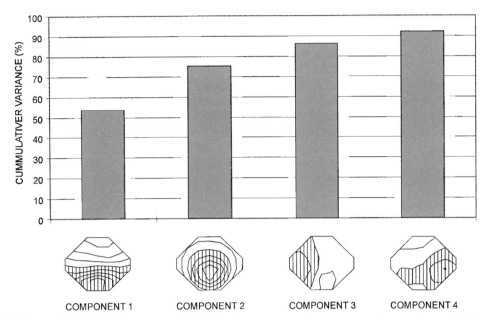

FIGURE 6   The maps illustrate the spatial distribution of principal components. These are basic field shapes with a component score of 1.0. The histograms show cumulatively the amount of variance explained. Component 1 explains more than 50%, and nearly 100% is explained by all four components. All component loadings were converted to microvolt values, and lines are in steps of 0.5 μV for components 1 and 2, and 0.25 μV for components 3 and 4. Hatched areas are negative, white areas are positive. Data from Skrandies *et al.* (1998).

patients with a wide variety of psychiatric disorders.

A Note on the Physiological Interpretation of Principal Components

The general problem of the reference location that applies to the analysis of evoked potential wave forms (i.e., the change of wave forms with a change of the reference location as described above) also applies to principal components. Changing the reference means to subtract a vector from the original data, and this procedure will cause some changes in the covariance and correlation matrix computed from the original amplitude measures. Because PCA reproduces the input matrix as a set of linear combinations, any change of the original data caused by different reference electrodes must also influence the derived solution, and PCA may not overcome problems with the original data.

In addition, it is important to keep in mind that PCA results in statistically defined components. Thus, the interpretation of components derived from PCA computations must always consider that a specific principal component reflects nothing more but a source of variance in the original data set. The pattern of component loadings depends on the covariation of potential amplitudes at various scalp locations over experimental conditions or recording time points. As shown above, different experimental conditions produce different principal components (see topographic component patterns in Figs. 5 and 6). In this example the differences in scalp distributions of component loadings are caused by the fact that different patterns of correlation between the recording electrodes on the scalp are produced when central or left and right hemiretinal areas are stimulated. Principal components are always directly influenced

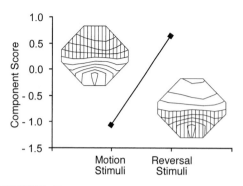

FIGURE 7 Scores on component 1 (shown in Fig. 6) elicited by motion (left) and pattern reversal stimuli (right) occurring 158 msec after stimulation. Note that an identical component contributes to the evoked potential field with different weighting scores and different polarity when experimental conditions are compared. Inset maps display the mean topographical distribution of the component appropriately scaled by the scores. Lines are in steps of 0.5 μV; hatched areas are negative, white areas are positive. Mean values computed on the data of 14 volunteers. Data from Skrandies *et al.* (1998).

by the variation in the data set caused by different experimental conditions. Thus, the temporal or spatial pattern of component loadings must not necessarily represent physiological components, and the relation between principal components and physiological mechanisms cannot be warranted by the statistical method.

It is well accepted that PCA is able to reproduce underlying components with a high degree of accuracy (Wood and McCarthy, 1984), but there may occur problems when component scores are analyzed in ANOVAs. The "misallocation" of variance across components described in a simulation study by Wood and McCarthy (1984) may be caused by the rotation of the component loadings. Möcks and Verleger (1986) and Rösler and Manzey (1981) have also drawn attention to possible problems of orthogonal rotations of principal components. We also note that the problem of misallocation of variance of component scores that occurs with overlapping com-

ponents in PCA (Wood and McCarthy, 1984) is certainly not restricted to PCA results. When analyzing amplitude measures of evoked potentials, component overlap certainly introduces similar problems. This is due to the fact that we are dealing with scalp-recorded data that are produced by the simultaneous activation of many intracranial neuronal generating processes.

On the other hand, PCA is a powerful tool when used as a means of data reduction. As obvious from Figs. 6 and 7, many amplitude measures can be reduced to a very small set of components that are meaningfully and strongly related to experimental parameters. This has been repeatedly reported by a number of researchers (Chapman and McCrary, 1995; Donchin, 1966; Skrandies, 1983; Skrandies *et al.*, 1998). Along a similar line, the finding that only three components (basic field distributions) may explain more than 95% of the variance when data are analyzed over time is in good agreement with the results of segmentation studies that showed the reoccurrence of similar spatial patterns over time when evoked potential maps series were segmented by topographical criteria (Lehmann and Skrandies, 1986; Skrandies, 1988).

OUTLOOK AND POSSIBLE APPLICATIONS OF TOPOGRAPHICAL BRAIN MAPPING

It is evident from many results and data that topographic mapping of brain electrical activity constitutes a means for the visualization of electric field distributions on the scalp, and for the adequate statistical and quantitative analysis of multichannel electrophysiological recordings. These methods may be applied for brain activity that occurs spontaneously or is elicited by sensory stimulation or psychological events. Electrical brain activity can be characterized in terms of latency (i.e., processing times), synchronous involvement and extent of neuronal populations (i.e., field strength), and topographical distribution of potential components.

Practical applications are twofold: much is to be learned from studies on functional states of the human brain, information processing, and motor planning in healthy volunteers, and clinical questions may be answered on the functionality and intactness of the central nervous system of patients suspected of central nervous system or psychiatric disease. Noninvasive experimental investigations are part of addressing contemporary neurophysiological questions on how global states affect brain functions such as processing of sensory or psychological information, movement planning and execution, or internal states related to cognition and emotion. In healthy people as well as in patients, such processes can be studied and characterized by spatiotemporal patterns of electrical brain activity.

In clinical settings, sensory evoked brain activity is recorded in order to test the intactness of afferent pathways and central processing areas of various sensory modalities in neurological, ophthalmological, or audiological patients. Event-related brain activity elicited during cognitive tasks has its main application in the fields of psychiatry and psychology, where perception, cognition, attention, learning, or emotional processes are under study. These fields profit from the application of topographic mapping and analysis of brain electrical activity in real-time. Future applications of topographic mapping of electrophysiological activity will include the coregistration of the high time-resolution EEG recordings with brain-imaging methods such as functional MRI. One may expect that the collaboration of the fields will lead to functional imaging of brain activity with high temporal and high spatial resolution.

Acknowledgment

Supported in part by Deutsche Forschungsgemeinschaft, DFG Sk 26/5–3 and DFG Sk 26/8–3.

References

Chapman, R. M., and McCrary, J. W. (1995). EP component identification and measurement by principal components analysis. *Brain Cogn.* **27**, 288–310.

Dillon, W. R., and Goldstein, M. (1984). "Multivariate Analysis Methods and Applications." John Wiley & Sons, New York.

Donchin, E. (1966). A multivariate approach to the analysis of average evoked potentials. *IEEE Trans. Biomed. Eng.* **13**, 131–139.

Glaser, E. M., and Ruchkin, D. S. (1976). "Principles of Neurobiological Signal Analysis." Academic Press, New York.

Harman, H. H. (1967). "Modern Factor Analysis," 2nd Ed. The University of Chicago Press, Chicago.

John, E. R., Ruchkin, D. S., and Vidal, J. J. (1978). Measurement of event- related potentials. *In* "Event-related Brain Potentials in Man" (E. Callaway, R. Tueting, and S. H. Koslow, eds.), pp. 93–138. Academic Press, New York.

John, E. R., Easton, P., Prichep, L. S., and Friedman, J. (1993). Standardized varimax descriptors of event related potentials: Basic considerations. *Brain Topogr.* **6**, 143–162.

Lehmann, D. (1987). Principles of spatial analysis. *In* "Handbook of Electroencephalography and Clinical Neurophysiology. Rev. Series, Vol. 1: Analysis of Electrical and Magnetic Signals" (A. Gevins, and A. Rémond, eds.), pp. 309–354. Elsevier, Amsterdam.

Lehmann, D., and Skrandies, W. (1980). Reference-free identification of components of checkerboard-evoked multichannel potential fields. *Electroencephalogr. Clin. Neurophysiol.* **48**, 609–621.

Lehmann, D., and Skrandies, W. (1984). Spatial analysis of evoked potentials in man: A review. *Prog. Neurobiol.* **23**, 227–250.

Lehmann, D., and Skrandies, W. (1986). Time segmentation of evoked potentials (EPs) based on spatial scalp field configuration in multichannel recordings. *Electroencephalogr. Clin. Neurophysiol.* (Suppl. 38), 27–29.

Möcks, J., and Verleger, R. (1986). Principal component analysis of event-related potentials: A note on misallocation of variance. *Electroencephalogr. Clin. Neurophysiol.* **65**, 393–398.

Nunez, P. L. (1981). "Electric Fields of the Brain." Oxford University Press, New York.

Rösler, F., and Manzey, D. (1981). Principal components and varimax-rotated components in event-related potential research: Some remarks on their interpretation. *Biol. Psychol.* **13**, 3–26.

Skrandies, W. (1981). Latent components of potentials evoked by visual stimuli in different retinal locations. *Int. J. Neurosci.* **14**, 77–84.

Skrandies, W. (1983). Information processing and evoked potentials: Topography of early and late components. *Adv. Biol. Psychiatr.* **13**, 1–12.

Skrandies, W. (1986). Visual evoked potential topography: Methods and results. *In* "Topographic Mapping of Brain Electrical Activity" (F. H. Duffy, ed.), pp. 7–28. Butterworths, Boston.

Skrandies, W. (1987). The upper and lower visual field of man: Electrophysiological and functional differences. *Prog. Sensory Physiol.* **8**, 1–93.

Skrandies, W. (1988). Time range analysis of evoked potential fields. *Brain Topogr.* **1**, 107–116.

Skrandies, W. (1989). Data reduction of multichannel fields: Global field power and principal components. *Brain Topogr.* **2**, 73–80.

Skrandies, W. (1995). Visual information processing: topography of brain electrical activity. *Biological Psychol.* **40**, 1–15.

Skrandies, W. (2001). Electroencephalogram topography. *In* "The Encyclopedia of Imaging Science and Technology" (J. P. Hornak, ed.), Vol. 1, pp. 198–210. John Wiley & Sons, New York.

Skrandies, W., and Lehmann, D. (1982). Spatial principal components of multichannel maps evoked by lateral visual half-field stimuli. *Electroencephalogr. Clin. Neurophysiol.* **54**, 662–667.

Skrandies, W., Jedynak, A., and Kleiser, R. (1998). Scalp distribution components of brain activity evoked by visual motion stimuli. *Exp. Brain Res.* **122**, 62–70.

Wood, C. C., and McCarthy, G. (1984). Principal component analysis of event-related potentials: Simulation studies demonstrate misallocation of variance across components. *Electroencephalogr. Clin. Neurophysiol.* **59**, 249–260.

F

Brain Imaging Techniques: Invasiveness and Spatial and Temporal Resolution

Alberto Zani, Gabriele Biella, and Alice Mado Proverbio

INTRODUCTION

In this appendix we provide some estimates of the spatial and temporal resolution, as well as of the invasiveness, of the most frequently used neuroimaging techniques. Before illustrating these estimates, it is important to remember that neuroimaging techniques may be subdivided into two broad categories according to their different aims: imaging of brain anatomy (*structural imaging*), or of brain function (*functional imaging*). Structural imaging is used to examine the static outlines of brain structures in both physiological and pathological situations. Functional imaging, on the other hand, is used to gain knowledge on (1) which structures are activated during a specific cognitive task, at sensory and/or cognitive levels, (2) the interactions between the structures that are activated, and (3) the way the functional activation of the brain is reorganized in individuals affected by neurological diseases, strokes, or head injuries.

Generally speaking, the structural category of neuroimaging techniques includes two well-known neuroradiological techniques: computerized axial tomography (CAT) and magnetic resonance imaging (MRI). As far as brain imaging capacity is concerned, both are far superior to their forebear, the X-ray technique.

Functional imaging includes a wide range of techniques, which are listed here in increasing order of spatial and temporal resolution: (1) 2-deoxyglucose cerebral blood flow (2-deoxyglucose CBF), a forerunner of hemodynamic techniques rarely used nowadays; (2) single-photon emission computed tomography (SPECT); (3) positron emission tomography (PET); (4) functional magnetic resonance imaging (fMRI); (4) electroencephalography and event-related potentials (EEG–ERP); (5) magnetoencephalography (MEG); and last, but not the least, (6) microelectrode single-unit recording, which involves recording electrophysiological signals from inside or outside the membrane of a single neuron body by means of microelectrodes.

Although the categorization of neuroimaging techniques into the two aforementioned approaches is generally sound, it should be mentioned that all these techniques have some limitations and attempts are being made to overcome these. Some very recently devised techniques combine both structural and functional imaging information and cannot be classified into either category. A rather interesting example of these combined techniques is the so-called CAT–PET.

SPATIAL AND TEMPORAL RESOLUTION

The accuracy with which the imaging techniques are able to provide definite images of the anatomy of the centers of the central nervous system (CNS), and/or the activation of these centers, in order to be able to localize them reliably, is defined as *spatial resolution*. Conversely, the speed with which the techniques can keep on scanning the CNS anatomy and physiology, taking into account all intrinsic limitations, i.e., the minimum time that must necessarily pass between the collection of a measure of one CNS activation and the successive one, is described as *temporal resolution*.

Figure 1 is a graphical representation of an estimate of the normal spatial and temporal resolution for each of the imaging techniques mentioned above. The spatial resolution, expressed in millimeters, is reported on the ordinate axis; the temporal resolution—here indicated in seconds on a logarithmic scale—is depicted on the abscissa. The height and width of the forms with which the different techniques are represented in the figure indicate the known range of spatial and temporal resolutions, respectively, for each of the techniques. The increasing saturation of the gray hue of the different shapes represents the increasing degree of invasiveness of the techniques.

Structural techniques currently have the most accurate spatial resolution or, in other words, localization capacity. Both CAT and PET techniques have a spatial resolution that is vastly superior to that of previous techniques. Indeed, their spatial resolution has become so good that it is now in the order of millimeters.

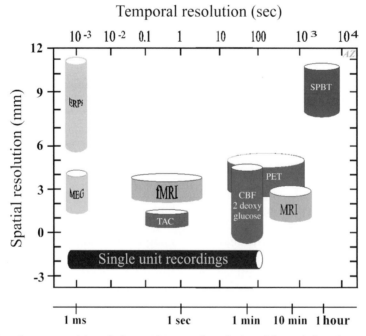

FIGURE 1 Invasiveness, spatial resolution, and temporal resolution of the main imaging techniques used in humans to investigate function and structure of the brain. The different sizes of the shapes representing the different techniques vary as a function of the level of both spatial resolution (in milimeters) and temporal resolution (in seconds). Note that the increasing level of saturation of the gray color represents the increasing levels of invasiveness of the techniques.

In PET, for example, the activated parts of the brain selectively take up a radioactive tracer previously administered intravenously to a patient or healthy volunteer. The gamma rays deriving from the emission of positrons by these activated structures allow a functional map of cerebral activation to be built; as illustrated in Fig. 1, such a map has a precision ranging between about 2 and 5 mm. fMRI, on the other hand, can reflect structural variations caused by increased local blood flow and dilatation of cerebral tissues with a mean precision of 3 mm, although the range is from 2 to 4 mm.

Notwithstanding their high spatial resolution, none of the functional imaging techniques, with the exception of MEG, can provide functional images that are also accurate in temporal terms. In fact, the temporal resolution with which they can provide accurate images of ongoing functional activation of the brain is rather poor. This resolution can reach the order of a tenth of second (~100–150 msec) with the most technologically advanced type of fMRI—that is, 3 or 4 tesla echo-planar fMRI (or *event-related fMRI*)—but still remains in the order of seconds with less powerful equipment. The temporal resolution of PET is tens of seconds or even minutes. The significance of this technical limitation to research can readily be appreciated by considering that an action potential originating in the pyramidal motor neurones of the premotor cortex propagating along the efferent pathways takes about 150 msec to reach the muscle bundles of the forearm, causing flexion of the terminal phalanx of the index finger, in order, for example, to press a button for measuring reaction times. Or consider that we can identify an object that enters our visual field within a few hundreds of milliseconds (~180–220 msec). It is clear that the velocity with which the above-mentioned neural processes occur means that their subprocesses escape measurement techniques because of the interval between successive sampling.

Given that the final aim of research on the mind and brain should be to construct a model of functional relations between the pathways and centers of the brain from which mental life comes, besides simple localization of these to particular areas of the brain, it is important to have a temporal resolution of milliseconds for the processes involved. The only imaging techniques that have such a good temporal resolution are the techniques used systematically or on single cells that measure the electromagnetic activity of the brain directly. As illustrated by Fig. 1, the maximal temporal resolution, as well as spatial resolution, is provided by single-unit recordings. Thanks to these it is possible to carry out neurofunctional investigations with a temporal resolution below the order of milliseconds ($<10^{-3}$), and with a spatial resolution under 1 mm. It is, however, unthinkable to use this technique for functional imaging of the human brain because of its invasiveness; it would require neurosurgery to implant the microelectrodes.

Unlike single-unit recordings, scalp recordings of voltages (EEGs and ERPs) that mirror the intracranial currents originating from neuronal sources in the brain cortex, and spreading by volume conduction throughout the brain and the scalp, can be used as tools for human research. Indeed, while having the advantage of 1-msec temporal resolution, or quite close to this level, the recording method is completely noninvasive. However, because of its irregularities, the skull is not a homogeneous conductor. The volume currents that come in contact with the electrodes over the scalp are distorted by irregularities such that the technique does not have sufficient spatial resolution to be able locate the real intracranial sources of the currents.

This difficulty translates into a spatial resolution that cannot be relied on for localization purposes. In the best cases, localization of the electric dipole ranges between a minimum of 6 mm and a maximum of 11 mm or even beyond, depending on a whole series of recording conditions and modeling parameters (see Fig. 1). Even then, there are some extreme cases, such as the so-called *far-field potentials*, in which the scalp site at which the largest signal is measured is actually far away from the source area; for example, sensory-evoked responses of the auditory cortex to unilateral stimuli, despite originating on the dorsolateral side of the contralateral brain hemisphere close to the ear, produce their largest amplitudes at the top of the scalp.

Although having the same temporal resolution as the EEG, magnetoencephalography is only minimally influenced by the nonuniform conductivity of the brain, skull, and scalp, and if the head is modeled using spherical geometry the recorded magnetic field can be considered completely independent of the conductivity of the head. Referring once again to Fig. 1 it can be seen that only MEG has high levels of both spatial and temporal resolution. In detail, the spatial resolution of this technique ranges from a minimum of 1.5 mm to a maximum of 4 mm for the cortical areas of the brain. Unfortunately, this resolution decreases dramatically to some centimeters for subcortical regions. This technique could, therefore, be the technique of choice for localizing activity in the superficial areas of the brain, i.e., the cerebral cortex, which is responsible for mental processes in general. Unfortunately, this technique is still too expensive to become as widely used as the ERPs.

In order to overcome the various limitations of each of the techniques presented here, strategies are being developed to use *combined methods;* for example, the images obtained by MRI, fMRI, or PET can be combined with those from microelectrodes, or those from MEG and ERPs. Combination methods can be based on a direct or an indirect approach. The former uses hemodynamic images to obtain a real structural basis of the estimates of functional activation acquired separately, whereas the latter

involves parallel recording of these parameters in a single experimental paradigm. Although it is certainly true that the different approaches are very useful individually, only integration of the techniques with different spatial and temporal resolutions can provide truly valuable information on the neurofunctional mechanisms of mental processes, and on their temporal course of activation.

INVASIVENESS

Techniques to investigate the function and structure of the nervous system can be classified as invasive, semiinvasive, and noninvasive. The difference between the invasive and semiinvasive techniques is that the former implies a surgical lesion (mechanical) and the latter involves a physicochemical stress (with radioopaque or radioactive substances).

Techiques that can be defined as noninvasive are MEG and EEG, both of which involve simple recordings of electrical potentials or natural magnetic fields produced by brain activity without experimentally introduced chemicostructural perturbations of the cerebral regions.

Semiinvasive techniques provide a means to observe dynamic and structural properties through images that are reconstructed on the basis of a principle of both active and passive detectability. In the first case, the products of rapidly metabolized compounds or radioactive substances with a short half-life are detected. The compounds are injected intravenously and, being distributed preferentially to certain regions of the brain, show in the various areas of the brain a differential distribution that is proportional to the state of activation of the area (PET, SPECT, and, when tracers are used, also fMRI and MRI). In the case of passive detection (e.g., CAT), the X radiations are delivered by the machine and hit the cerebral tissues *ab externo* (with the usual radiographic principle). Even MRI and fMRI, without injection of markers, induce changes in cerebral or spinal structures. In fact, applying a magnetic field causes a change, albeit transitory, in the characteristics of the spatiotemporal molecular organization, with realignment of the electromagnetic dipoles of charged molecules.

Mechanically invasive techniques belong to the realm of functional neurosurgery; this involves extra- or intradural recordings, or even recordings from deep structures (in the case of therapeutic placement of stimulatory electrodes). These techniques obviously involve surgery on specific nervous tissue and perforation or opening of the skull.

Mechanical or physicochemical invasiveness implies a different degree of danger for the patient. Naturally this creates a boundary; the economic costs and benefits of the results of the diagnostic or surgical intervention must be compared to not carrying out the procedure. On average, given precise conditions and the noninstrumental diagnosis, the indication for an invasive intervention is highly controlled and justifiable.

Suggested Reading

Single-Unit Recordings

Huguenard, J., and McCormick, D. (1994). "Electrophysiology of the Neuron." Oxford University Press, New York.

Llinás, R. (1988). The intrinsic electrophysiological properties of mammalian neurons: Insights into central nervous system function. *Science* **242**, 1654–1664.

Nicholls, J., Nartin, A., and Wallace, B. (1993). "From Neuron to Brain." 3rd Ed. Sinauer, Sunderland, Massachusetts.

Hemodynamic Functional Imaging

Bandettini, P. A., Rasmus M. B., and Donahue, K. M. (2000). Functional MRI. Background, methodology, limits, and interpretation. *In* "Handbook of Psychophysiology" (J. T. Cacioppo, L. G. Tassinary, and G. G. Berntson, eds.), 2nd Ed., pp. 978–1014. Cambridge University Press, Cambridge, Massachusetts.

Binder, J. R., and Rao, S. M. (1994). Human brain mapping with functional magnetic resonance imaging. *In* "Localization and Neuroimaging in Neuropsychology" (A. Kertesz, ed.), pp. 185–212. Academic Press, Orlando.

De Yoe, E. A., Bandettini, P., Neitz, J., Miller, D., and Winans, P. (1994). Functional magnetic resonance imaging (fMRI) of the human brain. *J. Neurosci Meth* **54**, 171–187.

Frith, C. D., and Friston, K. J. (1997). Studying brain function with neuroimaging. *In* "Cognitive Neuroscience" (M. D. Rugg, ed.), pp. 169–195. Psychology Press, Taylor & Francis Group, Hove, East Sussex, UK.

Josephs, O., Turner, R., and Friston, K.J. (1997). Event-related fMRI. *Hum. Brain Mapping* **5**, 243–248.

Perani, D., and Cappa, S. (1999). Neuroimaging methods in neuropsychology. In "Handbook of Clinical and Experimental Neuropsychology" (G. Denes, and L. Pizzamiglio, eds.), pp. 69–94. Psychology Press, Taylor & Francis Group, Hove East Sussex, UK.

Posner, M. I., and Raichle, M. E. (1994). "Images of Mind." W. H. Freeman, New York.

Reiman, E. M., Lane, R. D., Van Petten, C., and Bandettini, P. A. (2000). Positron emission tomography and functional magnetic resonance imaging. *In* "Handbook of Psychophysiology" (J. T. Cacioppo, L. G. Tassinary, and G. G. Berntson, eds.), 2nd Ed., pp. 85–118. Cambridge University Press, Cambridge, Massachusetts.

Rosen, B. R., Buckner, R. L., and Dale, A. M. (1998). Event-related MRI: Past, present, and future. *Proc. Natl Acad. Sci USA* **95**, 773–780.

Rugg, M. D. (1999). Functional neuroimaging in cognitive neuroscience. In "The Neurocognition of Language" (C. M. Brown and P. Hagoort, eds.), pp. 15–36. Oxford University Press, Oxford and New York.

Electromagnetic Imaging

Del Gratta, C., and Romani, G. L. (1999). MEG: Principles, methods, and applications. *Biomed. Technik* **44** (Suppl. 2), 11–23.

Hari, R., and Lounasmaa, O. V. (1989). Recording and interpretation of cerebral magnetic fields. *Science* **244**, 432–436.

Hillyard, S. A., and Picton, T. W. (1987). Electrophysiology of cognition. *In* "Handbook of Physiology, Sect. 1, Vol. 5, Higher Functions of the Brain" (F. Plum, ed.), pp. 519–584. American Physiological Society, Bethesda, MD.

Hillyard, S. A. (1993). Electrical and magnetic brain recordings: Contributions to cognitive neuroscience. *Curr. Opin. Neurobiol.* **3**, 217–224.

Kutas, M., and Dale, A. (1997). Electrical and magnetic reading of mental functions. *In* "Cognitive Neuroscience" (M. D. Rugg, ed.), pp. 197–242.

Psychology Press, Taylor & Francis Group, Hove East Sussex, UK.

Kutas, M., Federmeier, K. D., and Sereno, M. I. (1999). Current approaches to mapping language in electromagnetic space. In "The Neurocognition of Language" (C. M. Brown and P. Hagoort, eds.), pp. 317–392. Oxford University Press, Oxford and New York.

Näätänen, R., Ilmoniemi, J., and Alho, K. (1994). Magnetoencephalography in studies of cognitive brain function. *Trends Neurosci.* **17**, 389–395.

Regan, D. (1989). "Human Brain Electrophysiology: Evoked Potentials and Evoked Magnetic Fields in Science and Medicine." Elsevier, Amsterdam.

Scherg, M. (1992). Functional imaging and localization of electromagnetic brain activity. *Brain Topogr.* **5**, 103–111.

Scherg, M., and Ebersole, J. S. (1993). Models of brain sources. *Brain Topogr.* **5**, 419–423.

Swick, D., Kutas, M., and Neville, H. J. (1994). Localizing the neural generators of event-related brain potentials. *In* "Localization and Neuroimaging in Neuropsychology" (A. Kertesz, ed.), pp. 73–121. Academic Press, Orlando.

Vaughan, H. G. (1988). Topographic analysis of brain electrical activity. *In* "The London Symposia (EEG Suppl. 39)" (R. J. Ellingson, N. M. F. Murray, and A. M. Halliday, eds.), pp. 137–142. Elsevier, Amsterdam.

Combining Techniques

Dale, A. M., and Sereno, M. I. (1993). Improved localization of cortical activity by combining EEG and MEG with MRI cortical surface reconstruction: A linear approach. *J. Cogn. Neurosci.* **5**, 162–176.

Halgren, E., and Dale, A. M. (1999). Combining of electromagnetic and hemodynamic signals to derive spatiotemporal brain activation patterns: Theory and results. *Biomed. Technik* **44** (Suppl. 2), 53–60.

Luck, S. J. (1999). Direct and indirect integration of event-related potentials, functional magnetic resonance images, and single-unit recordings. *Hum. Brain Mapping* **8**, 115–120.

Wieringa, H. J. (1993). "MEG, EEG and the Integration with Magnetic Resonance Images". Doctoral Thesis." CIP-Gegevens Koninklijke Bibliotheek, Den Haag, Nederlands.

Index